A Model of
Human Occupation:

Theory and Application

A Model of Human Occupation:
Theory and Application

Edited by

Gary Kielhofner
Dr.P.H., O.T.R., F.A.O.T.A.

Professor and Head
Department of Occupational Therapy
College of Associated Health Professions
The University of Illinois at Chicago
Chicago, Illinois

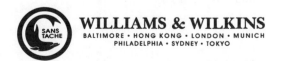

WILLIAMS & WILKINS
BALTIMORE · HONG KONG · LONDON · MUNICH
PHILADELPHIA · SYDNEY · TOKYO

Editor: John P. Butler
Associate Editor: Joseph E. Seitz
Copy Editor: Caral Shields Nolley
Design: James R. Mulligan
Illustration Planning: Wayne Hubbel
Production: Raymond E. Reter

Made in the United States of America

Library of Congress Cataloging in Publication Data

Kielhofner, Gary, 1949–
  A model of human occupation.

  Bibliography: p.
  Includes index.
  1. Occupational therapy. I. Title.
RC487.K54 1985   615.8'5152   84-12031
ISBN 0-683-04600-4

92 93 94   13 14 15

*To my wife, Nancy, and
my children, Kimberly and Kristian*

Preface

The publication of this book is the latest compilation of many persons' efforts to build and apply a theory unique to occupational therapy. It brings into print the results of the long, evolutionary development of occupational behavior theory begun by Dr. Mary Reilly. As two participants who were part of this developmental process, we will view how this occupational behavior theory began and grew, and how the model of human occupation fits into the development of this theory that emphasizes the health-building attributes of occupation.

Early in its history, the occupational therapy profession built upon principles from moral treatment of the mentally ill. Early founders of the profession, such as Meyer, Slagle, Barton and Tracy, stressed the health-restoring properties of occupation, habit training and a balance of work, play, sleep, and rest. However, during the two world wars, there was a rapid expansion of occupational therapy into the treatment of physical dysfunction. As the profession became more closely allied with the medical model of treatment in medicine and surgery, therapists were urged to become more scientific in line with the reductionist, basic science tradition in medicine. As a result, therapists' concerns became more narrow and the emphasis of treatment was on remediating discrete areas of physical and mental dysfunction.

From 1958 to 1977, in various presentations to the profession, Reilly (28–33) alerted occupational therapists to the realization that sole allegience to the medical model of practice would not sustain occupational therapy as a viable and unique service to patients. She stated that the medical model is designed to prevent and reduce illness and does not address the reduction of incapacity that results from illness. It is the occupational therapists' responsibility to activate residual adaptation of patients and to help deficit humans achieve life satisfaction through work and social involvement. Thus, Reilly urged a different conceptualization of occupational therapy which reflected the writings and ideas of the early occupational therapy founders and which borrowed from theories of the behavioral sciences to provide a rationale for the importance of occupation in human life and the need for humans to explore and master their environments. She argued further that occupational therapists should, accordingly, be concerned with the difficulties people have in coping with their occupations. Reilly termed the developmental continuum of play and work, occupational behavior, and proposed it as the unifying concept about which occupational therapists could develop a body of theory to support practice. The term, occupation, acknowledged the importance of patients' economic skills, attitudes and interests that motivated and enabled them to survive in an increasingly complex technological world.

Reilly thus initiated the development of a paradigm for practice in which occupational therapy could act on the healthy behavior of patients as well as solve problems of function that arose in association with the disease process. Furthermore, she urged therapists to make efforts to theorize about what occupational therapy is, so that the occupational therapy process could be systematically taught. Occupational behavior theory, she anticipated, would also provide additional explanations for the course of health and disease. Finally, she argued that the profession's theory should guide not only practice and education but also research in order to explain and measure the effectiveness of occupational therapy.

Reilly, using a psychiatric occupational therapy program as a testing and proving ground for her thinking about occupational therapy, developed a model to examine life roles and skills relative to community adaptation and to create an environment where relevant occupational behavior could be evoked and practiced. She sought to build a milieu that would acknowledge competency, arouse curiosity and develop appropriate skills and habits. Patients' daily living was to be balanced between work, rest and play. Occupation would thus be the integrating focus for improved patient behavior. The concept of role, which included the occupational roles of preschooler, student, worker, housewife and retiree, was also central to this model.

Under the guidance of Dr. Reilly, the curriculum at the University of Southern California (from 1966 to 1976) became a laboratory for the development of a theory to fit these specifications. Students, working with each other in small groups, and closely with Reilly, explored, researched, discussed, and refined concepts which made up a growing body of knowledge. While occupational behavior as reflected in the bio-psycho-social functioning of disabled patients was identified as the focus of occupational therapy services, human achievement in daily occupation was identified as the focal point for theory development. As the framework began to develop, the theoretical work of White, Erikson and McClelland, who introduced into the behavioral sciences the theme that humans had a need for competence and achievement, were identified as supporting concepts for the idea that humans needed to engage in occupation. This achievement phenomenon began in childhood play and continued through adult work and resulted in interests, abilities, skills, and habits of competence, cooperation and competition.

Case method was chosen as the clinical problem-solving technique, the way to handle the complex data on patient behavior and to plan treatment. The concept of role was used as a central perspective for organizing case data. Combining assessments of the person's past history and present function led to a role-function diagnosis; treatment emphasized adaptive skills and behavior necessary for role reconstruction.

The period of occupational behavior theory building at the University of Southern California resulted in many investigations which became available through publications and presentations. The following is an incomplete, but illustrative example of the studies which evolved from, and supported, occupational behavior theory. Case method was explained as the scientific form of clinical thinking and the method for gathering patient information (20). Specific components of occupational behavior were identified and explained; this included play as a facilitator of development (17, 24, 36), intrinsic motivation as the dynamic of occupation (6), interests as influences on choice and level of

activity (23), and the development of the worker role (25). Other students investigated related themes such as cultural influences on work and play (16), human adaptation (35) and time as an organizer of behavior (18).

During the middle years the students identified and studied more specific aspects of the basic concepts, relating them to the generic problems seen in occupational therapy practice. This included low motivation (3), competition (1), environmental concerns (5, 26), play skills (8), and family influence on patient behavior (22, 38).

Toward the end, a group of students refined the concepts of occupational behavior, addressed the historical antecedents and began to move the concepts more directly into treatment application, through description and application of the theory to case studies. They described occupational role development in retarded persons (37) and adolescents (2), occupational role acquisition of the critically disabled (7), play as a facilitator of competent behavior (34), temporal adaptation (9), and clinical perspectives on motivation (4).

In recent years, it is Kielhofner who has been most visible through publications in the continuing effort to explore concepts of occupational behavior therapy and to translate it into clinical practice. Kielhofner (12) and others sought to organize occupational therapy knowledge around the central concern for occupation in human life, thus contributing to the development of an occupational behavior paradigm for the profession. He has, through his guidance of graduate students and collaboration with colleagues, continued the work of refining this vast and complex body of knowledge through scholarly activity.

The model of human occupation was introduced several years ago by Kielhofner, Burke and Igi (10, 11, 14, 15) as a particular attempt to synthesize occupational behavior concepts into a practice and research model. In seeking to extend the model into clinical practice, Kielhofner, his colleagues and students (13) have developed and refined clinical instruments submitting them to studies to establish reliability and validity, and have carried out descriptive research to test and refine the model. But, also, he has made every effort to constantly apply them to practice for, as he says, "...the efforts of occupational therapists have value only in terms of what they do for clients and patients." (12, p viii). While originally thought by many to be esoteric, it is significant to note that occupational behavior has begun to be applied to specialized areas of practice (19, 21) and is being utilized by others who are neither Reilly's nor Kielhofner's students. For example, two therapists presented a paper at the 1983 Illinois Spring Conference about their application of occupational behavior concepts in their practice at the Rehabilitation Institute of Chicago; it is the conceptual model upon which the developing educational program at Thomas Jefferson University in Philadelphia is based.

Reed (27), in her examination of models of practice, considers that the model of human occupation is different from Reilly's occupational behavior theory, although she acknowledges that it grew out of Reilly's work. Her critique of occupational behavior centers around its lack of synthesis and exposition in a single publication. In our judgement, Kielhofner has been attempting to do just that and certainly accomplishes it with the presentation of this volume.

A Model of Human Occupation has continued to use the same major concepts of occupational behavior theory: role, interests, values, personal causation, intrinsic motivation, environment, and open systems, to name a few. Rather than centering on the medical model, it deals with occupational dysfunction, and it emphasizes case method as evidenced in this text. However, as with any evolving model, additional concepts and new elaborations have been added by those who have continued developing the theory. Whenever an extension of a theory is substantial, as this one is, the question arises as to whether the additions are a continuation or a new direction. Whether or not the shapers of A Model of Human Occupation have been "true" to the original theories of occupational behavior theory will, of course, be open to individual interpretation. In the eyes of these "beholders" the model is very definitely an extension and further evolution of occupational behavior theory and has much to commend it.

It must be acknowledged that Kielhofner and his associates have put a much heavier emphasis on empirical validation of theoretical concepts and assessments. His colleagues have validated previous work as well as further developed and clarified particular concepts for the model. While this empirical work is different from the heuristic approach used by Reilly, it strengthens the case for the use of these concepts. In addition, these concepts have been consolidated into

a model which can be used in many areas of practice, thereby providing greater specificity for treatment implications. Thus, therapists will now have, with this volume on the model of human occupation, more detailed guidance to operationalize occupational behavior theory into their own practice—be it in physical, psychosocial or developmental dysfunction.

Kielhofner and his associates have certainly followed Reilly's caveat to "... forge an orderly frame of reference from which we can treat, teach and do research" (30, p 224).

M. JEANNE MADIGAN
LILLIAN HOYLE PARENT

References

1. Bell CH: Competition as a motivational incentive. Am J Occup Ther 29:277 279, 1975.
2. Black MM: Adolescent role assessment. Am J Occup Ther 30:73–79, 1976.
3. Borys S: Implications of interest theory for occupational therapy. Am J Occup Ther 28:35–38, 1974.
4. Burke JP: A clinical perspective on motivation: Pawn versus origin. Am J Occup Ther 31:254–258, 1977.
5. Dunning H: Environmental occupational therapy. Am J Occup Ther 26:292–298, 1972.
6. Florey LL: Intrinsic motivation: the dynamics of occupational therapy theory. Am J Occup Ther 23:319–322, 1969.
7. Heard C: Occupational role acquisition: a perspective on the critically disabled. Am J Occup Ther 31:243–247, 1977.
8. Hurff JM: A play skills inventory: a competency monitoring tool for the 10-year-old. Am J Occup Ther 34:651–656 1980
9. Kielhofner G: Temporal adaptation: a conceptual framework for occupational therapy. Am J Occup Ther 31:235–242, 1977.
10. Kielhofner G: A model of human occupation, Part 2. Ontogenesis from the perspective of temporal adaptation. Am J Occup Ther 34:657–663, 1980.
11. Kielhofner G: A model of human occupation, Part 3. Benign and vicious cycles. Am J Occup Ther 34:731–737, 1980.
12. Kielhofner G: Health Through Occupation. Philadelphia, FA Davis, 1983.
13. Kielhofner G: An overview of research on the model of human occupation. Can J Occup Ther 51:59–67, 1984.
14. Kielhofner G, Burke JP: A model of human occupation, Part 1. Conceptual framework and content. Am J Occup Ther 34:572–581, 1980.
15. Kielhofner G., Igi, CH: A model of human occupation, Part 4. Assessment and intervention. Am J Occup Ther 34:777–788, 1980.
16. Klavins R: Work-play behavior: cultural influences. Am J Occup Ther 26:177–179, 1972.

17. Knox SH: A play scale. In Reilly M (ed): *Play As Exploratory Learning*. Beverly Hills, Sage 1974, 247–266.

18. Larrington GG: An exploratory study of the temporal aspects of adaptive functioning. (Unpublished thesis, University of Southern California, 1970.)

19. Lindquist JE, Mack W, Parham, LD: A synthesis of occupational behavior and sensory integration concepts in theory and practice, Part 2. Clinical applications. *Am J Occup Ther* 36:433–437, 1982.

20. Line, J: Case method as a scientific form of clinical thinking. *Am J Occup Ther* 23:308–313, 1969.

21. Mack W, Lindquist JE, Parham LD: A synthesis of occupational behavior and sensory integrative concepts in theory and practice, Part 1. Theoretical foundations. *Am J Occup Ther* 36:365–374, 1982.

22. Madigan MJ: Expectations of parents for their disabled children. (Unpublished masters thesis, University of Southern California, 1972.)

23. Matsutsuyu JS: The interest checklist. *Am J Occup Ther* 23:323–328, 1969.

24. Michelman SS: The importance of creative play. *Am J Occup Ther* 25:285–290, 1971.

25. Moorhead L: The occupational history. *Am J Occup Ther* 23:329–334, 1969.

26. Parent LH: Effects of a low-stimulus environment on behavior. *Am J Occup Ther* 32:19–25, 1978.

27. Reed KL: *Models of Practice in Occupational Therapy*. Baltimore, Williams & Wilkins, 1984.

28. Reilly M: Occupational therapy can be one of the great ideas of 20th century medicine. *Am J Occup Ther* 16:1–9, 1962.

29. Reilly M: An occupational therapy curiculum for 1965. *Am J Occup Ther* 12:293–299, 1958.

30. Reilly M: The challenge of the future to an occupational therapist. *Am J Occup Ther* 20:221–225, 1966.

31. Reilly M: The educational process. *Am J Occup Ther* 23:299–307, 1969.

32. Reilly M: The modernization of occupational therapy. *Am J Occup Ther* 25:243–246, 1971.

33. Reilly M: A response to defining occupational therapy: the meaning of therapy and the virtues of occupation. *Am J Occup Ther* 31:673, 1977.

34. Robinson AL: Play: the arena for acquisition of rules for competent behavior. *Am J Occup Ther* 31:248–253, 1977.

35. Shannon PD: Work adjustment and the adolescent soldier. *Am J Occup Ther* 24:111–115, 1970.

36. Takata N: The play history. *Am J Occup Ther* 23:314–318, 1969.

37. Webster PS: Occupational role development in the young adult with mild mental retardation. *Am J Occup Ther* 34:13–18, 1980.

38. Williams, J: Toward an occupational therapy assessment of family dynamics. (Unpublished masters thesis, University of Southern California, 1971.)

Acknowledgments

It is difficult to give adequate acknowledgment to those who, in some way, influenced the development of the model of human occupation and the various extensions and applications that occur in this volume. The model, as represented here and elsewhere, is truly a collective effort building on important earlier work and developing as many people elaborate its concepts, research its propositions and clinically apply it.

The earliest debt of the model is owed to Mary Reilly and the students who, over many years, developed the occupational behavior tradition at the University of Southern California. As a latecomer, I inherited a rich tradition in which important themes and concepts were already identified. The model first took shape in rudimentary form in the process of writing my master's thesis during which Linda Florey, Phillip Shannon and Nancy Takata were important influences. Later Janice Burke and Cynthia Heard Igi collaborated to refine and elaborate the model. Uncounted hours of conversation and debate between myself, Janice and countless colleagues and students resulted in shaping the model as originally published in 1980. Janice's original work on spelling out the dimensions of personal causation became exemplary for elaborating other concepts in the model. Roann Barris had an important dual role in first extending our understanding of the environment and later collaborating with me to extend and elaborate many of the concepts of the subsystems. Once again, many hours of helpful discussion with therapists and students lie behind the finished product. Beyond that stage, the contributions of others have become too numerous to fully account. Many of those efforts resulted in published works and the authors' efforts are appropriately visible. Others have worked behind the scenes supporting the development of the model in various ways. Notably, the rehabilitation staff at the National Institutes of Health, Clinical Center, have generously provided resources and support including the funding and manpower for development of the artwork for this text and related educational media.

A number of individuals gave generously of their time and efforts to comment upon portions of the manuscript. Thanks are owing to Margaret Antoine, Tammy Bean, Julia DeJean, Anne Fisher, Katie Heredia, Holly Holyk, Amy Leong, Muriel MacKallor, Louise Nakamine, Bonnie Oldham, Suzanne Poirier, Randy Reichler, Nancy Warner, Nancy Wilke, and Beth Wolfe for their helpful input and comments. No doubt there are many others of whom I am unaware. Each of the contributors to this volume worked under a tough timetable, and through their efforts have made elaborations and applications of the model which could never be imagined or effected by a single author. The sense of a community of therapists working on this idea has been especially heartening and has helped several of us through some tough periods when it seemed this volume might never be completed.

Contributors

Roann Barris, Ed.D., O.T.R.
Assistant Professor
Department of Occupational Therapy
University of Wisconsin
Madison, Wisconsin

Nancy Bledsoe M.S., O.T.R.
Director of Occupational Therapy
Winchester Memorial Hospital
Winchester, Virginia

Janice Posatery Burke, M.A., O.T.R.,
F.A.O.T.A.
Private Practice and Clinical Associate
 Professor
Department of Occupational Therapy
University of Southern California
Los Angeles, California

Florence Clark, Ph.D., O.T.R.,
F.A.O.T.A.
Associate Professor
Department of Occupational Therapy
University of Southern California
Los Angeles, California

Sally Hobbs Cubie, M.S., O.T.R.
Assistant Professor
Department of Occupational Therapy
College of Allied Health Sciences
Howard University
Washington, D.C.

Gloria Furst, M.P.H., O.T.R.
Consultant
Occupational Therapy Department
Clinical Center, National Institutes of Health
Bethesda, Maryland

Jana Green, O.T.R.
Occupational Therapist
Cancer Rehabilitation and Continuing
 Education Program
Medical College of Virginia Hospitals
Richmond, Virginia

Betty Herlong Harlan, M.S., O.T.R.
Captain, U.S. Army
Assistant Chief, Occupational Therapy
 Department

Landstuhl Army Regional Medical Center
Germany

Kathy L. Kaplan, M.S., O.T.R.
Occupational Therapy Consultant
Washington, D.C.

Marion Kavanagh, M.S., O.T.R.
Senior Occupational Therapist
Richmond Community Mental Health Center
Richmond, Virginia

Gary Kielhofner, Dr.P.H., O.T.R.,
F.A.O.T.A.
Associate Professor
Department of Occupational Therapy
Sargent College of Allied Health Professions
Boston University
Boston, Massachusetts

Ellen Kolodner, M.S.S., O.T.R.,
F.A.O.T.A.
Assistant Professor
Department of Occupational Therapy
College of Allied Health Sciences
Thomas Jefferson University
Philadelphia, Pennsylvania

Sue Hirsch Knox, M.A., O.T.R.,
F.A.O.T.A.
Private practice
Los Angeles, California

Ruth Ellen Levine, Ed.D., O.T.R.
Professor and Chairman
Department of Occupational Therapy
College of Allied Health Sciences
Thomas Jefferson University
Philadelphia, Pennsylvania

Mike Lyons, M.S., B. Occ. Thy., B. Econ.
Senior Tutor
Department of Occupational Therapy
University of Queensland
St. Lucia, Queensland, Australia

M. Jeanne Madigan, Ed.D., O.T.R., F.A.O.T.A.
Professor and Chairman
Department of Occupational Therapy
Virginia Commonwealth University
Richmond, Virginia

Zoe Mailloux, M.A., O.T.R.
Instructor
Department of Occupational Therapy
University of Southern California
Los Angeles, California

Carol Lee McLellan, M.S., O.T.R.
Occupational Therapist
Southside Virginia Training Center
Petersburg, Virginia

Anne M. Neville, Ph.D. (Cand.), O.T.R.
Chief Occupational Therapist
Veterans Administration Medical Center
Boston, Massachusetts

Peggy Neville, O.T.R.
Occupational Therapist
Gaebler Children's Center
Waltham, Massachusetts

Frances Maag Oakley, M.S., O.T.R.
Consultant
Department of Rehabilitation
Clinical Center
National Institutes of Health
Bethesda, Maryland

Joan Owens, M.S., O.T.R.
Occupational Therapist
St. Peter's Hospital
Albany, New York

Lillian Hoyle Parent, M.A., O.T.R., F.A.O.T.A.
Coordinator of Education and Research
Department of Occupational Therapy
The University of Texas Medical Branch
Galveston, Texas

Joan C. Rogers, Ph.D., O.T.R., F.A.O.T.A.
Associate Professor in Occupational Therapy
Assistant Professor in Psychiatry
University of Pittsburgh
Pittsburgh, Pennsylvania

Charlotte Brasic Royeen, M.S., O.T.R.
Assistant Professor
Department of Occupational Therapy
Howard University
Washington, D.C.

Cheryl Salz, M.S., O.T.R.
Supervisor of Occupational and Recreational
  Therapy
St. Luke's—Roosevelt Hospital
New York, New York

Jayne Shepherd, M.S., O.T.R.
Occupational Therapist
Occupational Therapy Department
Sheltering Arms Hospital
Richmond, Virginia

Teena L. Snow, M.S., O.T.R.
Clinical Instructor
Department of Medicine
University of North Carolina
Chapel Hill, North Carolina

Cynthia A. Stabenow, O.T.R.
Coordinator, Arthritis Rehabilitation Unit
Rehabilitation Research and Training Center
University of Virginia Medical Center
Charlottesville, Virginia

Janet Hawkins Watts, M.S., O.T.R.
Assistant Professor
Department of Occupational Therapy
Virginia Commonwealth University
Richmond, Virginia

Contents

Introduction

Gary Kielhofner

Occupational therapists daily face problems and challenges which call both for breadth of knowledge and for clarity and organization of perspective. The therapist must, therefore, have both a wide array of concepts and a means of synthesizing those concepts into a framework for efficient decisions and action. In this text, a model of human occupation is presented. The goal of this model is to address the needs of therapists for an integration of the concepts and techniques which characterize mainstream practice in occupational therapy.

The model seeks to provide explanations of the occupational functioning of persons, knowledge which all occupational therapists require to serve the occupational needs of human beings. This model, by focusing on occupational behavior, seeks to articulate the unique orientation and expertise of occupational therapists. At the same time, the model draws together interdisciplinary concepts from many fields. It also invites the use of concepts and practices from other compatible theoretical frameworks. As an integrative and systematic organizational device, the model should allow therapists to identify their concerns for patients and clients in a holistic fashion. Use of this model is intended to elevate clinical practice from a simple application of techniques to a professional process of conceptual problem-solving, planning and action.

THE NATURE AND USE OF A CONCEPTUAL MODEL

Since this text proposes to describe and elucidate a *model* of human occupation, it is important to consider first what is meant by a model and what is its purpose. A model is a conceptual or mental representation of some phenomenon (1). The purpose of a model is to organize and to make more efficient one's thinking about that phenomenon. Generally, models describe and explain very complex processes and/or structures and seek to make persons' thinking about

them easier and more systematic. The purpose of the model of human occupation is to provide a representation of various structures and processes that underlie occupational behavior. In human beings, occupation is a multifaceted phenomenon that involves the simultaneous operation of biological, psychological, social, and ecological factors. Without a means to synthesize these important variables and their relationships, the occupational therapist can be faced with an unwieldy morass of facts and concepts. The model of human occupation is a conceptual representation of the variables and their relationships that constitute and determine occupational behavior in humans.

CONCEPTUAL MODELS IN OCCUPATIONAL THERAPY

In order to understand where models fit into the overall knowledge of organization of occupational therapy, it is useful to think of theory as divided into two levels. The highest level is the gestalt knowledge of the field which incorporates *all* the field's concerns, concepts and technical expertise. This highest level of knowledge also defines the field, sets boundaries on its activities and specifies its values and goals. This gestalt level of knowledge in occupational therapy has been referred to as the *paradigm* of the field (2, 5, 9). While occupational therapy presently has no clearly defined paradigm, one is beginning to be developed which preserves the early themes and concepts of occupational therapy. It has grown out of the work of many contributors and represents the fundamental belief that occupational therapy is concerned with the occupational nature of human beings and with the use of occupations as therapy.

The second level of knowledge in occupational therapy is less global; it is the level of models of practice. Since the paradigm is broad and all encompassing, it is too global for direct application in practice. Rather, clinicians and researchers employ more simplified and encapsulated models. The model of human occupation organizes a number of key concepts but not all of the concepts from the emerging paradigm of occupation.

Ultimately the field may have several practice models, each of which is related to the broader paradigm and which guide practice and research for different types of populations and settings and even for different conceptual orientations of occupational therapists. As models develop and their practice and research applications are demonstrated, therapists may be able to choose the model which best suits their own situation and practice.

While some diversity of practice models is desirable, the field cannot have an unlimited number of such models. Thus, while models are not as encompassing as the paradigm, they should be broad enough to have a variety of applications. The model of human occupation has been applied in various types of clinical processes and with a variety of patient and client populations. This text seeks to give a representative view of the types of applications which are possible and to encourage readers to go on to make their own applications analogous to those demonstrated here.

The model of human occupation synthesizes major theories which have been used or developed by occupational therapists. Thus, the model does not exclude other legitimate theories, concepts and techniques in occupational therapy. For example, the chapter on child development seeks to illustrate how neurodevelopment is part of the development of occupational behavior and how the occupational behavior of the child facilitates sensory and motor development. A later chapter will illustrate how a therapist practicing under the model in pediatrics would also employ neurodevelopmental treatment techniques. Similarly, the chapter on physical disabilities will illustrate how biomechanical approaches are integrated into treatment guided by the model.

The model is intended to facilitate holistic thinking about a person's occupational dysfunction. The model cannot incorporate the details of many forms of biological and psychological disturbances which are aspects or correlates of occupational dysfunction; consequently, therapists using the model will necessarily draw upon existing concepts and practices relevant to understanding and remediating these more discrete aspects of dysfunction in individuals they serve. The model is intended as a way of bringing together these various facts and approaches into a single coherent perspective. It should provide a logical basis for including other concepts and practices and, at the same time, allow the therapist to avoid unnecessary reliance on a single technique or approach. The model is designed as a thinking tool to aid decisions about which concepts and techniques are relevant and warranted in a particular situation.

BACKGROUND AND GENESIS OF THE MODEL

The model of human occupation has grown out of the occupational behavior tradition first developed by Reilly (7, 8) and her colleagues and students. Over a period of many years, these persons engaged in exploratory research to identify appropriate concepts for understanding occupational behavior in human beings and for explaining why and how occupation could be used as a therapeutic measure. Since the number of concepts grew to be large and somewhat cumbersome, it became necessary to develop models of practice which integrated these concepts into a workable format. The model of human occupation began as one such model which sought to build upon the existing occupational behavior tradition. Over a period of several years, with the collaboration of many colleagues, the model has been elaborated, expanded and clarified. Since the time of its original publication (2–4, 6) helpful criticism, research, further theoretical exploration, and a variety of projects aimed at clinical application have resulted in changes which are reflected in this text. No doubt this model will continue to change and develop as it responds to criticism, empirical findings and needs for clinical relevance.

CONTENT AND ORGANIZATION OF THE VOLUME

This book is divided into several major sections that proceed from theoretical to applied in nature. The first section presents and discusses the model and its general implications for occupational therapy practice. The model is based on general systems theory and posits that human beings function as open systems. As elucidated in Chapter 1, this means that humans are recognized as spontaneous beings with unfolding potentials and that they maintain and change themselves by what they do. The concepts of open systems are presented as the basic structure of framework of the model. Open systems theory not only provides a cogent conceptual structure for the model, but also illuminates the nature of the therapy. That is, occupational therapy is recognized as an open system process in which therapists enable persons to maintain and change their function through facilitating their participation in selected occupations.

Chapter 2 builds upon the system framework introducing concepts which elucidate human occupation. Referred to as the components and determinants of occupation, the concepts introduced in this chapter seek to explain how persons choose, order and perform their occupational behavior. Concepts of personal causation, values, interests, roles, habits, and skills are central to this discussion. The role of neurological musculoskeletal, and symbolic phenomena in the process of skilled behavior is also covered. This chapter presents the internal patterns and components that characterize the occupational nature of humans. The following chapter focuses on the dynamic processes that are influenced by, and that maintain or change, these internal patterns.

Occupational behavior is directed to, and is influenced by, the environment. Chapter 4 presents a conceptualization of the occupational environments in which persons behave. It discusses the factors that influence persons' choices to enter settings that change their behavior once they interact with those settings. The final chapter in the first section most directly bridges the theory to clinical application. It utilizes the model as a way of conceptualizing function and dysfunction in occupational behavior. The aim of this discussion is to provide occupational therapists a unique way of viewing states of adaptation and maladaptation in clients and patients.

The second section of this book discusses occupational development. Using the model as an organizational framework, literature pertaining to development of occupational behavior in childhood, adolescence, adulthood, and later adulthood is synthesized into an overall conceptualization of the occupational behavior developmental continuum. This section of the book seeks to achieve a critical link between the field's concern for occupation in human life and the necessity of incorporating a developmental perspective into the understanding of occupational behavior.

The two following sections of the book present applications of the model in practice. In Section 3 treatment planning, occupational analysis (which is an expansion of traditional activity analysis), and program development are presented. These discussions cover generic applications of the model relevant to many areas of practice.

Section 4 presents applications of the model in specific areas of practice. The organization of chapters in this section corresponds to natural groupings of practice that have arisen in the field. They include physical disabilities, psychosocial disorders, pediatric dysfunction, mental retardation, and aging-related occupational dysfunction. The inclusion and grouping of disabilities are not intended as a statement on the potentials for application of the model or as an endorsement of any particular way of categorizing disabilities or areas of practice. They are simply based on practical considerations, including convention within the field and the state of the art, in applying the model to practice. The final sections of the book include practical resources and exercises to facilitate understanding and using the model.

THE MODEL IN THE CURRENT CONTEXT OF PRACTICE

Occupational therapy is in a period of rapid transformation fueled by a number of internal and external factors. Externally there is a growing expectation from consumers, health care administrators and policy makers, third-party reimbursers, and peer professions that occupational therapists demonstrate a sound rationale for, and efficacy of, their services. Internally, the field is responding to these expectations and challenges and moving toward a greater level of complexity and coherence in its knowledge and practice.

The various internal and external challenges to occupational therapy are requiring more sophistication and effort than ever before. The field must develop its own unique knowledge and translate that knowledge into viable practice. Occupational therapists can only do so if there is an active collaboration between those who generate and organize knowledge and those who operationalize it in clinical practice. This book is the product of such an alliance and seeks to present the kind of coalition of theory and practice that is needed to serve occupational therapy in the future.

References

1. Bors S: *The Art of Awareness.* (ed 2). Dubuque, Iowa, Brown Publishers, 1973.

2. Christiansen CH: Editorial: toward resolution of crisis: research requisites in occupational therapy. *Occup Ther J Res* 1:15–24, 1981.

3. Kielhofner G: A model of human occupation, Part 2. Ontogenesis from the perspective of temporal adaptation. *Am J Occup Ther* 34:657–663, 1980.

4. Kielhofner G: A model of human occupation, Part 3. Benign and vicious cycles. *Am J Occup Ther* 34:731–737, 1980.

5. Kielhofner G, Burke JP: A model of human occupation, Part 1. Conceptual framework and content. *Am J Occup Ther* 34:572–581, 1980.

6. Kielhofner G, Burke JP, Igi CH: A model of human occupation, Part 4. Assessment and intervention. *Am J of Occup Ther* 34:777–788, 1980.

7. Reilly M: Occupational therapy can be one of the great ideas of 20th century medicine. *Am J Occup Ther* 16:1–9, 1962.

8. Reilly M: The education process. *Am J Occup Ther* 23:299–307, 1969.

9. Shannon P: The derailment of occupational therapy. *Am J Occup Ther* 31:229–234, 1977.

Theoretical Tenets of the Model

Introduction

The five chapters in this section present the theoretical tenets of the model. Topics addressed are the open system theory basis of the model, the variables which compose and influence occupation, the dynamics of occupational behavior, the importance and influence of the environment, and the nature of adaptation and maladaptation in occupational behavior. Collectively these chapters constitute the basic theory of the model.

The chapters are punctuated with practical examples throughout in order to facilitate comprehension and appreciation of the concepts presented. The reader will encounter a large number of concepts which provide the foundation for later chapters. Thus, understanding of this section of the book is critical for appreciation of later chapters. While the reader will most likely find it necessary to return to this section from time to time to renew acquaintence with an idea or concept, the glossary which defines all the concepts introduced in this section should also be a valuable asset.

It should also be noted that a number of exercises in the workbook correspond to this section of the text. The first exercises, which invite the reader to apply concepts from the model to an understanding of self, should be particularly useful in facilitating a more in-depth comprehension of the model.

CHAPTER 1

The Human Being as an Open System

Gary Kielhofner

In this chapter we explore open systems theory and its application to the study of human behavior. Open systems concepts provide a basis in the model for understanding less abstract concepts such as the motivation for occupation and the interaction of the person with the environment. Thus, this chapter provides the conceptual foundation for the subsequent discussion of components and determinations of occupational behavior.

There is nothing new about thinking of phenomena as systems. For instance, occupational therapists study the nervous and musculoskeletal systems. The concept of a system is that certain objects (e.g. muscles and bones) have interrelationships which allow them to function collectively toward an identifiable purpose. A system occurs in nature where several structures constitute some kind of logical whole with readily apparent functions. Two or more systems can combine to form a more complex, yet still identifiably coherent and functional, entity (e.g. the neuromuscular system). In this case the systems that combine to form a larger system are referred to as subsystems. Thus, the concept of systems is simply a coherent way in which to approach understanding of complex phenomena.

While the concept of systems has long been accepted and utilized in science, the theory of open systems is a recent and innovative conceptualization (3, 21). The purpose of open systems thought is to explicate those characteristics and processes that characterize living phenomena. Thus, openness in a system implies exchange of information and/or matter with the environment and the actualization of potentials (21). These processes are basic to all life forms whether they be simple cells, plants, human beings, or social organizations. The relevance of open systems theory has been discussed in such diverse fields as biology (14, 22) psychology (1),

organizational theory (10), medicine (7), and nursing (18). This universality of open systems theory is not surprising since, as Boulding (3) notes, it is developing as a common conceptual language which can be shared by many fields. Occupational therapists will increasingly find that open systems concepts provide a point of exchange between varied clinical and administration personnel in health care. Because open systems theory exists at a level of abstraction beyond the usual substantive theory of disciplines, it serves as an integrative framework for the unique concepts within each field's domain of knowledge. The model which is explicated in this text uses open systems theory as a framework for integrating concepts which explain occupational behavior in humans.

TRADITIONAL CONCEPTS OF HUMAN BEHAVIOR

Throughout history human beings have viewed themselves in a host of ways. Various thought systems have stressed spiritual, animalistic, altruistic, hedonistic, and other diverse facets of the human character. However, one global view of human behavior has dominated both science and popular thought in the past two centuries. This perspective is variously called the mechanistic, closed system or reductionist orientation (13, 21). Mechanistic and closed system thinking refers specifically to the tendency to see all phenomena as machine-like in their operations. A closed system is one that does not interact with its environment or exhibit properties of life; machines are man-made closed systems. Reductionism refers to the methodological orientation which assumes that all phenomena, like machines, can be studied by taking them apart and examining how the pieces are fit together.

The predominance of such a conceptual orientation today is owed to the course of development of science and technology in the Western world. Physical sciences such as astronomy and physics were the first disciplines to achieve substantial success and status. The methodologies and concepts they developed were suited to the study of nonliving phenomena. Viewing the atom or the solar system as a machine-like system (i.e. as a miniature or giant clockwork) was a particularly fruitful enterprise.*

Much of the progress of the physical sciences was due to the methodology which accompanied the mechanistic perspective (6). Reductionist analysis involves the decomposition of phenomena into their constituents in order to study the discrete relationships between them. All phenomena are believed to be constituted by causal relationships among their parts. Accordingly, the doctrine of reductionism is that any system, no matter how complex, can ultimately be understood by reducing it to its least common denominators or building blocks and specifying the cause-and-effect relationships between them. This conceptual strategy has been a powerful tool for science.

The biological and behavioral disciplines began to mature only after the astounding success of the physical sciences. Seeking to replicate the scientific acumen of these classic sciences, the newer disciplines imported their perspectives and methodology. Mechanistic and reductionist thought thus became the basis for understanding living phenomena including the behavior of human beings.

Mechanistic thinking generated and was, in turn, abetted by the rise of the industrial revolution (6). The machine was the achievement par excellence of the industrial age. Not surprisingly the human mind and human body were popularly viewed in this same scientific and technical mode which had advanced civilization. Most readers will recall having learned about the body through the analogy of a factory or a machine; textbook diagrams and posters routinely portray this mechanistic image of humans. Even everyday language bears the ma-

chine analogy. For instance, thinking is described as the operation of cogs turning inside the head.

Bolstered by such trends in popular thought the psychological and social sciences adopted wholeheartedly the perspective of human behavior as a mechanistic phenomenon (6, 9, 19). They sought to understand it through the study of relationships between underlying constituents and their cause-and-effect relationships and, in turn, strengthened the everyday cultural view of people as machine-like.

OPEN SYSTEMS THOUGHT AS AN ALTERNATIVE TO CLOSED SYSTEMS VIEWS OF HUMANS

In many cases the mechanistic, closed system concepts of science advanced understanding of human performance. For instance, kinesiology applied the study of mechanics to understanding how the musculoskeletal system achieves movement. While such reductionism has been a helpful tool for science, it also has important limitations. One impetus for open system thinking was the recognition that, whatever humans (and other living phenomena) had in common with machines, humans were much more complex (1, 20). Thus, additional conceptual tools are required to understand them. Open systems theory offers new concepts to augment and replace incomplete and oversimplified explanations of human behavior. Differences between closed and open systems thought which will be discussed are illustrated in Table 1.1.

Mechanistic thinking has been criticized as resulting in a view of humans as robot-like, passive, seeking equilibrium, and functioning on purely utilitarian grounds (1, 3, 12, 21). In contrast to these closed system views, open system thinking stresses the degree to which human beings are active, spontaneous, and seek stimulation and tension. Further, they acknowledge that much of creative and constructive human thought and action exceeds utilitarian goals such as survival. These themes identify humans as having innate needs for action, stimulation, creation, and production which rank alongside needs for security and survival.

It is also recognized that analyzing constituent parts and their cause-and-effect relations is not an adequate method for sciences which study

---

* It is interesting to note that in modern physical sciences the mechanistic viewpoint is no longer tenable. Major scientific revision of physics rejected the classic newtonian mechanical view of the universe (6). The idea that even the physical realm of nature is like a giant clockwork is no longer considered a valid perspective.

Table 1.1.
A comparison of closed system and open system thinking

Closed system thinking	Open system thinking
Views all phenomena as machine-like	Recognizes special properties of living systems
Analyzes phenomena via reduction to components	Analyzes phenomena as gestalt wholes
Oversimplifies	Recognizes complexity
Results in a view of humans as passive automata seeking equilibrium	Stresses active, spontaneous, tension and stimulation-seeking properties of humans
Views behavior in utilitarian terms, such as survival	Acknowledges creative, playful and productive behavior which exceeds utilitarian requirements
Ignores uniquely human traits such as cognition, decision making, planning, self-awareness	Accounts for self-determination in human behavior stressing purposefulness, goal orientation, meaning, and other conscious processes

human phenomena. Open system theorists seek to study humans as gestalt wholes recognizing that human behavior cannot be understood solely by studying underlying components. Further, it is argued that not all relationships between components of human beings are cause-and-effect in nature. Consequently, new concepts for explaining varied types of interrelationships are proposed.

Many human functions which do not conform to the mechanistic model of behavior were overlooked or discounted by closed system thinking. For instance, free will and related themes such as cognition, decision-making, planning, and self-awareness were ignored or considered inconsequential artifacts of more basic processes (21). Open system thinking seeks to construct a more existential and humanistic view of persons. For instance, open system concepts elucidate self-determination, the ability for change and self-repair and the general capacity of humans to guide their courses of action through conscious awareness. Open system thinking is humanistic in that it stresses that the human being is a locus of spontaneous action and ability for self-direction.

Open system concepts are particularly relevant to occupational therapy. The field's philosophy has always stressed those aspects of human beings addressed by open system theory. Open system thought is also especially salient for the field's clinical practice. Occupational therapy is based on the premise that participation in occupation has the potential to ameliorate dysfunctional states (8, 11, 17, 23). As we will see in the coming discussion, open system concepts

provide a means of more clearly understanding how this therapeutic process works.

Characteristics of An Open System

Many definitions and properties of open systems are discussed in the literature (1, 3, 9, 14). They converge on a set of common themes which may be represented in the following definition of an open system:

An open system is a composition of interrelated structures and functions organized into a coherent whole that interacts with an environment and that is capable of maintaining and changing itself.

This definition can be better appreciated by contrasting the open system to the closed system. Closed systems are also sets of interacting structures and functions. However, they do not possess their own internal coherence which determines overall function, they do not interact with the environment, and they cannot maintain or change themselves. For example, clockworks consist of various cogs and springs (structures) which interact, impinging on each other, transferring movement along a continuum from spring to hand (function). The clock works because of a simple cause-and-effect chain of events by which movement is transferred from one part to another. Any coherence in the clock is that of the creator and fabricator and is, thus, externally imposed on the cause-and-effect operations. Each part and function of the clock is simply a step in a sequence of structures and functions. If a cog is removed or damaged the system breaks down. Clockworks do not interact with an environment and cannot maintain or change their function. Some external agency is needed to wind (i.e. to import energy into the closed system) or to alter the pace of the clock.

In contrast, even the simplest of open systems, the cell, has an overall coherence which allows it to survive despite disturbances or even disruption to a part (21, 22, 24). It maintains its much more flexible structure in the midst of exchanging matter with its environment. Finally, within certain limits, it can alter its structures and functions to accommodate changes in the environment. Open system concepts have been developed to acknowledge and explain these additional and very complex properties of the open system.

SPONTANEITY AND THE PRIMACY OF FUNCTION OVER STRUCTURE

Open systems exhibit two interrelated characteristics. The first is that they are spontaneous. Open systems do not rely on action or agency from the outside to initiate their behavior (21). The fundamental character of all open systems is their self-initiated and ongoing action. Related to this is that open systems have encoded in them informational processes which guide how their potentials will unfold over time. Thus the potential of becoming more complex is part of the spontaneity of the open system. Examples are the potential of the seed to become a plant and the potential of the human brain at birth to become a highly differentiated organ with a role in both physical action and mental activity.

OPEN SYSTEMS VERSUS STATE-DETERMINED SYSTEMS

Open systems also exhibit a predominance of function over structure. Closed systems are state-determined systems that function in a given manner *because* their structures are arranged in a particular way. Open systems are not state determined. That is, their function is not simply caused by the arrangements of structure (21). Function is, instead, influenced by the built-in or acquired goals of the system, the state of the structure, and the conditions in the environment. It is the interaction between these elements which results in the function of the open system.

The difference between state-determined functions and those in the open system is illustrated by the following example. If we observe chemical reactions in a living cell, its behavior will depend in part on various structures in the molecular make-up of the cell, but these various biochemical actions will be governed by the cell's overall purpose and needs (14, 22, 24). Conversely if the same chemicals which are represented in the cell are collected together, the chemical reactions which will take place will only be those determined by the state or structure of the chemical compounds involved, falling short of what happens in the cell. Thus, living systems build upon state-determined systems and integrate them into a more coherent yet flexible organization, and thus possess organizational properties that exceed the complexity of the chemical domain.

RELATIONSHIP OF STRUCTURE AND FUNCTION

As a consequence, the structure of the open system is not static. Rather, its continued existence depends on the underlying action of the system. The structure of the open system cannot endure without the function of the system. Both a cell which ceases to take in nutrients and a muscle which is not utilized undergo degeneration of their structure. Thus, the relationship of structure to function in the open system is much different and more complex than in the closed system.

ENTROPHY AND NEGATIVE ENTROPHY

In the closed system, function or process results in a wearing down of the system and in a movement toward a simple and homogeneous state (3, 21). Examples are the operation of a gasoline engine which eventually erodes parts of the engine and the movement of various gas molecules which results in an even distribution of gases throughout a container. The wearing down of the closed system toward simpler homogeneous states is called entropy.

In the open system, function of the system has the potential to move the system in the opposite direction. That is, the system's functions and processes can build up or make an open system more heterogeneous and complex. For example, action and practice increases muscle strength and motor coordination. Such processes are called negative entropy—that is, a reversal of the natural entropic tendency of closed systems.

Not only is it the case that an open system's function can have a positive organizing effect on the structure; the function also underlies the very existence of the structure. An example that might facilitate understanding of what is meant by this aspect of primacy of function over structure is the plant—a fairly simple open system. In the various phases of a plant's existence its structure may take on very different forms: a seed, a sprout, and a grown plant with leaves, branches, flowers, and fruit. The structure is time-limited and clearly the result of an enduring process. What is more definite about the plant than any particular structure it assumes is that it is part of a cycle of processes that have their own built-in spontaneous order.

CIRCULARITY

We have argued that there is a primacy of function over structure so that function is responsible for maintaining and changing structures in the open system. This is due to the circularity of function in the open system (21). Circularity refers to the fact that the action of the open systems acts back on itself. Another way of saying this is that the open system increasingly becomes what it does. A plant becomes larger because it grows. A muscle becomes a more capable working organ because it is used to do work. A person becomes a better problem solver by virtue of engaging in problem solving. This process of becoming (8) is used in therapy to induce changes in the underlying structure used for action (11).

PHASES OF THE OPEN SYSTEM CYCLE

The way in which function maintains and changes structure can be better understood by delineating the phases of process in the basic cycle of the open system. They are: intake, throughput, output, and feedback (21).

Intake† is the process whereby the open sys-

tem imports energy and information from the environment (1). Eating and reading are examples of intake. The importance of the environment is apparent here since the system can only take in what is available in the environment. The environment of the human being is those objects, events and people with which the person comes into contact.

Throughput is the process by which the system converts what was imported into some other form and incorporates or uses it for its own maintanence or as a resource for generating output (21). Digesting food and incorporating it into cellular structure is an example of throughput. Similarly, visual impressions taken from this page are converted into meanings, understandings and insights that can be used later for thinking about other topics.

Output is the action or production of the system (9). In short, it is what the system does in and to the environment. Output is made possible by the conversion and storage of energy and information in the throughput phase. For example, food that is taken in is converted to energy for movement; information taken in through reading is converted to personal knowledge which can be used to discuss a topic.

Feedback is the return of information by which the system learns about the process or consequences of its action. This returning information becomes part of the intake of the system. Referred to as a feedback loop, it forms a connection between output and intake and completes the open system cycle. Figure 1.1 diagrams the basic cycle of the open system.

Let us consider an example that illustrates this cycle. One is listening to a conversation and reacts to something being discussed. One then enters a comment, listening to oneself as one speaks to monitor how well one expresses the idea and observing the reaction of the other conversants. In this example listening is the intake. The reaction to the conversation is a process of throughput whereby one converts the information to an opinion or idea as it is interrelated with what one already knows or thinks. Expressing a comment is output. Monitoring oneself while talking and noting the reactions of others are examples of feedback. Other persons' responses will, in turn, be taken in, evaluated and reacted to (throughput) and may lead one to give yet another comment (output). As the example illustrates, the cycle of the open system is a constant and ongoing process that subtly shapes and directs how we think and behave.

---

† The term "intake" is used here because it is more adequately descriptive of the active and selective process of importing energy and information than a more frequently used term, "input." Open systems do not passively receive energy and information from the environment but actively seek out and select what they require.

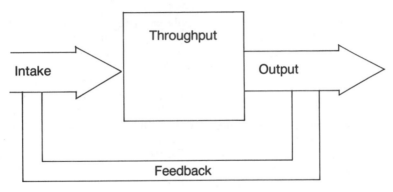

Figure 1.1. The open system cycle.

It is important to note that while the environment provides information necessary for the system, output is not an automatic or passive response to the environment. Before the system intakes information it must have a reason for doing so. Thus, the built-in, or acquired, purposes or goals of the system are critical. Some interest in the topic of conversation or in the conversants is a prerequisite before one pays attention to, and takes in, what is being said. Both intake and output of the system are often in response to the purpose or goals of the system. The output of the system involves changing or manipulating the environment. The interaction between system and the environment is thus a dynamic and complex process, whereby both shape and change each other.

PURPOSEFULNESS

We have noted that open systems exhibit an overall coherence and that they act in response to inner goals. This is referred to as the property of purposefulness in open systems (3, 21). Some of the purposes of open systems are universal. For instance, living systems seek to maintain and prolong their existence. Other purposes can be secondary and acquired. For example, an animal can come to seek water at a given place because it fulfills a need related to survival. Human beings are unique in that they pursue many purposes which are apparently unrelated to such basic things as survival. That is, they may do things simply because they are attractive or meaningful. This is not so surprising if we consider that life itself is an improbable phenomena. Spontaneous living action of the simple open system unfolds in humans as the creation of complex ends and means referred to as culture.

STEADY STATE

In addition to pursuing goals, open systems also maintain themselves in certain optimal conditions. This is referred to as the steady state of the system. This does not mean that open systems seek to be constant or homeostatic. Homeostasis has classically been used to refer to a tendency to return to constant and unchanging states. At one time this was the predominant view of living things—i.e. that they sought to minimize disturbances and changes, always returning to an original state of affairs (21). In contrast, the concept of a steady state recognizes that systems seek to keep certain equilibria, but that the process may involve constantly changing states. The system, the environment, or both, may be in a state of constant change. Maintaining a steady state in the midst of such change is much more complex than homeostasis. For instance, a steady state that humans seek is to be aroused and challenged (2). Too little challenge leaves persons understimulated and they will experience discomfort as in sensory deprivation experiments. Too much challenge may create fear. In order to maintain this steady state of arousal, humans undergo constant change (16). For example, when one begins a new activity, what might pose a reasonable challenge initially, becomes a boring task once one's skill is improved. One takes on more challenging tasks with the result that skill is even further argumented and consequently even greater challenges must be sought. Thus in order to maintain a steady state of arousal the system finds itself undergoing constant transformation and seeking ever greater stimulation. The system maintains a steady state in the midst of changing.

EQUIFINALITY

Open systems, we noted earlier, embody spontaneity and potential. Spontaneity results in the initiation and continuation of the open system cycle when environmental conditions are appropriate. The open system cycle maintains and changes the system, thus allowing the unfolding of potentials. The openness of the open system is represented in the ability of the system to achieve different states and to achieve them through different pathways, a property referred to as equifinality (21). That is, unlike chemicals in a test tube which arrive at equilibrium through a series of predictable chain reactions, the open system is able to unfold its potentials in a wide variety of directions and through different sequences. For example, the human infant has the potential for communication through language but, depending on the environment, any language can become the child's means of communicating. The infant further has the capacity to acquire perceptual motor skills, but experience (i.e. the open system cycle over time) will determine whether that potential unfolds as the ability to fabricate a basket, play a violin or perform surgery. Such flexibility is critical to the ability of the human to adapt to varying environments.

The ability of the system to achieve end states through various pathways is also important for adaptation under conditions where the structure of the human system is interrupted through disease or trauma. For example, blind persons can read—ordinarily a visual function—through touch. Such adaptations of alternative processes to achieve a given end are open system properties that characterize the human capacity for repairing itself and for achieving a desired state or function through flexible means. If humans were state-determined systems, adaptation after disability would be impossible.

DIFFERENTIATION, MODULARIZATION AND CENTRALIZATION

Open systems not only undergo change, but generally the direction of their change is one of increasing complexity (21). Open systems typi-

cally begin in an amorphous state and evolve toward being multifaceted and highly integrated entities. In human beings this pathway is from the fertilized ovum to the adult who possesses not only a highly complex body, but a staggering mental capacity. Open systems become more complex through three interrelated processes: differentiation, modularization‡ and centralization (21).

Differentiation refers to the change from homogeneous to heterogeneous states. That is, when the open system's potentials unfold, various parts take on different sets of characteristics and different functions. Returning to the example of the fertilized ovum, as the cell divides and subdivides, it results not in millions of identical descendent cells, but in highly differentiated cell groups whose structure and function vary from that of other groups of cells. As a concomitant to this evolving diversity in form and function, differentiated parts of an open system exhibit a division of labor. Neuronal and epithelial cells that evolve have vastly different roles to play in the overall functioning of the system.

While differentiation is influenced by innate programmed features (potentials) of the system, it is also highly impacted by the function of the system. Earlier we discussed how the underlying processes of open systems maintained and changed their structures; it can further be specified that differentiation of structure is also influenced by the system's function. For example, differentiation of movement in the hand in order to achieve a variety of grasps is a function of developmental experience in which the child learns to perceive objects and tasks that require a given grasp, and to successfully execute that grasp.

Lest the differentiation of open systems result in highly heterogenous but totally nonfunctional entities, there must be processes of integration where the divergent structures and processes are related to each other and to the purpose of the whole. Modularization and centralization are the processes that facilitate the integration and regulation of differentiated functions.

Modularization refers to the establishment of

---

‡ The term "mechanization" often is used instead of "modularization," a term proposed by Bruner (5). The latter term is used here because it has less connotation of a closed system operation.

a pattern of relations between components of the system (5). Once the patterns are established, the components function semiautonomously as integrated wholes (12). For instance, in the nervous system when pathways of excitation become facilitated, certain actions and reactions occur quite automatically and coherently. The patterns of action are referred to as modularized patterns. Through modularization, some functions of the open system do occur automatically and unconsciously almost as though they were parts of a machine. However, the critical difference is that modularized functions of the open system are created through the action of the system and they may also be changed through the action of the system. Koestler (12) discusses this concept pointing out that humans are not by nature machine-like, but that some people, when they are maintained in unchanging circumstances, do become more and more like automata. Such a process results in persons becoming maladaptive.

Like differentiation, modularization is a process which relies on the function of the system. Establishing a habit is an example of this process. Repeated performance of a behavior is required before it becomes a stable pattern. Modularization allows the structures and functions of differentiated parts of the system to become integrated into functional relationships which endure within the system. Modularization is an important process since it allows parts of the open system to function semiautonomously freeing up the system to concentrate on other functions. In an adaptive open system there is always a balance between structures and functions which are open and changing and modularized ones which are stable and enduring.

Modularization alone is not sufficient to allow integration of levels of function throughout the system. Consequently, a third process, centralization (21), comes into play. When several parallel patterns have been established, the system may find it necessary to coordinate these functional subunits under a single governing entity. This centralization occurs throughout the open system. For example, in the human body, the brain governs and coordinates many body functions. This centralization, that establishes leading parts which rule over other parts of the system, results in the existence of higher levels in the system—that coordinate and govern lower levels. These levels of subsystems are referred to as a hierarchy.

HIERARCHY

One of the most important aspects of the open system is that it exhibits a hierarchy of structures and functions (25). Not all components of a system are parallel to each other. Most parts of a system are governed by other leading parts and, in turn, govern yet lower components. For instance, muscles govern action at joints, while they are in turn governed by the action of the nervous system which is commanded by the conscious choices of the person. When one "wills to move a little finger" a series of commands operate through this hierarchy from conscious thought to neurological excitation, to muscular contraction, and, finally, to mechanical action moving the appendage.

It is important to recognize that this is a much more complex process than the kind of causal chain which operates in mechanical systems with one part affecting the other and so forth. Here very different systems must translate one form of energy into another. Mental energy translated into electrochemical energy must become mechanical energy as levels of the hierarchy are crossed.

RESONATION

Because the relationships between different levels of the hierarchy of a system are not cause and effect in nature, system theorists have an alternative language for referring to their functions. Moss (15) refers to the process of components of a system impacting each other as resonation. This term acknowledges that as a disturbance, change or action makes its way through the system, it interacts with the particular set of conditions which exist in a given part. When the electrochemical impulses passing through the nervous system reach the muscle tissue, they are transformed into the physiological processes which occur in muscles.

COMMANDING AND CONSTRAINING

The interaction between two components of a hierarchical system is more than a linear cause and effect process (25). Two terms, commanding and constraining, are used to describe the interaction between a higher component and a lower component of a system. Higher levels command lower levels (i.e. nervous system physiochemical signals give commands to muscles to contract). On the other hand, lower levels constrain the higher levels. An example of this is that the nervous system cannot command movement over the full range of motion at a swollen, painful and deteriorated arthritic joint. The control signals of higher levels and the constraints of lower levels are important characteristics of open systems which have many clinical implications. For instance, movement at a particular joint is ordinarily thought of as a function of joint integrity, muscle strength and the ability of the nervous system to give appropriate signals to the latter. Less frequently do persons consider the mental state of the patient as a component of joint movement. And the impact of the social environment on such discrete phenomena as moving a joint is usually out of the range of clinical considerations. Yet such simple functions of movement are affected by the cognitive processes of the actor and by social surroundings.

HIERARCHICAL PHENOMENA IN HEALTH CARE

Like many other disciplines, health care professionals have been guilty of ignoring these hierarchical effects (4). This is owed to another important aspect of mechanistic thinking, its materialistic orientation—i.e. giving ascendancy or prime status to the material level of reality over all over levels (6). Because of such thinking of mechanistic science we have concentrated on physical causes of physical disturbances, failing to recognize that causation may be much more complex. We are only beginning to recognize the complex resonation between social, psychological and biological levels. For example, ulcers are physical problems that have their genesis in the social realities of high standards of competition which are mediated though the intermediate levels of the hierarchy, mental stress and parasympathetic nervous system excitation. Nevertheless, we still tend to recognize the disruptions caused by illness primarily at the physical level. This is evident in occupational therapy when a therapist treats an injured or disabled hand, or paralyzed limb with minimal or no consideration of the complex reverberations of disturbances at one level on the other levels of the hierarchy.

Influences of a disturbance at one level of the hierarchy of an open system may resonate throughout several levels. The consequences may be exaggerated or magnified; they may be delayed or so diverse in nature that we fail to recognize their interconnectedness. Therapists who have worked earnestly attempting to increase a patient's strength and range at a joint affected by disease or trauma are often dismayed to find that all their efforts were for naught. Patients sometimes go home only to brood in depression; begin drinking; have families decompensate around them; and return to the hospital with decreased or lost function and with some additional problem such as an addiction or decubiti. Realizing the intense interconnectedness of different levels of the open system, we should not be surprised that attempts to correct or ameliorate problems at one narrow level almost invariably fail because their consequences at other levels were ignored. One of the major thrusts of the model we are constructing in our discussions will be to make the clinician aware of the many levels of function that are potentially involved in any disability.

SUMMARY AND DISCUSSION

In the preceding pages we have examined open systems theory exploring its relevance to human behavior and to occupational therapy. We noted that open systems concepts are being chosen as replacements for traditional mechanistic concepts that tend to oversimplify human behavior and ignore many important human traits while creating a picture of humans as passive automata. Open systems concepts, on the other hand, were shown to view humans as self-directing and capable of making planned change. This orientation, it was argued, is more suited to occupational therapy.

We discussed open system concepts examining the properties of the open system and the processes involved in change in the open system. We identified open systems as spontaneous and as having intense commerce with their environments through a cycle of intake, throughput, output and feedback. This cycle was recognized as responsible for the basic process of self-maintenance and change in the open system. Open systems were described as purposive and oriented to maintaining steady states. Equifinality, or the ability to achieve various states through multiple routes, was described as a manifestation of openness in a system. Change in the open system was examined as a process involving differentiation, modularization and centralization. It was noted that open systems typically develop from amorphous entities to hierarchically arranged systems with complex interrelationships between their different parts. We saw that the complex relations between parts was not limited to cause and effect but included hierarchical processes of resonating, commanding and constraining.

This chapter offered an introduction to open system theory. The following discussions will employ open system concepts as the foundation for talking about human occuptional behavior. As we begin to apply open system concepts to an explanation of how and why persons engage in occupation we will elaborate several themes introduced here. Subsequent chapters examine how the human system is organized, identifying its parts, and their hierarchical relationships. We will examine how circularity is exhibited as persons interact with the environment through their occupational behavior. We will also examine how occupational characteristics of the individual are differentiated, modularized and centralized over the course of development. In short, the abstract open system concepts we have introduced here will be applied to specific topics in the study of human occupation.

Another thrust of future discussions will be to employ open system concepts to explain disability in the system. The current discussion offered a way of understanding how an open system was organized. In future sections we will examine how disease and environmental stresses can produce disorganization in the system. We will consider how one assesses the disabled person as a system exhibiting problems in its self-maintenance and self-change and how to use open system concepts to conceptualize therapy. Occupational therapy will be proposed as an open system process wherein a person engages in therapeutic tasks and activities and thereby maintains and changes functional capacity.

The present discussion began construction of a model of human occupation. Open system concepts provide the conceptual foundations of the model. They are a set of abstract ideas to which we can attach more concrete and substantive concepts directly pertinent to human occupation.

References

1. Allport GW: The open system in personality theory. In Buckley W (ed): *Modern System's Research for the Behavioral Scientist*. Chicago, Aldine, 1968.
2. Berlyne D: *Conflict, Arousal and Curiosity*. New York, McGraw Hill, 1960.
3. Boulding K: General system theory—the skeleton of science. In Buckley W (ed): *Modern Systems Research for the Behavioral Scientist*. Chicago, Aldine, 1968.
4. Brody H: The systems view of man: implications for medicine, science and ethics. *Perspect Biol Med* Autumn:71–92, 1973.
5. Bruner J: Organization of early skilled action. *Child Dev* 44:1–11, 1973.
6. Capra F: *The Turning Point: Science, Society and the Rising Culture*. New York, Simon & Shuster, 1982.
7. Engel G: The need for a new medical model: a challenge for biomedicine. *Science* 196:129–126, 1977.
8. Fidler G, Fidler J: Doing and becoming: the occupational therapy experience. In Kielhofner G (ed): *Health through Occupation: Theory and Practice in Occupational Therapy*. Philadelphia, FA Davis, 1983.
9. Hall AD, Fagen RE: Definition of a system. *General Systems* 1:18–28, 1956.
10. Katz D, Kahn R: *The Social Psychology of Organizations*. New York, Wiley, 1966.
11. Kielhofner G: General system theory: implications for the theory and action in occupational therapy. *Am J Occup Ther* 32:637–645, 1978.
12. Koestler A: Beyond atomism and holism—the concept of the holon. In Koestler A, Smithies JR (eds): *Beyond Reductionism*. Boston, Beacon Press, 1969.
13. Koestler A, Smythies JR: *Beyond Reductionism*. Boston, Beacon Press, 1969.
14. Miller J: *The Living System*. New York, McGraw-Hill, 1978.
15. Moss G: *Illness, Immunity, and Social Interactions*. New York, Wiley, 1973.
16. Reilly M: *Play as Exploratory Learning*. Beverly Hills, Sage, 1974.
17. Rogers J: Order and disorder in medicine and in occupational therapy. *Am J Occup Ther* 36:29–35, 1982.
18. Roy C: *Introduction to Nursing: An Adaptation Model*. Englewood Cliffs, NJ, Prentice Hill, 1976.
19. Skinner BF: *Beyond Freedom and Dignity*. New York, Knopf, 1971.
20. von Bertalanffy L: General system theory and psychiatry. In Arieti S (ed): *American Handbook of Psychiatry*, New York, Basic Books, 1966.
21. von Bertalanffy L: General system theory—a critical review. In Buckley W (ed): *Modern System's Research for the Behavioral Scientist*. Chicago, Aldine, 1968.
22. Warren C, Allen M, Haefner JW: Conceptual frameworks and the philosophical foundations of general living systems theory. *Behav Sci* 24:296–310, 1979
23. Webster PS: Occupational role development in the young adult with mild mental retardation. *Am J Occup Ther* 34:13–18, 1980.
24. Weiss PS: The living system: determinism stratified. In Koestler A, Smythies JR (eds): *Beyond Reductionism* Boston, Beacon Press, 1969.
25. Weiss PS: *Hierarchically Organized Systems in Theory and Practice*. New York, Hafner, 1971.

CHAPTER 2

Components and Determinants of Human Occupation*

Gary Kielhofner and Janice Posatery Burke

The previous chapter described human beings as complex open systems who interact with the environment and who maintain and change themselves through their output or action (Fig. 2.1). All functions of the human organism are open system functions. For instance, the biological integrity of the body is maintained through the intake of nutritional substances, the throughout process of digestion and the output or excretion of waste. Psychological functions such as feelings of belonging are similarly affected by the intake of affection from others and the output or expression of warmth and caring.

The model of human occupation which is being elucidated here offers an explanation of only one facet of the human beings, their occupational behavior. Therefore, the more general concepts of open systems which are relevant to all aspects of human beings are applied only to specific structures and processes related to occupation. There is no attempt to incorporate or explain aspects of human beings beyond the scope of their occupational nature (e.g. sexual or spiritual aspects).

While the model itself will elaborate what is meant by occupational behavior, the following definition serves as a starting point:

Occupational behavior is an activity in which persons engage during most of their waking time; it includes activities that are playful, restful, serious and productive. These work, play and daily living activities are carried out by individuals in their own unique ways based on their beliefs and preferences, the kinds of experiences they have had, their environments and the specific patterns of behaviors that they acquire over time.

* Adapted from and reprinted with permission of The American Occupational Therapy Association, Inc., © 1980 *The American Journal of Occupational Therapy*, 34:572–581.

As the definition suggests, a theory of occupational behavior must account for several aspects of human activity. It must explain why humans choose to spend most of their time in occupation; and it must explain how persons are able to perform work, play and daily living activities and how those occupations are organized into the routines of everyday life. These are the themes to which this theoretical model is directed.

THE SUBSYSTEMS

In the previous chapter, it was noted that any system can be composed of a number of subsystems and that these subsystems may be hierarchically organized. For instance, the neuromuscular system is composed of a nervous subsystem and a musculoskeletal subsystem. The two subsystems constitute a hierarchy with the nervous system governing the musculoskeletal system.

To explain how occupational behavior is *motivated*, *organized* and *performed* this model conceptualizes the human system as composed of a hierarchy of three subsystems. They are: volition, habituation, and performance (Fig. 2.2). The volition subsystem governs the overall operations of the system and is responsible for choosing and initiating occupational behavior. The habituation subsystem is a middle level subsystem which organizes occupational behavior into patterns or routines. At the bottom of the hierarchy is the performance subsystem which is responsible for producing occupational behavior. These three subsystems work together in an integrated fashion to allow the human system to output occupational behavior. They represent a continuum in the human being from the automatic performance of routine everyday behavior to the conscious choices for occupational roles. Thus, we conceptualize the human being as an open system composed of three hierarchically arranged subsystems that func-

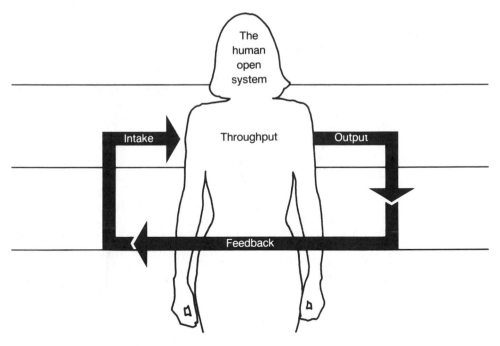

Figure 2.1.   The human being as an open system.

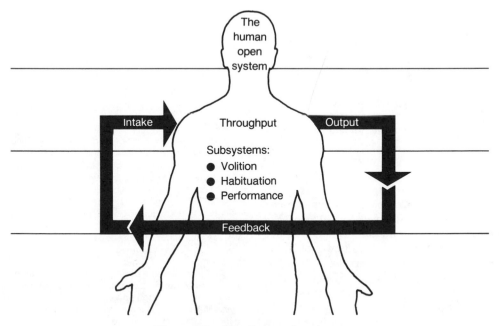

Figure 2.2.   The three subsystems.

tion to choose, routinize, and produce occupational behavior.

The Volition Subsystem

The volition subsystem is conceptualized to address the question of how occupational behavior is motivated. The volition subsystem is defined as *an interrelated set of energizing and symbolic components which together determine conscious choices for occupational behavior. The energizing component is a generalized urge for exploration and mastery. The symbolic components are images (i.e. beliefs, recollections, convictions, expectations) which include, personal causation, values and interests* (Fig. 2. 3).

The term, volition, connotes willing or choosing. Conceiving of motivation as a process of willing behavior is a departure from the classic concepts of motivation. Traditional definitions such as those found in psychoanalysis and behaviorism, began with the assumption that behavior was caused by underlying drives. These drives operated like built-up pressure demanding release or expression (a closed system concept) (11, 14, 17, 54). Drives were also conceived of as viscerogenic—that is, arising from tissue needs (e.g. hunger, thirst, sex). In the presence of the need state, the organism was motivated to seek and gain satiation. Behavior was conceptualized as a function of the organism's action enacted for the purpose of relieving the tension that arose in association with these drives. Acquisition of skills and other learned behaviors was seen as a by-product of such tension-releasing behavior. The idea of conscious choice of behavior was largely considered irrelevant to the topic of motivation. Indeed, humans were viewed as being at the mercy of their drives and free will was considered an illusion (50).

It is now understood that motivation is a more complex, open system phenomena that involves rational and emotional choices for behavior. Not all energy underlying a system's action is like built-up pressure. Rather, it can be manifest in the open system's spontaneous tendency to express or use itself. Reilly (41, p 6) captured the essence of this idea in the phrase "the power to act creates the need to use the power." The essence of a living system is that, inherent in it, is a spontaneous energy which moves it to action. Because it is alive, the open system seeks to act.

Occupation is motivated by humans' need to explore and master themselves and their world.†
The concept of an urge to explore and master is based on the observations and theories of a number of writers (1, 11, 14, 36, 41, 49, 51, 54, 55) all of whom stress that humans have an urge to be aroused, to seek sensory stimulation, to act, and to be effective. The underlying urge toward exploration and mastery has a biological basis. It is viewed as the need arising from the complex nervous systems of human beings which requires sensory stimulation and the opportunity to act. In contrast to viscerogenic drives which motivate short-term tension-reducing behavior, this neurogenic energy is manifest in persistent tension-seeking behavior (1, 54). It guides human beings to investigate, to create, to fabricate, to celebrate, to compete and cooperate, and to engage in the whole range of acts which constitute occupational behavior.

Volition is thus conceptualized as beginning with this powerful neurogenic urge toward exploration and mastery which provides the basic energy and desire for choosing action. Behavior energized by this urge is chosen for its own sake—it is intrinsically motivated as opposed to behavior which is done in order to satisfy some external motive (14).

While the concept of a powerful and persistent neurogenic urge to explore and master offers an explanation of why persons would spend a great deal of their time in interaction within their environments, it does not explain how persons make selections for their interactions. Thus, it is also recognized that volition is composed of

---

† The phase, "exploration and mastery," was chosen as a descriptor for the urge which was conceptualized to underlie occupation because the phrase was thought to capture the range of behaviors and needs that authors concerned with intrinsic motivation discussed. As with any set of terms, these words may convey colloquial meanings not intended as part of the concept. "Mastery" is a term which is associated by some with the idea of dominating or exploiting. For example, mastery of the environment may convey to persons the connotations of exploitation and spoiling of the environment and its natural resources. Similarly, it may connote unfair domination of other persons. This is not the connotation intended by the present concept. "Mastery" was chosen as a descriptor for the global human urge to gain control over personal action and over the demands and challenges posed by the physical and social environment. Thus, mastery is used here to connote fitness and responsiveness to external demands and to personal desires for competence.

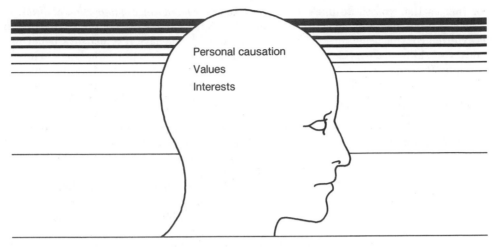

Figure 2.3.   Volition subsystem.

images or symbols (40) that the person holds about exploring and mastering the world. These images concern the person's awareness and beliefs about self as an actor in the world. Forming the symbolic component of the volition subsystem, they are values, personal causation and interests. These images are continuously generated and modified through experience as the person interacts with the environment.

The human infant comes into the world with this powerful and global urge to explore and master. Initially such exploration is evidenced by the child's emerging visual awareness of, and interest in, objects and people, and by undifferentiated kicking and swiping at objects. With time and maturation, vocalization, object manipulation and play with others provide continued opportunities for interaction with and information about behavior and its effect on the environment. As the child so encounters the material and human world, an internal image about self as an agent in the world is built-up. This image, which begins as primitive awareness, differentiates into three sets of images: values, personal causation, and interests.

As these images develop throughout life they influence the choices a person makes. That is, the individual is energized by the urge to explore and master, but the urge is influenced by what the person perceives to be interesting and valuable, and by what the person believes himself or herself capable of doing. In this way personal causation, interests and values interact with the urge to explore and master shaping the person's choices of occupational behavior. Ongoing en-

actment of occupational behavior provides new experiences and feedback that generate continuous images of personal causation, values and interests leading to new choices, and so forth. Thus, the open system cycle provides opportunities for constant differentiation of these images throughout the course of development.

PERSONAL CAUSATION

One of the first discoveries of life is the connection between personal intention, action and its consequences (4, 11). Throughout early development individuals become increasingly aware that they can command their bodies to act and that acting on the environment can have effects. Once the link between intention and its external consequences is established, the individual has developed a sense of personal causation (11).

Personal causation refers to an individual's personal knowledge of self as a cause who creates observable changes in the environment. As experience accumulates, individuals develop this sense that they can affect their own behavior and changes in the environment. Personal causation is thus a set of convictions about self that influences personal choices. In the context of examining how choices for behavior could be therapeutically elicited, the concept of personal causation was elaborated to identify four dimensions of this personal knowledge (6). Personal causation is defined as *a collection of beliefs and expectations which a person holds about his or her effectiveness in the environment*. The collection of images that constitute one's sense of personal causation includes belief in internal versus external control, belief in skills, belief in the efficacy of skills, and expectancy of success versus failure (6) (Fig. 2.4).

Internal Versus External Orientation

Experience encountering the environment yields a generalized sense of one's degree of autonomy. This belief in internal versus external control is *the individual's conviction that outcomes in life are related to personal actions (internal control) versus the action of others, fate or luck (external control)*. An adaptive perspective includes the general belief that one is in control with an appreciation for those things which are beyond personal control. A sense of being in control is associated with the tendency of a person to seek out appropriate opportunities in the environment, to pay attention to feedback as a means of correcting performance and to engage in a moderate amount of risk taking (43). Persons who feel externally controlled often take unreasonable or very few risks, ignore or distort feedback and do not pay attention to opportunities in the environment—behaviors consistent with their belief that it doesn't make any difference what they do since the outcomes in their lives are beyond their personal control. External orientation is also associated with general feelings of alienation (6, 11, 19).

Belief in Skill

The second aspect of personal causation is belief in skill which is *a person's conviction that he or she has a range of important abilities*. These convictions about areas of skills often determine choices for behavior. A person's belief in skill generally is reflected in the types of work and play chosen. Adaptive persons recognize which skills they perform exceptionally well, adequately and poorly. Ask an accomplished carpenter what he or she is good at and one will likely get the response "I'm good with my hands." In contrast, the successful accountant is more likely to respond with "I'm good with figures."

In hospitals and rehabilitation settings, patients may not recognize or believe that they have skills. Many persons with disabilities have a distorted belief in skill. Among the reasons for this distortion may be trauma or disease which has significantly impacted on one or more aspects of functional ability. Limited opportunities to engage in activities that give feedback on performance may also contribute to a skewed sense of skill. When a person's belief in skills is distorted, behavior may reflect either a failure to use capacities or attempts to perform tasks that are beyond abilities. Only when a disabled person begins to rebuild a realistic belief in skill is a more adaptive pattern of behavior likely to emerge. Thus, gradual experiences in a safe and playful environment contribute to increased belief in skill.

Belief in the Efficacy of Skill

In addition to belief in skill, persons also possess an image of the efficacy of skill which is the *belief that one's abilities are useful and relevant in one's life situation*. Most persons can

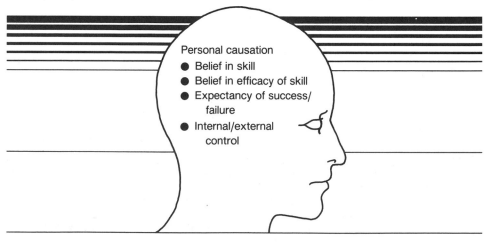

Figure 2.4.   Personal causation.

recall some childhood challenge such as a tree to climb or a street to cross which was beyond their capacity. They stood before the obstacle knowing they could climb, jump or cross a street, but this particular challenge was one for which their skill was not yet efficacious. With time and experience skills develop and are used to successfully meet such challenges. This perceived match between one's capacity and the demands and resources of the environment leads one to make positive choices for encountering the environment through occupational behavior. Because skill is developed in terms of one's environment and its characteristics, there is generally an ecological match of personal capacity to one's surroundings.

Expectancy of Success or Failure

Because of their awareness of time, persons' beliefs about control and skill also lead to perceptions of what future action will yield. The expectancy of success or failure is *one's anticipation of future endeavors and whether their outcomes will be successful or not.* Experience teaches one whether one is likely to succeed or fail and where such outcomes are likely. The expectancy of success is closely linked to a sense of hope—a positive feeling about the future. Without expectancy of success it is difficult for a person to apply effort and sustain present action. A person who expects failure will attempt to avoid the tasks or settings that require performance. When persons are asked to perform in therapy, they may refuse or resist because they cannot see the possibility of success. Fear of failure is, in itself, a paralyzing condition which prevents persons from encountering their environments.

PERSONAL CAUSATION AND THE PROCESS OF CHOOSING

As persons interact with their environments, they generate images about their effectiveness. This is the view of self as a causal agent, or personal causation. This complex of convictions about the self as a cause greatly influences choices for action. If an individual consistently achieves desired outcomes and experiences self as capable of successful action, a positive sense of effectiveness develops. Experiences yield complex images of the more specific aspects of one's capacity for action, its environmental relevance and its potential for success. This self-knowledge is continually influenced by one's ongoing stream of actions, experiences, and feedback (52).

Personal causation represents a continuum of behaviors exemplified on the one end by persons who believe they are in control and have relevant skills and potential for success (origins) and on the other end by those who lack belief in their own control and skills and who are more apt to expect failure (pawns) (11). Most individuals demonstrate a combination of origin or pawnlike behavior in different situations they encounter depending on their degree of experience and knowledge. In general, an experience of freedom and commitment to self-improvement is associated with positive personal causation while feelings of constraint by outside influences and consequent failure to commit oneself to action and growth is associated with negative images of personal causation (6, 11, 32).

Both because the personal convictions one holds are the result of action and its consequences, and because this personal causation influences choices for action, personal causation is self-augmenting. Origins believe in their essential freedom and ability to control their lives; they take action, experience control and further develop their belief in control. Pawns remain convinced of their helplessness, will not decisively act, give up control, and receive the feedback that they are constrained by circumstance and inability.

Belief in internal control and in skill are, of course, not the same thing as actual control and skill. Consequently, a person's image about self is not necessarily accurate. One may have had the experience of feeling as though one were especially good at something until confronted with someone whose skills were far superior. Such experiences usually cause one to adjust and maintain a realistic view of personal abilities. If one develops an underestimation or overestimation of control and skill, adaptation problems may follow. In order to adapt a person need not have a complete and unfailing belief in personal causation. Rather, a realistic appreciation of capacity founded on some degree of control, skill and success is optimal.

VALUES

From earliest childhood experiences, persons interact with an external cultural milieu that embodies certain values relevant to occupation. Values are *images of what is good, right and/or important.* They are principles which guide human conduct (20, 24, 28, 31, 51). As individuals interact with various environments, they generally assimilate the values of those environments, acquiring convictions about what actions are good, right and important. These internalized value images influence choices for occupational behavior. Persons perceive value when they see a course of action as the only proper way to act (31). The process of acquiring values begins in early childhood development when adults' reactions to children's behavior communicates the perceived worth or appropriateness of behavior. It also continues throughout adulthood as individuals are confronted with new life situations, either natural or traumatic, which demand that one acquire, give up or change values.

Values represent a blending of biology and culture (33). That is, humans inherit the biological urge to explore and master, which finds its expression in human culture. The culture, in turn, defines potentials and boundaries for how that urge will be expressed. Thus, in one culture, environmental mastery may mean seeking harmony with nature and, in another, it may signify dominating nature.

Cultural values can shape human behavior in either adaptive or maladaptive directions. For instance, a strong work ethic may be indirectly responsible for individuals who overstress themselves by demanding unnecessarily high quantity in all aspects of their work.

Since values are commitments to performing in culturally sanctioned ways, one experiences a sense of belonging when one operationalizes values. Strong emotions are also associated with values. Values are perceived as obligatory in nature and thus exert a strong influence on choices that persons make. Since values determine one's view of the worth of various occupations, they influence the degree of satisfaction and sense of self-worth that one derives from performing various occupations.

While human values span a wide spectrum of both secular and spirtual concerns, there are four components of values relevant to occupational behavior: temporal orientation, meaningfulness of activities, occupational goals, and personal standards (Fig. 2.5).

Temporal Orientation

Human beings are unique in their ability to be aware of, and oriented to, time. Temporal orientation is *the way in which an individual interprets and views his or her own placement in time; it includes the degree of orientation or concern with past, present or future, and beliefs about how time should be used.* Humans bear a complex image of themselves located in time (2); it is composed of memories of the past, present awareness, and anticipation of the future. Consequently, behavior is not always chosen solely on the basis of present contingencies, but can reflect both past lessons and future goals (9, 10, 26).

Both cultures and individuals vary greatly in their degree of orientation to past, present and future, and temporal orientation also changes with development. The child is present oriented, while the older adolescent and the young adult are more future oriented.

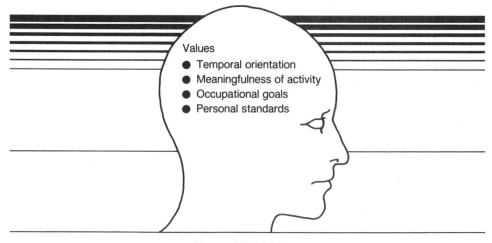

Values
- Temporal orientation
- Meaningfulness of activity
- Occupational goals
- Personal standards

Figure 2.5.   Values.

In addition to concern with past, present and future, an individual also holds values about how time should be used (21). For most Westerners time is viewed as a commodity which can be sold, wasted and allocated. Persons in this cultural milieu tend to feel an obligation to fill time with activity, preferably work. Thus, they schedule time for efficiency and feel guilty when they waste time.

Temporal orientation exerts an important influence on how persons choose occupational behavior. Persons with a strong future orientation and a belief that time is a finite commodity will tend to delay gratification and to work more than play. Persons who are unable to orient themselves to the future because they have not learned to do so or because disease may have interfered with future plans may have difficulty choosing occupational behaviors in the present.

Meaningfulness of Activities

An individual's experience and participation in the environment results in the building up of certain images about various activities or occupations which are very personal and evoke strong emotions. This phenomena, the meaningfulness of activities, is *an individual's disposition to find importance, security, worthiness, and purpose in particular occupations.*

The search for meaning is a distinct characteristic of humans (15). While one can experience meaning through love and suffering, participation in occupation is also an important source of meaning (15). Meaning in occupations is built-up through life experiences in which the relationship of occupations to the social milieu and the larger human condition is appreciated. For instance, one's work can take on meaning because one understands how it contributes to other's well-being or to the production of some commodity needed by others. Occupations can also take on meaning because of states they evoke. For instance, recreational or hobbyist activities can take on meaning because they provide a time to reflect on one's life and to experience a sense of calm and relaxation. Activities may also have meaning because of their particular association with past life situations. For instance, a person may value baking because it was a particularly fulfilling aspect of being a homemaker and is associated with childhood images of pleasure and security.

Thus, the relationship of occupation to meaning is a complex one. Persons achieve meaning in their lives by performing those occupations which have come to bear a certain significance or importance. Developing occupations which have personal meaning and incorporating them into one's life-style is critical since a lack of meaning in life produces anxiety and depression (15).

Occupational Goals

The next components of values are occupational goals; they are *objectives for personal accomplishments or for future occupational activities or roles.* Goals are plans of action and are important for competent performance in that they sustain behavior when it is not immediately gratifying (9, 26). For instance, students will engage in onerous studies in order to achieve a degree or entry into an occupation.

Goals interrelate with an individual's orientation to time. By having future objectives for activities, roles or accomplishments, a person is enabled to find greater satisfaction and meaning in everyday life. A lack of goals for the future can lead to a sense of helplessness and disorientation and to depression (37). Such a state often follows the onset of some physical trauma that appears to destroy an individual's plans for the future.

Personal Standards

In addition to attaching meaning to various occupations, individuals develop personal standards for how occupations ought to be performed. Personal standards are *commitments to performing occupations in moral, excellent, efficient, or otherwise socially sanctioned ways.* Each individual acquires a personal set of standards that sets priorities for how occupations are to be carried out. Some persons value being quick and efficient while others prefer being slower, more deliberate and exact. Some persons value independent, solitary activity while others feel it is important to cooperate as part of a team. Such valued styles of performing not only determine how an individual will choose to conduct a particular activity, but also influence what occupations will be more likely to be chosen.

There are also some general standards of performance reflected in each culture. Within a culture, activities tend to have their own related standards for performance. In some activities, grace and beauty matter (e.g. karate and figure skating); in others, almost any means that achieves an end is suitable (e.g. boxing and ice hockey). Competent performance requires that, to a degree, an individual incorporates as a personal value the standards of performance of a given culture, setting or activity.

It has been clinically observed that physically disabled adults may put as much effort into appearing to sit and hold their extremities in a natural position as they put into efficient performance of motor behaviors, sometimes sacrificing the latter to maintain the former. For example, it was observed that while quadriplegics had to use alternative grasps and movements to handle cards in a game of poker, they still managed to slap the cards on the table (a stylized movement inherent to many card games) although it involved some additional risk that a card would be dropped or misplaced. In therapy, considerations of efficiency may need to be tempered and understood in terms of the individual's own preferred styles of performance. On the other hand, disabled persons may have to examine activities to determine what is most important about performing them, or to realize the necessity of performing in new ways that may not meet old standards of performance.

An individual who maintains very low standards of performance may produce substandard work that offers no sense of pride or worth, while an individual with excessively high standards of performance may feel chronically frustrated or may be unable to complete activities. Thus, standards of performance should be realistic, taking into consideration the ambience of the environment, the particular occupation being performed and one's own abilities.

THE PROCESS OF VALUING AND CHOOSING

In the previous discussions it has been argued that values relevant to occupation concern the importance persons place on past, present or future as a time for performance, the relative goodness or badness of ways of occupying time, the importance of occupations in and of themselves or for accomplishing future goals, and the right way to perform when engaging in occupations. These values are guidelines for personal performance. What a person chooses to do generally reflects in some way what he or she values.

Value change is central to human development. Throughout life persons set new priorities, find new sources of meaning, achieve goals and set out to accomplish new ones. Persons are

typically only aware of values on reflection, and sometimes must systematically evoke and examine what is important to themselves when making major decisions. Since values are shaped in the social surround, history is a significant force in what persons find important. Thus, over the life span, persons may find themselves making different choices for new and emerging reasons. Discovering and acknowledging value in one's occupations is important for a sense of well-being. Persons judge their own worth by the occupations in which they engage and the importance they attribute to them. Self-esteem and life satisfaction thus accrue when persons pursue occupations of value.

INTERESTS

The final realm of self-knowledge in volition is interests. Interests are *dispositions to find occupations pleasurable*. Three dimensions of interest represent one's orientation to pleasure and satisfaction in occupations: discrimination, pattern, and potency (Figure 2.6).

Interests are generated from action (34). For instance, when persons say they are interested in music or in tennis, they are indicating that they experience pleasure in listening to music or in playing the game of tennis. Interests are thus based on self-knowledge about how one experiences various occupations.

Interests represent not only a person's disposition to find pleasure and enjoyment in occupations, but also influence what occupations a person will tend to choose (34). Because interests represent one's image or awareness of enjoyability of occupations, they influence those choices persons make when they are most free. For that reason, leisure or play activities are often based almost entirely on interest, whereas work may involve a combination of interest, value and other reality factors such as ability and environmental constraints (18).

Many factors influence how one experiences interest in activities. There may be certain biological predispositions that make information or experience related to particular senses more or less pleasurable. For example, one may innately enjoy the experience of sound over tactile experience. Whatever biological propensities exist, they are shaped early in life and throughout the course of development by the physical and social environment that provides the opportunities for the experience of pleasure or displeasure in action. Specifically, interest formation is influ-

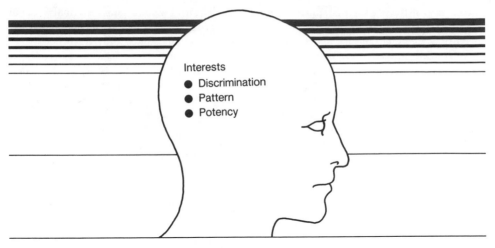

Figure 2.6. Interests.

enced by culture, family, economic and educational resources, and by peer groups (34).

Discrimination

Implied in the concept of interests is the notion that persons do not experience all occupations equally; they develop preferences for certain occupations over others. Discrimination of interests is *the degree to which one differentiates a liking or expectation of enjoyment in certain occupations*. Discrimination of interests includes both the degree of interest which various occupations represent to a person and what aspects of an activity are pleasurable. For example, persons who have experience with crafts may find themselves more interested in woodworking than ceramics. Although they may find that they enjoy the products of their efforts equally, the difference in their interest may be in the process. The tools used in ceramics are minimal and there is more direct contact with the material. Clay is soft and moist and changing. Woodworking involves a number of complex tools and the material is hard and constant. Some people may find that the olfactory experience of clay is bland while woodworking may seem to involve pleasant and sweet smells of wood and finishes. The temporal sequence and timing of ceramics is somewhat dictated by the properties of clay— i.e. how fast it dries, what can be done with it at different stages of drying, whereas wood allows more freedom of temporal organization. All of these differences may contribute to one's degree of interest in woodworking versus ceramics.

Discrimination represents an accumulated sense of what is more or less enjoyable to do. It can be quite fluid depending on the degree of openness an individual has to new experiences, on the person's developmental level and on available environmental opportunities.

The acquisition of new interests may be influenced by some underlying, more stable, forms of discrimination. For instance, a preference of slow paced, private activities with concrete outcomes versus fast paced activities involving other people may influence a person's tendency to find painting more pleasurable than racketball.

The ability to discriminate interests is very important for choosing occupations. Interests are priorities in effect; some rank higher, some lower, on one's internal scales of desirability. Preferring certain activities or objects over others, allows one to choose. Persons who lack interests or who cannot discriminate interests may have difficulty choosing or maintaining occupations. Without a clear sense of interest, occupations are less likely to be enjoyed. On the other hand, when one can discriminate interests, one is more likely to experience a sense of general pleasure in occupations and will be more disposed to future action.

Pattern

Collective experiences generally result in a pattern of active interests. The pattern of interests refers to *a configuration of occupations one is disposed to enjoy*. While certain underlying dispositions may influence the discrimination of interests, the overall pattern of interests may be influenced by a need for balance and variation. For instance, while an individual may in general prefer solitary, creative, activities with products, it may be important to have an interest that involves people, or one without a concrete outcome which is experienced primarily for fun.

Certain interest patterns are indicative of normal development and historical changes. One can speak of typical adolescent interests which are often influenced by a variety of fads and changing peer ideas about what is an acceptable interest. Adult interests are also influenced by popular notions; for example, more adults today are interested in running and other forms of exercise than 10 years ago. Interest patterns may signal a lack of balance in daily life such as a pattern centered exclusively around the worker role.

Potency

The final aspect of interests is their potency. Potency is *the degree to which interests are based on past experiences and influence present action.* Potency is the link between interest and action. Interests lead to action and they are generated out of action (34). The strength of a particular interest depends not only on the individual's perception or report of enjoyment in the occupation, but also on the degree to which that perception is based on past experience. Some persons indicate interests which are merely a wish for involvement or a vicarious sense that an occupation would be fun, but which are not based on experience in the activity. Such stated interests lack the potency of past experience.

The degree to which a person's expressed interest is actually linked to choices for action is another aspect of potency. Many factors may influence the potency of interests in the present and future. For instance, one pilot study found that alcoholics had significantly less pursuit of interests than normal peers although the overall interest patterns of both groups were similar (47). In another situation, potency may be adversely affected when a person retains a strong interest in activities that require motor performances lost through disability.

THE PROCESS OF INTEREST FORMATION AND CHOOSING OCCUPATIONAL BEHAVIOR

As with values and personal causation, interests are both an influence on, and a consequence of, action. Persons come to learn about the potentials for enjoyment in occupation through experience and, once they have acquired these images, their choices for action are influenced by them. Because interests are largely a personal matter, they may be freer of outside influences than values and personal causation, both of which may be more influenced by how others respond to one's peformance.

Interests also appear to be fairly stable for some persons and quite variable and changing for others. Change in ability and energy over the course of development may influence change in interests or in the way they are enacted.

It appears that some persons generally find more enjoyability and pleasure in what they do than others. Some people experience a global lack of interest in the world about them. Taken as a whole, one's interests are an influence on choices for action, maintenance of effort and intensity of involvement. As persons have a variety of occupations which they perceive to be enjoyable and which they routinely pursue, their overall conviction in the possibility of pleasure in activity is abetted. The reverse is equally true.

Interests are important for human freedom and quality of life. When a person does something purely out of interest, he or she freely chooses. The degree that one's occupational behavior reflects interest will influence satisfaction with life.

VOLITION AND CHOICE

The previous sections described and discussed the volition subsystem. Volition explicates the process of choosing occupational behavior. The volition subsystem is conceptualized as a collection of biological and symbolic components that provide the basic underlying energy and personal knowledge for choosing occupational behavior (Fig. 2.7). The biological component is energy arising from the complex nervous system of humans manifest as an urge to explore and master. Unlike behaviors which release tension and thus satiate needs quickly, occupational behaviors are engaged in persistently for their own sake (e.g. for the excitement, challenge, enjoyment, and feelings of competence that they provide).

Along with the biopsychic urge to explore and master, humans have the ability to form symbols or personal images about their past experiences, their present existence and their future potentials. These are a complex collection of parallel and interrelated images of personal causation,

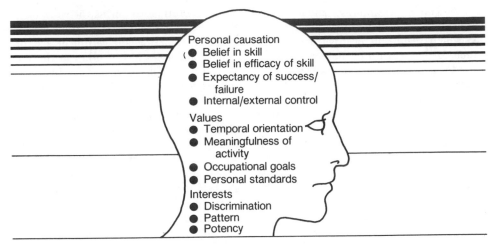

Figure 2.7.   Components of the volition system.

values and interests. These images, combined with the urge to explore and master, shape the choices an individual makes for occupational behavior. The individual is motivated to explore and master via those occupational behaviors which are perceived to allow expression of personal causation, value and interest.

Since personal causation, interests and values are parallel and interrelated images, one cannot fully understand an individual's volition without considering all three aspects. For example, people cannot consider themselves to be truly competent if they cannot do things that they value. In turn, one will tend to value those things which are attainable through personal effort. Similarly, it is unlikely a person will develop interest in an activity for which he or she is chronically unfit.

These volitional images together allow one to discriminate what things are fun but frivolous and what things are onerous but important— and one behaves accordingly. Thus, while some choices are based on a blending of interest, capacity and value, other choices may involve a struggle against incapacity because of a personally held value. The way in which persons employ their images of interest, value and competence is complex and presents a vast unknown area for future exploration. The study of these images should yield understanding of why some persons fail to struggle and become disabled and how others struggle in spite of overwhelming disability. Without knowledge of the images persons carry that inform them about their action potentials in the world, one cannot understand their choices to engage in, or to avoid, occupational behavior. Further, one cannot effectively

lead, encourage, or support them to participate in occupation without such information.

The volition concept does not argue that all decisions are explainable by the urge to explore and master and the images of personal causation, value and interest. However, it does specify that adaptive choices, reflect a strong influence of volition, or willing, in occupational behavior. Choices for behavior often incorporate necessary compromises and persons may sometimes choose because they are responding to constraints or expectations from internal factors and the external environment. In other cases components of volition may be insufficiently formed to guide choices, or may represent conflicts that prevent healthy choices. This may occur, for example, when a person lacks well formed values or when external values of others prevail over one's value system. When choices are made because of such constraint or disorganization, they may lead to maladaptive occupational behavior.

Inasmuch as volition is conceived of as a process of willing or choosing courses of action, it expresses a belief in the possibility and importance of human freedom. Within the opportunities and constraints imposed by the environment and by personal abilities, the individual can and must choose to be adaptive. The self-images of personal causation, values and interests either constrain or enhance the person's acting on the urge to explore and master. Because the maintenance and unfolding of these self-images is a product of the open systems cycle, the course of volition is either self-enhancing or self-destructive. A person who makes choices based on values, interests and a positive sense of personal causation tends to behave in a manner which results in positive experiences and which further augments these self-images. An opposite cycle of events can occur when the self-images are negative and poor courses of action or inaction are chosen. Additionally, disease, trauma or other life changes can affect volition.

Because the volition subsystem is the highest and ruling subsystem in the open system representing the occupational nature of humans, it is the most important one for determining the course of adaptive or maladaptive occupational behavior. Choices made by the individual can either enhance or disorganize the lower habituation and performance subsystems.

The Habituation Subsystem

The volition subsystem offers a way of understanding how humans make conscious choices for occupational behavior. Additional concepts are needed to explain how the human system maintains everyday patterns of behavior without ongoing conscious choices. The habituation subsystem is conceptualized as a middle-level subsystem which regulates this patterned behavior.

The habituation subsystem is *a collection of images which trigger and guide the performance of routine patterns of behavior.* Two sets of these images exist and interrelate in guiding everyday occupational behavior. They are roles and habits (Fig. 2.8). Roles and habits interrelate to guide performance. For instance, one's worker role

guides performance during the work-day, and a habit of self-care guides the routine performance of rising, grooming, and getting dresed for work. Habits and roles also overlap in the way they impact and guide behavior. For instance, work role performance is influenced by the individual's habits of workmanship.

As with volition, the habituation subsystem is differentiated over time through the open system cycle. The child comes into the world without internal regulators of patterned behavior save, perhaps, certain biorhythms. Soon, he or she begins to acquire routines of day and night, sleeping and waking. Over the course of development, very complex routines of self-care, work and play are developed. For periods of time roles and habits may be relatively stable. At certain developmental stages (e.g. entering the student role, the work role or retirement) changes take place in both roles and habits, requiring reorganization in the habituation subsystem.

ROLES

In the course of development one begins to perceive that others in the social surround recognize one as filling certain positions. Persons learn that they have positions in social groups but also that they are expected to behave in certain ways because of their statuses. (20, 25, 53). This procss is one of internalizing roles; it involves coming to see self as a student, worker, parent, and so forth. Internalized roles are *images that persons hold of themselves as occupying certain statuses or positions in social groups and of the obligations or expectations that accompany*

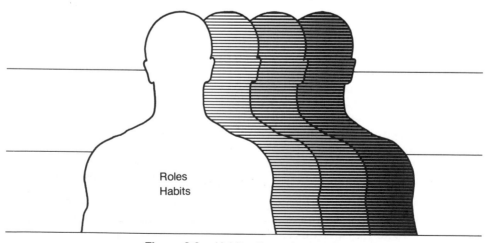

Roles
Habits

Figure 2.8. Habituation subsystem.

being in these roles. Internalized roles have three components: perceived incumbency, internalization of expectations, and balance (Fig. 2.9). When a role is internalized it becomes part of one's self-image. A role defines who one is, and specifies a range of attitudes one must exhibit and tasks one must perform. Roles thus serve as a source of identity (8, 44, 45, 53). Persons are recognizable to others and come to think of themselves in terms of the roles they occupy.

Roles, Society and Socialization

Just as the culture provides an individual with a range of values which can be internalized, the social group provides the roles which a person may enter. The social group is a system composed of roles (25). For example, in the family there are roles of parents, children, siblings, and spouses that define specific functions within the family organization.

Because roles are necessary for the functioning of the social system (25), others in the social group come to define what they expect of the person in a given role. For example, the instructor or teacher fulfills a specific role in the classroom which is aimed at facilitating learning and imparting information. Students, parents and principals recognize this and expect the person in the role to engage in behaviors which achieve its purpose. Only by the teachers conforming to these expectations can the social organization of the classroom be maintained. The process of communicating role expectations to the individual is referred to as socialization (3). As children develop, parents begin to give them expectations

for being a family member. These expectations involve where and how the child plays, the emergence of helping behavior and self-care, and conformity to family routines. These expectations for performance as a family member are much more informal and loosely constructed than the role expectations that come with later life. Thus, there is a developmental progression from informal to formal roles. This role progression parallels the child's ability to internalize role expectations and to use them to guide behavior.

Types of Roles

The types of social roles that an individual may internalize have been categorized as personal-sexual, familial-social and occupational roles (23, 25). Originally, only the latter were considered to be of concern to occupational therapy (35). Occupational roles included player, student, homemaker, worker, and retiree. Now it is recognized that a single role may have personal-sexual, familial-social, and occupational dimensions (38). A role is defined as having an occupational dimension if it provides an avenue for expression of play or leisure, or if it requires productive behavior. Thus, for example, the role of spouse would incorporate *both* opportunities and expectations for familial behavior and occupational behavior. A number of roles which provide opportunities for, and which expect, occupational behavior have been delineated (38). Table 2.1 illustrates these roles and their definitions.

In addition to these roles which allow expres-

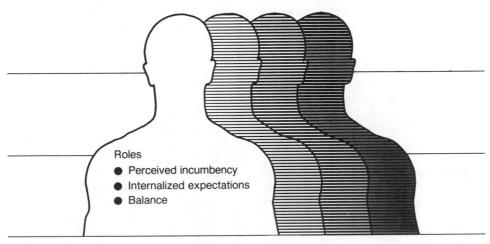

Figure 2.9. Roles.

Table 2.1.
Roles with occupational dimensions

Role	Occupational behavior within the role
Student	Attending school on a part-time or full-time basis
Worker	Part-time or full-time paid employment
Volunteer	Donating services to a hospital, school, community, neighborhood, political campaign, or similar benefit
Care giver	Responsibility for the care of someone such as a child, spouse, relative, or friend
Home maintainer	Responsibility for the upkeep of a home such as house-cleaning or yardwork
Friend	Visiting or doing something with a friend
Family member	Spending time or doing something with a family member such as a spouse, child, parent, or other relative
Religious participant	Participation in activities sponsored by a religious organization
Hobbyist/amateur	Involvement in a hobby or amateur activity such as sewing, playing a musical instrument, woodworking, sports, theater, or participation in a club or team
Participant in an organization	Involvement in an organization such as the American Legion, National Organization for Women, Parents Without Partners, or Weight Watchers

sion of occupational behavior, there are also roles which can convey expectations for passiveness or negative performance. Such roles are generally recognized as deviant since the person in the role is seen by society as diverging from normal behavior (16). Two kinds of deviant roles are relevant to consideration of persons with disabilities, the sick role and the invalid role. The sick role allows a certain degree of legitimated and controlled deviance (39). For instance, when a person is sick and formally recognized as such, the normal expectations for the worker role are suspended and the person is expected instead to conform to the administrations and advice of medical personnel in order to get well. Generally the sick role requires passivity and compliance. This sick role can be counterproductive when rehabilitation efforts are aimed at giving the individual more responsibility for self and requiring more productivity (7).

The person with a permanent disabling condition can enter into a further stage of deviance, the invalid role. Though many terms have been used to describe this role [e.g. the disabled or impaired role (12, 30)] the term "invalid" most clearly indicates the status and expectations of the role. A person in this role is not considered able to validate self through participation in society. The role status is one of helplessness and worthlessness and the role expectation is that behavior will be insufficient for contributing to society.

Perceived Incumbency

While individuals are not typically preoccupied with the roles they are filling (44), they do have a subliminal awareness of when they are in a role and, on reflection, persons can identify their life roles. Perceived incumbency is *the belief that one has the status, rights and obligations of a role and that others also perceive one to be in the role.* It also includes the image one holds of when, during the day, week, and so forth, one is typically in a given role. Recognition that one is entering or leaving a role is often demarked by change in dress, manner of speech and ways of relating to others. In addition, different performances or tasks are recognized as part of each role. One does certain routines each day as one goes to work, comes home to family and the like. Subliminal awareness of being in a role acts as a framework to guide such behavior. This does not mean that the role causes or determines the behavior. Rather, a useful way of phrasing it is that awareness of being in a role "colors" behavior. Persons may take on an air of authority when they are acting as parents, therapists and teachers, and more of an egalitarian air when acting as spouses and colleagues. Roles serve as backdrops that influence how one behaves and experiences one's own and other persons' behavior (25).

Internalized Expectations

Since roles represent functional units within a social system each role carries with it a related set of performances that are necessary or important for the maintenance of the social system (3). When the individual has incorporated this information about the demands of each role, he or she has acquired internalized expectations of the role. Internalized expectations are *images that one holds of what others expect one to do by virtue of being in a role.* When expectations are internalized, they are also accepted as obligatory and become self-imposed rules (3).

Parents in the family system must provide a source of income; maintain the household; and provide instruction, guidance and authority for children. The other parent, children, relatives, neighbors, and the community at large are affected when someone in the parent role does not perform his or her share of the functions necessary for maintaining the family system. Parents who do not discipline their children may receive negative feedback from relatives, neighbors and school officials, because failure to perform this function affects those in associated social systems. In order to maintain orderly interactions in social life, social members thus make known their expectations for performance to those who are in roles as well as those likely to take on such roles in the future. For example, childhood and adolescent phases of development incorporate many experiences that inform developing individuals about what will be expected, when they become parents or workers. Further, once persons enter the roles, others in the social system give even more specific information about what is expected. The process of internalizing expectations of a role may never be complete. As one performs in a role new contingencies or changes in the social system may raise new demands for performance.

A person entering a new role generally goes through a period of negotiation in which his or her own perceptions of the obligations of the role are either brought into conformity with the expectations of others or in which expectations of the others are altered (23, 45). This is usually a give-and-take process. Each new person filling a role does it differently than any other person. As long as the individual's performance entails conformity to the more important expectations, the individual will likely be judged competent in the role. However, if an individual continues to enact a role based on expectations that are at variance with those in the social system, he or she is likely to be judged unfit for the role. Furthermore, the individual will create strain in the social system to which that role belongs: the system itself will have to change, someone else will have to fill the obligations which are not being fulfilled, or the system will falter. Such situations evoke resentment or even fear on the part of others and inevitably result in a negative view of, and negative feedback to, the individual. While we tend to think of role failure as an adult phenomena, persons may also fail to meet expectations of early life roles. For instance, the child with developmental delay may fail to meet parents' expectations of what a child should do.

Role Balance

The final aspect of internalized roles is balance. Role balance is *integration of an optimal number of appropriate roles into one's life.* Every role carries with it different avenues for expression of needs—some roles allow one to explore, others to pursue competence or achievement. Roles also place demands on persons for task performance and time use. A balance of roles provides some rhythm and change between these different modes of doing (48) and allows sufficient time and effort for performing tasks associated with each role. Role balance thus exists when roles are not conflicting or competing for time and when there are adequate roles to structure one's use of time. At one time or another, everyone feels role strain as they are torn between two incompatible sets of demands and time conflicts.

Another form of role imbalance is a lack of roles or role loss. Roles not only serve as guides to behavior that shape performance in ways that society expects, they also provide structure and purpose to everyday occupational behavior. Persons who have not acquired sufficient life roles tend to experience a lack of identity, purpose and structure in their everyday life.

Role loss can also lead to imbalance in life roles. It can be accompanied with a feeling of disorientation because one has lost a source of identity and a guiding format for behavior. Ordinarily, the succession of life roles provides a replacement for the lost role. For example, the student role is typically followed by the worker role. In some cases, however, persons' roles may end abruptly without definitive roles to replace them. This may happen in old age when the spouse or worker role is lost. Persons more easily adapt to the loss of roles if they have other roles which can take on more importance. For example, the person with a friendship role or hobbyist role may more easily adapt to loss of a spouse or worker role.

Maintaining role balance thus requires that persons achieve an overall integration of roles despite ongoing changes in specific roles. Role balance is maintained as long as the individual is provided with a sense of identity and purpose and with sufficient expectations and structure to guide time use.

THE TAKING ON OF LIFE ROLES

Roles provide a means for the needs of both the individual and society to be met. Roles provide avenues of defined behavior with established purposes and boundaries within which a person can enact the urge to explore and master. Roles also provide a means of channeling a person's action into patterns and tasks required by various social systems. By engaging in role behavior, the individual thus satisfies the demands of both volition and the environment.

Role change is a feature of all human life. Roles change as one moves from one organizational setting to another—e.g. going from work to home. Roles also change as an individual progresses through the course of development. Persons enter and leave these roles both because they choose to do so and because social expectations constrain persons to enter and exit roles at various life stages. For example, roles such as that of spouse and parent are expected of persons by a certain age in many social groups. Within the constraints and expectations imposed by society, persons have freedom to chose entry and exit from roles.

Generally the process of development is one of achieving a series of different role configurations. For instance, when the child begins the the student role, his or her sibling and child roles are also affected. When a parent returns to the student role, relationships to children, friends and relatives are also affected. Thus,

taking on a new role or relinquishing a role always has implications for overall role balance. Other roles must be adjusted to accommodate a particular role change.

HABITS

The concept of role provides an understanding of how people perform within positions in a social group and thereby tend to exhibit patterned behavior conforming to role expectations. Other aspects of an individuals's routine performance are regulated by habits. Routine behaviors during the day when an individual is not in a socially defined role are regulated by habits (26, 46). In addition, within roles, individuals have latitude to express their role performance in personal ways reflecting their own ambience and style. Routine behavior within a role, but not specifically required or expected by the role, is regulated by habits. Thus, habits and roles are interwoven in daily life and reciprocally organize routine behavior.

Habits are *images guiding the routine and typical ways in which a person performs*. Habits refer to both the temporal structuring of behavior and to the style and manner of performance. Like roles, habits are images that trigger and guide performance (26). The habit serves as an intermediary which organizes skills into larger purposeful routines that constitute a gestalt and often automatic action sequence. The more complex the routine is, the more likelihood there is that the person will need to consciously monitor at least part of the habit sequence to insure a desired outcome. However, simpler, regularly performed habits tend to be automatic. The adaptiveness of a habit pattern is reflected in three dimensions: degree of organization, social appropriateness and rigidity/flexibility (Fig. 2.10).

Degree of Organization

As noted earlier, habits provide a consistency in the pattern of time use in everyday occupational behavior. The degree of organization in habits is the *degree to which one has a typical use of time which supports competent performance in a variety of environments and roles and provides a balance of activity*. While no two days are exactly the same, most persons have and can identify a routine which is typical for a day of the week. In this society persons generally have patterns that characterize workdays and alter-

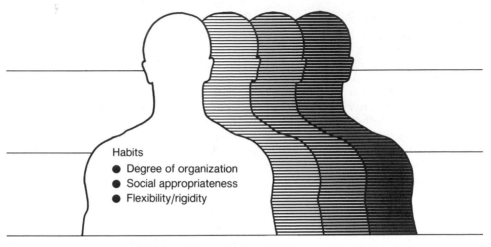

Figure 2.10. Habits.

nate patterns that characterize weekends or days off from work. The optimal degree of consistency in a habit pattern depends on the individual's roles and environment. Some worker roles demand a fairly stable routine of showing up for work, taking lunch and breaks, and terminating the work day. Routines within the job may be fairly stable and defined. Other forms of work may require a much more flexible pattern of behavior. In such cases, it is not doing the same thing at the same time each day which reflects organization in habits, but an individual's awareness of, and organization of, behavior to respond to typical kinds of tasks and problems that arise. Analyzing the organization in anyone's habit pattern thus requires an awareness of the social and task environment for which routine behavior is organized. When the patterns of behavior allow the person to respond to either stable or recurrent facets of the environment, then habits are sufficiently organized to satisfy environmental demands.

In addition to satisfying external demands, habits should organize behavior to allow a balance or rhythm of activity in the day and week (48). Thus, while the adult generally has habits organized around requirements for productivity, habits must also allow time for rest, play and sleep. In the case of play and rest, it may be less important that what the individual does is routine than that a routine of setting aside time for rest and recreation exists. Thus, persons may have a time each day in which they choose what to do depending on their mood. Some days one may engage in a hobby, other days watch television, still others meet with friends to play

cards at a local bar. The absence of time routinely set aside for choosing behavior could reflect a lack of organization in habits.

The presence of routines is also important for children; even the small child has typical days characterized by rising, morning hygiene and dressing, breakfast, playtime, nap, lunch, and so forth. Since these routines are largely executed by caretakers, it is often less apparent that the child has habits. Yet, children display anticipation of routine events and may become upset at departures from the routine.

Social Appropriateness

Habits mold behavior to the features of the social environment. Since habits guide how a person will routinely perform, their pattern must be in harmony with the social environment (8). The social appropriateness of habits is *the degree to which one's typical behaviors are those expected and valued by the environments in which one performs.* The norms for behavior provided by the social environment are incorporated into adaptive habit patterns. For example, habits of punctuality and industriousness reflect typical expectations of Western society for persons to be at work, meetings, and appointments at the scheduled time and to focus on the task at hand during periods of time so designated. If a person routinely fails to be punctual or to attend to the work tasks, the habit pattern will be out of synchrony with the environment and the person will be in danger of not fulfilling social demands for performance. Habits thus allow a person to be integrated into the smooth functioning of society. While not all habits are, of themselves, regulated by social norms, most habitual behavior impacts on an individual's ability to conform to societal expectations. For example, the routine of hygiene and dressing is not a matter of great social concern; one can choose how to get bathed and dressed. However, if one's routine is such that one appears dirty and inappropriately dressed or one that causes consistent lateness for work, the habit will have negative social repercussions. Since one's routine behavior is interwoven in a complex interrelated set of daily and weekly actions, performance of any routine behavior is likely to affect others.

Rigidity/ Flexibility

While habits are predicated on consistency in the environment and on the demands for role performance, variable contingencies and periods of change and disruption may periodically occur. Thus, an optimal habit pattern is one stable enough to provide consistency in behavior but flexible enough to accommodate such changes or contingencies. Ridigity/flexibility of habits is *the degree to which a person is able to change routines of behavior to accomodate periodic contingencies.*

The degree of ridigity/flexibility that will be adaptive for any particular individual depends, once again, on the particular environment and role demands of the individual. Little children can be extremely flexible in the way they spend their time during play since very few role demands are placed on them; the same is largely true of the retiree. The student must have a more stable set of habits since most of the everyday tasks and problems of school are highly structured and consistent. On the other hand, a farmer or freelance writer must have highly flexible routines to regulate behavior. Unusual circumstances like a storm which destroys a new crop or a breaking news story may demand quick response and reorganization of routines. For some persons demands for work are seasonal. This is true for teachers, students, farmers and other workers whose tasks are tied to recurrent annual patterns.

THE PROCESS OF HABIT FORMATION

Habits are formed through the process of modularization. As behaviors are practiced they tend to become more automatic and autonomous and do not require the conscious attention that they required during the early practice phase (29, 46). Habits require information in the form of images that the individual first consciously employs when performance is fitted to the purpose of the overall task and to environmental conditions (27). Later the images become latent or preconscious, so that one's performance becomes second nature. For instance, driving to work when one has moved to a new city or taken a new job at a different location requires conscious effort during the first few performances. Soon, it becomes so automatic that one need not think about the route to work so long as the usual conditions of traffic obtain. The habit of driving to work operates so autonomously that should one be driving along the route to work with a different destination, one may inadvertently pursue the route to work rather than to the intended destination.

Because habits function as somewhat autonomous wholes, they allow more efficient performance in daily life. This is for two reasons. First, habits organize skills into routines suitable for the particular environment in which they will be used. For example, work-related skills become organized into a work routine. Second, because habits function largely without conscious intervention, they free up the individual to do other things. Because the information within the habit structure is oriented to a particular purpose and set of environmental conditions, change in either requires the intervention of conscious decision making. Thus, a change in life plans, role change, or changes in the environment precipitate a time of habit change in which conscious behavior takes over until practice under the new set of conditions yields new habits.

THE HABITUATION PROCESS

The habituation subsystem serves the individual's need to perform in consistent and typical ways that are fitted to the characteristics and expectations of the environment. Both roles and habits function as collections of images that trigger and monitor behavior (Fig. 2.11). That is, both contain information about the purposes and processes of various occupational behaviors; they automatically receive feedback and use it to adjust ongoing behavior.

Habits and roles differ in several respects. Roles are publicly recognized positions that allow some social system to continue to operate

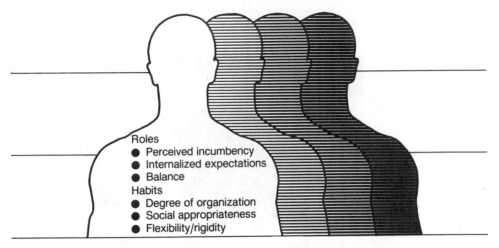

Roles
- Perceived incumbency
- Internalized expectations
- Balance

Habits
- Degree of organization
- Social appropriateness
- Flexibility/rigidity

Figure 2.11. Components of the habituation process.

and, thus, both the status and expectations of roles are a public matter. In turn, roles are an important source of self-identity. Habits are more private in nature regulating patterns of behavior during times persons are not in social roles and regulating patterns of behavior which support role performance.

In this way roles and habits form a network of organizing images that supervene in everyday life to trigger and guide performance. Roles and habits are not directly responsible for the performance of skilled behavior; this is the function of the performance subsystem. Thus, existing skills are organized into routines and typical performances by roles and habits. Habituation must organize skilled behavior into routines of behavior that reflect the characteristics of volition and that allow behavior to fulfill demands in the environment. For this reason the habits and roles one possesses are important determinants of one's degree of positive adaptation.

The Performance Subsystem

The previous discussions of volition and habituation attempted to explain how individuals make choices for occupational behavior and how behavior is organized into consistent and efficient routines. Now we come to the critical topic of how persons are able to perform occupational behavior. Whether it be simply walking or executing a movement in ballet, writing a song or whistling a tune, balancing a checkbook or deriving a mathematical theorem, stacking blocks or building a house, the human capacity for performance is astounding and complex.

The performance subsystem is conceptualized as that subsystem which directly makes possible the production of behavior. It is *a collection of images and biological structures and processes which are organized into skills and used in the production of purposeful behavior.* The images in the performance subsystem are those internalized rules which inform the individual about how to perform (4, 5, 22, 42). These rules are learned through exploration, imitation, and repetition. They are the internal maps for traversing external reality. The biological constituents of the performance subsystem are the neurological and musculoskeletal structures and processes which are used in the performance of occupational behavior.

CONSTITUENTS OF SKILLS

The symbolic images or rules and biological structures and functions are organized into gestalts referred to as skills. Thus, they are considered the constituents of skills (Fig. 2.12). The symbolic constituent is made up of those symbolic images or rules which an individual acquires through experience and that serve as guides for performance. The neurological constituent refers to the nervous system. And the musculoskeletal constituent refers to skeletal and muscular phenomena underlying human movement.

SKILLS

Because occupational behavior involves complex interaction with an environment of objects,

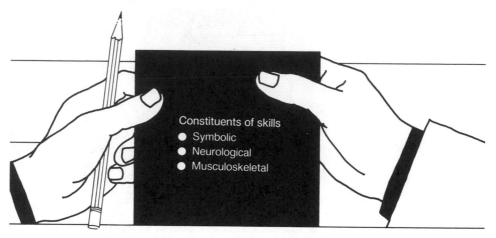

Figure 2.12.   Constituents of skills.

events and people, it requires the employment of organized units of behavior. These organized units of behavior are skills and they constitute the basic component of the performance subsystem. Skills are *abilities that a person has for the performance of various forms of purposeful behavior*. Ability means that there is an internal, organized, set of relationships between the constituents of skill that allows one to perform desired behavior.

Elements of this internal organization that support skill enactment have been identified as (*a*) perceiving the goal and features of a task and the appropriate means for accomplishing the task, (*b*) a means of translating this information into appropriate action and (*c*) a means of obtaining feedback on the action, comparing it to the goal of the task and making appropriate modifications (4, 5). A skilled act is composed of subroutines of behavior that are organized into a hierarchy. By virtue of this hierarchial configuration, the subroutines no longer exist as separate parts, rather they are integrated into a gestalt which employs the subroutines for a larger purpose. For instance, the act of reaching for a coin involves several subroutines of movement of the upper extremity and of the head and eyes. These various subroutines are organized into an act of reaching and performing a pincer grasp on the coin. Since the actions occur simultaneously or overlap in time, they are not performed as a simple chain of acts, but as a gestalt or whole organized at a higher level of function. In this case, the musculoskeletal movements are commanded by a central coordinated

pattern of motor neurons connected to afferent neurological pathways as proprioceptive, visual and tactile feedback are used to monitor and execute the skilled act. In addition, all of these neuromuscular processes are governed by an image or set of rules held by the person which define the nature and purpose of the act, its goals, the means by which it is accomplished and criteria for adjusting behavior to achieve the task (5). This becomes even more evident if we consider the skill involved in catching a ball. Here, complex coordination of proprioceptive and visual information results in moving the hand not to where the ball is, but to where it will be when the hand and the ball get there. Clearly, an internal image is needed whereby a person can interpret the trajectory and speed of the ball and positioning of the hand so that the two will meet in space. Movement is based on internal calculations and predictions about an event occurring in the environment (22).

A skill can be performed under varying conditions (4, 13). One can pick up a small coin or large stone. One can catch a fast flying ball or floating Frisbee. Flexibility is predicated on the integrity of the internal image and its ability to formulate from incoming information accurate interpretations and expectations that will guide the neurological and motor processes. This anticipatory feature of the image is illustrated when one picks up an empty container which one expected to be full; the resulting overexertion is because neurological excitation and force of contraction is based on the expectation of the weight of the object. The symbolic image, nervous excitation and musculoskeletal action thus combine in a delicately balanced and integrated fashion to support performance.

There is a complex interplay of musculoskeletal, neurological, and symbolic phenomena in the execution of any skilled act. Consider a carpenter using a simple plane to shape the surface of wood. The light waves impinge on the eye producing neurological impulses, these are transformed into symbols as the carpenter perceives the wood grain and makes a judgment about the direction of the grain and how the plane should be applied to the wood to achieve a desired result. The intention and purpose of planing is now transformed again to neurological energy which triggers muscular action producing complex movements to apply the plane to the wood. Visual and tactile feedback inform the carpenter how to adjust the force and angle of the plane. The symbolic, neurological, and musculoskeletal constituents are delicately organized into an overall coherent schema that constitutes an ability to plane and allows its application in any particular act of planing. Every human skill, no matter how simple or difficult involves these complex biosymbolic relationships.

Types of Skill

The three types of skills that are directly related to occupational behavior are: perceptual-motor, process, and communication/interaction skills (Fig. 2.13). Perceptual motor skills are *abilities for interpreting sensory information and* *for manipulating self and objects.* They incorporate all three constituents of skills. The nervous system takes in sensory information which is translated into images or perceived. Perception involves images developed to allow interpretation of sensory information. Perceptual data guided by one's intentions or purposes is used to monitor and alter motor output.

Process skills are *abilities directed at managing events or processes in the environment.* Process skills include problem-solving and planning abilities. Problem-solving abilities are directed at some process already begun which presents an obstacle or a set of unusual task demands that require control or solution before proceeding. Planning is the process of determining in advance how one will execute a series of acts or how different events will tie together in future time to achieve a desired result. Both types of process skills aim to find a course of action which is not explicit in the set of task demands and which requires creative imagination about alternatives and their consequences.

Communication/interaction skills are used with other persons. They are *abilities for sharing and receiving information and for coordinating one's behavior with that of others in order to accomplish mutual activities and goals.* Communication/interaction skills are diverse and may be those used in such varied occupations as playing a game, or working on a road construction team. These are skills needed in situations that require that one communicate intentions and needs in order to perform a task or participate in a mutual activity or those that allow one

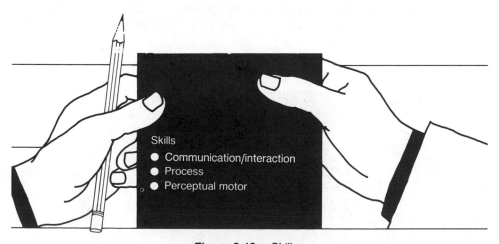

Figure 2.13. Skills.

to engage in mutual playful or productive occupations with others. Communication/interaction skills used in the course of occupation may include the sharing of emotions and thoughts related to self and others as they pertain to accomplishing productive tasks or engaging in leisure. So, for instance, letting a spouse know that one is tired of going bowling every Wednesday night or telling a colleague that one would like to have more responsibility on the job are communication/interaction skills related to occupation. Other examples of communication/interaction skills are giving instructions and supervising, getting information needed for task accomplishment, making intentions for a next step in a job or game known, playing to win and losing gracefully, and pitching in to help a group effort.

Communication/interaction skills involve all three constituents of skills. Internal images guide the intention to send messages and the interpretation of messages received. The nervous system takes in sensory information and gives the appropriate signals to the musculoskeletal system for the production of speech, gestures, and other bodily movements used to interact with persons.

Perceptual motor, process and communication/interaction skills are often used in combination. Playing a basketball game involves complex perceptual motor performances; requires quick problem solving and planning; and is predicated on a complex process of communicating to teammates, cooperating in passing the ball and carrying out plays, and competing with the members of the other team. Similarly, a work task as abstract as writing a book involves not only process skills of planning and problem-solving skills for how to organize information, but also communication skills for rendering ideas into words, perceptual motor skills for getting the words on paper via typing or handwriting and interaction skills for cooperation with colleagues who help to write and critique the book.

THE PERFORMANCE PROCESS

The performance subsystem is most directly linked to output of the system. All occupational behavior represents some level of skills and calls upon the symbolic, neurological and musculoskeletal constituents of skill (Fig. 2.14). The performance system is also critical for adaptation since it constrains and supports the two higher subsystems. Habits and roles can only build upon preexisting skills available to be organized into patterns or routines of behavior. The volition subsystem can only enact those behaviors that the performance subsystem can produce.

At the same time, the performance subsystem is organized by the higher level subsystems. The volition subsystem guides the process of choosing behavior and influences the types of action the system outputs and the types of feedback recognized. This, in turn, influences what new rules will be incorporated or what neuromuscular changes will take place; i.e. it determines how skills will be learned, maintained and changed through the open system cycle.

SUMMARY

This chapter introduced the three subsystems which are conceptualized as determinants and components of occupation (Fig. 2.15). Each subsystem is responsible for a different aspect of

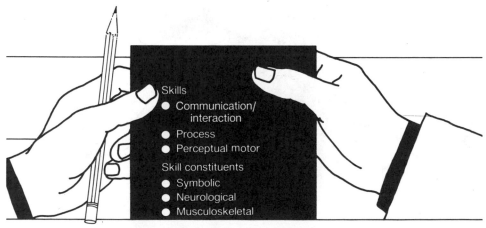

Figure 2.14. Components of the performance process.

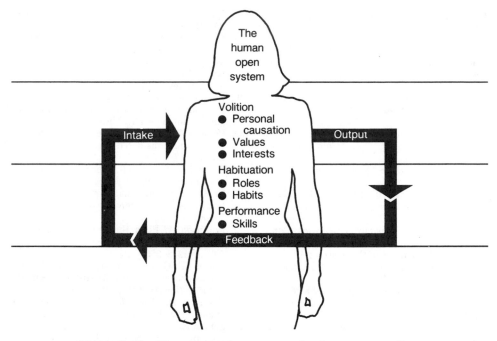

Figure 2.15. The open system representing human occupation.

occupational behavior. Volition guides the choices for occupational behavior, habituation regulates behavior into patterns and routines, and performance contains the components which allow the person to produce behavior. Within the subsystems, personal causation, values, interests, roles, habits, skills, and their musculosketal, neurological and symbolic constituents of skills were identified as important dimensions of occupational behavior. This internal organization of the system is responsible, along with the environment, for that occupational behavior the human system outputs.

Because the subsystems are part of an open system, they are not static structures determining behavior. Rather they are patterns of organization manifest in a living system and they change throughout the history of that system's existence. The open system cycle is responsible for shaping the internal organization of the subsystems. Further, because the subsystems are hierarchically arranged they interrelate according to hierarchial principles. In the following chapter the hierarchical and open system principles which explain the underlying dynamics of organization and change in the three subsystems are examined.

References

1. Berlyne DE: *Conflict, Arousal, and Curiosity.* New York, McGraw-Hill, 1960.
2. Boulding K: *The Image: Knowledge in Life and Society.* Ann Arbor, University of Michigan Press, 1973.
3. Brim OJ, Wheeler S: *Socialization After Childhood: Two Essays.* New York, Wiley, 1966.
4. Bruner J. Organization of early skilled action. *Child Development,* 1973 44:1–11.
5. Bruner J: The skill of relevance or the relevance of skills. *Sat Rev* 1970, April:66–73.
6. Burke JP: A clinical perspective on motivation: pawn versus origin. *Am J Occup Ther* 1977, 31:254–258.
7. Burke JP, Miyake S, Kielhofner G, Barris R: The demystification of health care and demise of the sick role: implications for occupational therapy. In Kielhofner G (ed): *Health Through Occupation: Theory and Practice in Occupational Therapy.* Philadelphia, FA Davis, 1983.
8. Cardwell JD: *Social psychology: a symbolic interaction perspective.* Philadelphia, FA Davis, 1971.
9. Cottle TJ: Time's children: Impressions of Youth. Boston, Little, Brown, 1971.
10. Cottle TJ, Klineberg SL: *The Present of Things Future: Explorations of Time in Human Experience.* New York, Free Press, 1974.
11. DeCharms RE: *Personal Causation: The Internal Affective Determinants of Behaviors.* New York, Academic Press, 1968.
12. De Jong G: Independent living: from social movement to analytic paradigm. *Arch Phys Med Rehabil* 1979, 60:435–446.
13. Elliott J, Connolly K: Hierarchial structure in skill development. In Connolly K, Bruner J (eds): *The Growth of Competence.* New York, Academic Press, 1974.
14. Florey LL: Intrinsic motivation: the dynamics of occupational therapy theory. *Am J Occup Ther*

1969, 23:319–322.

15. Frankl V: *The Unheard Cry for Meaning.* New York, Simon & Schuster, 1978.

16. Freidson E: Disability as social deviance. In Freidson E, Lorber J (eds): *Medical Men and Their Work: A Sociological Reader.* Chicago, Aldine-Atherton, 1972.

17. Freud S: *The Ego and the Id* (J. Riviere, translation). New York, Norton, 1960 (originally published, 1937).

18. Ginzberg E: Toward a theory of occupational choice: a restatement. *Voc Guid Q* 1972, March:169–176.

19. Goodman P: *Growing Up Absurd.* New York, Vintage Books, 1960.

20. Grossack M, Gardner H: *Man and Men: Social Psychology as Social Science.* Scranton, Pa, International Textbook Co, 1970.

21. Hall ET: *The Silent Language.* Greenwich, Conn. Fawcett Publications, 1959.

22. Hayek, FA: The primacy of the abstract. In Koestler A, Smythies RJ (eds): *Beyond Reductionism.* Boston, Beacon Press, 1969.

23. Heard C: Occupational role acquisition: a perspective on the chronically disabled. *Am J Occup Ther* 1977, 41:243–247.

24. Kalish RA, Collier KW: *Exploring Human Values.* Monterey Calif. Brooks/Cole, 1981.

25. Katz D, Kahn RL: *The Social Psychology of Organizations.* New York, Wiley, 1966.

26. Kielhofner G: Temporal adaptation: a conceptual framework for occupational therapy. *Am J Occup Ther* 1977, 31:235–242.

27. Kielhofner G, Barris R, Watts JH: Habits and habit dysfunction: a clinical perspective for psychosocial occupational therapy. *Occup Ther Men Health* 1982, 2:1–21.

28. Klavins R: Work-play behavior: cultural influences. *Am J Occup Ther* 1972, 26:176–179.

29. Koestler A: Beyond atomism and holism—the concept of the holon. In Koestler A, Smythies JR (eds): *Beyond Reductionism.* Boston, Beacon Press, 1969.

30. Larson DL, Spreitzer EA: The disabled role, affluence, and the meaning of work. In Stubbins J (ed): *Social and Psychological Aspects of Disability.* Baltimore, University Park Press, 1977.

31. Lee D: Culture and the experience of value. In Maslow AH (ed): *New Knowledge in Human Values.* Chicago, Henry Regnery, 1971.

32. Magill J, Vargo J: Helplessness, hope and the occupational therapist. *Can J Occup Ther* 1977, 44:65–69.

33. Mathes EW: *From Survival to the Universe.* Chicago, Nelson-Hall, 1981.

34. Matsutsuyu J: The interest check list. *Am J Occup Ther* 1969, 23:323–328.

35. Matsutsuyu, J: Occupational behavior—a perspective on work and play. *Am J Occup Ther* 1971, 25:291–294.

36. McClelland D: *The Achieving Society.* New York, Free Press, 1961.

37. Melges FT. *Time and the Inner Future: A Temporal Approach to Psychiatric Disorders.* New York, Wiley, 1982.

38. Oakley F: *The Model of Human Occupation in Psychiatry.* (Unpublished master's project, Virginia Commonwealth University, 1982.)

39. Parsons T: The sick role and the role of the physician reconsidered. *Health and Society,* 1975, Summer:257–278.

40. Polanyi M: *Personal Knowledge.* Chicago, University of Chicago Press, 1958.

41. Reilly M: Occupational therapy can be one of the great ideas of 20th century medicine. *Am J Occup Ther* 1962, 16:1–9.

42. Robinson A: Play: the arena for acquisition of rules for competent behavior. *Am J Occup Ther* 1977, 31:248–253.

43. Rotter JB: Generalized expectancies for internal versus external control of reinforcement. *Psychol Monogr: Gen Appl* 1960, 80:1–28.

44. Ruddock R: *Roles and Relationships.* London, Routledge & Kegan Paul, 1976.

45. Schein EH: The individual, the organization, and the career: a conceptual scheme. *J Appl Behav Sc* 1971, 7:401–426.

46. Seamon D: Body-subject, time-space routines, and place-ballets. In Bultimer A, Seamon D (eds): *The Human Experience of Space and Place.* New York, St. Martin's Press, 1980.

47. Scaffa M: *Temporal Adaptation.* (Unpublishd master's project, Virginia Commonwealth University, 1981.)

48. Shannon PD: The work-play model: a basis for occupational therapy programming in psychiatry. *Am J Occup Ther* 1970, 24:215–218.

49. Shibutani T: A cybernetic approach to motivation. In Buckley W (ed): *Modern Systems Research for the Behavioral Scientist.* Chicago, Aldine, 1968.

50. Skinner BF: *Beyond Freedom and Dignity.* New York, Knopf, 1971.

51. Smith MB: *Social Psychology and Human Values.* Chicago, Aldine, 1969.

52. Smith MB: Competence and adaptation: a perspective on therapeutic ends and means. *Am J Occup Ther* 1974, 28: 11–15.

53. Turner R: Role taking: process versus conformity. In Rose M (ed): *Human Behavior and Social Processes.* Boston, Houghton Mifflin, 1962.

54. White RW: Excerpts from motivation reconsidered: the concept of competence. *Psychol Rev* 1959, 66:126–134.

55. White RW: Competence and the psychosexual stages of development. *Nebraska Symposium on Motivation,* 1960.

CHAPTER 3

The Open System Dynamics of Human Occupation

Gary Kielhofner

The previous chapter presented the structures and processes that constitute the human system's inner organization and workings and that underlie occupation. They were represented as three subsystems that choose, maintain and produce occupational behavior. In this chapter we turn attention to how these inner structures and functions are part of the dynamics of a hierarchically organized open system.

CHANGE AND THE OPEN SYSTEM

The three subsystems and their components are not rigid structures, but rather they are organized and stable patterns. These subsystems are the result of differentiation, modularization and centralization processes and they are maintained and changed by the open system cycle of intake, throughput, output, and feedback. When viewed in the context of these open system processes, the dynamic order of the three subsystems becomes more apparent.

Output

Occupation is the output of the open system. As noted in the previous chapter, occupation is the playful and productive activity in which persons engage during most of their waking time. Occupational behavior is motivated by an urge to explore and master the environment and is chosen on the basis of values, personal causation and interests. It is organized into a set of internalized roles and habits, and it requires underlying skills and their symbolic, neurological and musculoskeletal constituents. Output, or occupational behavior, is thus an overt expression of the patterns of internal organization within the system.

WORK, DAILY LIVING TASKS AND PLAY

Occupational behavior is important to both self-maintenance and to the maintenance and shaping of the physical social and cultural environments. Three forms of occupational behavior are work, daily living tasks and play. Through their work, persons offer a product or service which is necessary or helpful to social environment. Whether it be growing a crop, mining coal, teaching children, writing a poem or nursing an ill person, work adds some value to the human condition. Human needs are met, a new commodity is created, new ideas or feelings are evoked, and so on. For this reason, work is highly valued; it is considered a fact of life (2).

Daily living tasks include those occupational behaviors necessary to maintain oneself biologically, to make oneself presentable as a recognizable member of one's culture or subculture, and to maintain a household with its physical and economic dimensions.

Play includes the exploration of the young, the recreation of adolescent and adult, and the leisure of the elderly. While play is often considered a frivolous human occupation, it is essential to both individual and collective human wellbeing. The play of the young serves as a preparatory time in which children acquire an internal organization that supports performance of more serious tasks later in the course of development (7). Adult play provides an arena in which persons can recreate themselves for work; express the values of the culture; explore themselves and their physical and social world; and discover new interests, values and areas of skills (3, 4).

The output or occupational behavior of the individual is important since it shapes the internal organization of the system. What persons do when they perform occupational behaviors influences what they become. This self-maintenance and self-change is mediated through the process of feedback.

Feedback

Feedback is the return of information to the system about the process and consequences of action (8). There are two types of feedback, internal and external. Persons receive internal feedback when they experience enjoyment in an activity, when they feel competent, when they see their own progress toward a goal, and so on. Such feedback informs persons about the processes of their own action. For example, when one goes out to the garden in the evening or to the local bowling alley with the expectation of enjoying the activity, the reflective experience of "I'm enjoying this" or "this is boring" is internal feedback about the process of the activity. Internal feedback can be used to monitor and adjust performance. For example, quizzing oneself after a period of studying provides feedback that may lead one to try studying differently or to concentrate on some areas over others. Feedback can also lead to permanent adjustments; a person may for instance, take on new study habits as a result of ongoing feedback. Internal feedback evaluates performance and its outcomes against personal criteria allowing one to temporarily or permanently alter courses of action to better achieve purposes and goals.

External feedback represents others' evaluations of one's occupational behavior, its processes and consequences; for example, a friend comments on one's bowling, or an "A" is received on an exam. Others may also evaluate one's progress toward mutually accepted goals. An example of this is the feedback therapists give to patients concerning progress toward treatment objectives.

The combination of internal and external feedback serves as a beacon or guidepost to monitor present behavior and future choices. When the individual is open to receiving feedback, it becomes part of the intake process of the open system cycle. Persons can choose whether to pay attention to internal or external feedback. We exhort others to pay attention to internal feedback when we say, "listen to your feelings," and to external feedback when we request that they "hear what we are saying."

Intake

Humans are surrounded by a complex environment of objects, events and people. Intake may come from the properties of these objects, events and people, or it may be information specifically created for one's own benefit—such as a grandparent's story about hard times and the importance of working for a living or an author's presentation of a concept.

As one takes in such information, one becomes knowledgeable about possibilities for action and constraints on action. The flow of information into the human system includes complex images about potentials, limitations, expectations, experience, and success and failure. What an individual takes in determines what information is available to the throughput of the system and consequently influences the system's organization.

Throughput

Throughput completes the open system cycle—it is the process whereby information is transformed and integrated into the system and in which the system is influenced or changed by this incoming information. Throughput is, thus, what happens when information flows into the three subsystems and interacts with existing information in them. In order to better understand how this works, each subsystem will be considered separately.

THROUGHPUT AND VOLITION

The volition subsystem is responsible for decision making. Energized by an urge to explore and master, this subsystem makes choices based on values, personal causation and interests. Information coming into the system via intake has the potential to influence choice, and to modify existing images of value, personal causation and interest. For the young child, whose volitional images are very new and fluid, each new experience provides information that influences and shapes these images. For instance, if a child picks up and tosses a rubber ball for the first time, having only thrown blocks and food before, the exaggerated response of the ball gives the child feedback that his or her action created a large effect in the environment and one which was amusing and interesting. When this feedback is taken in, it serves in the throughput process to intensify interest in throwing, to reinforce belief in the efficacy of throwing as a behavior and to identify the ball as a particularly interesting object to throw. The action and consequent experience thus operates through the open system cycle to shape images in volition. This will, in turn, increase the likelihood that a child will throw objects in the future and, in particular, it will enhance the likelihood of throwing a ball. As such experience is coupled with parental feedback about which behavior is valued (i.e. throwing the ball is, but throwing food isn't), the child develops complex images about what is good or bad to do, what he or she does well and what is enjoyable. Throughput in this case includes the use of incoming information to make a decision for action (i.e. seeing the ball and recognizing that it can be acted upon like other objects previously thrown) and incorporating information about the consequences of action (e.g. what the ball does when it is tossed and what parental reaction is to throwing the ball) into existing images of personal causation, value and interest.

THROUGHPUT AND HABITUATION

The role of habituation is to coordinate behavior into patterns or routines that reflect environmental conditions and volitional characteristics. When persons make new choices for behavior or when they enter new environments, new information must be integrated into the habituation subsystem. For example, as the young adult leaves school for the workplace, old patterns of behavior organized around the student role and related habits are changed and new patterns emerge as the individual internalizes the expectations of the worker role and learns new work-related habits. Information taken in from feedback on performance and information available in the environment augments, invalidates or replaces old information which guided roles and habits. When this new information is integrated into the role and habit images which trigger behavior, new patterns of performance become automatic and routine.

THROUGHPUT AND PERFORMANCE

Within the performance subsystem, behavior enhances, maintains or changes skills. Constant feedback to the system is used to monitor and guide skilled performance. For example, coloring in a coloring book involves the taking in of information about the picture to be colored, matching that information with knowledge about what colors the object could or should be, choosing a crayon, manipulating it to color the spaces, and using feedback to determine where the crayon should move next to fill in the space or to avoid coloring outside the line. The skilled act is guided by a constant cycle of visual, tactile, proprioceptive and other information which is used to adjust the skilled act of coloring. As the child performs, feedback about what works and

what doesn't is incorporated into the image that guides skilled performance. This image, in turn, may alter neurological signals so that the child puts more or less pressure on the crayon, moves it more carefully, and so forth. Through this cycle, skills and their underlying symbolic, neurological and musculoskeletal constituents are honed toward a more precise and efficient organization of subroutines for performance. That is, the child learns how to better match visual, tactile, proprioceptive and other feedback to achieve control over execution of the behavior. Throughput is thus a process of using incoming information not only to guide the performance of the skilled act but also to augment and modify the symbolic images and the neuromuscular phenomena involved in skilled performance.

ORGANIZATIONAL CHANGES IN THE OPEN SYSTEM

Over the course of development, the human open system becomes more complex and organized. As the open system cycle generates, imports and incorporates information from ongoing experience, it must be organized into various patterns or the system would simply overload with information. This organization is made possible by the processes of differentiation, modularization and centralization.

Differentiation

Differentiation, the process whereby system components evolve from simpler homogeneous forms to more complex heterogeneous forms, is made possible by the open system cycle (8). Differentiation is manifest in the emergence of a complex set of values, the discrimination of interests, and the formation of images about one's effectiveness. It is also reflected in the development from the single player role of childhood to the multiple roles of adulthood and in the emergence of complex habits for routine behavior. The differentiation of skills is a well documented process in which the child begins with only the primitive basis for perception and movement and progresses toward complex cognitive abilities and the capacity for a multitude of coordinated patterns of purposeful movement.

Differentiation occurs as simple behaviors generate feedback which, along with information from the environment, is incorporated into the system. Each cycle of the open system brings new information into the system; the information is matched to existing information and results in either an intensification, expansion or modification of existing entities. For example, a person who has formed an interest in running participates in a race and finds that competing with others is not as enjoyable as running alone. The interest is thus further differentiated. Similarly, a person who uses an existing motor skill to engage in a new behavior incorporates new information which shapes the skill to the demands of the new task so that it is differentiated from the earlier skill. Again, the system becomes more complex and more heterogeneous through this process.

Modularization and Centralization

Because differentiation generates new entities resulting in more diverse parts they must be integrated into functional units. This process, modularization, occurs when subroutines of coordinated movement are integrated into a manual skill or when skills, such as the abilities to read and write, are coordinated into study habits. Modularization makes the system more efficient by coordinating internal patterns to correspond to the features and demands of the environment.

Centralization occurs when leading parts emerge in the system. For example, the volition subsystem is recognized as the leading part which governs the other two subsystems. This centralization allows the organized patterns of skills, habits and roles to be guided and shaped by the conscious decision-making of the system.

HIERARCHICAL RELATIONSHIPS IN THE SYSTEM

The three subsystems constitute a hierarchy: the volition subsystem is the highest ruling subsystem; habituation, the intermediary; and performance, the lowest subsystem. Laws of hierarchy (1, 5, 8, 9) specify that the volition subsystem commands the habituation and performance subsystems, that the habituation subsystem commands the performance subsystem, that performance constrains habituation and volition and, finally, that habituation constrains volition. This set of relationships shapes both the performance of the system and how change can take place in the system.

Commanding and Constraining

Constraining means that the higher level subsystems cannot exercise functions beyond a range made possible by lower subsystems. For example, an individual cannot successfully enter a role unless he or she has the basic skills and habits that will be expected for role performance. If a person chooses a role for which he or she is not prepared, the system will be unable to produce the necessary skilled behavior and carry out the routines of the role.

At the same time that lower level systems constrain higher ones, the higher systems command and organize the lower ones. For instance, one can decide to obtain appropriate training and/or experiences that will allow development of skills and habits necessary for a particular role. This, of course, presumes that the underlying symbolic, neurological, and musculoskeletal constituents of skill are capable of supporting the level of skill for the role.

Resonation

Whenever changes take place in any part of a system, they resonate, or are felt throughout the system (6). Examples of resonating effects of change are found in association with disease and trauma. For instance, a hand injury may impact the musculoskeletal and the neurological constituent of skill. Loss of skills such as the ability to actively move digits will resonate throughout the entire system. The injury, if it creates a permanent limitation of skill, may require the individual to develop new habits. If the hand-injured individual is a truck driver, the impact on role behavior might be slight; if the individual is a professional musician, it could be devastating. In the same vein, the effects on personal causation and values might be slighter for the former but disastrous for the latter. What the example illustrates is that how a change resonates through a system will vary depending on how various subsystems are organized. A moderate disturbance to performance may have a major impact on habituation or volition.

Harmony and Balance

Because an open system is composed of many structures with complex interrelationships, there must exist an overall pattern of organization which is balanced or harmonious. When a system is balanced, the status of one component positively interacts with the status of other components. In addition, because the open system is basically an active system, balance must exist in the action or output of the system. An imbalance in output can lead to disorganization or distortion of the system's internal organization.

A system is in balance when the commands given by higher subsystems lead to proper use of lower subsystem potentials and when the constraints imposed by lower subsystems do not interfere with the choices and routines of the higher subsystems. An example of imbalance related to the first condition is an individual who consistently chooses to engage in tasks for which he or she is not adequately skilled.

A case in point is a young man who had developed physical work skills and enjoyed and valued this type of work. However, he had also internalized the value system of his professional parents who placed more importance on academic performance and a career. Because of this value conflict, over several years he periodically interrupted or combined his work with returning to college. Each return to college was experienced as highly stressful and resulted in failure in the schoolwork and an eventual breakdown of his worker and/or homemaker role followed by psychiatric hospitalization.

SELF-REPAIR OF HARMONY IN THE OPEN SYSTEM

An open system can respond to disharmony and repair it. Consider children who are congenital upper extremity amputees. Despite the disharmony created by this missing component of the musculoskeletal constituent of skill, such children learn to generate images for skilled action and achieve the neurological programming and anatomical flexibility to use their lower extremities to take over what are normally manual skills. Energized by an urge to explore and master, these children can still choose to encounter their worlds and learn to organize and to use their performance subsystem for the things they value and find interesting.

In the case of an acquired disability in later life, an individual often has to achieve a reorganization and restoration of harmony across the subsystems and their constituents. For example, the person with cerebrovascular accident and subsequent hemiplegia may have to learn to substitute a nondominant for a dominant hand to produce fine motor acts, and to employ process skills to deal with problems that arise in motor performance for daily living tasks. The same person may have to generate new habits, roles, interests and values and develop a new sense of personal causation based on new skills. Reorganization and self-repair must always be in terms of the entire system.

THE OPEN SYSTEM TRAJECTORY

Because change results from the open system cycle, an open system is always on a trajectory or path of development (8). Even if there is no gross change taking place in a person, experiences are being accumulated which reinforce or weaken existing traits and conditions.

The trajectory of change in any person is an extremely complex process. It may involve periods of cumulative and progressive change, periods of relative stability, and periods of disorganization followed by self-repair. Overall, the pattern of change throughout the lifespan should be one of moving toward greater and greater self-enhancement and integration. The trajectory of the individual is one that is shaped by the environments in which the person performs. It is manifest in the development of occupational behavior over the lifespan, and it may be either an adaptive or maladaptive course of change. These topics are taken up in subsequent chapters.

References

1. Boulding K: General system theory—the skeleton of science. In Buckley W (ed), *Modern Systems Research for the Behavioral Scientist*. Chicago, Aldine, 1968.
2. Chapple E: *Rehabilitation: Dynamic of Change*. Ithaca, N. Y., Center for Research in Education, Cornell University, 1970.
3. Cox H: *The Feast of Fools*. New York, Harper Row, 1969.
4. Huizinga J: *Homo Ludens*. Boston, Beacon Press, 1955.
5. Koestler A: Beyond atomism and holism—the concept of the holon. In Koestler A, Smithies JR (eds), *Beyond Reductionism*. Boston, Beacon Press, 1969.
6. Moss G: *Illness, Immunity, and Social Interactions*. New York, Wiley, 1973.
7. Reilly M: *Play as Exploratory Learning*. Beverly Hills, Calif., Sage, 1974.
8. von Bertalanffy L: General system theory—a critical review. In Buckley W (ed): *Modern System's Research for the Behavioral Scientist*. Chicago, Aldine, 1968.
9. Weiss PS: *Hierarchically Organized Systems in Theory and Practice*. New York, Hafner, 1971.

CHAPTER 4

Occupation as Interaction with the Environment*

Roann Barris, Gary Kielhofner, Ruth Ellen Levine, and Anne M. Neville

A distinguishing feature of the open system is its continual interaction with external surroundings. Humans, as open systems, willfully encounter and perform in various environments. This chapter examines the process of interaction between persons and environments, and environmental factors which influence this process.

In examining this interaction, the chapter conceptualizes the environment as four concentric circles or layers (Fig. 4.1). The core layer consists of objects, the materials and artifacts of daily life. The next layer corresponds to tasks, or the projects and activities that comprise play, work and self-care, and determine one's use of objects. Surrounding the layer of tasks are social groups and organizations. These groups delineate certain roles, relationships between roles and essential tasks necessary to the group's functioning. The final layer, culture, consists of the beliefs that tie together and govern the actions of groups of people. Together, these layers represent an environmental hierarchy which influences both the decisions to encounter one's surroundings and subsequent performances in these surroundings.

PERSON/ENVIRONMENT INTERACTION

Process of Choice

Throughout life, individuals choose to explore and master their surroundings (29). Decisions about which environments to explore reflect a combination of factors and circumstances. Infants, obviously limited in their physical mobility, must choose among those things that can be brought within their reach or the range of their

---

senses. Adults' decisions are limited by transportation, finances, inability to secure admission to certain settings, and so on. However, although decisions are influenced by constraints, they are also volitional.

Volition components collectively influence the manner in which a person enacts the innate urge to explore and master the environment. Personal causation influences the degree of challenge that one is willing to seek from the environment (9, 29), while values and interests determine the types of settings that will attract a person. *Arousal* is a concept that links these volitional traits with properties of the environment.

AROUSAL AND CHOICE

Arousal is an *internal state of an organism, with physiological (e.g. pulse rate and catecholamine output) and subjective (level of alertness and feelings of excitement) manifestations* (5, 33, 37, 59). One's level of arousal generally changes in response to environmental conditions unless one is already extremely underaroused (i.e. asleep or in a coma) or extremely overaroused (highly anxious or stressed) (59).

States of over- and underarousal affect one's mood, ability to perform and consequent desire to stay in a certain place or situation (5, 14, 31, 37, 43). People who are underaroused find themselves bored. To counteract this, they often fantasize or daydream, and under extreme conditions, may hallucinate. When individuals are overaroused, they feel anxious, out of control, and ineffective. In both cases, they may also make a more adaptive response of either trying to change the setting or leaving.

Environmental Characteristics Evoking Arousal

Various features of the environment have been identified as being arousal-inducing (5).

---

* Adapted from and reprinted with permission of The American Occupational Therapy Association, Inc., © 1982 *The American Journal of Occupational Therapy*, 36: 637–644. The organization and conceptual development of this chapter represent the primary work of the first author.

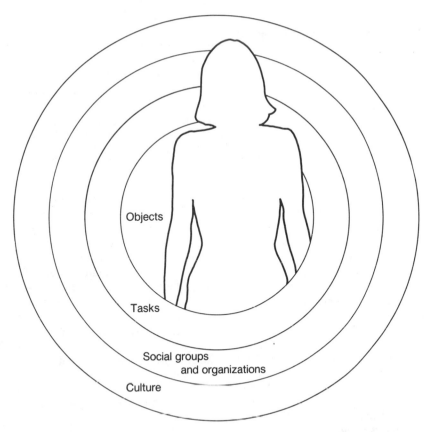

Figure 4.1.   Environmental layers and the human system.

Psychophysical properties refer to *physical characteristics of the setting and their intensity or quality.* A disco, for instance, is highly arousing partly because of the loud music and flashing lights. Ecological properties are *events that either directly or indirectly threaten survival or well-being.* A summer storm which uproots trees and causes a power outage can be overarousing to many people because of the knowledge of potential injuries to people and property. Collative properties of the environment are not physically identifiable; rather, they are *discrepancies between a person's past experiences and present perceptions of the environment* (5). Novelty, surprise and complexity are examples of collative properties. People experience novelty when their *surroundings are new to them, or discrepant with previous experience.* Surprise derives from the unexpected; *something happens that one has not been prepared for by previous experience.* Complexity relates to the *potential for continual discovery of ways to experience the environment.* Chess, for example, is a more complex game than checkers because different types of pieces are used, there are more options for moving them, and there are more possibilities for the use of sophisticated strategies. Table 4.1 summarizes the environmental properties contributing to arousal and provides further examples.

Collative variables generate feelings of uncertainty, a sense that one doesn't know precisely what will happen next. Because one wants to resolve these feelings, collative variables provoke a desire to explore the surroundings, and to find out more (5, 18). A familiar example is that of moving to or traveling in a new city. Generally, one's response to a new place is to want to explore, learn street names, see the sights, and to discover what makes this place different from where one lived before. But, because too much novelty or complexity can be overarousing and stymie the impulse to explore, people who grew up in rural communities are often uncomfortable in large cities, and overwhelmed by the crowds, noise, subways, and so on.

Whereas overarousal may be very stressful,

Table 4.1.
Arousal-inducing properties of the environment

Variable	Example
Psychophysical properties	Loud music; bright colors; intense heat
Ecological properties	Severe storms; extreme pollution; possibility of public failure
Collative properties	Novelty—learning a foreign language; surprise—a child's jack-in-the-box toy; complexity—a 35-mm camera versus an Instamatic

prolonged underarousal may be enervating and lead to uninvolvement in one's surroundings. The marked apathy and indifference of board-and-care residents may partly be a symptom of mental illness, but it is also the result of living in an underarousing environment.

VALUES AND INTERESTS IN THE ENVIRONMENT

Although arousal is involved in all one's decisions to enter or leave environments, environmental choices also reflect a search for a match between personal interests and values and the climate of interests and values in the environment (10, 29, 36). Environments embody interests and values largely because of a history of use that grows up around them, and the communication of this history from one generation to the next. Whether the setting is an avant-garde urban community or a country-western bar in a small town, those who enter settings recognize a match between their own interests and values and those of the persons who shaped and maintain the setting.

The climate of values and interests is enduring (39); therefore, people who perceive a large disparity between the values of the setting and their own will tend to leave or avoid the environment. However, if they do not leave, they are prone to shift toward greater congruency with the setting's prevalent values (40, 44). This shift toward congruency enables cohesiveness to develop among users of the environment and maintains the setting's characteristic climate of values and interests.

THE DENIAL OF CHOICE

At times, because of illness, age or other constraints, individuals are not able to freely choose their environments. When decisions concerning environmental entry, exit and interactions are denied to the individual, feelings of helplessness and a decreased sense of personal causation are likely to result (35, 53). These feelings of helplessness can be more devastating than illness. Older people, for instance, who are involuntarily relocated, have a higher mortality rate than individuals who retain control over where they are to live (32). Cardiac patients who are not given control over certain aspects of their environment (such as choosing when to have visitors and what form of leisure to engage in) have longer hospital stays than patients who are given these choices (52).

Performance and Press

The search for novel, interesting settings, and the attempt to find a match between one's interests and values and the interest and value climate of the environment culminate in a decision to encounter, in some way, a particular environment. Having chosen to interact with the environment, one then produces occupational behavior that reflects a match or mismatch between one's level of competence and perceptions of environmental press (32).

Press refers to environmental expectations for certain behavior (32). Although press is a property of the environment, a person must recognize it in order to feel obligated to perform in certain ways. When settings are familiar and umambiguous and the people within are similar, there will be greater consensus as to these environmental demands.

Press may be felt for varying behaviors and in varying degrees of strength. Consequently, it is an important phenomenon because it influences which skills and habits one will develop, and affects one's organization of them into coherent patterns of behavior or roles. For example, the press of a street gang is likely to be for macho, risk-taking behaviors, while the press of a sensitivity group will be for physical and emotional openness. Table 4.2 provides examples of settings and the types of press that might be experienced in them.

Individuals' reactions to press vary with their abilities and experience in that type of setting (32). A newly hospitalized patient, for instance, may find the press for passive, dependent behavior to be unfamiliar; however, as the person becomes habituated to the sick role, these behaviors will begin to seem natural.

PRESS AND AROUSAL

Maladaptive performance and affect result from too little or too much press for behaviors relative to an individual's level of competence (32, 52, 61). If the press is for a behavior that hasn't been learned, the person will experience the setting as either novel, challenging, or overarousing. For instance, a new therapist might find the press for working rapidly and independently in a large clinic where patients are scheduled every half-hour to be highly stressful; the experienced therapist, on the other hand, may find the press associated with performing as a staff clinician not to be challenging enough.

Expanding the Range of Settings

The cycle of choice, entry and interaction with the environment ultimately spirals into involvement with an increasing number of environmental settings (7). The process of expanding one's environmental range is influenced by several factors. Through the development of the volition subsystem, the person identifies settings relevant to plans for continued and future occupational performances. In so doing, the person also identifies the need to conform one's behaviors to the demands of these settings or to modify choices of settings. As competence develops in these settings, the individual becomes capable of choosing and encountering additional settings.

Table 4.2.
Press

Setting	Expectations
Classroom	Notetaking, listening to the teacher
Nautilus club	Exercising
Church	Sitting in pews; whispering; praying

The expansion of one's range of environments is also influenced by culture, age and geographically-related expectations (3, 38). For example, because many American women currently work, a large number of young children and infants are placed in day care centers. A geographic influence on range would be the expectation that children growing up in a large city should learn to negotiate subways and buses at an early age.

ENVIRONMENTAL LAYERS

Until now we have been describing the open system/environment interaction as a series of processes that occur in relationship to the environment as a whole, without differentiating among the layers of the environment. However, each layer of the environment (objects, tasks, social groups, or culture) has special attributes that illuminate the system/environment interaction. In the next part of this chapter we will examine properties or dimensions of each environmental layer and their contributions to the open system processes of arousal-seeking, matching interests and values, adapting to press, and range expansion. Table 4.3 presents a summary of this discussion.

Objects

In carrying out everyday activities, we interact with both people and objects. These objects may range from necessary tools or implements to frivolous adornments and are *the materials of everyday life.*

DIMENSIONS OF OBJECTS

Objects can be described in terms of four dimensions: availability, complexity, flexibility, and symbolic meaning (Fig. 4.2).

Availability

This refers to *the presence or absence of objects in one's surroundings.* Objects make an environment more arousing and more interesting just by virtue of being there; hence, people tend to maintain objects of interest around them. Although people vary in the extent to which they collect and save objects, it would nevertheless be rare for someone's surroundings to be entirely devoid of objects (11). While not necessarily being complex themselves, the presence of objects can increase the complexity of a setting by

Table 4.3.
Environmental layers and arousal and press

Dimension	Contribution to arousal and press
Objects	
Availability	Complexity, novelty, and interest in setting
	Development of certain skills
	Expectations for doing certain tasks
	Search for alternatives when necessary objects are not present
Complexity	Overall unfamiliarity and complexity of the environment
	Development of special skills
Flexibility	Changing levels of complexity
	Specific or variable use expectations
Symbolic meaning	Changing importance of objects
	Changing requirements for use
Tasks	
Complexity	Complexity of setting
	Development of higher level skills
	Fear of inability to perform
Temporal boundaries	Ecological threat (deadlines)
	Uncertainty and ambiguity
	Development of habits
Rules	Complexity and flexibility of task
	Need for conformity or originality
Seriousness/playfulness	Exploration and experimentation versus competence and achievement
	Development of habits of practice and industry
	Consequences attached to success and failure
Social	Novelty or uncertainty
	Ecological threat
	Performance standards
	Flexibility in habits
	Group roles
Social Groups and Organizations	
Size	Role definition and specialization or role blurring
	Social involvement
	Degree of ambiguity and novelty
Function	Degree of playfulness
	Role behaviors
	Temporal organization
Permeability	Similarity to members (novelty of setting)
	Complexity
	Skill development
	Role internalization
Structural complexity	Uncertainty and ambiguity versus clear-cut role definitions
	Social involvement
Culture	
Nature of work and play	Ecological threat related to failure/success in a valued activity
	Complexity of lifestyle
	Internalized roles
	Occupational opportunities

Table 4.3. (*continued*)

Dimension	Contribution to arousal and press
Space/time	Routine versus novelty in daily life Meaning of places Temporal organization Physical organization of environment
Transmission of knowledge and values	Ambiguity, threat, or complexity, related to learning right and wrong Ritualization versus awareness of nuances Development of values Logical behavior

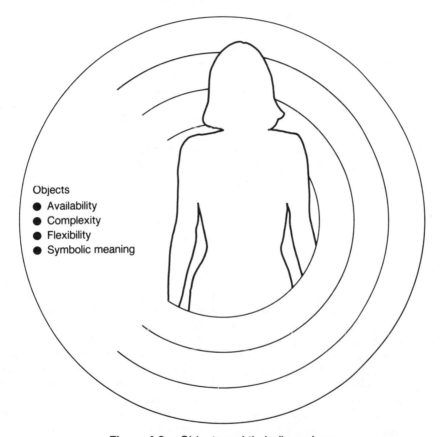

Figure 4.2.   Objects and their dimensions.

offering more possibilities for exploration and learning than might otherwise exist. Certainly, this is part of the basis for the popular belief that more is better.

The presence or absence of objects also contributes to press for certain types of behaviors or activities. Children, for instance, will engage in more solitary play when toys and play equipment are available, unless the toys are explicitly designed for social play (27, 46). However, an abundance of certain materials will not always lead to their use if no one present knows what to do with them (17, 62), or if they are not relevant to the person's life style. Gifts often share the fate of being forgotten in a dark closet when they seem useless or irrelevant to the receiver. Contrariwise, the scarcity of objects also influences the environmental press because when one lacks certain materials, one must look for alternatives to them, often to the point of becoming truly innovative with what is available.

Complexity

An object's complexity reflects *the amount of skill and learning required for its use.* When objects do not change over time, they become familiar and taken for granted by persons in the environment. If these objects are difficult to use, however, they do not rapidly become familiar. Therefore, the complexity of objects in the setting will affect its overall potential for inducing arousal. An environment with unchanging, simple and familiar objects will not usually be arousing, while a setting that is filled with uncommon, intricate equipment will be.

In addition to increasing the potential for arousal, complex objects place demands for engaging in specialized and skilled behaviors. In the past, bedrooms have usually been designed to be low arousing environments. Pastel colors, little furniture apart from a bed, chest of drawers, dressing table, and perhaps a television, along with lamp lighting created a low arousal setting that pressed for sleeping and intimacy. A recent social phenomenon, however, is the transformation of the bedroom into "the place to hang out" (13, p C-8). A trend toward keeping exercise equipment, home computers, small refrigerators, and other accoutrements in the bedroom, has made this room no longer a place to unwind but, instead, a place that maintains the pressures and expectations of an already overstressed lifestyle.

Flexibility

This dimension pertains to *the potential for using objects in a variety of ways, i.e. the degree to which objects lend themselves to manipulations and changes by the user.* Manipulability and malleability of objects lead to changing levels of complexity in the environment. The degree of flexibility similarly presses for specificity in the way something is used or, conversely, allows for unlimited possibilities. For example, objects that are important to children are often "raw" materials (boxes, sand, tires) that lend themselves to active exploration and involvement. What they are is not as important as what one can *do* with them (11). On the other hand, the fixed equipment found in many playgrounds can rapidly become boring because it can be used only in certain ways (26).

Symbolic Meaning

This is *a cumulative dimension that reflects objects' complexity, flexibility, and availability.*

Objects become symbols of power, prestige, independence, and so on, by virtue of such conditions as what one can do with them or how accessible they are. For example, objects that become symbols of wealth and status typically are rare or unusual in some respect. Owning a home video recorder may be a status symbol if most of one's peers can't afford to do likewise. Sometimes the absence of an object is also a status symbol. In the corporate world, *not* carrying a briefcase may indicate power since the person without a briefcase is not transporting information but making the decisions (30).

Complex objects often signify special powers. As society has become more technologically sophisticated, operating or manipulating complex machines frequently brings more status to certain jobs.

The potential of objects to be used or manipulated to achieve particular goals also contributes to their symbolic meaning. Adolescents, for example, frequently mention musical instruments, journals and stereo equipment as being their most prized possessions because they allow them to express their feelings and values in a socially competent manner (11). In adulthood, possessions are often a manifestation of power and independence. Adults prize certain objects because they make possible some activity; they enhance one's options within the environment (20). In a rural setting, a large pick-up truck may be a symbol of power because it enhances the owner's potential to haul wood, traverse mountain roads, or have a camper.

Objects also symbolize interests and values, thereby communicating important messages about one's identity. Adults use objects to identify their "trade"—both work and leisure (11). Religious icons and artifacts in one's house indicate a commitment to religious values, while tapestries and the presence of a floor loom communicate that one is a weaver.

Symbolic meaning contributes to arousal by changing the perceptions and importance attached to objects. Simultaneously, it also changes behavioral requirements for their use. Once a car is no longer merely a car but also a symbol of independence and responsibility, the owner must adapt to increased demands for competence in understanding its maintenance. This is especially true for women, who quickly lose the symbolic status of independence if they must rely on a mechanic's help for seemingly trivial car problems.

INTERACTING WITH OBJECTS

Interactions with objects are complex and diverse. People choose to have certain objects around them and to enter certain settings because of the objects they contain. At times one deliberately manipulates objects to accomplish particular goals or to reflect some personal belief; at others, the objects themselves induce certain experiences or attitudes and press for the learning of new skills. These interactions that occur reflect interrelationships among the four dimensions of objects, as well as individual differences in people and their occupational goals. An example is the ways in which people respond to and use computers.

Although small computers are rapidly becoming available to the public, most people still find them to be unfamiliar, novel parts of the environment. Nevertheless, individuals encounter computers in many parts of their daily lives. The reaction of many adults to increasing computerization is one of overarousal and discomfort with the impersonalization and technicalization they represent. Many children, however, are becoming familiar with computers early in their lives during school and leisure, and respond to computers as they do to a television set or pinball machine. Computers are also becoming a manifestation of interests and values, and a symbol of belief in progress and innovation. Owners of home computers communicate that they believe in, enjoy, and value a technologically complex life-style. Adults who share these beliefs experience and respond to a press for competency and fluency in the use of computers.

Tasks

"Task" is a common term, often calling to mind some chore, such as taking out the garbage. On the other hand, developmental psychologists frequently write of major life tasks, such as choosing a career or starting a family. Although we are less apt to speak of playful tasks than work tasks, in this chapter, task will be used to denote any occupational activity—work, play or daily living tasks.

The task environment consists of those *sequences of actions in which one engages to satisfy either external societal requirements or internal motives to explore and be competent.* These action sequences or projects (34) are organized toward the accomplishment of some goal and governed by certain rules for acceptable performance.

DIMENSIONS OF TASKS

Tasks consist of an aggregate of demand characteristics that emanate from several dimensions or features. These dimensions include complexity, temporal boundaries, rules or structure, degree of seriousness/playfulness in performance, and the social nature of the task (Fig. 4.3).

Complexity

Task complexity derives from *the level of skill and the number of steps required to execute the task.* Although complex objects generally lead to complex tasks, the range of complexity in a task can expand even though the user has become more familiar with the object. In fact, object familiarity may be prerequisite to increasing task complexity. For instance, a person must first acquire a basic familiarity with the piano keyboard before beginning to improvise jazz or play sonatas. Task complexity will contribute to arousal if the participant's skills are at a lower level than the task requires. At the same time, it presses for the development of higher levels of skill as a step toward alleviating this arousal.

Temporal Boundaries

Tasks may be *time-limited and performed in a discrete unit of time, or they may be continuous, occurring over a long interval with no identifiable point of conclusion.* Preparing dinner is an example of the first; restoring an old house, of the second. This is not to say that the latter task will never be concluded, but that the amount of time involved is not easily determined. In addition, tasks may be *bound to certain times of the day or to certain seasons, or they may be performed at an individual's discretion.* Preparing a departmental annual report is both time-limited and seasonal; ongoing supervisory activities are somewhat more discretionary.

Temporal requirements can be arousing because they may pose an ecological threat—one will not meet a deadline and may therefore lose a job or fail some sort of test; or they may contribute to the uncertainty of a situation—not knowing how long something will take renders the task ambiguous and complex. The temporal dimension presses for the development of habits. Working on an ongoing project, for example, requires an ability to budget time for the task and yet to be able to leave and return to it

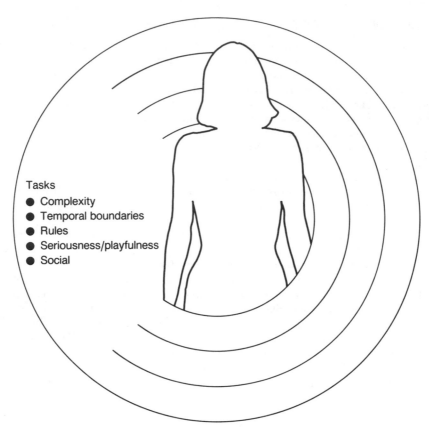

Figure 4.3. Tasks and their dimensions.

at another time without losing a sense of continuity and purpose in the activity.

Rules

The rules or *internal organization of a task* provide standards for its performance. Task structure is determined by the clarity and flexibility of these rules. In some tasks the rules are readily apparent, as are criteria for success and failure. Taking an exam, for instance, requires someone to be in a particular place at a particular time, and to answer a previously prepared set of questions. Success in this task is contingent upon correctly answering a preestablished percentage of these questions.

Creative endeavors generally have more flexible rules. Sometimes, the rigidity with which a task must be performed changes as the person becomes more competent and knowledgeable of the rules. Using a potter's wheel initially requires that one conform to certain rules regarding the properties of clay, the mechanics of the

wheel, and laws of gravity and balance. With mastery, these rules become subordinate to the artist's creativity and imagination.

Many tasks are so customary that their rules do not become evident until they are broken. One ordinarily does not think of a social conversation as being a rule-bound task; yet, many psychiatric patients break these taken-for-granted conventions. Engaging in conversations necessitates making eye contact, taking turns speaking, sticking to appropriate subject matter, and so on; not following these rules will likely disrupt a conversation. Interestingly, most games also have strict rules that must be followed by players. Thus, even seemingly simple and common tasks have standards of performance that must be adhered to.

The type of rules that govern a task will determine the level of task complexity. Rules press for recognition of certain conventions and a willingness to incorporate them into one's behavior.

Seriousness/Playfulness

The degree of seriousness/playfulness in a task is not always inherent in the task itself—the playful or serious nature of a task *reflects both the context in which it is performed and the consequences that are contingent upon successful performance.* The belonging of a task to a work or leisure role, the importance attached to the task by a cultural group, and the individual's ability to carry out the task all contribute to its playfulness or seriousness. For example, woodworking as a hobby will be performed more playfully than the woodworking of a carpenter; singing in church will be more serious than singing at a party. Further, although many activities generally fall into the domain of either work or play, people can still take their play tasks seriously or carry out their work tasks playfully.

Playful activities, because they lack consequences, are arousing enough to initiate exploration, but also unthreatening enough to permit error and to be fun. Although most persons' leisure is approached and maintained at a playful level, some leisure tasks do provoke the intensity and anxiety of high arousal. Chess or bridge can be played as social events or with extreme seriousness, and the skilled, serious player would probably find a social, low arousal match to be boring.

Work tasks can also vary in their playfulness. A conversation with one's co-workers can be serious, concerned with critical decisions, and highly goal-oriented; it can be concerned with work-related problems but involve joking and humor; or it can be concerned with matters that have nothing to do with work and yet be necessary to the maintenance of good relationships with one's colleagues. When work tasks are very serious, the injection of humor and playfulness into the activity is often necessary in order to defuse some of the arousal engendered by the activity. In this case, the playfulness is experienced as a temporary release from the seriousness of the task.

When tasks are playful, they press for experimentation, trying out new behavior and skills. As the nature of the task becomes more serious, the press changes toward demands for improved skill and more accomplished performance (competence). In addition, there is an increased press for habits of practice, industry and style. For example, when a child learns to swim, he or she will probably first simply play and get used to holding his/her head under water. Later, the child will begin to develop basic strokes and may even practice these strokes on dry land. Eventually, the child may begin to swim distances and to concentrate on form.

Social Dimension

This dimension incorporates two important aspects of tasks: its public or private nature, and the degree to which it is cooperative or competitive. Tasks are public or private depending on whether *the outcome is intended solely for oneself or for an audience.* For many people, the more public an activity is, the more arousing it is likely to be because of the threat of failing in front of a large group. Consequently, writing in one's journal may be relatively low in arousal, whereas writing a book chapter may be a task of much higher arousal because it must meet the approval of many other people.

The second aspect of the social dimension, competition and cooperation, concerns *the extent to which tasks involve the measurement of one's performance against another person or some recognized standard,* and *the degree to which two or more people must work together to accomplish some goal.* Competition and cooperation can coexist in an activity, as when one team competes against another. Both can be arousing, depending on the person's previous experience in either type of task. Thus, people who are accustomed to working alone may find the demands for sharing and social interaction in a cooperative task to be very arousing. While some people find competition to be overarousing, others are more highly motivated under competitive conditions (4). Professional athletes, for example, find that the arousal of competition induces them to higher levels of performance than they believed possible.

A task can be both competitive and public, such as a race or music competition, or it can be competitive and private when one is competing against personal standards of performance—for example, the runner who wants to achieve a certain speed or distance. A task can be cooperative and public when a joint endeavor is required for a performance, such as a group of actors putting on a play.

The social dimension of tasks presses for excellence in performance when public or competitive standards must be met, and it presses for the development of interaction skills when cooperation is necessary. Cooperation additionally presses for flexibility in one's habits in order to accommodate the working styles of other participants. The social dimension can also press for the development of group membership roles—i.e. being an initiator, following someone else's lead, monitoring and evaluating group progress, and so on.

INTERACTING WITH TASKS

People engage in a variety of tasks throughout their lives. Usually one's initial involvement is tentative and exploratory, but over time a great many tasks become relegated to habitual, routine parts of one's life. Habitual tasks cease to command one's attention until some change in either the person's ability or the parameters of the task occurs. For example, most people perform their daily self-care without ever being fully aware of what they are doing. However, a new graduate, preparing to go on a first job interview, may believe the consequences of choosing what to wear for that day to be so much more momentous than usual that he or she becomes paralyzed with indecision.

Tasks that do not become routine may continue to attract one because the individual sees them as leading toward a future goal. The ability to relate a current endeavor to a future goal keeps one involved in tasks that may be unpleasant or anxiety-provoking, and can impart meaning to activities that otherwise may seem unnecessary or boring.

The task environment directly influences the development of specific skills and habits. In fact, it is knowledge of this that contributes to the occupational therapist's ability to use tasks therapeutically. For instance, craft activities require the mastery of particular materials, problem solving, creative expression, and the development of habits of craftsmanship (45).

Tasks also influence learning in less direct ways. In play, for example, children may imitate the behavior of adults and begin to learn the roles they will assume later in life (48), they learn to interact with objects and peers (49) and they learn how to problem solve and take risks (8). Yet, much of this learning is subliminal and secondary to the task at hand—playing.

Social Groups and Organizations

People belong to and interact with many types of social groups and organizations throughout

their lives. These *collective units of individuals* range from informal social groupings, such as a lunch table group at work, to naturally occurring groups (e.g. the family), to formalized organizations developed for the explicit purpose of achieving some goal (16, 28). The groups that exist in a society create opportunities for people to assume occupational roles.

DIMENSIONS OF SOCIAL GROUPS AND ORGANIZATIONS

Although groups and organizations can be described in terms of numerous dimensions, those that appear most relevant to understanding how this layer of the environment contributes to the development of occupational performance are: the size of this group, its function or goals, the permeability of its boundaries, and the complexity of its structure (Fig. 4.4).

Size

This dimension pertains to *the number of people* involved in the group. The smallest unit that can exist in interpersonal relationships is the dyad. Dyadic relationships include such pairings as parent/child, mentor/protege, tutor/pupil, and coach/athlete. Upper limits to the size of a group or organization are usually determined by its purpose. Political organizations strive for large memberships, multinational corporations employ thousands of workers, but a staff meeting may involve less than 20 people.

The size of a group may press for either role specialization or role blurring. When fewer people than necessary are available to carry out group functions, people are frequently called on to perform in multipurpose capacities, with role blurring or a sharing of skills. For instance, professionals in community mental health settings are more likely to share aspects of their role with one another than professionals in a large psychiatric institution. In addition, there is often more pressure in smaller organizations to become centrally involved and to assume active, responsible positions (3, 60). Members of small churches, for example, are more involved in church-related activities than members of large congregations (60). In large groups, the press is more likely to be for role specialization. Thus, a large occupational therapy department may have a coordinator of fieldwork education, a clinical supervisor, senior therapist, staff therapists, and a department director. In large

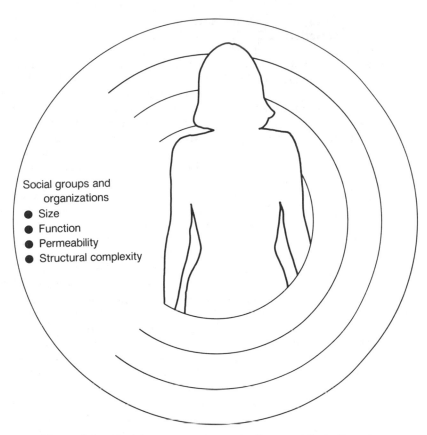

Figure 4.4.   Social groups and organizations and their dimensions.

groups it is also possible for people to remain on the fringes, in roles of only minimal involvement.

Both large and small groups can be arousing. Large groups often evoke tension in participants because the expectations of individuals may be ambiguous. However, role blurring can be equally anxiety provoking, since one's job loses its original definition and the parameters of the job become uncertain. Dyads can be unarousing when individuals are familiar with each other's expectations and style of performance, or overarousing when the relationship is new and members are uncertain of one another's standards.

Function

A group's function is its *dominant purpose.* Work organizations may be concerned with manufacturing or providing services, education, maintenance of the social order or the creation of knowledge (28). Groups whose primary purpose is play may include teams for organized sports, informal networks of people with shared leisure interests and groups that provide services or entertainment for other people.

A group's predominant concern with play or work will establish a climate that is more or less arousing for participants. Generally, for members to continue in a playful group, the atmosphere will be one that is optimally arousing; therefore, players will seek to manipulate their surroundings and tasks so that the organization is neither boring nor threatening. For example, a monthly poker group may have an unwritten rule that discussion about family problems or stresses is taboo. Further, although stakes may be modest so that losses are not catastrophic, occasionally outrageous bets may vary the level of risk involved (23).

Because the consequences of work are often more crucial to one's survival than those of play, the environment of work groups can potentially be overarousing to members. In addition, strategies for changing the arousal level may focus more on changes within the person than within the environment since workers do not always have control over the work organization. Despite this potential for overarousal, many work settings are low arousal environments—in many cases because role expectations are mundane and repetitive. Some organizations attempt to deal with the lack of novelty for workers by offering transfers to new roles or retraining individuals for different tasks.

The function of a group presses for the investment of a certain amount of time. For instance, many work organizations require members to work 40 hours a week, from 9:00–5:00, for approximately 11 months of the year. However, elementary and high schools may require teachers to be present from 7:30 until 3:00, for 9 months of the year, while hospitals may require 1st year residents to be on call for 72 hours in a row. Leisure groups generally press for less structured time commitments and may allow for individual variation in how members allocate their time to the group. Thus, two members of Roadrunners may not only run at different times of the day, but one may attend all the club meetings and the other may not.

Organizations also press for a certain level of commitment and role internalization. If the press for involvement is low, an organization may attract members who do not become fully committed to it. When an organization requires substantial involvement, members must make a greater effort to internalize the role, frequently through special training or initiation of some sort. As a result, however, such organizations may exhibit low turnover rates and high member cohesiveness. Fraternal lodges, for example, are often closely-knit groups that rarely lose their members.

Permeability of Boundaries

This dimension refers to *how easy or difficult a group is to join, and how susceptible it is to pressures from outsiders.* Membership requirements for an organization may be predicated solely on some homogeneous characteristic such as age (e.g. beginning elementary school) or a sharing of interests, or they may be more stringent and require a period of preparation, learning, and practice. In work organizations, in particular, different entry requirements may exist for different positions (51).

When entry requirements are based primarily on sharing a homogeneous trait, joining a group is likely to be low in arousal because one either has or does not have the trait. With more demanding membership requirements, arousal increases since successful entry is less certain.

As entry requirements become stringent, the press for developing specific skills, knowledge and attitudes is likely to increase. Joining a professional baseball team requires more expertise as a baseball player than does joining a local softball league. Also, as it becomes more difficult to enter an organization, the demand for commitment to the group tends to increase.

An organization's boundaries also vary in how open or closed they are to influences from the external environment. A group that has relatively stable goals (15, 54) and rigid entrance requirements may be very closed to outside forces (28). Until recently, the army has been an example of a highly-insulated organization. Extremely radical or conservative political factions are another example. Groups that are very open to environmental influences usually have less homogeneity in their membership requirements and give individual members more opportunities to participate in strategic decision-making. Free schools, in the late 1960s and early 1970s, were open groups highly susceptible to changes in community attitudes and in the beliefs and goals of their students and staff (56).

Insulated groups are often less arousing than more permeable groups. The latter, because of their openness to environmental changes, may be unstable (15, 54, 56), and thus considerably more arousing to members. In fact, the unpredictability of such groups can lead to burn-out of the members.

Impermeable groups press for unquestioning conformity to standardized behaviors, whereas more permeable groups press for frequent redefinition of the group's mission and for innovative problem solving (56).

Structural Complexity

This dimension is an aggregate of the dimensions of size, function and permeability and pertains to *the type of networks and relationships among a group's members.* For instance, increasing organization size tends to lead to increasingly hierarchic structures. Witness the organizational charts for many large hospitals, with their numerous chains of command (e.g. director of medical services, director of adjunctive services, director of dietary services, and so on) emanating from a powerful but removed administrator at the very top. In addition to hierarchical structures, large organizations are usually characterized by networks that link people with similar roles, statuses or interests (54). For example, within a university there may be a network of women faculty, a network of allied health faculty, and a network of department heads. Leisure groups and organizations are likely to have informal, lateral structures, based on networks of common interests. For example, a group of employees who go to the same bar after work once a week may have been formed by a common interest in drinking and relaxation, and will probably not contain differentiated membership statuses.

The complexity of groups has interesting implications for arousal. Hierarchically organized groups often have clear-cut role descriptions, thereby decreasing uncertainty and ambiguity in role performance. Groups that consist of loosely linked networks of individuals may also be unarousing, because they afford members the opportunity to settle into relatively peripheral and unthreatening roles. However, the potential for novelty and arousal increases when individuals have the opportunity to move in and out of a variety of positions and interrelationships with other members.

Group structure, in concert with size, presses for how centrally involved members will become and how specialized their roles will be. However, whereas the size of a group indicates how many people will become central to the group's functioning, structure indicates who these people will be. For example, positions at the bottom of a hierarchy generally carry with them minimal responsibility and power. In laterally organized groups, the press may be more variable, as individuals can seek and negotiate their level of responsibility.

INTERACTION WITH SOCIAL GROUPS

Social groups and organizations have a major impact on the development of role behavior. Because roles are learned in the context of groups (58), the groups that are available to a person will directly influence the roles available to that person as well. An infant's role repertoire is limited primarily to family-derived roles in dyadic or small group relationships—daughter, son, niece, sister. A child participates in larger groups—school, clubs, after-school sports—assuming the roles of player, friend and student. Eventually, the range of groups open to a person

narrows, as decisions to join one group naturally exclude other groups from one's future.

The process of occupational choice essentially involves the delineation of a series of leisure and work groups an individual will attempt to become qualified for and to enter. At the same time, other groups will become irrelevant or inaccessible to the person. For example, the individual who goes to college and studies journalism is delineating a future in which he or she will primarily be involved with media production groups (e.g. publishing companies, newspapers, communications industries) or educational organizations, but will probably not be a member of groups concerned with providing rehabilitative services. Similarly, in developing one's skills as an amateur bowler, a person becomes prepared to join bowling leagues in the future but probably not other sports groups.

Culture

Although culture has been defined differently by various writers, most writers agree that culture consists of *the beliefs and perceptions, values and norms, and customs and behaviors that are shared by a group or society, and passed from one generation to the next through both formal and informal education* (1, 47). Two implications are embedded in this definition. First, one's culture leads to a characteristic way of perceiving and acting in the world (47). Second, because of this characteristic way of acting, a culture results in particular representative lifestyles that embody accepted notions of success or competence in society (6, 41, 47).

Defining culture in terms of coherent, recognizable lifestyles points to the fact that cultural groups may contain within them *subcultural* groups, which conform to some of the prevailing cultural conventions while preserving unique characteristics of their own. Thus, in American society, there may be urban, rural, ethnic and other subcultural groups.

DIMENSIONS OF CULTURE

Many dimensions can be used to compare and describe cultures; three are particularly relevant to the relationship between culture and occupational performance and will be the focus of this section. They are the nature of work and play, the space/time dimension in which work and play occur, and how knowledge and values about work and play are transmitted from one generation to the next (Fig. 4.5).

The Nature of Work and Play

The meaning and value of work and leisure, the activities that are considered acceptable forms of each, and the extent to which a culture dichotomizes these behaviors allow one to understand the nature of work and play for a given cultural group.

Although work has always been necessary for subsistence, the precise form of this work and the extent to which different forms are valued vary historically and culturally. At one time the relationship between work and subsistence was quite direct—the product of work was food and shelter. Today, although food and shelter are still obtained by working, most people do not directly engage in the activities of locating food or creating their shelters. In fact, when these things are actually done, they are often performed in the guise of hobbies (e.g. baking bread,

studying herbal lore) or to make improvements in one's lifestyle beyond what is actually necessary for survival (e.g. building an addition to one's house, redecorating the interior, planting a garden). Because the relationship between ends and means is less direct, and because a larger number of people can use their wages for more than just subsistence needs, both work itself and the many forms of working have a range of meanings for people.

These meanings reflect the underlying value system of a culture and its historical trends and innovations. For example, in the United States, a country shaped by rebellion, westward expansion, and a pioneering spirit, the qualities of independence and individuality are highly valued. However, the occupations that have come to signify or "mean" these qualities differ according to geographic region, ethnic group and other subcultural groupings. In the rural South, being a tobacco farmer or being self-employed in a small business are occupational roles of status, whereas for Jewish-Americans, occupa-

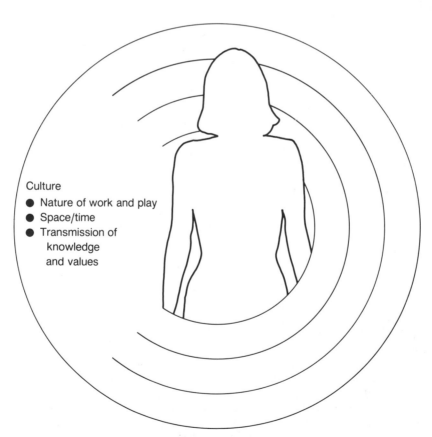

Figure 4.5. Culture and its dimensions.

tions that require high levels of education (e.g. doctors, lawyers, professors) are typically valued. Although these occupations may represent a plethora of meanings to the people who enact them, they are also particular cultural representations of independence, uniqueness and success.

Another aspect of the meaning of work is the centrality and importance of work in an individual's lifestyle. Among the Greeks and Romans, to be seen working was a sign of inferiority (2). In cultural groups that are dominated by the Protestant work ethic, however, one's entire lifestyle may be shaped around work. Nevertheless, within different occupational subcultures, work assumes greater or lesser degrees of centrality in people's lives. Many industrial workers recognize the primacy of the workplace in their lives, but derive more satisfaction from the parts of their lives carried out away from the workplace (12). For other occupational groups, work may penetrate into all aspects of members' lives (21, 42). Doctors may use free time to catch up on professional reading, their friends may be other doctors, and they tend to be actively involved in their professional organization.

The meaning and importance of leisure also vary with cultural groups. In many primitive cultures, and prior to the industrial revolution, there was no sharp distinction between work and leisure. Play was part of work, not separate from it (2). In industrialized societies, however, work and play have become dichotomized activities, with play or leisure referring to discretionary, freely chosen activity. But, although many people share this view of work and play as contrasting ways to use time, typical forms of leisure vary widely.

People experience a range of individualized meanings in their leisure as well; however, certain meanings or attitudes toward leisure inhere in the cultural group at large. In the 1960s and 1970s, in reaction to increasingly technological and consumeristic life-styles, many Americans began to value hand-crafting products. Leisure came to mean a chance to demonstrate one's relatedness to natural materials, and to show that one could survive without relying on mass-produced commercial artifacts. Today leisure is assuming another cultural meaning. In a highly competitive society, many people are seeking to gain achievement and status in their leisure, whether or not they are doing so in their work.

Culture also prescribes what forms of work and play are expected of, and acceptable for, different members of society. This is most easily seen in the changing options for women in the United States. Prior to the 1960s, American society expected most women to be housewives and mothers. Their leisure time was somewhat amorphous, since it fell at peculiar times of the day, and since "free" time was likely to involve sewing (e.g. making clothes), baking or other family oriented activities. Women were not expected to work outside the home, but if they did, socially acceptable forms of work included teaching, nursing and being a secretary. With the impact of the women's movement, however, the options available to women have broadened. Many women both work and raise families, and although most women who work still find employment in female-dominated occupations, more and more women are entering traditionally male arenas of employment. Further, because current American values include the pursuit of fitness and self-fulfillment, many women, in addition to their homemaker and worker roles, are members of health clubs, jog or participate in some other form of exercise on a routine basis.

An interesting example of how culture influences work or leisure expectations is provided by a study of the culture of a black urban ghetto (41). Because conventional employment opportunities for the black adults in this study were either menial jobs or nonexistent, work roles that are considered deviant by white middle-class American culture were deemed normal and successful. Hustlers, pimps, preacher-hustlers, and entertainers were all models of competent occupational performance. This cultural influence extended downward to affect the ghetto child's approach to the traditional prework role, that of student. By the time children had entered school, many had already begun imitating and internalizing behaviors that would lead to success in the urban ghetto culture but which were antithetical to the student role—such behaviors as verbal manipulativeness, resourcefulness, self-reliance, and mistrust of authorities. In doing so, these adolescents were assuming more culturally relevant prework roles of cool cats, jesters, and so on (41).

The nature of work and play has two major implications for arousal. First, the meaning of work and play in general, and of different occupations in particular, determines the value attached to worker and player roles and to various forms of work and play. When activities are highly valued, it becomes increasingly important to succeed at them. Arousal increases as well, because the possibility of failure in a highly valued role is a form of threat to the individual.

Second, the variety of socially-sanctioned forms of work and play contributes to the complexity of individuals' lifestyles. For example, because more roles are available to women today, the increasing expectations for their role participation has led to a more complicated and complex existence, as women try to balance and succeed in work, home, and leisure.

The press of this dimension lies in expectations for internalized roles and values. A culture or subculture demands that its members engage in certain approved activities and communicates certain attitudes or values that one should hold about these activities. Further, the nature of work and play in a cultural group creates the opportunities or range of activities that one can choose from. Although occupational decisions are predicated on identifying one's interests and values, these decisions bear the influence of one's cultural background. It takes tremendous, deliberate effort to make choices that defy this background. Such choices, however, may be made more easily when one can envision oneself as a member of another subcultural group. Thus, young adults of the 1960s who rebelled against their parents' middle-class cultural values, often did so as members of a cooperative or communal group. Similarly, women who defied conventional beliefs about female occupations often found the support of feminist organizations to be invaluable.

Space/Time Dimension of Work and Play

Cultures organize the use of space and time by prescribing *what activities should take place in what locations and when these activities should occur* (1, 24, 25, 47). In the United States today we generally have separate spaces for work, play, family life, spiritual activities, and so on; however, the boundaries between these places and activities were not always so well-differentiated. In preindustrial America, work and home life were carried out in the same place. With the advent of factories, people began to "go to work" in a place outside their home, a pattern that eventually gave rise to the dominant middle-class life-style of commuting to the office, carrying out one's job, and then commuting home again to resume the rest of one's life. Today, however, occupational roles such as investment counselor, psychotherapist, and professor cross the boundaries between home and work, and

such technological trends as the growth of satellite media capacities and increasing ownership of home computers are making the centralized office building less necessary (55).

Cultural differences can also be found in the extent to which play space is separate from home life. In rural subcultures, for instance, the home is likely to be the setting for many leisure activities, whereas in urban areas such as New York, people are more likely to leave their apartments in search of leisure (22).

Away from home, play may be carried out in formal spaces that exist solely for that purpose (e.g. health spas, tennis clubs, bowling alleys) or in informal spaces that serve a multitude of purposes. Cultures differ in their use of both formal and informal space for leisure. For example, a study in Taipei, Taiwan, found that middle-class families did not permit their children to play in the streets whereas working-class parents did (50).

The use of time for work, play, and other parts of life is also culturally distinct (25, 47). One difference in the use of time occurs in the extent to which people in a cultural group are oriented to doing one thing at a time (completing one sequence of events before beginning another) or to doing several things at once (25). Although most Western cultures are sequentially oriented, some subcultural groups are not. Farming, for example, requires an ability to attend to overlapping crops, to balance time-limited tasks with ongoing tasks, and so on. Sequentially oriented cultures easily lend themselves to sharp distinctions between work and play time. The 9:00–5:00, 5-day workweek dominates much of American life. But, just as the geographic separation of work from the rest of life is weakening, so, too, are the boundaries of work time weakening (55).

Sequentially oriented cultures also make a strong distinction between doing *something* and doing *nothing*. Doing something is characterized by visible activity; sitting, meditating, daydreaming and other "passive" situations are considered to be doing nothing. Because doing nothing has a negative connotation, these cultures communicate a message that one must always appear to be busy.

Space and time moderate arousal levels by routinizing certain aspects of daily life. Once people are used to allocating time in certain ways, disruptions in their routines—such as oversleeping, being late to work, or an appointment that takes too long—can be stressful and overarousing. Misusing or using places in a different (novel) way can also lead to arousal because people must revise or reframe their notions of what to do in these spaces.

The cultural use of space and time creates a press for organizing one's life in a certain way. People who might naturally be "night" people force themselves to be "day" people in order to meet the cultural expectations for working from 9:00 until 5:00. This aspect of culture further prescribes how much time one should spend doing things and where one should do them. In addition, because people recognize common uses for certain places, they may experience a strong press to reorganize the physical environment when changing the function of a setting.

The Transmission of Knowledge and Values

Cultures transmit knowledge and values about work and play through *informal, formal and technical processes of teaching and learning* (25). Informal learning involves imitation of role models, trial and error and other imitative processes that tend to be difficult to describe or pin down (25). For example, a young man entering the business world may begin to dress in the style of his boss, use similar mannerisms, and so forth. Formal learning generally occurs in situations where right and wrong ways of doing something are so taken for granted that explanations are not given (even if they exist) (25). Much of the behavior that is customarily associated with boys and girls is learned formally— girls don't fight, boys don't hit girls, etc. Technical learning involves the use of reason and logic to discriminate between right and wrong (25). Technical, formal, and informal learning are generally used in conjunction with each other. The army, for instance, involves a combination of formal and technical learning. New army recruits engage in a heavily ritualized basic training, but many of the skills for using equipment or for carrying out military procedures require technical learning. Some occupational subcultures that are seemingly dominated by technical knowledge actually highly value informal learning. For example, the medical subculture considerably devalues academic (technical) knowledge in favor of informal knowledge gained through clinical experience (19).

Formal, informal and technical learning can each be arousing, although for different reasons. Formal learning, because it involves rigid situations, can be very threatening. It is particularly arousing to a new member of a subculture. The new worker, anxious to avoid mistakes but not knowing why one thing is right and another wrong, may be afraid to do anything at all. Technical learning is likely to be arousing because it may involve complex procedures and reasoning processes. Informal learning is potentially the least arousing of all three kinds of learning, but it, too, can induce arousal when one chooses a role model who seems hopelessly impossible to emulate. Informal learning can also be arousing because the boundaries of behavior are more ambiguous; there is no clear delineation of right or wrong when one is learning intuitively.

Formal learning presses for the development of ritualized behaviors, the inculcation of certain values, the continuity of tradition, and suspension of questioning. Informal learning presses for flexibility and sensitivity to the nuances of daily life, and technical learning presses for logical behavior and following directions by rote. Technical learning does not, as a rule, press for creativity; one follows certain steps in order to arrive at a predetermined result.

INTERACTION WITH CULTURE

By prescribing acceptable forms of work and play, attitudes toward these occupations, and place and time boundaries to them, culture describes a collection of situations or events that form a recurring part of people's lives. For example, situations common to a college student subculture might include a Saturday football game, a fraternity party and final exam week. The cultural expectation for a person's participation in particular situations provides a framework for anticipating and predicting the range of settings important to that person's life.

Unlike objects, tasks and social groups, one's cultural heritage is relatively circumscribed—a person is born into a particular cultural group. However, one may later in life choose to become part of a subcultural group. This choice is made on the basis of holding certain values about lifestyles and rejecting others. One may also become a member of an occupational subculture because of choices of occupational roles and organizations. Nevertheless, these subcultures exist in relation to a larger cultural group. The subculture of nursing, for example, is more likely to attract women than men in the United States because of prevailing beliefs in this country about proper work roles for men and women.

Hierarchy in the Environment

Because the environment is hierarchically organized, each level influences and organizes the levels below. Quite simply, this means that culture determines the groups that are available to and valued by persons, groups select and organize the tasks that people will perform when they become members, and tasks dictate what objects will be used and how they will be used. For example, in Chillum, a Washington, D.C. suburb with a large Fiumedinisi Italian community, membership in the Fiumedinisi Lodge is an important means of providing cultural continuity for these families. Certain social events occur at the Lodge on a regular basis; dances, for example, involving all generations of family members, are frequently held to the music of a local Italian band. The family is another highly valued social group in this community. Some activities that are commonly shared by the Fiumedinisi families include listening to a weekly radio show broadcast from Italy and an annual wine-making and tasting party. In addition, these families have held onto and passed down certain trades that were learned and practiced in Italy: barbering, shoemaking and cabinetry. Thus, children who develop skill in the tasks and use of objects associated with these trades do so partly because of their membership in a family group that is part of a culture which values these trades (57).

Lower levels of the environment also constrain higher levels. Therefore, without certain objects, tasks may need to be modified or will go undone. Without the performance of certain tasks, groups may either radically change in nature or fold. And, with large scale changes in organizations, culture will likewise undergo change. Thus, for example, the scarcity of gasoline several summers ago has led to an increase in car-pooling groups; many leisure industries suffered economically from a decrease in tourism as a leisure activity; and small, fuel-saving cars became highly valued by many Americans.

IMPLICATIONS OF PERSON/ ENVIRONMENT INTERACTION

Understanding occupational performance as the outcome of person/environment interaction has two major implications for occupational

therapists. The first is that all persons seen for therapy are inextricably a part of their native environments, and the second is that occupational therapy is, itself, an environment with which patients and clients interact.

Because persons both shape and are shaped by their environments, occupational function and dysfunction reflect the individual's history of environmental interactions. As a result, no attempt to understand a person's behavior will ever be complete without some understanding (or assessment) of the environments from which the person came and the behavior patterns that were encouraged and discouraged by those environments. Institutionalized children, for example, may not freely explore their surroundings through play because there may be little of novelty or interest to explore. Later in life, this lack of exploration may be reflected in a timidity about engaging in new occupations or in a relatively limited repertory of problem-solving behaviors. Without understanding the institutional context of their development, however, their timidity or poor problem solving may inappropriately be attributed to lethargy, neurological deficits, depression, or some other factor.

Another aspect of understanding the person's history of environmental interactions is recognizing that people who come to therapy as clients or patients bring with them environmentally encouraged values about what groups, objects and tasks are important and meaningful to them. For example, an elderly black man with right hemiplegia had become completely dependent on his wife following his stroke. Despite a previously vigorous life-style, he now experienced no feelings of competence in his life. In exploring his occupational history, the home therapist discovered that he had grown up around textile industries and enjoyed doing things with his hands. Therefore, in addition to a regimen of strengthening, balance and self-care activities, the therapist introduced her client to Turkish weaving. Completing this rug as a gift to his wife became his motivation for staying alive.

The second implication is that the overarching process of occupational therapy is the creation of environments for clients' exploration, competence and achievement. These environments are created by the objects or devices given to clients to help them carry out tasks, through the social groups maintained in the clinic, and through the attitudes and values conveyed by the clinic. For example, an occupational therapy group of clients who meet every morning in a large kitchen with industrial equipment to prepare lunch for the entire day center is an environment in which food preparation is being learned as a vocational trade. The use of efficient but complex objects, the routinization of tasks, the size of the group, and the need to maintain commercially acceptable standards of performance (being on time, and not deviating from certain ways of carrying out tasks) all serve to differentiate this environment from that created by a small group which meets to prepare and eat a special meal as an occasion for leisure and peer interaction.

A number of principles can be derived from the previous discussions of environmental layers to maximize one's use of occupational therapy as an environment. First, to create a setting that is optimally arousing to clients, one may need to create conditions that will either decrease or increase the person's arousal level. Removing distractions, simplifying tasks, lowering criteria for success, and decreasing the number of people in the setting are ways to lower arousal. Providing a variety of activities to choose from, increasing task complexity, increasing interactions with other people, and setting higher criteria for success are all approaches to raising arousal.

Second, the environment can help foster a client's sense of internal control by increasing the number of decisions open to the person, making information available to clients, and in some cases, increasing the predictability or certainty of the program's expectations.

The third principle concerns the interests and values inherent in the clinic. The setting of occupational therapy should create opportunities for clients to pursue former interests, and it should provide continuity with their cultural backgrounds.

The environment should convey expectations for behaviors that are relevant to clients' needs. This can be achieved by using objects in familiar, socially acceptable ways, by setting performance demands that are commensurate with the client's level of ability, by expecting the client to actively participate in developing goals and strategies for change, and by giving clients opportunities to maintain or assume the roles that they will perform upon discharge from the hospital.

Finally, the client should have the opportunity to perform competently in a variety of settings.

Treatment should therefore be visualized on a continuum that extends from the acute phase of hospitalization through community reintegration.

Because the open system of human occupation is maintained through the cycle of interaction with the environment, it is not enough for therapists to know only about the person. The therapist must also understand the process of person/environment interaction and the way in which it influences the open system cycle. The most effective therapy will be that which is informed by a sensitivity to, and understanding of, clients' environments and which skillfully manipulates and arranges environments to facilitate occupational behavior.

References

1. Altman I, Chemers M: *Culture and Environment.* Monterey, Calif, Brooks/Cole, 1980.
2. Anderson N: *Dimensions of Work.* New York, David McKay, 1964.
3. Barker RG, Wright HF: *Midwest and Its Children.* Hamden, Conn, Archon Books, 1971.
4. Bell CH: Competition as a motivational incentive. *Am J Occup Ther* 1975, 29:277–279.
5. Berlyne DE: *Conflict, Arousal, and Curiosity.* New York, McGraw-Hill, 1960.
6. Brake M: *The Sociology of Youth Culture and Youth Subcultures.* London, Routledge & Kegan Paul, 1980.
7. Bronfenbrenner U: *The Ecology of Human Development: Experiments by Nature and Design.* Cambridge, Mass, Harvard University Press, 1979.
8. Bruner JS: On coping and defending. In Coleman J (ed): *The Psychology of Effective Behavior.* Glenview, Ill, Scott, Foresman & Company, 1969.
9. Burke JP: A clinical perspective on motivation: pawn versus origin. *Am J Occup Ther* 1977, 31:254–258.
10. Chapin SF: Activity systems and urban structure: a working schema. *J Am Inst Plann* 1968, 34:11–18.
11. Csikszentmihalyi M, Rochberg-Halton E: *The Meaning of Things.* Cambridge, Cambridge University Press, 1981.
12. Dubin R: Industrial workers' worlds: a study of the "central life interests" of industrial workers. In Smigel EO (ed): *Work and Leisure.* New Haven, Conn, College and University Press, 1963.
13. Dullea G: The busy bedroom. *New York Times,* July 10, 1980, pp C-1, C-8.
14. El-Meligi AM, Surkis J: The scientific study of "inner" experience: a general systems approach. *J Orthomol Psychol* 1977, 6:219–230.
15. Emery FE, Trist EL: The causal texture of organizational environments. *Hum Relat* 1965, 18:21–31.
16. Etzioni A: *Modern Organizations.* Englewood Cliffs, N.J., Prentice-Hall, 1964.
17. Fietelson D: Cross-cultural studies of representational play. In Tizard B, Harvey D (eds): *Biology*

of Play. London, William Heinemann Medical Books, 1977.

18. Franken RE: *Human Motivation.* Monterey, Calif, Brooks/Cole, 1982.

19. Freidson E: *Profession of Medicine: A Study of the Sociology of Applied Knowledge.* New York, Harper Row, 1970.

20. Furby L: Possessions: toward a theory of their meaning and function throughout the life cycle. In Baltes PB (ed): *Life-Span Development and Behavior,* NY, Academic Press, 1978, vol 1.

21. Gerstl JR: Leisure, taste and occupational milieu. In Smigel EO (ed): *Work and Leisure.* New Haven, Conn, College and University Press, 1963.

22. Giovanninni J: I love New York and L. A., too. *New York Times Sunday Magazine,* September 11, 1983, pp 144–148.

23. Goodman W: The luck of the draw. *New York Times Sunday Magazine,* August 7, 1983, p 54.

24. Hall E: *The Hidden Dimension.* Garden City, NY, Anchor Books, 1966.

25. Hall E: *The Silent Language.* Garden City, NY, Anchor Books, 1973.

26. Haywood DG, Rothenberg M, Beasley RR: Children's play and urban playground environments. *Environ Behav* 1974, 6:131–168.

27. Johnson MW: The effect on behavior of variations in the amount of play equipment. *Child Dev* 1935, 6:56–68.

28. Katz D, Kahn RL: *The Social Psychology of Organizations.* New York, Wiley, 1966.

29. Kielhofner G, Burke JP: A model of human occupation, Part 1. Conceptual framework and content. *Am J Occup Ther* 1980, 34:572–581.

30. Korda M: Status marks: a gold-plated thermos is a man's best friend. In Katz AM, Katz VT (eds): *Foundations of Nonverbal Communication.* Carbondale & Edwardsville, Ill, Southern Illinois University Press, 1983.

31. Lancy DF: Play in species adaption. *Annu Rev Anthropol* 1980, 9:471–495.

32. Lawton MP: *Environment and Aging.* Monterey, Calif, Brooks/Cole, 1980.

33. Leff HL: *Experience, Environment and Human Potentials.* New York, Oxford University Press, 1978.

34. Little BR: Personal projects. *Environ Behav* 1983, 15:273–309.

35. Magill J, Vargo JW: Helplessness, hope and the occupational therapist. *Am J Occup Ther* 1977, 44:65–69.

36. Matsutsuyu JS: The interest check list. *Am J Occup Ther* 1969, 23:323–328.

37. Mehrabian A: Public places and private spaces. *The Psychology of Work, Play, and Living Environments.* New York, Basic Books, 1976.

38. Moore RG, Young D: Childhood outdoors: toward a social ecology of the landscape. In Altman I, Wohlwill JF (eds): *Human Behavior and Environment,* vol 3, *Children and the Environment.* New York, Plenum Press, 1978.

39. Moos RH: *Evaluating Treatment Environments: A Social Ecological Approach.* New York, Wiley, 1974.

40. Newcomb TM: *Personality and Social Change.* New York, Dryden Press, 1943.

41. Ogbu JU: Origins of human competence: a cultural-ecological perspective. *Child Develop* 1981, 52:413–429.

42. Orzack LH: Work as a "central life interest" of the professional. In Smigel EO (ed): *Work and Leisure.* New Haven, Conn, College and University Press, 1963.

43. Parent LH: Effects of a low-stimulus environment on behavior. *Am J Occup Ther* 1978, 32:19–25.

44. Pervin LA: Performance and satisfaction as a function of individual-environment fit. *Psychol Bull* 1968, 69:56–68.

45. Pezzuti L: An exploration of adolescent feminine and occupational behavior development. *Am J Occup Ther* 1979, 33:84–91.

46. Quilitch HR, Risley TR: The effects of play materials on social play. *J Appl Behav Anal* 1973, 6:573–578.

47. Rapoport A: Cross-cultural aspects of environmental design. In Altman I, Rapoport A, Wohlwill JF (eds): *Human Behavior and Environment.* New York, Plenum Press, 1980, vol 4.

48. de-Renne-Stephan C: Imitation: a mechanism of play behavior. *Am J Occup Ther* 1980, 34:95–102.

49. Robinson AL: Play: the arena for acquisition of rules for competent behavior. *Am J Occup Ther* 1977, 31:248–253.

50. Schak DC: Determinants of children's play patterns in a Chinese city. *Urban Anthropol* 1972, 1:195–204.

51. Schein EH: The individual, the organization, and the career: a conceptual scheme. *J Appl Behav Sci* 1971, 7:401–426.

52. Schultz R, Hanusa BH: Environmental influences on the effectiveness of control- and competence-enhancing interventions. In Perlmutter LC, Monte RA (eds): *Choice and Perceived Control.* Hillsdale, NJ, Lawrence Erlbaum Associates, 1979.

53. Seligman M: *Helplessness.* San Francisco, Freeman & Company, 1975.

54. Tichy N: A social network perspective for organization development. In Cummings TG (ed): *Systems Theory for Organization Development.* New York, Wiley, 1980.

55. Toffler A: *The Third Wave.* New York, William Morrow, 1980.

56. Torbert WR: Pre-bureaucratic and post-bureaucratic stages of organization development. *Interperson Develop* 1974/5, 5:1–25.

57. Valente J: A piece of home. *The Washington Post,* January 3, 1984, pp A-1; A-6.

58. Versluys HP: The remediation of role disorders through focused groupwork. *Am J Occup Ther* 1980, 34:609–614.

59. Walker EL: *Psychological Complexity and Preference: A Hedgehog Theory of Behavior.* Monterey, Calif, Brooks/Cole, 1980.

60. Wicker AW: *An Introduction to Ecological Psychology.* Monterey, Calif, Brooks/Cole, 1979.

61. Wohlwill JF, Kohn I: Dimensionalizing the environment. In Wapner S, Cohen SB, Kaplan B (eds): *Experiencing the Environment.* New York, Plenum Press, 1976.

62. Yi-Fu Tuan: Children and the natural environment. In Altman I, Wohlwill JF (eds): *Human Behavior and Environment,* vol 3, *Children and the Environment.* New York, Plenum Press, 1978.

CHAPTER 5

Occupational Function and Dysfunction

Gary Kielhofner

As a profession seeking to influence the occupational well-being of human beings, occupational therapy must have an approach to conceptualizing function and dysfunction (11). The previous chapters discussed the open system characteristics and occupational nature of human beings providing a foundation for such a conceptualization. These concepts will now be directed to delineating a view of occupational function and dysfunction.

Classical concepts of health viewed it as merely the absence of disease and disability (4). A person was considered healthy when no acute or chronic pathological condition was present. More recent conceptualizations of health recognize the importance of being able to actualize values and do what one wants to do (4), to engage in activity commensurate with one's abilities and limitations (6), to participate in work and play and other aspects of life (9), and to meet the challenges of the environment (4).

This emerging view of health stresses the importance of function over structure. It reflects a movement from a closed system to an open system conceptualization of health. In a closed system perspective, the human being is viewed as a machine and well-working is assumed as long as all parts are in order; when a part is defective or disrupted, it is assumed that the machine cannot function. Open system concepts not only stress the importance of function as a criterion of health but also allow consideration of how a system can continue to function in spite of damage to its parts. This is particularly important for occupational therapy since practitioners mainly work to enhance the lives of persons with permanent disability.

The concept of adaptation has been proposed as a way of viewing individual well-being (4). It is broader than the traditional concept of health and incorporates an open system's view of humans. The concept of adaptation acknowledges that human life involves the person's struggle to adapt to, and to control, environmental conditions (4). A person is considered adaptative who is able to meet the challenges, expectations and opportunities of the environment and who behaves so as to maintain and enhance personal integrity and potentials.

Just as open system concepts may apply to all aspects of human function, adaptation is a broad concept which may encompass many aspects of human life. Therefore, while adaptation is a useful interdisciplinary concept for understanding health, a more specific conceptualization is needed to delineate occupational therapy's view of function and dysfunction.

OCCUPATIONAL FUNCTION AND DYSFUNCTION

In an earlier chapter, we noted that occupational therapy's concern is with the occupational nature and behavior of human beings. It follows that the field is concerned with the adaptation of persons *in terms of their occupational function and dysfunction.* Occupational functioning is a subcategory or specific sphere of the larger domain of human adaptation.

It has been proposed that the occupational nature of the human being can be represented as an open system energized by an urge to explore and master and composed of three subsystems and their components. It was further specified that occupational behavior consists of efforts to maintain self, to contribute productivity to society and to participate in the playful events of the culture. Recalling the criteria of adaptation, we can identify more specific criteria for occupational function and dysfunction. That is, persons are occupationally functional when they: (*a*) act so as to satisfy society's expectations and need for productive and playful participation, and (*b*) act so as to allow expression of exploration and mastery, and maintenance and enhancement of personal causation, values, interests, roles, habits, and skills and their constiuents. Conversely, a person is occupationally dysfunctional when: (*a*) societal demands and expectations for productive and playful participation are not met and/or (*b*) behavior does not fulfill the urge to explore and master or threatens the disruption of the system's components. These criteria of occupational function and dysfunction do not refer to static states in the system but rather to *processes*—that is, to the person's occupational behavior and how it affects the human system.

An Occupational Function/Dysfunction Continuum

In addition to specifying criteria of occupational function and dysfunction, it is also necessary to recognize that persons exhibit degrees of adaptive or maladaptive occupational functioning. To this end an occupational function/dysfunction continuum is proposed (Fig. 5.1). It comprises six levels of adaptation/maladaptation in occupational behavior. Achievement, competence and exploration represent levels of occupational function; inefficacy, incompetence and helplessness are levels of occupational dysfunction.

Although the following discussions will discuss these as discrete levels of function and dysfunction, they should be recognized as points on a continuum. Further, it should be noted that any individual's behavior may include features from more than one level.

Levels of Occupational Function

The continuum of occupational behavior is represented in three levels of arousal and accomplishment: exploration, competence and achievement (10). This continuum of occupational functioning includes behaviors ranging from free experimentation with the environment in order to learn what one can do, to performance according to personal standards and environmental demands. Figure 5.2 illustrates the three levels of occupational function.

ACHIEVEMENT

Achievement is a striving to maintain and enhance one's performance in occupational roles where standards of performance and excellence are identifiable (8). It represents the fullest mastery over self and the environment. Persons achieve when they have developed sufficient skills and habits to allow control over their own performance and over factors in the environment.

Values are extremely important for achievement level performance. Persons commit themselves to persistently put forth efforts toward maintaining their behavior to standards of performance. A person's level of achievement depends on what standards he or she internalizes. Achievement requires a future orientation, an ability to envision goals and to direct oneself toward accomplishing ends or toward maintaining a level of performance over time. Achievement goals may be focused and ambitious, such as seeking to make a promotion at work or to win an award. Or, achievement goals may be global, such as a goal to maintain balance in one's life by seeking to be a consistently good parent, worker, homemaker, and volunteer. Achievement behavior ordinarily involves taking on occupational roles. Achievement may be public as in the worker role or more private as in some amateur or leisure role.

Achieving persons have a belief in internal control and in personal skills, which they seek to monitor and improve. Their expectancy of success is predicated on self-development, a degree of calculated risk-taking and constant application of effort. Achievement allows one to turn one's interest into creative, productive, and sometimes competitive behavior. Interest is generally intensified as persons have opportunity to do what they do well and to be recognized for it by others. The major reward of achievement is the pleasure achieved in the activity itself. High levels of achievement are associated with intense involvement and a sense of complete control and oneness with the activity (2, 3).

Disabled persons achieve not only by strug-

Levels of occupational function	Levels of occupational dysfunction
Achievement------ Competence------ Exploration---	---Inefficacy------ Incompetence------ Helplessness

Figure 5.1.   An occupational function/dysfunction continuum.

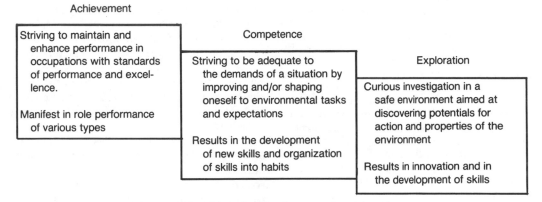

Figure 5.2.   Three levels of occupational function.

gling with the demands and expectations of achievement level performance, but also by overcoming the limitations or difficulties they experience as a result of their disability. This is aptly illustrated in the following example.

Alice: Career Professional. Alice is a 32-year-old assistant professor in a large urban university. She was born with spina bifida and related problems of a neurogenic bladder, sensory loss in one lower extremity, and generalized motor weakness of both lower extremities. Throughout her life, she has been hospitalized numerous times for surgeries which included amputation of a portion of her foot and an ileostomy. Currently, she ambulates independently but must limit her physical activity to safeguard her lower extremity against further injury, taking special care to monitor the noninnervated areas.

As a child and adolescent, Alice was playful and outgoing. Her family encouraged her to explore her potentials and achieve despite her physical limitations and frequent illness and hospitalizations. Often rejected by peers in school in games and sports, she responded by developing skills for managing others' reactions to her disability.

Despite her operations and after having to attend high school and college recuperating on crutches, Alice continued to achieve as a student. She completed a degree in biology and later obtained a graduate degree in a medical profession. She worked with psychiatrically disabled patients and later became director of a psychiatric program while simultaneously maintaining a private practice and working toward a doctoral degree.

Today, Alice is a teacher, researcher and clinician. She has a number of hobbies including painting and sewing. The hobby of sewing was originally important to Alice as she made and modified clothes which enhanced her physical appearance. She has a wide variety of friends with whom she regularly recreates. Her interests also include frequent excursions to a nearby large city on weekends for shopping, visiting friends and eating out.

While Alice acknowledges that she has clearly attained achievement in her professional career, she notes that it is especially challenging to do so as a handicapped person. Interestingly, Alice manages to achieve at work not so much despite, but in terms of, her disability. Many of her skills such as learning to get along well with others, managing their impressions of her and making them feel comfortable, reflect her desire to both explore and master her condition and to live in terms of who she is. Even her chosen career reflects having turned her disability into an asset.

She has developed efficient habits which allow her to maintain control over her physical problems, to perform at a high level in her career and to build a leisure and homemaker role into her life-style as a single professional woman. She managed to maintain her productive roles despite having from time-to-time to return to the patient role. Alice describes the importance of mastering the patient role so that she can demand and secure proper medical care, allowing herself to experience periods of depression during an acute problem and yet rebound to her waiting occupational roles. As evidence of this, Alice recently was hospitalized the week before she left her home of 11 years to assume a new teaching position. She was out of the hospital one day, moving the next, and assuming her professional role within a week. Alice has maintained a belief in internal control by taking situations which threatened personal causation and developing skills to achieve control over them. Her success in academic roles allowed her to develop a strong belief in her abilities and their efficacy in achieving her goals of becoming a professional. Alice's values are very much influenced by her experience as a disabled person. Her strong feelings of the importance of allowing individuals to develop their potentials, her view of the importance of caring, intellectual achievement and interpersonal openness are all reflective of the life experiences of a person who has developed an adaptive occupational life-style while having a permanent disability. Table 5.1 illustrates a conceptualization of Alice's occupational functioning via the components of the model.

COMPETENCE

To be competent is a universal motive energized by the desire to be recognized as adequate by one's peers. Competence requires and builds upon prior exploratory experiences. Being competent means being adequate to the demands of a circumstance or task (13). The aim of competency is to be able to deal effectively with the environment and to improve and shape oneself and one's ability to perform according to feedback on performance (10). Persons performing at a competency level focus on attaining, improving and organizing skills into habits that allow consistent, adequate performance (10, 12). Thus, persons internalize information about the environment shaping their behavior into patterns that reflect social norms and requirements of task performance.

Competency affords the individual a sense of gaining greater personal control. The efficacy of skills is improved as they are organized into routines of competent behavior. As one acquires these routines and develops their relevance to the environment, the expectancy of success is enhanced.

The value of competency lies in the person's sense that he or she is approximating the standards of performance inherent in tasks and in society. Competency signifies a process of becoming, growing and arriving at a greater sense of personal mastery. Competency requires an orientation to the future manifest in delay of gratification and commitment to goals. Objects and processes which are interesting to an individual are made even more pleasurable as one achieves a degree of mastery over them. Competency is a natural developmental level of occupational functioning beginning in childhood and continuing throughout life as people prepare for new roles. Competency level occupational functioning is also reflected in the efforts of persons to adapt to disability. The following case illustrates this.

Harold: Adjustment to Hand Injury. Harold is 42 years old, married and has one child. Several months ago he began work as a correction officer for a federal prison. He was

Table 5.1.
Alice: a career professional

Personal causation	Has a strong belief in internal control and expectancy of success from having developed skills to overcome liabilities and from positive experiences in academics
Interests	Has well-differentiated interests compatible with limitations
Values	Is committed to excelling; has high standards of performance and strong future orientation. Values the importance of persons achieving their potentials
Roles	Achieves in the work and homemaker roles and has regular pursuit of a satisfying leisure role
Habits	Habits are well organized to accommodate expectations of roles, physical limitations and time for leisure
Skills	Despite limitations to the kinesiological and neurological constituents, skills are highly developed. Process and communication/interaction skills are developed specifically to overcome problems related to the disability
Open system cycle	Output includes a high level of achievement and a full active schedule of occupational behavior which is balanced and satisfying. Is positively assessed by friends, colleagues and professors. Pays careful attention to the environment so as to meet challenges and overcome obstacles

engaged in on-the-job training, preparing to take a series of physical and mental exams which would certify him for the job. At the same time he rented and farmed several acres of land. During the spring wheat harvest he accidentally caught his right, dominant hand in a combine mechanism, resulting in a crush amputation of his thumb, ring, index, and middle fingers at the metacarpophalangeal level. Following surgery and a continuing course of therapy in a hand clinic he has been able to develop a marginally functional grasp using his thenar eminence and the remaining fifth digit which is restricted in active flexion and extension.

From the beginning of his rehabilitation, Harold identified that he wished to continue his training and pursue his goal of permanent employment as a correction officer and would make necessary adaptations in his performance. Of major concern is his ability to physically respond to prisoners in an emergency. He has secured a placement as the officer in charge of a main gate so that direct contact with prisoners is minimized. However, he has to do additional paperwork related to prisoners' coming and going and to unusual events in the prison compound. While Harold has a prosthesis which allows him to write with the dominant hand, he feels that wearing it inside the prison is a liability as it might put him at a disadvantage against a potential assailant. Thus, he has chosen instead to change dominant hands, learning to write with his left hand. Because prison reports must be error-free and completed quickly he has developed a new habit of composing the report in his head until he feels it is appropriate and then taking the time to write it down. This reduces loss of time from having to redo reports.

Harold has had to make similar adaptations to a number of routines necessary for his job and for preparation to take certification exams. Taking notes from books to prepare for exams now takes much longer, so that he must devote more time to studying. Partly because of this, he has decided not to attempt to farm during this period. He has secured permission to taken written exams under altered conditions so as not to be penalized by his slow writing.

To pass the certification exam he must also be able to deliver a number of accurate shots to a target within a given time period with both a shotgun and a .38 caliber revolver. The test involves firing two rounds of ammunition which means that he must reload the guns once during the timed test. Thus, he is faced not only with changing handedness in discharging the firearms, but with acquiring a routine for unloading and loading them. He has managed to develop a process for loading the shotgun without trouble, but getting small bullets in and out of the revolver is more problematic. The test requires delivering a number of accurate shots out of 12 possible shots (two rounds). Thus, he developed a routine of firing six shots which the chamber holds, then loading and firing only an additional four bullets to save time. Ten well placed shots within the same time period yields a passing score.

He is making similar adaptations in his hobby of cutting firewood with a chain saw. He sold his larger chain saw to purchase a smaller one which could be handled more safely. He relies on good planning to avoid unsafe situations in which he might lose control of the saw.

Overall, Harold expresses confidence in his ability to adapt to his injury. He has been able to maintain a sense of control by alternating many of his habits. Harold expects to successfully complete the certification process and to secure a permanent job as a correction officer. He has been able to maintain the efficacy of his former skills by organizing them into new routines.

He has had to learn new skills, especially ways of using the injured limb functionally. He speaks of having to think more before he uses it demonstrating his substitution of process skills for lost motor capacity. Finally, he describes having developed new skills for dealing with persons' reactions to his stigmatized upper extremity. Children react most strongly to it, some expressing fear. He relates with some pride how he is able to assuage children's fears, inviting them to touch it and doing such things as offering them soda and candy with the affected hand.

Harold is assuring his potential to continue his occupational behavior by engaging in a competency process of developing new habits and skills. Feedback from colleagues and superiors is positive and he recognizes his own success in being able to adapt to the hand injury. Table 5.2 illustrates features of Harold's occupational functioning.

EXPLORATION

The earliest and least arousing level of occupational behavior is exploration. Childhood play begins with this curious manipulation and observation of the environment (5, 10). Exploration is a behavior that requires a safe and nurturing environment (10). Persons' belief in the benign nature of the environment is just as

Table 5.2.
Harold: adjustment to hand injury

Personal causation	Maintains sense of internal control by modifying routines to perform old tasks and by substituting process for motor skills. Realistically expects success in the future
Values	Has maintained a committment to work goal; is able to internalize and meet high standards of performance
Interests	Has modified both work habits and personal habits to allow pursuit of interests in work and pastimes
Roles	Relinquished farming role to concentrate on current work-trainee role
Habits	Major readjustment of routines to accommodate lost motor skills to role demands
Skills	Development of new process skills and communication/interaction skills required by the disability
Open system cycle	Is learning a new line of work. Pays careful attention to the demands of the environment so as to make use of resources and adjust behavior to requirements of environment. Is aware of his own success and receives positive feedback from peers and supervisors

important as their belief in personal ability. Exploration is largely made fail-safe because it has no objective or performance standard beyond satisfying one's curiosity (1).

Exploration provides opportunity for learning, for discovering new modes of being, and for new ways of expressing ability (7). Exploratory behavior does not typically demand a high level of skill but it nurtures the development of skills. An individual may also seek new avenues to employ existing skills in exploratory behavior. Sometimes exploratory behavior of this sort emerges after a traumatic episode in which some aspect of skills are lost and the individual seeks to find ways of employing remaining skills in new areas. Exploration is often an important aspect of adult behavior when the individual is pursuing new avenues of occupational behavior, making role changes, reexamining ways of accomplishing old tasks, or discovering new sources of meaning.

Exploration generates a sense of curiosity and excitement and renews hope and trust in the environment and in the possibilities of finding interest and meaning in action (7, 10). It thus serves a "re-creactive" function for human beings and often exists in the domain of play, recreation and leisure. The following example illustrates the importance of exploratory behavior in the life of a person with a disability (2).

Arthur: Learning to Explore. Arthur is a 13-year-old who was hospitalized with a diagnosis of adolescent adjustment reaction.

He was unable to perform in school and exhibited behavioral problems at home. He was a highly anxious young man, deeply concerned with failure. He avoided novel situations and tasks in which he might fail, and he tended to become disorganized during unstructured periods of time.

Arthur lacked gross and fine motor skills; he was inept at interacting with peers; and he was a poor planner and problem solver. He had never successfully entered into exploratory behavior and could not now function at a competency level. Arthur's entry into a state of occupational function at the exploratory level was abetted by therapeutic intervention.

Having been slowly introduced to new activities without demands for performance and without threat of failure, Arthur has become able to enjoy exploration. Although he is chronologically beyond the stage of sensorimotor exploration, he takes a great delight in exploring textures, properties, smells, and colors of various objects he encounters. These are opportunities he did not fully exploit in the past. After thoroughly investigating characteristics of new materials, he has some interest in finding out what he can do with them or make out of them. Arthur is also exploring new social behaviors; he is beginning to interact with peers, to share materials, to initiate conversation, give and receive compliments, and join in simple games and sports.

Arthur is beginning to develop some confidence in his ability to negotiate the physical and social world. Just as importantly, he is developing trust that the world can be a relatively safe place. He is discovering interesting aspects of objects, tasks and persons in the environment. He is now able to value and find meaning in exploration because it offers opportunities for enjoyment and control and because others in the environment (therapists, staff, family) value his exploratory behavior.

The skills he gains through exploration will enable him to more successfully fulfill his roles as player, student and family member. He has begun to establish a routine of exploration during scheduled therapies and to structure some of his own free time. He is enhancing his capacities, achieving satisfaction and pleasure in his behavior, and moving toward fulfilling the expectations of others. His current exploratory behavior will help yield the necessary skills for competency behavior. Table 5.3 illustrates Arthur's exploratory level occupational functioning.

Profiles of Adaptive Occupational Behavior

Development from childhood to adulthood is a pathway from exploration to achievement. The continuum from exploration to achievement is also the pathway for organizing any new behavior or for making changes in one's occupational life-style. Persons return to exploratory and competency levels of performance when they move into new roles, encounter new settings or make drastic life-style changes. Thus, achievement is not the exclusive level of occupational behavior in adult life. For instance, achieving persons in mid-life may reenter an exploratory phase in order to seek a new life-style or find renewed meaning in work.

An individual's life-style may be dominated by one level of occupational behavior but incorporate others. Thus, an adult who achieves by maintaining several roles, may at the same time be exploring some new behaviors and organizing new habits for a role about to be entered. Indeed, maintaining an adaptive occupational life-style generally requires incorporation and balance of different levels of occupational function.

Levels of Occupational Dysfunction

Occupational function represents states of optimal arousal and involvement in the environment. The dysfunctional end of the continuum represents opposite tendencies. Thus, occupational dysfunction represents stress and a lack of involvement in the environment. The three levels of maladaptation in occupation are inefficacy, incompetence and helplessness (Fig. 5.3).

INEFFICACY

An individual's occupational dysfunction is at the level of inefficacy when there is an interference with performing meaningful activity accompanied by dissatisfaction with performance. Sources of inefficacy may be environmental constraints, disease processes, or imbalanced life-styles. The elderly person placed in a nursing home without access to lifelong occupational behaviors of cooking and homemaking may enter such a maladaptive cycle of occupational behavior. The person in early stages of chronic disease may be having difficulty maintaining or returning to previous occupational patterns and, consequently, be concerned over ability and like-

Table 5.3.
Arthur: learning to explore

Personal causation	Is developing trust in the safeness of the environment and in his potential to interact positively with the environment
Values	Is beginning to value and find meaning in exploring the environment
Interests	Has largely sensorimotor interests in objects and is beginning interest in peers and games
Roles	Is taking on the player role in solitary and peer-game play and gaining experience to prepare him for other roles
Habits	Ability to structure free time and routine of regular exploration is emerging
Skills	Perceptual motor and communication interaction skills are developed as he explores objects and persons
Open system cycle	Output consists of exploration. He attends to and takes in information about objects and people in the environment. He is eliciting positive responses of peers and adults

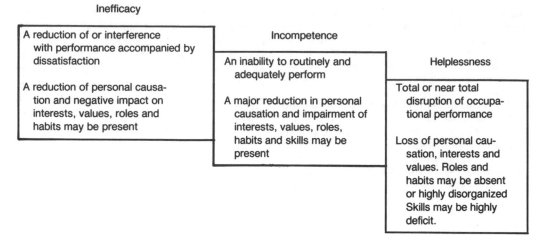

Figure 5.3. Three levels of occupational dysfunction.

lihood of success. A person who has rigidly pursued achievement may experience extreme burnout, no longer able to feel satisfied and competent.

Persons at the inefficacy level experience a reduction of personal causation and may question the likelihood of achieving future goals or finding meaning in their lives. They may be prevented from or find themselves unable to maintain the same level of investment and interest in valued occupations.

These persons may experience moderate anxiety or depression over the risk of further failure and/or dissatisfaction. Roles may be temporarily disrupted or role performance may decrease. An imbalance or disorganization of habits may reduce performance and life satisfaction.

Bob: Residuals of Cancer and Its Treatment. Bob is 22 years old and was diagnosed as having sarcoma of the jaw 3 years ago. He studied automobile mechanics during the latter part of high school in a vocational training program. Bob chose mechanics as an occupation because he enjoyed working with his hands and found the problem solving in mechanics challenging and attractive. He worked briefly as a mechanic before being diagnosed with cancer. At the time he still lived at home but was engaged to be married and planned to support a family.

Bob's treatment over a 2½-year period included surgical removal of part of his mandible and surrounding tissue, chemotherapy, and radiation therapy. The disease process and subsequent extensive treatment necessitated Bob's leaving his work. In addition, his fiance broke off their engagement. He has received no medical treatment for 6 months and the cancer may have been brought under control.

Bob expresses a strong desire to return to work and to get an apartment, but he also experiences a great deal of anxiety and lacks confidence about doing so. For the past several months, his daily routine has consisted of self-care, long meals during which he watches television, routine chores around his parent's home where he still lives, and occasional excursions to a store or to a movie. He has few active friends because, as he describes it, their lives went on while his essentially stopped for 3 years. Old buddies are married, have families and jobs, and live in their own homes.

Bob still possesses the skills to do mechanics and he has occasionally worked on a friend's car in the past few months. He is concerned over whether or not he will be able to manage the routine he had in the past. In his own words he has "gotten a lot of bad habits" and he refers to having gotten accustomed to "doing nothing all the time." He is dissatisfied with his current performance, but remains hesitant and apprehensive about returning to work, living on his own and beginning to engage more regularly in normal leisure pursuits. Since neither his upper nor lower extremities were affected by the cancer, he still has the musculoskeletal constituents necessary for work; he previously had good process and communication skills and continues to exhibit them. His major problem is that both his roles and habits have eroded. He is overwhelmed by the demands and expectations of the roles of worker and homemaker to which he wishes to return.

Although Bob still values the roles of automobile mechanic and living independently; his view of the future has been sharply affected by the uncertainty of survival. He is just beginning to reorient himself to the possibility of having a future and to being able to resume meaningful activities. His personal causation has been eroded; while he still believes he has the appropriate skills for homemaking and work, he is uncertain about the potential for success and lacks conviction about his ability to control his life. He continues to have the same interests as in the past, but the disease and treatment have disrupted their routine enactment.

Bob's cycle of behavior threatens to lead to further occupational dysfunction. His everyday behavior is marginally competent; that is, he takes care of himself and contributes to chores in the home. However, he is not performing at a level he desires or that is developmentally appropriate. The longer he continues in his present behavioral pattern, the more distant seems the possibility of returning to worker and homemaker roles. His skills as a mechanic may begin to erode if the period of nonworking is continued. Table 5.4 illustrates Bob's occupational dysfunction.

INCOMPETENCE

A major loss or limitation of skills, a failure or disruption of self-confidence and satisfaction, and inability to routinely and adequately perform the tasks of everyday living associated with occupational roles is characteristic of a state of incompetence. It may result from marginal learning due to poor environments, from disease or from a life-style which erodes system organization. Persons may experience a major reduction in personal causation including a sense of loss of control over their situations and fear of failure. Substantial feelings of anxiety or depression can arise over the inability to adequately fulfill life roles and the negative feedback which results. Persons find themselves distanced from values and interests. Life looses its attractiveness, meaning and potential for satisfaction.

Individuals may be unable to adequately maintain role performance. Along with a disruption of skills, there may be a distortion of habits so that behavior is disorganized, rigid, or imbalanced. The following case illustrates occupational dysfunction at the level of incompetence.

Larry: Unable to Enact Occupational Roles. Larry is 30 years old; he has mild cerebral palsy and is mildly mentally retarded. The cerebral palsy affects his performance and gait and also his speech production. He lived for several years in a state hospital and was discharged to a residential facility about 7 years ago. At that time, he was placed in a sheltered workshop but found the work boring and below his capacity. So he quit. Since

Table 5.4.
Bob: residuals of cancer and its treatment

Personal causation	Believes in skills and, in the past, felt internally controlled. Presently unsure about his ability to control his life, organize his day and succeed in the future
Values	Continues to value his chosen occupation. Feels he should be performing to standards and organizing time appropriate for someone his age, but cannot operationalize these values
Interests	Retains old work and leisure interests, but is unable to enact these interests at his premorbid level
Roles	Lost worker and leisure roles during treatment. Behavior is reorganized to suit a chronic patient role. Experiences difficulty regaining past roles and concern over meeting role expectations. Currently experiences a paucity of occupational roles
Habits	Routine of daily behavior has become much less productive. Has acquired "bad habits" of inactivity and inefficiency
Skills	Still has past skills, but they are threatened now from disuse
Open system cycle	Level of activity is greatly reduced with much time spent in passive activity. Use of the resources in the environment is greatly decreased. Feedback includes self-devaluation and dissatisfaction with performance

leaving the sheltered workshop, Larry has had no productive role save his marginal homemaker activities. Larry lives in a room with three other men; in that setting he attempts to do self-care and minimal maintenance of his living space. Infrequently, when he has money, Larry may go to a movie, ride the bus or eat out. He also takes walks in the neighborhood using the occasion to window-shop. However, much of his day is spent, as he describes it, "passing the time." Most of the time he sits unoccupied or sleeps or watches television. Along with this inactivity, he complains of chronic fatigue. He is bored, listless and overtly depressed. He expresses a strong desire to return to the worker role for more activity. He also feels a strong concern that he is going nowhere in his life and reports feeling like he is "going crazy." His prospects for finding work are poor as he is both unskilled and mentally and physically impaired. Further, he has no idea of how he might enter a worker role and considers it an unattainable goal. His lack of activity is stressful both because it leaves him with long periods of unsatisfying passive behavior and because it signifies stagnation in his life. Indeed, he refers to his past in the state hospital as more desirable than his present life. He sees the community as an uninviting place with fewer opportunities than the state hospital.

Larry feels totally externally controlled. He complains that he lacks privacy and that his belongings are stolen by his roommates. He lacks money to finance activities he might enjoy and there are no resources in the residential facility for carrying out activities. He also hesitates to frequent the community because of his stigmatized speech and gait; he is acutely aware of the whispers, glances and uncomfortable giggles that inevitably occur when he ventures into a new setting.

He has been unable to establish a satisfying and meaningful routine of behavior and has no major occupational role to organize his time and provide him a positive sense of identity. He expresses few interests and is unable to pursue any interest on a regular basis.

Feeling externally controlled and alienated from the community, he tends to withdraw into passiveness and inactivity which further erodes his skills, routine and confidence. His feelings of anxiety and depression are likely to increase if his present cycle continues. Table 5.5 illustrates Larry's occupational dysfunction.

HELPLESSNESS

A person who experiences total or nearly total disruption of occupational performance coupled with extreme feelings of ineffectiveness, anxiety and/or depression is in an extreme state of occupational dysfunction, helplessness. A state of helplessness may result from some traumatic episode which suddenly renders a healthy person totally dependent or from a lifelong series of negative experiences.

Because of the overwhelming threat to self that characterizes a major traumatic episode or an accumulation of lifelong negative experiences, persons in a state of helplessness are totally alienated from values, or totally unable to relate past values to their present condition. They see the future as foreboding and the present as onerous. Such persons may have no belief in skill, feel totally controlled by external forces and are overwhelmed with fear of failure. Such persons cannot direct or control their own behavior, may be unable to express or enact interests and may be unable to fulfill any life roles. Skills and habits may be totally disrupted so

Table 5.5.
Larry: unable to enact occupational roles

Personal causation	Feels externally controlled, lacks belief in interpersonal skills; fears that skills will erode from inactivity; and expresses concern over stigma in public
Values	Sees work as important and meaningful but unattainable
Interests	Has few interests and is unable to routinely pursue interests
Roles	Has a minimal homemaker role and is unable to fill other occupational roles
Habits	Everyday behavior is characterized by inactivity and few identifiable routines
Skills	Cerebral palsy negatively affects motor performance; intellectual limitations and poor past experiences constrain other skills
Open system cycle	Activity level is minimal and lower than in the past. He does not seek out resources and opportunities in the environment

that performance is minimal or absent. The dysfunction may be so marked that persons are unable to care for themselves. The following case is illustrative of someone at the dysfunctional level of helplessness.

Elizabeth: Chronic Psychiatric Problems. Elizabeth is 70 years old and was recently admitted to a psychiatric hospital. She had become severely depressed and unable to care for herself in the nursing home where she lived. Elizabeth has a diagnosis of major depression and has a long history of psychiatric hospitalization and placement in community residential facilities.

In the hospital Elizabeth has progressed to the point of being able to do basic self-care and to eat with minimal supervision. When not occupied with these activities she sits in her room doing nothing. She does not spontaneously interact with either staff or other patients.

Elizabeth expresses a feeling of being unable to direct her own behavior. She values the possibility of having more independence, but does not expect to be able to care for herself in the future. She has no specified goals and cannot identify any activity which is meaningful for herself. She did indicate an interest in walking, which she did at the nursing home, and in being around younger people. Mostly, she liked to watch younger people engaged in recreation; she did not interact with them. Presently, neither of these activities is part of her routine schedule. There are ample grounds for her to walk about on, but there are no younger people accessible in the

hospital. She has no relatives with whom she has been in contact for the past several years.

Elizabeth does not see herself in any occupational role. On the other hand she has been in the passive patient and chronically impaired role for many years. She has internalized the expectation that others will regulate her life and look after her, because she is unable to do so herself.

Elizabeth has difficulty planning and problem solving in activities. She is sometimes confused and cannot concentrate. She tends to be socially isolated and cannot effectively communicate spontaneously. She has minimal skills for basic self-care, but has no leisure skills. Her present lack of walking appears related to a fear of becoming disoriented on the hospital grounds. Overall, Elizabeth exhibits a withdrawn, helpless demeanor which is very dissatisfying to her and which apparently is affected by, and abets, her depression. Without external support her occupational behavior would likely degenerate even further as it had in the nursing home where she became incapable of self-care. Table 5.6 illustrates Elizabeth's occupational dysfunction.

OCCUPATIONAL DYSFUNCTION AS AN OPEN SYSTEM PROCESS

Because human beings are open systems they must engage in a cycle of output, feedback, intake, and throughput to maintain and enhance themselves and to meet environmental requirements. Occupational dysfunction is a disruption of the open system cycle that manifests itself in

Table 5.6.
Elizabeth: chronic psychiatric disability

Personal causation	Feels almost no sense of control over life. Can identify few skills and has no real hope for control in the future
Values	Identifies more independence as a value; cannot identify meaningful activities or goals
Interests	Acknowledges an interest in walking and being around younger people; these interests are not currently being enacted
Roles	Has no appreciable role except the chronic psychiatric patient role
Habits	Appears to be able to regulate her self-care alone, but is unable to structure her time outside of that activity, relying instead on the institutional schedule
Skills	Has basic self-care skills, but has no leisure or work-related skills. She has difficulty planning and problem solving, and communicating and interacting with others
Open system cycle	Activity level is minimal. The environment is not conducive to supporting occupational behavior and she does not make use of available opportunities for activity

a decrease, cessation or imbalance of output and in a consequent disorganization of the internal subsystems and their components.

Occupational dysfunction thus describes a malfunction in the interface of a person and the environment. The factors which contribute to any dysfunction are assumed to emanate from the environment as well as the person. Thus, identification of an occupational dysfunction requires acknowledgement of environmental factors.

THE ROLE OF THE OCCUPATIONAL THERAPIST IN OCCUPATIONAL FUNCTION AND DYSFUNCTION

Occupational therapists may offer services to persons who are at risk for, or who are experiencing, occupational dysfunction. An individual at risk may require occupational therapy services to maintain a state of occupational function. Persons who are experiencing occupational dysfunction require intervention to move them toward occupational functioning. The process of therapy is one of providing opportunities for occupational function until individuals can maintain an adaptive open system cycle of their own.

Since change in an open system only occurs through changing the cycle of behavior, the patient or client is not only the focus but also the instrument of therapy. Through engaging in directed occupations, the person begins to change the entire cycle, to organize or reorganize the internal components of the system and to increase the potential for adaptive output in the future.

Treating the Person as a Whole

It is sometimes argued that occupational therapists treat the whole person. This is not accurate. As noted earlier, adaptation and maladaptation involve many aspects of the person. The administrations of several professionals is required for the complex biological, occupational, spiritual, and other factors involved when a person is maladaptive.

While occupational therapists do not treat the whole person, they should treat the occupational person holistically. In addition, the therapist treats the occupational person in concert with, and with consideration for, other forms of treatment and other aspects of the person's maladaptation. Treating the individual holistically means that the occupational therapist takes into consideration all subsystems, the open system cycle and the environment. For example, focusing only on the performance subsystem by providing a functional splint or adaptive equipment without concern for the patient's priorities and what he or she wants to control could result in the person's failure to follow through on using the splint or equipment. If the equipment does not become part of a functioning cycle then it does not enhance the system's potential for adaptation. By the same token, focusing solely on personal causation by providing experiences which provide success and increase feelings of internal control without enabling the person to develop needed skills will result in failure.

CONCLUSION

This chapter offered an approach to conceptualizing occupational function and dysfunction. It is proposed as a way of classifying persons as adaptive or maladaptive in respect to occupational therapy's special area of concern. Six levels of a function/dysfunction continuum were identified. While they were discussed as discrete levels, they should be recognized as points on a continuum from highly organized to highly disorganized occupational behavior. They should serve as useful guides for identifying persons' approximate degrees of dysfunction. It is not anticipated that all persons can be neatly placed on one of the levels; individuals may exhibit characteristics from more than one level. Persons may also be functional in some aspects of their occupational behavior and dysfunctional in others.

By identifying approximate present levels of function or dysfunction and desired levels of function the therapist can better identify what kinds of reorganization may be required for a person. The continuum may also be useful in identifying appropriate types of programming for persons whose occupational dysfunction appears predominantly characteristic of one level.

The schema proposed in this chapter is a beginning to the process of developing a taxonomy of function and dysfunction for use in occupational therapy. Because the conceptualization uses open systems concepts of the model, it locates function and dysfunction not in static states of the individual but in the dynamics of the system's organization or disorganization and in the cycle of interaction with the environment.

This conceptualization calls attention to the need to treat persons in a holistic fashion and to recognize the centrality of personal action in maintaining or regaining occupational function.

References

1. Bateson G: *Mind and Nature: A Necessary Unity.* New York, Bantam Books, 1980.
2. Csikszentmihalyi M: Play and intrinsic rewards: *J Hum Psychol* 1975, 15:41–63.
3. Csikszentmihalyi M. The concept of flow. In Sutton-Smith B (ed): *Play and Learning.* New York, Gardner Press, 1979.
4. Dubos R: *The Mirage of Health: Utopias, Progress and Biological Change.* New York, Harper Row, 1959.
5. Florey L. Intrinsic motivation: the dynamics of occupational therapy theory. *Am J Occup Ther* 1969, 23:319–322.
6. Kass LR: Regarding the end of medicine and the pursuit of health. In Adler M (ed): *The Great Ideas Today.* Chicago, Encyclopedia Britanica, 1978.
7. Kielhofner G: *Health Through Occupation: Theory and Practice in Occupational Therapy.* Philadelphia, FA Davis, 1983.
8. McClelland D. *The Achieving Society.* Princeton, NJ, Van Nostrand, 1961.
9. Montagu A, Matson F: *The human connection.* New York, McGraw-Hill, 1979.
10. Reilly M (ed): *Play as exploratory learning.* Beverly Hills, Calif, Sage, 1974.
11. Rogers J: Order and disorder in medicine and occupational therapy. *Am J Occup Ther* 1982, 36:29–35.
12. White R: Excerpts from Motivation Reconsidered: The concept of competence. In Proshansky HM, Ittelson WH, Rivlin LG (eds): *Environmental Psychology.* New York, Holt, Rinehart Winston, 1970.
13. White R: The urge toward competence. *Am J Occup Ther* 1971, 25:271–272.

SECTION 2

Occupational Development

Introduction

The five chapters in this section examine the nature and course of development in occupational behavior throughout the life span. This section of the book represents a blending of the occupational behavior and developmental perspectives in occupational therapy.

The chapters in this section seek to provide a focused and coherent description of only one aspect of development, the development of occupational behavior. The reader should find these chapters useful as a perspective on the continuity of development throughout the life span and as a discussion of those elements of development for which the occupational therapist requires expert knowledge. Some aspects of occupational development (for example, neurodevelopment) were not given detailed treatment both because of space limitations and because of the availability of excellent discussions of these topics elsewhere in occupational therapy literature. Additionally, the therapist working with persons from a particular developmental stage will, no doubt, wish to be familiar with other aspects of development in that stage than those covered here. The references at the end of each chapter should be a useful resource for accessing additional information. Only the information relevant to concepts in the model of human occupation were integrated from the references into each chapter. Many of the references contain excellent discussions of other aspects of development.

The reader should find these chapters a resource for understanding the changing role of occupation in human life over the entire developmental continuum. Additionally, many of the challenges and difficulties of occupational development are highlighted. Comprehension of the course of development is necessary background to understanding function and dysfunction in the occupational behavior of persons that occupational therapists serve.

The chapters contain a wide array of information and should be a helpful reference on various details of occupational development. A corresponding exercise in the workbook allows the reader to apply concepts from this section to self-analysis.

CHAPTER 6

The Development of Occupational Behavior

Gary Kielhofner and Roann Barris

In the previous section it was argued that the human being is an open system in constant interaction with an external environment. It was further noted that this interaction, termed the open system cycle, results in the system changing itself. The accumulation of feedback and experience from ongoing environmental interaction combined with innate biological-based potentials propels the human system into a trajectory of change. For each human being that trajectory is unique, full of possibilities and stresses, and punctuated with both positive and negative events. Still it is possible to speak of a typical pattern of change throughout the life span. This is the topic of the present chapter and other chapters in this section.

The trajectory of change throughout the life span is referred to as development. Development is a complex process involving changes in biological, psychological, social, spiritual, and other dimensions of the human being. The following chapters explore the course of development of occupational behavior. Their discussions are necessarily focused on those phenomena most directly related to the unfolding of occupational capacity and of the occupational career or lifestyle of the individual.

PROCESSES INVOLVED IN DEVELOPMENT

In the Chapter 1 discussion of open systems, it was noted that, in the living system, processes were important and dominant over structures. The course of development in the human being most fully illustrates this. Development is a pattern of change, a process that is recognizable for all humans. Throughout the developmental process underlying structures are changed and transformed (1, 2, 6).

The open system cycle of intake, throughput, output, and feedback is the basic dynamic underlying development. Development also involves the open system process of differentia-

tion, mechanization and centralization. These processes contribute to an overall trend toward increasing complexity in the system. Take, for example, development of a child's capacity for coordinated motor action. Through the child's cycle of output (motor action), feedback (e.g. proprioceptive, tactile and other feedback about consequences of action), intake (e.g. perceptual information about the environment) and throughput (integration of this information into the system of rules which guides motor behavior), the basic skills or capacities for motor behavior are changed (5). They first change by differentiation. For example, the child learns to use various grasps for holding on to and picking up things. These patterns then become mechanized (e.g. a succession of motor acts can be integrated into patterns of motor performance for using various tools) (4). Once these patterns have been established, the child no longer has to attend to the specifics of how to move his or her body, what grips to use or how to organize movements of the hand into coordinated sequences. When this happens, a new level of function emerges (1). As perceptual-motor behaviors are differentiated and mechanized, new centralized functions of creative imagination and planning come into play and rule or govern the more primitive behaviors. This process of differentiation, mechanization and centralization allows the developmental progression from sensorimotor to constructive play. This developmental sequence is recognizably one in which new emerging forms of behavior build upon and integrate behaviors previously learned. The hierarchical nature of development is reflected in this building upon previous levels of learned behavior to affect new performances (1, 2, 5).

HIERARCHY IN DEVELOPMENT

Because development organizes the system hierarchically, any previous difficulties or problems in the organization of behavior will affect the emergence and organization of new levels. Thus, the completion of learning and experience at one level of development is important not only so that an individual attains appropriate experiences and abilities, but so that later learning and change will not be negatively affected (5, 6).

Hierarchical development is not a smooth progression or accumulation of experience leading to discrete change. It involves periods of slowed and greatly accelerated change, and periods of major transformation and reorganization which may be preceded by turbulent and disorganized states (4). In the same vein, not all events which contribute positively to the course of development are experienced as pleasurable events when they occur. Stress and life crises can be major stimulants to growth and change in the course of development (6, 7).

Development involves changes, refinements and unfolding of potential in each of the subsystems. Two principles describe the interrelationships of the subsystems in development. First of all, development never takes place in any one system without the influence of other subsystems. For example, the child cannot acquire changes in performance that are not accompanied by, or that do not affect, changes in volition. As new skills are acquired the child also gains an awareness of those skills which enhance personal causation. Similarly, adults who wish to increase their feelings of skillfulness must work to increase actual skills in the performance subsystem.

The second principle is that the period for development of each subsystem lengthens as one ascends the hierarchy. The child has mastered a wide range of perceptual motor skills, before he or she takes on several differentiated roles and long before a personal system of complex values is shaped.

INTERNAL AND EXTERNAL FACTORS IN DEVELOPMENT

In Chapter 1, it was noted that the behavior of any open system was a function of three factors: (a) the internal organization of status of the system, (b) the system's goals and (c) conditions in the environment. This is no less true for the course of development. Internal conditions refer to the biological and symbolic status of the system—such phenomena as the maturation of the nervous system and the emergence of abstract thinking are internal conditions that influence the course of development.

The decision-making of the system guided by volition is also a critical determinant of the course of development and becomes more and more important as the human being matures. Occupational choice, the process of making major decisions for entry into, and exit from, occupational roles is a major process in the development of occupational behavior (3). Finally, resources and conditions in the environment have an important role in maturation of occupational behavior. Within certain limits, the human infant can readily become a Wall Street businessperson or mineworker. The organization of the culture and the occupations it provides, the values about types of work and their appropriateness for a person of a certain class, sex or race, the family climate, and the physical environment of the home are just a few of the many environmental factors which can influence what course an individual's occupational life will take. In the end, development is an interplay of internal biological and symbolic factors, environment and individual choice, although at some stages, one factor may become more important than others. For instance, in childhood, biological changes make possible the entire course of skill acquisition and play a dominant role in the unfolding of one's capacity. On the other hand, a major life change in adulthood may be precipitated by value changes as an individual ceases to find satisfaction in achievement for its own sake, and begins to ponder the meaning of his or her work.

DEVELOPMENT AS ACTUALIZATION OF POTENTIALS: OPENNESS IN DEVELOPMENT

Occupational development represents an actualization of potentials related to the occupational sphere. Most basic is the potential for effectively using one's symbolic and neuromuscular constituents to accomplish tasks. This is the potential to become skilled. The second potential is that of organizing one's performance into a coherent pattern that becomes the reality of life, and reflects one's position in society. This is the potential for forming habits and roles. Finally, there is the potential for self-determination—for choosing one's course of living according to values, personal causation and interests. This is the potential to will one's life and behavior.

Not only is the human neonate a locus of tremendous potential for development over the course of life, but development itself is also a phenomenon which appears to have a vast degree of openness. In discussion of each stage of development, authors point out that particular developmental phenomena may vary from generation to generation as affected by historical changes or that development may vary across different cultures. Development is now recognized more and more as a process with many degrees of freedom influenced by particular sets of circumstances in which any group of individuals find themselves. Occupational life-styles over the span of development may thus change dramatically in the course of human civilization. This is, of course, more true beyond early infancy when biological factors appear to play a predominant role in the nature and pace of changes. By the time persons reach old age, however, who they have become is clearly a function of when and where they have lived, who their predecessors and colleagues were and what local and world events impacted on their lives.

TRANSFORMATION OF WORK, PLAY, AND DAILY LIVING TASKS

The most obvious outward manifestation of occupational development is that persons do different things at different stages of development. We thus recognize younger children as players, older children and adolescents as students, adults as workers, and older persons as retirees. As we will see later, the transformation of behavior is actually more varied and multi-faceted. But the fact remains that as the individual develops, what he or she does in everyday life changes.

The transformation of work, play and daily living tasks in the life span reflects an underlying order to development. This order is manifest not only in the individual, but in society as a whole. The transformation of play, and its purpose and meaning, provides an example. The child who is primarily a player also happens to be doing a great deal of learning through that play. Helpless at birth, the child achieves through his or her play experiences mastery of the perceptual motor, communication/interaction and process skills necessary for survival in later life (5). The adult in modern society is expected to, and generally does do, the work of the culture, which includes creating and maintaining a safe and nurturing environment for the new generation of children who are learning to be competent in their play. Another growing

phenomenon in western culture is the assumption of financial and other responsibilities for retired parents by their adult children. Because of this pattern the adult has less free time for play than either the child or the elderly person. For the child, play is a preparatory time whereas, for the adult, it is a source of relaxation and recreation from work. For the elderly person without access to work, it is a source of self-worth and self-identity. The patterns of work, play and self-care over the life span and the ways they influence the individual to perform, to find meaning and worth and to change are of considerable importance in development of humans.

NORMAL VERSUS ADAPTIVE DEVELOPMENT

Many discussions of development carry with them the implicit or explicit theme that the particular courses or process of development described are normal. However, it is important to consider what is meant by "normal" development. In many cases normal is a reference to what is normative or average. For example, most discussions of childhood development describe various attainments that on the average have occurred by a particular age. Normative decriptions are, perhaps, most helpful in very early childhood where changes are, to a large degree, governed by innate biological factors. However, normative descriptions are increasingly problematic as the individual ages. Great variation may occur across persons, and very discrepant behaviors might be described as normal in the sense of not being "abnormal" or pathological. In fact, what is average for a particular group of adults may not represent what is most adaptive or healthy.

What may be a more useful concept than normal development is adaptive development. Using the criteria posed in Chapter 5, adaptive development would be recognized as a course of life change which results in fulfillment of the individual's urge to explore and master, maintaining and enhancing the viability of the systems' organization, and which allows the individual to meet reasonable environmental demands. Such a definition also allows the concept of development to be more reasonably applied to persons with disability. Most persons with a chronic disability will, in some ways, deviate from the normative or average course of development. Yet they may develop in adaptive ways.

The course of development as described in the following chapters should thus be viewed not so much as a yardstick against which to measure adaptation in an individual, but rather as descriptions of courses of adaptive development which characterize many people and from which implications for alternative developmental courses may be drawn.

References

1. Bruner J: Organization of early skilled action. *Child Dev* 1973, 44:1–11.
2. Bruner J: On voluntary action and its hierarchical structure. In Koestler A, Smithies JR (eds): *Beyond Reductionism*. Boston, Beacon Press, 1969.
3. Ginzberg E: Toward a theory of occupational choice. In Peters HJ, Hansen JC (eds): *Vocational Guidance and Career Development*, ed 2. New York, MacMillan, 1971.
4. Koestler A: Beyond atomism and holism—the concept of the holon. In Koestler A, Smithies JR (eds): *Beyond Reductionism*. Boston, Beacon Press, 1969.
5. Reilly M: *Play as Exploratory Learning*. Beverly Hills, Calif, Sage, 1974.
6. von Bertalanffy L: General system theory and psychiatry. In Arieti S (ed): *American Handbook of Psychiatry*. New York, Basic Books, 1966.
7. von Bertalanffy L: General system theory—a critical review. In Buckley W (ed): *Modern System's Research for the Behavioral Scientist*. Chicago, Aldine, 1968.

CHAPTER 7

Childhood

Peggy Neville, Gary Kielhofner and Charlotte Brasic Royeen

AN OVERVIEW OF CHILDHOOD

Childhood is a period of tremendous growth and change. The child's interactions with the physical and social environment in combination with the innate biological program direct and shape the course of change after birth.

During the period of gestation neurological and musculoskeletal constituents of skills become differentiated and, to a degree, modularized. At birth only rudimentary constituents of skills exist in the form of reflexes; volition and habituation are largely undifferentiated. After birth the highly plastic nervous system and musculoskeletal system of the child are greatly changed and organized through the open system cycle. Symbolic abilities emerge out of the interaction of the child's nervous system with the environment.

The course of child development is one of generating, differentiating and modularizing system components. The newborn's volition subsystem consists of the neurogenic urge to explore and master which leads the child to engage the environment, thus generating skills. As skills emerge, the child's volitional awareness also increases so that there is a harmony or synergy in their co-development. For example, the newborn's physical activity creates sensory feedback that modifies the innate reflexes. Information is taken in, and integrated into, the central nervous system in the throughput process. This sensory information is organized and neurological structures are modified so that more complex behaviors can be enacted (25). At the same time the child also gains a rudimentary awareness that these responses occur and can be willed. Consequently, through advances in representation and mastery of the body, the child can choose more and more complex behavior.

The open system processes of the child are driven by the output of play (33). Play is the dominant role of childhood and the dynamic vehicle processing maturation of the subsystems. Early play is largely exploratory and focuses on seeking and generating sensory, motor and affective experiences. During middle childhood there is further refinement of skills and exploration gives way to concern with competence. At this stage a productive family member role emerges and the child becomes capable of and responsible for some self-care and chores. In late childhood play makes room for the student role and increased productivity in family roles. During this period the achievement level motive emerges as the child learns to compete and to perform according to standards. Elements of all three levels of occupational functioning can be found at all stages of childhood; the transformation from exploration to achievement refers only to the dominant mode of each stage.

This chapter will discuss development of occupational behavior during the three stages of childhood: early childhood (0–2 years), middle childhood (2–6 years) and late childhood (6–11 years).* These stages of childhood development are continuous and are influenced by culture, family, and other environmental variables. While there may be variation in the ages and stages of development, the central reality of childhood is that the interaction between the child and environment results in the differentiation and co-development of the subsystems.

EARLY CHILDHOOD, THE SENSORIMOTOR PERIOD (0–2 YEARS)

Infants' development in the sensorimotor period is one of rapid transformations. They ini-

---

* Because the goal of this chapter is to present an overview of how occupational behavior develops in the child, it cannot provide an in-depth description of neurological or sensory integrative development in childhood. A list of Suggested Readings is provided at the end of the chapter for those readers wanting more specific information on neurological development and sensory integration.

tially receive and respond to information in a global and undifferentiated manner (i.e. "yes," there is a sensory input or "no," there is not a sensory input), lacking discrimination or qualitative responses to sensory input. For example, infants react to being touched, but cannot discriminate where they are being touched. They show visual recognition of familiar objects and people, but their focus is vague and they cannot differentiate complex shapes (3).

Active playful participation within the environment, rather than passive experience is of paramount importance in the infant's development. Sensory integration occurs, for example, only as the infant actively interacts, explores and experiments with the environment. The infant actively takes in varied sensory information and organizes it in the throughput phase. As this information becomes part of the system's neurological and symbolic structure it allows more sophisticated output. Such dynamic transformation underlies all development. In the following sections, developmental changes in each subsystem during early childhood are discussed.

Performance Subsystem

Development of the performance subsystem is paramount in early childhood. The performance subsystem is a collection of almost endless potentials which are activated and organized by the child's ever changing interaction with the environment.

DEVELOPMENT OF SKILL CONSTITUENTS

The tremendous plasticity and learning potential of the infant is owed to the incomplete maturation of the nervous system at birth (2, 7). The nervous system plays a central role in early development. It is the governing system which must coordinate use of the still maturing musculoskeletal system. It is the substratum out of which symbolic capacities emerge (8) and, importantly, it embodies a self-activating principle or inner drive (2, 3) which is the basis for the urge to explore and master.

The newborn has only a rudimentary organization in the neurological constituents of skills. The gross structure of the nervous system is basically present at birth; however, it has yet to be refined and differentiated beyond reflex patterns. Reflexes are inherited species' preadaptations to sensory information taken in from the environment (35). Eventually, through the open system cycle, the nervous system is reprogrammed to allow higher cortical control and more complex adaptations to the environment.

As primitive reflexes are integrated into the central nervous system, and the higher cortical centers are able to exert their influence on the lower centers, the infant becomes capable of more voluntary control. For example, when under the influence of the asymmetrical tonic neck reflex, babies have difficulty keeping their heads in midline. Further, due to lack of higher level inhibitory influences, voluntary control of reaching movements is limited. Later, through development of the neuromuscular system, the child can voluntarily turn his or her head in a desired direction and shows more purposeful reach and grasp.

Development of the symbolic, neurological and musculoskeletal constituents of skills is highly integrated. The course of early development is marked by the differentiation and creation of symbols, neuromuscular units, and synergistic patterns which underlie the emergence of perceptual motor skills.

The infant in the first few months is already responding to many sensations. Gentle movements and touch are taken in by the tactile and vestibular receptors, a process crucial for organization of the brain. Infants respond to the sensation of gravity by making attempts to lift their heads. From every movement, sensations and feedback are received from the muscles and joints, and are organized in the throughput phase so that neural patterns are formed which allow more controlled and higher level adaptive responses.

Integration of the various sensory input also helps the child develop a symbolic awareness of personal actions. For example, when an infant reaches to grasp a mobile, proprioceptive and kinesthetic feedback provide information about where his or her hand is in space. The attempt to grasp or manipulate the mobile generates tactile feedback, as well as corollary discharge or a signal that a motor message has been sent to the muscles by the brain. Visual information is received as movements and colors are observed. This provides the child information not only about the object, but also about how his or her hand feels when it is moved and when it is used to act on objects in the environment, and how movements can have environmental results. It also serves to help the child set up a "library" of motor skills. This information is integrated into the system in throughput providing the child information in the form of symbols which will help guide future reaching behaviors. As the child acquires symbols he or she begins to literally "feel" what a movement is like and this aids in the development of motor planning. An increase in awareness of action and its consequences, and in the level of skill, occur. In the future, the child will reach toward the mobile with greater accuracy.

The symbolic constituent of skills emerges from an "internal organizational principle" in the brain (8). Symbols not only emerge from the nervous system to constitute a new hierarchical level but they also supervene in or govern neurological events (38, 39).

Thus once symbols emerge, motor commands emanating from the central nervous system are also intentions emanating from the child's awareness. The intention to move and the neuronal command from the central nervous system are simply two aspects of one complex phenomenon. Symbols emerge when the nervous system processes sensation into meanings which results in an internal model of self and of the external world (33). The ability to symbolize provides the child with a fund of knowledge gained from previous events and actions which can be applied to present situations to enable more competent actions (33). This class of symbols is referred to as rules (33, 34). Rules of action, objects and people are learned in play and guide behavior since they inform the child of how one can act on the environment.

The genesis of symbols is in the child's action; mental symbols initially involve motor actions (29, 31) and are highly dependent upon motor planning. Such symbolic representation is accomplished by generating a neuronal model of the symbol. Thus, symbol use is achieved via the mechanism of establishing and modifying neuronal models (4). As the child develops, the malleable neuronal models become more and more sophisticated and abstract. However, such subsequent symbolization is developmentally based upon adequate symbolization of the first neuronal model, body scheme. Therefore, body scheme is the developmental paradigm for symbol use during childhood. Since body scheme is dependent upon sensory integration, the relationship between symbolization, neurological and musculoskeletal constituents of skills is obvious. This interaction is apparently critical in the development of more complex perceptual

motor skill actions. That is, once a child has mastered a particular perceptual motor act it is "supplanted by a 'higher order action' that usually encompasses it as a subroutine" (Ref 8, p 4). The higher order action is a more complex perceptual motor task which can only occur because the child has processed information to combine two or more perceptual motor tasks which are used to accomplish some new purpose (8). As an example, a child who has learned to reach out and grasp an object and to bang his or her hands on a surface making noise will then use these motor behaviors later as part of a more complex routine in which an object is held and banged against a surface. Thus, the relationship between symbolization and neuromuscular action is one in which symbolization enables the planning and execution of perceptual motor acts based on well-learned perceptual motor behaviors that are combined into new actions (8). In turn, as these new perceptual motor acts are executed and practiced they become modularized allowing the process of symbolization to deal with yet more complex actions.

Over time symbolization becomes dissociated from action. For example, the child can imitate things internally rather than through overt behavior. The child also begins to use objects in play for symbolic purposes (31). This ludic representation is based on the child's ability to treat an object as if it were something else (e.g. pretending a broom is a horse). Thus the development of skill constituents represents a long pathway from primitive reflexes to symbols. As these underlying constituents of skills are transformed, the child's perceptual motor, process and communication/interaction skills develop.

PERCEPTUAL MOTOR SKILLS

Early perceptual motor development shows a gradual progression of the child's ability to dissociate movements; this is a process of differentiation which allows more isolated and refined movements, or what is called superimposing mobility upon stability (18). For example, ability to separate head/eye movements will enable increased visual skills and dissociation of shoulder from arm and hand allows more mature reaching and prehension patterns. At the same time integration or modularization of perceptual motor skills is continuously occurring. The child receives feedback about his or her actions and is able to use it to further coordinate perceptions and actions to execute a skilled act. Major gross motor developments in this period are increased head control, development of equilibrium reactions, and increased mobility. The child's major accomplishment is being able to conquer gravity by rising up to a standing position, and beginning independent ambulation. Simultaneously with these developments the child is also expanding skills in the fine motor area, demonstrating more isolated finger use, developing voluntary grasp and release, and exploring toys in more varied ways (3, 17).

In the sensorimotor stage, spatial perception increases as the child moves through space and gains knowledge about space and his body in relation to space. Increased body awareness will facilitate motor planning for both gross and fine motor tasks. Increased visual control of the eyes to direct the hand and maturing fine motor abilities permit the child to engage in such play activities as beginning scribbling, manipulating varied switches as on a surprise box, completing simple puzzles, and beginning block building. During the latter part of this stage the child can be observed in play activities intensely involved with taking or putting things in and out of containers. These play activities, in turn, foster the development of new perceptual motor skills.

PROCESS SKILLS

The infant's ability to engage in means-end behavior is the beginning of process skills. At about 10–12 months the infant uses familiar internal schemes, rather than inventing new means for dealing with an encountered obstacle (32). However, the infant can solve simple problems such as removing an obstacle to attain a goal, illustrating that the infant's behavior is fully intentional and intelligent (19). At this early age of development the child does not possess a full variety of alternatives since his ability to invent new means is limited. Thus, early process skills do not show much novelty or creativity. Between approximately 12 and 18 months, more complex problem solving occurs as the child begins to experiment with variation and novelty. Knowledge of alternatives is gained which will assist the child later in more advanced tasks requiring problem-solving skills.

COMMUNICATION INTERACTION SKILLS

The ability to symbolize also becomes important in development of the child's communica-

tion/interaction skills. The newborn is able to respond to sounds but vocalizations are meager and nonexpressive. Except for crying the infant is almost inarticulate. Vocalizations increase as the oral and respiratory apparatus develop. By 28 weeks the infant has become familiar with facial expressions, gestures and postural attitudes of persons in the environment. The young child initially makes needs known through crying, gestures or squeals. By 40 weeks the child tends to imitate gestures, facial expressions and sounds, and has a vocabulary of one or two words. At this age there is also a new social responsiveness. This is seen in the child's enjoyment of having people around and in his participation in games such as pat-a-cake and peek-a-boo (17).

The 1 year old becomes more adept at repeating words and begins to understand simple directions. Significant changes occur between 1 and 2 years in communication/interaction skills. At 1 year the child shows perception of emotions of others and is becoming capable of influencing and adjusting to these emotions. The 18 month old can use words with, and instead of, gestures and communicate to others a wide range of emotional states, although the expressions are egocentric. By age 2 the child's vocabulary has remarkably expanded and he or she is able to relate experience, although the sense of time in speech has not yet been mastered (17).

Habituation Subsystem

Acquired skills are eventually organized into habits and roles. The newborn's internal regulation is biologically determined by such states as hunger. Most patterned behavior is first externally regulated and then internalized as the child develops. Gradually a pattern of internally regulated patterns of sleeping, waking, eating, and so on, emerge; over time these regulating patterns become more complex and are shaped into player and family roles.

ROLES

Internalized role expectancies are limited in early childhood. Parents universally recognize the young child as being in the role of a player. Parents tend to see the behaviors in play as reflective of development and thereby value and expect the child's performance in play. Parents are also critical for initiating the child into the player role by setting up situations or contexts for play, beginning with the brief interludes of exaggerated speech and motor stimulation, and extending into simple games of peek-a-boo and the like (41). Beyond parental expectations that the child be lively and cheerful when playing, there are initially few expectations. Later, parents set boundaries on what objects the child can play with, what types of behaviors are allowed and with whom the child can play. Thus, the player role comes to have its own demands and expectations.

Around the age of 2 the family member role first emerges as parents expect and value productive contributions of the child to the routines of family life. About this time the child has generated the skills to allow participation in dressing, toy clean-up, and even doing small chores. Initially, during this stage these behaviors are seen by parents as "cute," yet indicative of the child's emergence as a full-fledged productive family member.

HABITS

The biological regulation of internal functions such as breathing, digestion, heart rate, and the perception of sensory intake provide the child's first patterns of consistency and organization. Developing familiarity with sensations and learning to rely on the consistency and continuity of providers appear to be important for development of the child's internal sense of order and organization. The child begins to anticipate and predict events and behaviors of others and to feel the security which is necessary for exploration and experimentation in play.

Gradually more patterned behaviors are developing as the child begins to sense routines related to times for sleeping, waking, bathing, eating, playing, and so on. By the age of 40 weeks the infant has internalized a sense of the routines of everyday life (17). For example, a 1 year old will show recognition and need for a bedtime routine, insisting that a series of regular behaviors be carried out before going to bed such as getting a favorite stuffed animal and having a story read. By age 2 the young child can routinely perform some simple self-help skills such as drinking from a cup, spoon feeding, and assisting in washing and dressing, and shows recognition of the organization of these skills into a sequential routine. The child is thus learning habits of self-care and is becoming a more autonomous person.

Volition Subsystem

The capacity for intention or volition exists at birth. Behavior that occurs in the form of reflexes is "converted into intentional action when the infant has had an opportunity to observe the results of his own acts."(Ref 8, p 2). In other words the child becomes aware that he or she can be a cause by experiencing self having effects, and from this experience is able to desire having various effects (10). Neuromuscular maturation contributes to the differentiation of the volition subsystem as the child becomes capable of exercising more choice in increasingly complex behaviors. Feedback from these actions contributes to development of personal causation, interests and values.

PERSONAL CAUSATION

Through play the child develops a sense of personal causation. The experience of control is something which is felt rather than visually perceived, and therefore is derived more from touch and kinesthesis, rather than vision (11). Sensory integrative functions are thus seen to be important in the ability to experience self as a cause—personal causation. In time childrens' increased skills and their play allow them to experience themselves as being able to cause an event, although it may be as simple as making a noise or changing body position.

In infants' initial undifferentiated state they are unable to separate themselves from the environment and are centered about the self (32). Through a process of decentration the child gains an increased awareness of the existence of self as separate from the environment. This sense of self as a distinct being will also contribute to the child's ability to know one can have an impact on the environment.

VALUES

Cultural values also begin to infuence the child early in life. Studies have shown sex differences in toy preferences as early as 13–14 months (23). Although biological factors may be one part of this difference in interests, it also appears to be due to social learning of cultural values. The child begins to internalize value images of what is acceptable or unacceptable and this guides his choice of play. Parental approval and disapproval of certain actions also guide the child's understanding of what behaviors are appropriate and thus socially valued.

INTERESTS

Children's interests and how they choose play activities closely relate to neuromuscular development and the resulting maturation of skills. The child's interest in objects is first with their sensory aspects such as color, texture and noise, and later with their potential for use in action such as stacking blocks or throwing a ball. Interests are reflected in play behavior consisting first of simple, repetitive actions which are carried out for the pleasure of the action. For example, a child who is developing increased stability and is practicing this new control of movement may repeatedly squat and then resume a standing position, demonstrating immense enjoyment and showing pride in this accomplishment. Such functional play is pleasurable because it gives a feeling of power that comes with the mastery of a new action (15).

During the first 4 months when the infant's behavior by chance produces an interesting or advantageous result, he or she immediately attempts to repeat this behavior through a process of trial and error (32). Interest at this stage is in producing actions centered about the body. The sensory intake which the infant's behavior provides is pleasurable and contributes to the desire to repeat these actions (31). Later, the child's interests have expanded so that these behaviors now tend more to involve events or objects in the external environment. Through the trial and error process of discovering how to repeat events, skills become more precise and effective. At approximately 12–18 months, infants' behaviors reflect interest in novelty, and in producing variations in the event. Thus the child seeks out new ways of acting on objects by experimentation (19, 32).

During this period the child's interest in the external world is primarily modulated by the principle of arousal. The child will seek novelty and complexity slightly beyond that with which he or she is familiar. As skills and information increase the child's interest in the environment will change accordingly, being directed to newer and more complex objects and events such as walking, gross and fine motor capacities, and beginning abilities to problem solve and communicate. Early childhood is largely an explor-

atory period for the child paving the way for the next stage of development.

MIDDLE CHILDHOOD (2–6 YR)

The growth and drive toward competency become a dominant feature during middle childhood. Play continues as the major occupational behavior facilitating development of performance skills for mastery during middle childhood and it further differentiates volition and habituation. The child begins to regulate his or her behavior internally, enter roles and become a more fully volitional being, capable of differentiating choices based on inner images.

Performance Subsystem

During middle childhood the performance subsystem is characterized by the refinement of existing skills and the continued rapid acquisition of new skills. Thus, the child gains increasing competence for interacting with the environment and is more able to actively seek complex situations and novel experiences.

DEVELOPMENT OF SKILL CONSTITUENTS

Due to continuous maturation of the neurological and musculoskeletal constituents of skill, the child's motoric capacities become more controlled and differentiated. Reflexes continue to be integrated as the central nervous system functions to coordinate skilled action. Higher level functions can occur within the cerebrum as postural mechanisms become more automatic (12).

As an example, the child's ability to ride a bike reflects these changes in skill constituents which enable more complex skills. Through differentiation of neuromuscular functions and structures the child can isolate movements. Lower extremities are used to pedal the bike, while upper extremities and visual and vestibular perception are used to control its direction. These actions would not be possible without the centralized role of the central nervous system in coordination of sensory input with behavioral output. In the developing child sensory integration is vital to these processes for producing change in the system. For example, integration of tactile, proprioceptive and vestibular input will contribute to postural control and body awareness which will assist in differentiation of movements and motor planning.

During this stage there is also much growth in symbolic functions, based upon the initial neuronal models generated in early childhood. There is an elaboration of multiple representational systems which includes mental images, imitation, symbolic play, symbolic drawing, and language (30). The child in this stage has a strong attachment to symbols (13). The child's use of symbols moves towards a closer representation to reality (31). For example, in constructions the child seeks a more exact imitation, and in imaginary play there is greater concern to have props and outfits to simulate reality.

PERCEPTUAL MOTOR SKILLS

In early skills constituent acts are clumsily organized in a loosely ordered sequence (8). Feedback later shapes these awkward patterns and higher order acts evolve. This progression is seen in the child's acquisition of motor skills. For example, feedback from planning and executing movement (i.e. internal feedback such as vestibular and proprioceptive information and feedback on the consequences of action) are used by the central nervous system to refine movement strategies, balance and motor control.

At this age, the child actively seeks out vestibular play activities such as, spinning around a pole, merry-go-rounds, slides, jungle gyms, and rolling down a hill. These provide the sensory input and elicit a somatomotor adaptive response necessary for higher level sensory integration. Other forms of play such as rough and tumble games, sandbox activities and fingerpainting enhance proprioceptive and tactile system functions. Integration of all of these refined sensory processes contributes to basic skill acquisition regarding attention, sequencing and behavioral control, and to further development of perceptual motor skills.

Development in the perceptual motor area enables the child to have an increased command of tools as seen in beginning drawing skills and play involving tool use and constructive toys. Knowledge gained from exploration of objects during the sensorimotor period is now used for tool manipulation in more goal-directed perceptual motor behavior. Thus, the growth in tool use reflects the incorporation of earlier subroutines into higher level acts.

PROCESS SKILLS

During this period process skills evolve to a higher level as growth in symbolic functions continues. In addition, as skills require less attention to execute due to the process of modularization, more capacity for information processing is made available for task analysis (8).

The 3-yr-old is in a transitional stage when much differentiation of perceptual abilities occurs, but by 5 the child is able to solve perceptual problems without relying solely on the kinesthetic trial and error process of earlier ages (17). Advances in cognitive thought now enable the child to begin to be able to plan ahead, such as having an idea about what he wants to paint or build. Process skills are also being developed as the child has more opportunities for decision making in play behaviors and as the child begins to initiate and operationalize coherent themes in play, such as playing house, and in participation in early simple games which require planning and strategy.

COMMUNICATION/INTERACTION SKILLS

During middle childhood language development in terms of structure and form is essentially complete (17). Interaction skills increase during this stage as vocabulary expands and the child can now use words to express feelings, desires and problems, and to describe motoric actions, phsyiological needs and basic plans. Increased ability to communicate is observed even in the 2-yr-old who will dramatize the emotional expressions of those in his social mileu. For example, in pretending to carry on a phone conversation, the young child will imitate facial expressions and voice intonations of adult models. The child also begins to seek information from others. Typical during this period is the frequent asking of questions which become more meaningful as development progresses. Development of communication/interaction skills assists in the child's cultural adaptation. The child has now become quite talkative and will sit and converse readily during mealtimes. Thus, these skills are contributing to a more defined role as a family member and again demonstrates the co-development of the subsystems.

Interaction skills are also seen to change as the child moves from solitary or parallel play, to a growing interest in playing with other children.

The child begins to develop the ability to wait one's turn or share possessions and becomes capable of more associative and cooperative small group play (24). This growth in communication/interaction skills will serve as a preparation for meeting later social expectations in school and play.

Habituation Subsystem

As the child is becoming capable of more independent actions, expectations for role enactment are more defined. Roles during middle childhood are informal and may include the following: family member, player, preschooler and, towards the latter part of this period, role of friend. Skills that were learned earlier are now integrated into routines as the child models his or her behavior on observed patterns in the social surroundings (8). During this stage imitation, practice of routines and molding behavior to the environment serve to yield greater internalization of behavior regulation.

ROLES

The child's consciousness of family group and his or her role as a family member increases. By age 3 the child shows conformity to the requirements of home life (17). As a family member who has gained in independence, the child is given more responsibility to carry out self-care tasks and help with chores such as setting the table, washing dishes and taking out the trash. Participation in chores is the child's initial experimentation with the work role (36), as well as an expansion of the family member role. The child's participation in birthday and holiday celebrations also strengthens awareness and association with the role of a family member. As the child becomes capable of more associative play, the role of player now requires more effective communication/interaction skills to guide behavior in this role. During middle childhood a capacity for developing friendships begins and thus the role of friend emerges.

Role expectations are internalized as the child observes adult models in the environment, and then enacts these roles in sociodramatic play (25). Through sociodramatic and imitative play, the child is able to enter the world of adults and experiment with varied work roles. Understanding of behaviors and attitudes associated with a role is enhanced. Games also become an arena

for role taking and the child learns to understand the function of roles within groups through games (28, 33). The child gradually comes to perceive of him or herself as occupying a specific role, first showing recognition that certain behaviors characterize different roles. For example, the child uses dress ups, props and verbal dialogue and gesturing to simulate models and environmental settings (9). Thus, in middle childhood the child both tries out various roles in play and begins to internalize a family role and later a friend role.

HABITS

Routine behavior is still somewhat determined and guided by caretakers, and the child's pattern of time use is mainly around the role of player and family member. Maturation of skills in the performance subsystem enables the child to acquire habits of self-care and contributes to the child's growing conformity to societal expectations. The child increasingly becomes aware of routines and is more and more able to organize behaviors in time to accomplish chores and routines of dressing, toileting and eating. The child also comes to rely on repetition of the routines as a source of security, predictability and comfort (6).

Beginning work habits, such as cleaning up after a task or doing a daily chore are being formed. As social contacts increase the child learns patterns of behavior which will be necessary for adjustment to the standards of society. In sociodramatic play the child learns intellectual discipline, self control and tolerance and sensitivity to demands of peers (37). These will be important habits for the child's successful entry into school and for his or her growing role in the peer group.

Volition Subsystem

The child's growing competence and widening range of interaction with the environment serve to further differentiate the volition subsystem. From the selection of sensory information (16) to decisions to participate in games and other play forms, the child's volitional image increasingly guides and influences choices of behavior.

PERSONAL CAUSATION

Self-concept has become more developed and contributes to the child's ability to perceive self as a causal agent. The child's increased awareness of selfhood is seen in the importance attached to his or her name and the adamant use of the words "me" and "mine."

Awareness of skill capacities is gained from engaging in the environment. In the early years the child desires to be autonomous but does not yet have a realistic sense of his or her abilities. The child will often insist on helping with tasks which are beyond his or her competencies, saying with fervor, "I can do it." "Testing" is also a form of play in which the child discovers what he can do (i.e. "I can climb up here") (40). Through this experimentation the child learns efficacy of skills to guide future choice of behavior.

Play serves in a variety of ways to enhance personal causation. Play experiences which enhance sensory integration provide the child with increased mastery over sensory intake and motor output, increasing a sense of confidence and control over the environment (3). The ability to choose in play (i.e. where one will play, with what and so on) provides a sense of internal control. Finally, in play children reenact events which may previously have been overarousing and thus achieve a sense of mastery or control over experiences wherein they may previously have felt out of control (14, 31).

Throughout all the child's experiences in play and in relation to tasks in the home, success and recognition by others increases the image of effectiveness. The combination of success and failure, control and the lack thereof also differentiates the personal causation image so that it becomes more reality based. The child learns to translate the unbounded sense of autonomy into a realistic sense of internal control, skill and possibility of success.

VALUES

In middle childhood the child begins to be more value oriented. The sense of temporal awareness and ability to understand time and duration increases (17) so that the child becomes more future oriented. This orientation is reflected in the ability to carry a play project over from one day to the next, to set short term goals and to delay gratification.

As the child's interactions with adults and peers become increasingly sophisticated, he or she begins to understand the value of certain norms of behavior such as taking turns and sharing. The child also shows a growing awareness of which behaviors are negatively or positively valued by parents, siblings and others, so that values increasingly are a factor in decisions for behavior.

INTERESTS

As in early childhood interests are mainly guided by the child's changing skills. Action-oriented activities continue to be enjoyed and increased hand dexterity enables the child to engage in play requiring fine motor control, such as constructing simple projects. Growth in language ability results in interest in exploring verbal humor, chanting rhymes and so on (42).

Interests at this age are also influenced by the child's need to feel competent. Children will tend to center interests on those activities that provide optimal arousal. The child also begins to show an interest in activities that extend over longer periods of time. For example nonselective collections may become an interest during this time (42).

The availabiltiy of various objects and events in the environment now become more critical for shaping interests since the child's increasing abilities allow pursuit of a wide range of options for action. Generally, it is the environment now and not the child's abilities that are limiting what he or she will like.

Summary

The child strives towards gaining competency during middle childhood and there is a growing differentiation of the subsystems. Due to developments in the performance subsystem the child has a wider range of alternatives available for engaging the environment and has become a more social person. Play has moved from exploration to symbolic, dramatic, constructive, and pre-game play (42). The emergence of independence in daily living tasks has increased the child's sense of autonomy and contributed to the development of habits and roles. The child can now more effectively interact and adjust to demands of the social environment. Growth in competence further modifies volitional images as a sense of personal causation is experienced, interests are expanded, and values relevant to standards of society are internalized. These developments are preparing for the entry into late childhood which requires more advanced skills and organization of habits for adjusting to new roles.

LATE CHILDHOOD (6–11 YEARS)

Major changes occur during late childhood when the social environment of the child expands enormously. There is a movement away from the home as the central focus of the child's activities. The level of achievement in occupational function is introduced as the child enters the student role. During late childhood there is greater concern with standards of performance and environmental demands such as assuming more responsibility at home, performing successfully in school and relating to peers and adults in varied situations. More mature expectations and performance are demanded as a result of the differentiation in the components of the subsystems. Extrafamilial influences increase as the child's environment now includes teachers and a greater number and variety of peers and social events. Participation in more formal social organizations begins during this period.

The child now learns to master and confront a growing sphere of social environments involving more complex interactions. The effectiveness of interactions used to meet demands of these situations and resulting images of personal causation which are formed will affect the way later challenges are encountered in adolescence and adulthood.

Performance Subsystem

Skills attained during late childhood relate to the requirements for successful performance in the new and expanding roles of the child. There is also a desire to refine previously learned skills.

DEVELOPMENT OF SKILL CONSTITUENTS

During late childhood there is a refinement of the neurological constituent and continued growth of the musculoskeletal constituent as proficiency in skills is gained. Maturation of these constituents now enables greater speed, accuracy and coordination. The technological complexity and specialization of modern society require that the child acquire multiple skills in order to adapt. A high level of skills development is needed to meet the social and task requirements confronting the child. For example, fine motor skills of writing must be adequately developed so that the child can efficiently do homework, copy notes, fill out test forms, and so on, without using unnecessary cognitive effort.

The increase in symbolic functions is manifest in the child's attainment of concrete operational thought (32), occurring at approximately age 7. At this point the child has the capacity to learn and operate according to rules, and this ability makes formal education possible (13). At this level of thought the child can check symbols against experience, and therefore can distinguish between fantasy and reality (13).

Advancements in imagery during late childhood enhance process skills. Prior to this the child was only able to produce an approximate mental image of a static situation. The child can now attune to transformations which occur, recognizing intervening steps between beginning and end states. Imagery now has a more dynamic nature. This progression in imagery is seen, for example, in the child's increased ability to correctly solve tasks involving the concept of conservation. Thus, advances in imagery permit the child to have a greater understanding of the world and assist the process of reasoning (19).

PERCEPTUAL MOTOR SKILLS

The emergence of student role brings new requirements for perceptual motor competence. Sensory motor experience from early and middle childhood have provided the foundation or building blocks necessary for academic skills (3). The refinement of gross motor skills now enables the child to engage in more socialized play such as group games and sports. Play again serves as an avenue where perceptual motor skills are further practiced and advanced, and at the same time greater neuromuscular control is achieved. For example, the focus now on speed and coordination is seen in the enjoyment of games which challenge the child to finish in a certain amount of time.

Fine motor skills are developing more precision. The child can use a greater variety of tools and is thus capable of making more complex products in constructive play.

PROCESS SKILLS

Problem solving skills are enhanced due to the progression in mental representational abilities and advancements in cognitive thought. The range of alternatives which the child can explore when dealing with a situation is also expanded. When perceptual motor skills reach a higher level of development and regularity the child can focus more on problem solving and decision making (22).

COMMUNICATION/INTERACTION SKILLS

Communication skills evolve as vocabulary increases rapidly and further syntactic and semantic advances are made. The meanings assigned to words become more adultlike as development progresses. Mastery of language both in terms of expressive and receptive skills becomes vital with the increase in social play and the child's exposure to more situations where it is necessary to communicate needs and desires in order to successfully engage in an occupation with others. Growth of communication/interaction skills leads to a strengthening of friendships in the school age child. Issues can be discussed with peers and the child becomes more aware that others may share the same view or have divergent views. Through school and cooperative play, interaction skills such as learning how to relate to a leader, and how to lead others, are acquired.

Changes occurring in the ability to follow rules are also part of interaction skills since rule following is a necessary characteristic of social life and important in occupational performance. During the years from approximately 7–10 the child is able to agree and cooperate with a partner on a common set of rules and at the same time compete to win. By approximately 11 or 12 years of age there is a fascination with rules. The child enjoys inventing new ones or elaborating on preexisting rules (19, 32, 42).

The child engages in more organized play such as team sports. Also common during this stage is the formation of clubs or gangs where children participate in choice of leader and members, design of rules, select special passwords, and plan for mutual activities.

Habituation Subsystem

As the child proceeds through late childhood internal regulation of patterned behavior increases steadily. Both roles and habits are significantly differentiated and modularized during this period.

ROLES

The range of roles which a child may enter increases markedly. The major role change is entry into the student role. This requires reorganization of the habituation subsystem as new habits must be formed to guide occupational

behavior in this role. Previous childhood roles as family member and player are affected, and require adjustment to adapt to the requirements of student role. The role of friend assumes more importance with the growing interest in strengthening peer relationships. The child's identity may now include a role in the social organizations such as the Brownies, Cub Scouts, Little League, and so on. Greater responsibility for performing household chores is now given to the child, resulting in an increased awareness and understanding of the worker role. For example, the school age child may be given specific "jobs" to perform such as safety patrol, cleaning erasers and delivering messages. Toward the end of this stage, the child may also be given responsibility to care for younger children. In all these instances, certain expectations for performance are learned and habits formed to guide behavior in these roles.

Awareness and understanding of other occupational roles is enhanced when social contacts increase to include teachers, club leaders and families of peers. Thus, more role models are provided for the child to imitate in play and continue the development of internal expectations for varied roles. The enculturation process is advanced as social horizons expand and more information related to societal expectations is acquired.

In late childhood realization of being in roles increases dramatically. The child's perception of being in the student role is seen in comments such as "I'm in the first grade," or "I go to school now." Recognition of entering this role is also illustrated in the child's desire to have certain items which are associated with a student such as a lunch box, pencil case and bookbag. The use of baseball or Scout uniforms and specific tasks which are associated with a role, such as homework, reciting pledges and attending regular meetings, also serve as means to solidify the child's perception of self as being in a specific role.

Though role of student becomes a prime focus during this stage, the general role of "child" also appears to become more clear with the child's growing interaction with the peer group and participation in the "culture of childhood" (13). The child shares with peers a common way of viewing and dealing with the world. Oral tradition passes the learning of certain jokes, sayings, riddles, and superstitions. Thus the child learns certain behaviors and language associated with the role of childhood.

HABITS

Formation of habits is centered around the support of routines in the home, school and social organizations. Previous development of self-care habits and earlier patterned behaviors assist the child in acquiring routines needed for occupational behavior during late childhood.

Habit patterns show a marked change since use of time is not confined primarily to roles of player and family member. The many hours of free play give way to a more structured time pattern as adjustment to the student role occurs. It is now required that one wake up at a certain time to be prompt in arrival at school. Self-care habits must be well organized so morning routine can be carried out efficiently. Setting aside necessary time for homework, while also allowing for time to pursue play interests requires the child to organize time to achieve a balance in activities. Parents initially guide this organization and gradually the child assumes more responsibility for time management.

Many habits which will be essential for later entry into the worker role are fostered through home, school and play environments of the child (5, 22, 26, 27, 36). Habits such as regular attendance, punctuality, industry, neatness, attention, and perseverance are acquired in school and elsewhere. Play activities promote habits of craftsmanship and sportsmanship. The enculturation process is furthered as habits are acquired which reflect the values and expectations of society. Development of these habits will be necessary for future work occupations.

Volition Subsystem

Through childhood there has been a gradual increase in the individual's ability to exercise choice in occupational behaviors. The open system cycle of the child has resulted in continuous differentiation of the volition subsystem as feedback from interactions evolves new images of personal causation, values and interests.

PERSONAL CAUSATION

New demands for performance arise and the child is confronted with the challenge of continuing to feel capable in the face of these demands. Earlier experiences of competency will be important in the child's ability to master the more complex tasks and social situations which are introduced during this period.

The child is facing new experiences which may involve competition with peers, higher skill levels, and increased feedback from adults regarding performance. This could potentially be an arousing time for the child. Expectancy of success and belief in one's skills will be important to enable the child to meet these demands. Skills developed earlier in the family and play environment will now be relevant to experiences in school and other social settings, and assist the child in believing that he or she can encounter the environment in a positive way. Erikson discusses the danger of developing a sense of inadequacy at this stage if the child "despairs of his tools and skills" (14, p 260). Efficacy of skill is important in the child's feeling that previous experiences in home and play have prepared for the entry into new environments.

Through achievements in school and participation in more varied play activities an awareness of skills is gained. Report cards may be seen as a type of information contributing to the child's belief in academic skills. Through experiences with craft projects the child may acquire a sense of having skills for tasks requiring use of tools and hand manipulation skills. Feedback from peers in activities where there may be acceptance or rejection based on skill further develops the concept of self regarding one's strengths and weaknesses.

When the child successfully meets challenges in the new roles encountered during late childhood, the development of belief in internal control is increased. Parental behaviors will also affect belief in internal control. As there is less dependency on family and as social contacts increase, the child moves toward a growing awareness that adults do not possess the absolute authority and that there are other opinions and choices of behavior which are different from those in one's own family. Thus, as the child grows older, a perception of being more equal to adults develops, along with a belief in the capacity to make one's own decisions.

VALUES

During late childhood more sources are available for acquiring cultural values relevant to occupation. Growth in symbolic capacity and the expanding social circle of the child play a role in the development of values. Rather than focusing on the external or objective aspect of a situation the child can now take into account the subjective aspect or intent, and can consider needs and desires of the group.

The child is still primarily present oriented. Towards the latter part of this period play may involve an interest in crystal balls and the Ouija board (1). Although playful activities, they show a beginning concern about the possibilities which the future may hold.

In school one is required to learn skills and master information which may not be initially rewarding and the purpose or result of this learning may be unclear. Thus, through school, a greater sense of future orientation and ability to delay gratification is gained. The child learns that society values an orientation to the future and certain requirements are necessary in the present as a preparation for future occupations. This reflects the relationship between occupational goals and orientation to time.

The child also begins to learn the meaningfulness of work and productivity. During this stage the child learns that producing things will gain recognition from others and he or she begins to internalize a sense of pleasure in work performance (14). The child may also begin to attach meaning to work through participation in chores where greater responsibility is given. For instance, small jobs such as shoveling snow or cleaning the car, will give the child a sense of being a productive individual. Meaningful leisure time occupations may include enrollment in a class for swimming or music lessons to achieve greater skill. Certain scholastic and atheletic activities, or a special activity with a friend may become meaningful as the child shows a concern to become competent and accepted in these areas.

There is a growing concern with standards of performance centered on tasks in school, social organizations and peer relationships. Standards such as neatness in work are acquired in school. The value of working together and learning to lose gracefully and not carry a grudge are standards of performance that define for the child how one should engage in varied activities.

INTERESTS

Interests become further differentiated during late childhood and the child exercises more choice in developing an interest pattern. There is less dependency on others in the environment to provide opportunities for exploration of interests. Activities can now involve more complex interactions with people and objects in the environment. This is the stage where interests revolve around games with rules, gross motor sports, finer constructions, selective collections, curiosity with nature, participation in activities with peers and membership in formal organizations (21, 42). The change in play interests also reflects the child's increased adjustment to reality. A decline in symbolic play occurs as the social world of the child expands and the child becomes more intent on adaptation to the work situation (31).

A pattern of interests begins to emerge as interests become differentiated. For example, enjoyment of music may lead the child to pursue guitar or dance lessons, and leisure time is spent rehearsing these new skills. A child's interests in a school subject may be carried over to the home environment where more time is spent reading or discussing a certain topic. A greater balance in interest pattern is now possible. The child can explore interests which provide challenge and competition such as involvement in a sport and also have interests which are more relaxing and solitary—reading.

Interests are also reflected in the stage of fantasy occupational choice which occurs during late childhood (20). Play is used as the opportunity to choose and project self into varied occupational roles. These choices are based on interests and do not take into consideration capacities and limitations.

SUMMARY

Through the course of childhood development the differentiation and integration of the three subsystems takes place. Table 7.1 summarizes these processes in the three stages of childhood. Development of performance skills has enabled the child to engage the environment in increasingly complex ways. Skills have become organized into habits to guide occupational behavior in the emerging roles of child, family member, player, friend, organizational participant, and student. The child's active engagement with the environment has resulted in images of personal causation and the development of values and interests. In turn, as development has progressed, the child can now exercise more choice in occupational behaviors which reflect his or her interests and values.

The information which the child receives from the environment, the manner in which it is processed and the behavioral response reflect the dominant motive of each stage: exploration, competence or achievement. Play is vital as a vehicle for the differentiation of the subsystems. Sensory integrative processes have also influ-

Table 7.1.
Developmental changes in childhood occupational behavior

Early childhood	Middle childhood	Late childhood
VOLITION		

Personal causation

Early childhood	Middle childhood	Late childhood
Sensory experiences in play serve as a foundation for a feeling of control. The child increasingly forms an image of self as distinct and, therefore, capable of having effects on the environment	Increased awareness of selfhood results in an image of personal abilities. Choices in play provide a sense of increasing internal control Experiences of success and failure differentiate personal causation making images of ability more realistic	Increasing expectations for performance demand increased belief in skills, and provide opportunities to further test and develop a sense of ability. Developing a sense of adequacy is central at this age. While play is still important, school and other activities become arenas for peformance, testing skill, and receiving feedback about capacities and limitations

Values

Early childhood	Middle childhood	Late childhood
Parental expectations and values shape childhood play, and images of what behavior is acceptable and unacceptable	Value orientation begins to emerge, manifest in a sense of time, and awareness of the value of social norms and peer and parent values. Values are increasingly a factor in decisions for behavior	Growth in symbolic ability and increased social contact allow the child to grasp values more fully, including an increasing orientation toward future goals. The child begins to encounter meanings related to occupation and internalize standards of performance relevant to school and other settings

Interests

Early childhood	Middle childhood	Late childhood
Interests are closely tied to neuromuscular development since the child enjoys practicing and exploring his/her capabilities. Interests first center on sensory motor experiences, producing actions centered around the body, and later having effects in the environment	Increases in perceptual motor and communication skills lead to a broadening of interests. Interests which extend over time begin to emerge. Interests are still related to optimal arousal and feelings of competence. Environment becomes more critical in shaping interests	Interests are further differentiated as the child's opportunities for choice expand. Growing activities lead to interests in more complex activities. Interests also become more refined and specific. Occupational choice is now dominated by interests

HABITUATION

Roles

Early childhood	Middle childhood	Late childhood
Child is recognized as being in the role of a player. Parents are critical for initiating and fostering this role. Expectations are few initially, and later center on where, how and with what the child can play. Family role emerges toward the end of this period, but expectations are minimal	Consciousness of family role increases with conformity to home life routines. Family role responsibility increases with growing partipation in chores. Observing role models and sociodramatic play enhances understanding of roles. Games become arenas for role taking. Realism in roles becomes an in-	Range of roles increases markedly, including the student role and roles in social groups such as clubs and spontaneous peer groups. Increased responsibility at home moves the child toward greater understanding of the worker role. Role identity increases and the child has concern for the

Table 7.1.—Continued

Early childhood	Middle childhood	Late childhood
	creasing concern in the child's play. Friendship role begins to emerge	objects associated with roles. The role of being a child becomes clearer as the child participates in the culture of childhood

Habits

There is a gradual trend from biological and parental regulation of patterned behavior. A sense of routine is internalized. Behaviors show recognition of daily routines. The child begins to internalize self-help routines	Increased self-regulation of everyday behavior and growing conformity to social norms is manifest. Beginning work habits emerge and through social contacts and play child learns habits of intellectual discipline, self-control and so on	Habits are formed around routines of school, home and social organizations. Habits change with initiation of new roles and their demands for time use and behavior. Habits essential to the worker rule as punctuality, attention and perseverance emerge. Societal expectations are increasingly reflected in habits

PERFORMANCE

Skill constituents

Nervous system is central in early childhood, serving as the governing system for the musculoskeletal system and the substratum of symbolization. Reflexes become integrated into the central nervous system allowing cortical control and more complex adaptation. Neuromuscular and symbolic constituents co-develop, each contributing to the other's organization and maturation	Reflexes continue to be integrated into the central nervous system allowing more coordinated action. The child can isolate movements and coordinates movements and perceptions into more complex performances such as riding a bike. This is made possible by the integrative role of the central nervous system and sensory integration processes	Maturation of neurological and musculoskeletal constituents allows greater speed, accuracy, and coordination. Increase in symbolic functions is manifest in the child's attainment of concrete operational thought at about age 7.
Symbolic constituent emerges as nervous system interacts with the environment and symbols begin to supervene in nervous system functions. Symbolization is initially linked to, and later dissociated from, action.	Symbolic functions continue to develop with elaboration of multiple representational systems such as imitation, mental images, symbolic play, and so on	Imagery now has a more dynamic nature allowing the child to attune to transformations and steps between beginning and end states

Perceptual Motor Skills

Child gradually comes to dissociate movements, which allows greater control in gross and fine motor actions. Child progresses from head control to ability to stand and ambulate. Spatial perception and body awareness increases, facilitating perceptual motor skills	Child seeks out vestibular play activities leading to further development of perceptual motor skills. Perceptual motor development is reflected in increased command of tools and use of constructive toys	Refinement of gross motor skills allows participation in group games and sports. Focus of development is on speed and coordination and precision in fine motor skills.

Table 7.1.—Continued

Early childhood	Middle childhood	Late childhood
Process Skills		
Means-ends behavior represents emergence of process skills. Child begins simple problem solving such as removing obstacles. Since exploration is limited, early problem solving does not show substantial creativity or novelty	As basic skills require less attention more information processing can be used for task analysis. Advances in cognitive thought now allow the child to plan ahead. Child has more opportunities to make decisions, use strategies, and operationalize themes in play	Problem solving and ability to explore alternatives is greatly expanded.
Communication/Interaction Skills		
Newborn responds to sounds, but vocalizations are not articulate. By 28 weeks the infant is familiar with facial expressions, gestures and postural attitudes. The child progresses from crying to making needs known through gestures, facial expressions and words. Participation in early simple games is the beginning of more complex social interaction. At 1 year the child can repeat words, understand simple directions, and at 2 can relate experience and has a remarkably expanded vocabulary	Structure and form of language become essentially complete. With increased communication ability, interaction becomes complex involving play with other children in which social skills such as taking turns and sharing are acquired and practiced.	Communication becomes more sophisticated in terms of syntax, semantics and vocabulary. Increased communication ability allows participation in more complex occupations requiring ability to convey desires, plans and so on. Rule-following ability progresses. Later there is a fascination with creating rules. Team sports provide opportunities for complex interactions in various roles. Knowledge and ability to cooperate with others on rules increases.

(At this age children still have trouble fully understanding rules—how they're decided and why they can be changed in different situations, etc. Ability to be more reflective in rules will come with adolescence) |

enced the child's occupational performance by contributing to the development of more complex skills and fostering positive emotional development. Experiences in childhood have provided many of the foundations for future entry into more formal occupational roles. The effectiveness of interactions and competence developed during childhood will contribute to the child's ability to adapt to the developmental tasks and roles of adolescence.

References

1. Arnaud SH: The dramatic play of six-to-ten year olds. In Engstrom G (ed): *Play: The Child Strives Toward Self-Realization*, (Proceedings of a conference). Washington, D.C., National Association for the Education of Young Children, 1971.
2. Ayres AJ: *Sensory Integration and Learning Disorders*. Los Angeles, Western Psychological Services, 1972.
3. Ayres AJ: *Sensory Integration and the Child*. Los Angeles, Western Psychological Services, 1979.
4. Ayres AJ: *Sensory Integration Theory Workshop*. Cincinnati, Ohio, June, 1981.
5. Bailey DM: Vocational theories and work habits related to childhood development. *Am J Occup Ther* 25:298–302, 1971.
6. Brown NS: Three-year-olds' play. In Engstrom G (ed): *Play: The Child Strives Toward Self-Realization*, (Proceedings of a conference). Washington, D.C., National Association for The Education of Young Children, 1971.

7. Bruner J: The nature and uses of immaturity. *Am Psychol* 27:687–708, 1972.
8. Bruner J: Organization of early skilled action. *Child Dev* 44:1–11, 1973.
9. Curry NE, Tittnich E: Four-year-olds' play. In Engstrom G (ed): *Play: The Child Strives Toward Self-Realization*, (Proceedings of a conference). Washington, D.C., National Association for the Education of Young Children, 1971.
10. DeCharms R: *Personal Causation: The Internal Affective Determinants of Behavior.* New York, Academic Press, 1968.
11. DeCharms R: Personal causation and perceived control. In Perlmutter LC, Monty RA (eds): *Choice and perceived control.* Hillsdale, NJ, Lawrence Erlbaum Associates, 1979.
12. DeQuiros JB, Schrager OL: *Neurophysiological Fundamentals in Learning Disabilities.* San Rafael, Calif, Academic Therapy, 1978.
13. Elkind D: *The Hurried Child.* Reading, Mass, Addison-Wesley, 1981.
14. Erikson E: *Childhood and Society* (ed 2). New York, Norton, 1963.
15. Frost JL, Klein BL: *Children's Play and Playgrounds.* Boston, Allyn & Bacon, 1979.
16. Gardner DB: The child as an open system: conference summary and implications. In Engstrom G (ed): *Play: The Child Strives Toward Self-Realization*, (Proceedings of a conference). Washington, D.C., National Association for the Education of Young Children, 1971.
17. Gesell A, et al: *The First Five Years of Life.* New York, Harper Row, 1940.
18. Gilfoyle EM, Grady AP, Moore JC: *Children Adapt.* Thorough-fare, NJ, Charles B. Slack, 1981.
19. Ginsburg H, Opper S: *Piaget's theory of intellectual development* (ed 2). Englewood Cliffs, NJ, Prentice-Hall, 1979.
20. Ginzberg E: *Occupational Choice.* New York, Columbia University Press, 1956.
21. Hartley R, Goldenson M: *The Complete Book of Children's Play.* New York, Crowell, 1957.
22. Hurff JM: A play skills inventory: a competency monitoring tool for the 10-year-old. *Am J Occup Ther* 34:651–656, 1980.
23. Jacklin CN, Maccoby EE, Dick AE: Barrier behavior and toy preference: sex differences (and their absence) in the year-old child. *Child Dev* 44:196–200, 1973.
24. Knox SH: A play scale. In Reilly M (ed): *Play As Exploratory Learning.* Beverly Hills, Calif, Sage, 1974.
25. Lindquist JE, Mack W, Parham LD: A synthesis of occupational behavior and sensory integration concepts in theory and practice, part 1. Theoretical foundations. *Am J Occup Ther* 36:365–374, 1982.
26. Matsutsuyu J: Occupational behavior: a perspective on work and play. *Am J Occup Ther* 25:291–294, 1971.
27. Mauer P: Antecedents of work behavior. *Am J Occup Ther* 25:295–297, 1971.
28. Mead GH: *Mind, Self, and Society.* Chicago, University of Chicago Press, 1934.
29. Michelman S: Play and the deficit child. In Reilly M (ed): *Play as Exploratory Learning.* Beverly Hills, Calif, Sage, 1974.
30. Newman B, Newman P: *Infancy and Childhood.* New York, Wiley, 1978.
31. Piaget J: *Play, Dreams and Imitation in Childhood.* New York, Norton, 1962.
32. Piaget J, Inhelder B: *The Psychology of the Child.* New York, Basic Books, 1969.
33. Reilly M (ed): *Play as Exploratory Learning.* Beverly Hills, Calif, Sage 1974.
34. Robinson AL: Play, the arena for acquisition of rules for competent behavior. *Am J Occup Ther* 31:248–253, 1977.
35. Sarnet HB, Netsky MG: *Evolution of the Nervous System.* New York, Oxford University Press, 1974.
36. Shannon PD: Occupational choice: decision-making play. In Reilly M (ed): *Play as Exploratory Learning.* Beverly Hills, Calif, Sage 1974.
37. Smilansky S: Can adults facilitate play in children?: Theoretical and practical considerations. In Engstrom G (ed): *Play: The Child Strives Toward Self-Realization*, (Proceedings of a conference). Washington, D.C., National Association for the Education of Young Children, 1971.
38. Sperry RW: A modified concept of consciousness. *Psychol Rev* 76:532–536, 1969.
39. Sperry RW: An objective approach to subjective experience: further explanation of a hypothesis. *Psychol Rev* 77:585–590, 1970.
40. Sutton-Smith B: The playful modes of knowing. In Engstrom G (ed): *Play: The Child Strives Toward Self-Realization*, (Proceedings of a conference). Washington, D.C., National Association for the Education of Young Children, 1971.
41. Sutton-Smith B: A "sportive" theory of play. In Schwartzman HB (ed): *Play and Culture.* West Point, NY, Leisure Press, 1980.
42. Takata N. Play as a prescription. In Reilly M (ed): *Play as Exploratory Learning.* Beverly Hills, Calif, Sage, 1974.

Suggested Readings for Sensory Integration Theory

Ayres AJ: Learning disabilities and the vestibular system. *J Learn Dis* 11:18–29, 1978.
Ayres AJ: *Sensory Integration and the Child.* Los Angeles, Western Psychological Services, 1979.
Ayres AJ, Tickle LS: Hyper-responsivity to touch and vestibular stimulation as a predictor of positive response to sensory-integrative procedures by autistic children. *Am J Occup Ther* 34:375–381, 1980.
Ayres AJ, Mailloux Z: Influence of sensory integration procedures on language development. *Am J Occup Ther* 35:383–390, 1981.
Larson K: The sensory history of developmentally delayed children with and without tactile defensiveness. *Am J Occup Ther* 36:590–596, 1982.
Montgomery P (Ed): *The Vestibular System: An Annotated Bibliography.* Los Angeles, Center for the Study of Sensory Integrative Dysfunction, 1981.
Price A, Gilfoyle E, Meyers C (eds): *Research in Sensory Integrative Development.* Rockville, Md, American Occupational Therapy Association, 1976.
Royeen CB, Lesinski G, Ciani S, Schneider D: Relationship of the southern California sensory integration test, the southern California postrotary nystagmus test, and clinical observations accompanying them to evaluations in otolaryngology, ophthalmology, and audiology: two descriptive case studies. *Am J Occup Ther* 1981, 35:443–450.

CHAPTER 8

Adolescence

Roann Barris and Gary Kielhofner

AN OVERVIEW OF ADOLESCENCE

Traditionally, adolescence has been viewed as a unique period of stress and turmoil. Classical views of adolescence as a time of storm and stress have focused on both the intrapersonal and sociocultural factors as influencing this stage of development (1, 24). Psychodynamic theories, for example, emphasize the processes of disengagement from the family and the increasing individuation of the adolescent, concomitant with psychosexual development, as contributing to the turmoil of this period, while sociological theories describe adolescence as a social problem, created by industrialization and technologicalization of modern society (1, 20, 24, 35). Such writers argue that the period of adolescence is an unnecessary artifact of complex modern society in which the transition from childhood is prolonged by extensive schooling, a lack of clear rites of passage for entry into adulthood, and an economic system which does not require adolescents to be highly productive (20, 35). Historians support this perspective by marking the change from the preindustrial practice of sending out young people to apprentice with and work for other families, to the post industrial revolution identification of teen-age boys with the outside work world and girls with home, to an increase in years of mandatory schooling as a partial response to child abuse at work and, finally, to the prolonged schooling so characteristic of many middle-class adolescents today (59).

However, to view adolescence as being both a developmental stage involving intraindividual changes as well as the result of social and historical conditions may have the most validity, and similarly be most useful in understanding why some adolescents make the transition from childhood to adulthood with ease while others do not. That is, different social and psychological issues may be central to different persons at various points in their development, and different means of resolving these issues will also be available to them. For example, an adolescent may experience stress because he or she feels ready and wants to assume adult roles, yet these roles may not be expected of or available to the adolescent (24). Stress may also arise when the adolescent has a limited conceptualization of the possibilities or opportunities for growth and development (42).

Recognizing adolescence as both a developmental and sociocultural phenomenon makes it difficult to establish boundaries around it. Most people associate the beginning of adolescence with both biological (prepuberty) and institutional (junior high school) changes (21, 39). Others suggest that adolescence begins when the individual believes he or she should be accorded adult privileges but is nevertheless still denied these (49). The end of adolescence is also equivocal, and may coincide with entry into the worker role or with other typical social markers of adult social status (e.g. voting rights) (21, 39, 49). The ambiguities surrounding the beginning and end of this period are apparent in such examples as a 15-year-old mother, the adolescent who contributes to the family income and helps bring up the youngest children, and the 30 year old who is still in graduate school and uncommitted to a worker role. The themes of this chapter concerning adolescence are summarized in Table 8.1.

The Volition Subsystem

Adolescence is characterized by a push for autonomy or self-assertion (35, 48). Self-assertion involves the development of a personal philosophy or set of values, of interests, and of increased responsibility for decision-making, and reflects feelings of mastery in one's life (35, 48). This urge for autonomy reaches its peak during adolescence because intellectual, cognitive and emotional capacities for the first time allow the person to experience greater depths of awareness, to see things in terms of good *and* bad, rather than either/or, and to comprehend the world through one's own perspective as well as that of others (35, 48).

Table 8.1.
Adolescent development

VOLITION

Personal Causation

The adolescent must maintain confidence in self while facing new demands and challenges

The adolescent strives toward greater control both in present and future in terms of long-term goals

There is generally a transformation from external to internal control in adolescence, but environmental factors, especially parental styles, can affect feelings of control

New demands for skills in new settings may raise both present and future uncertainties over personal skill and potential for success

Women may have less expectancy of success in adolescence because of socialization practices which tend not to prepare young women for the challenges of a work world and, instead, communicate expectations for a more passive homemaker role

Feelings of ability are critical for occupational choice; external factors such as unemployment may raise fears about skills and control and affect the choice process

Values

Maturation of values in adolescence is influenced by growing capacity for abstract thought resulting in concern with universal ethical guidelines

Central to adolescence is the formation of a values system based on value exploration

Family, peers and historical events influence the adolescent's value system

The adolescent becomes increasingly future oriented, develops a sense of ownership of life and feels responsibility for personal destiny

Coupled with the increasing awareness of time may be a sense of urgency and of the demand for responsibility in the future

The adolescent must achieve a sense of meaning in work and play, realizing the purpose of productive activity and the significance of leisure

The lack of worthwhile work for the modern adolescent serves as an impediment to achieving a sense of the meaning of work

The adolescent must develop a growing sense of standards that pertain to work and to the demands others will make of him/her in the worker role; this is at first general and then more specific during preparation for a particular line of work

The most important goal for adolescents is the eventual acquisition of a worker identity and role

Interests

Interests change as the adolescent attempts to develop the wisdom and skills to enjoy leisure

Interest change focuses on movement out of family-centered activities and reflects the influence of peers and fads

Adolescent interests represent a degree of experimentation with risk in an attempt to achieve a sense of self and of control

Social environment, geography and culture are influences on the pattern of interests developed

Adolescents require actual experience with activities in order to fully discriminate and realize potency of interests

HABITUATION

Roles

Adolescence is a time of role transition, role ambiguity and, above all, role experimentation as the adolescent leaves the roles of childhood and moves toward adult roles

An overall adolescent role influences all other roles of the adolescent, leading to transformation characterized by an increased expectation for autonomy and responsibility in continuing roles such as the family, friend, and student roles

The adolescent may also face and have to deal with discrepancies between expectations for responsibility and freedom

New roles become available to the adolescent for experimentation as the adolescent has access to dating, student government, organized sports, work, volunteerism, and so on

With increasing roles and role demands the adolescent faces the task of balancing and integrating roles

Table 8.1.—*Continued*

Habits

New habits must be developed as the adolescent enters a new school system and begins preparation for the demands of work

With increased autonomy the adolescent must develop more organized habits for time use

Adolescents must also learn habits of industriousness and efficiency for adequate performance in adult roles

PERFORMANCE

Skills

The musculoskeletal constituent of skills undergoes a period of rapid growth

Nervous system maturation allows emergence of the final level of symbolic capacity as the adolescent reaches the stage of formal operations, fully capable of abstract thought

Changes in school and other environments make demands for new skills; additionally, the adolescent may begin to develop skills specific to a line of work

OCCUPATIONAL CHOICE

Adolescence is dominated by the need to choose an occupation and thus enter adulthood

Environmental factors including family, social class, school, and adults in all settings potentially influence occupational choice

---

As the adolescent is seeking increasing self-direction in his or her life, various social groups, such as family, school and other organizations, begin to expect the adolescent to take more initiative and responsibility for actions. Adolescents must successfully learn to make choices which bring personal satisfaction and meaning and which also satisfy others in the social surround. Responsible self-determination, the product of a successful adolescence, accrues from a number of transformations in the volition subsystem as the adolescent becomes more acutely aware of both the freedom to choose his or her life-style, and the need to define values and interests, and to feel competent. In this way, adolescence poses both an opportunity for tremendous personal growth and transformation and a potential threat as one strives for identity (15).

PERSONAL CAUSATION

The development of personal causation during the period of adolescence involves maintaining confidence in oneself while facing new demands and challenges, experiencing a desire and need for more personal control, and having to acquire new skills and perform tasks in new settings. The adolescent's sense of personal causation must also be oriented to future circumstances—success can no longer be measured only in short-term goals, but must begin to incorporate goals of performance in future roles.

Locus of Control

A transformation from external to internal control characterizes adolescence (27, 28). The subculture in which adolescents live has a significant impact on the development of an internal locus of control. Social class, for instance, may affect the development of an internal locus of control because of the types of family experiences open to the adolescent. Children of more affluent families tend to have more opportunities for self-determination of their leisure activities, whereas children in less affluent families may be limited to more family-centered and, consequently, less self-determined leisure (32). Child-rearing practices can influence locus of control; e.g. parents who combine a high degree of support with a high degree of control tend to raise children who are conforming and submissive (55). Geography can also influence locus of control through the degree of independence which can be assumed by the adolescent. Thus, adolescents who live in isolated areas and must rely on their parents to drive them to settings and activities which interest them may feel more externally controlled than those with easy accessibility to places of interest (43).

Expectancy of Success and Belief in Skills

In addition to the more general task of achieving internal control, adolescents face a number of new situations which influence their expectancy of success or failure, and their belief in skill and its efficacy. Even adolescents who have generated a sense of belief in skill and found their repertoire of skills relevant to family, school and other settings may now experience a number of uncertainties. The adolescent begins to encounter new settings (e.g. an intensive peer group, junior high, high school, college, and job training) all of which demand the performance of old skills under new conditions or the acquisition of new skills. These circumstances focus attention on the issue of personal causation. Although the successes of childhood provide a foundation for feelings of competence, the adolescent is confronted with the task of remaking a sense of skillfulness and efficacy.

The transition from elementary to junior high school may be particularly critical in terms of the adolescent's belief in skill and efficacy. Self-esteem, which includes one's belief in the likelihood of success, has been shown to decrease significantly in 11- and 12-year olds (50). In a large scale study children who did not change to a junior high school at the same age did not show a comparable drop in self-esteem; thus, this decrease seems more probably related to the changed social environment, rather than to such factors as the onset of puberty (50).

Female adolescents may have lower expectations for success than do males (48) and, to some extent, they may be socialized to become incompetent, or at least to view themselves as incompetent, in certain types of tasks (48). In high school, for instance, the attitude that girls should not be smart and, in particular, that they should not be smart in math or science, continues to be communicated by many teachers and textbooks (5). A large percentage of bright, capable young women in college also appear to revise downwardly their occupational goals toward "acceptable" female occupations (25). However, this characteristic, which has been labeled a "fear of success," may occur *not* because these women lack belief in their abilities but because they think they *can* succeed, and they fear the consequences that success might bring (25).

The expectancy of success in adult occupational roles is especially important. Awareness of factors such as high unemployment or high skill levels needed for a desired occupation may evoke feelings of concern over the possibility of future success. In fact, concern over success may lead many adolescents to choose a work role that does not represent their ideal but seems more within reach of their capabilities (36).

As the adolescent faces the sometimes foreign arena of work he or she may wonder about the efficacy of his or her skills. Even when one has acquired skills and is aware of it, one cannot help but wonder whether skills used in hobbies, in chores, or on the basketball court will have any relevance to the factory or the office. Adolescents' concern over the relevance of their education and/or job training to the skill demands of anticipated occupations is sometimes reflected in a focus on technical aspects of the job. This, however, may be discrepant with the goals of educators and/or trainers who stress professional, judgmental, client-oriented, or ideological aspects of the job (36).

VALUES

A central aim of adolescence is the formation of a value system (31, 35, 38, 52). Although the commitment to a particular set of values cannot be accomplished without a period of conflict, this crisis and resulting choice ultimately lead to the achievement of a personal identity (38, 52).

The maturation of values during adolescence is influenced by the growing capacity of the adolescent for abstract thought (i.e. a symbolic component of the performance subsystem). Because the adolescent can perform more complicated mental judgments, he or she can internalize a clearer and more personal sense of values. Another major force influencing adolescent value formation is the movement of the adolescent beyond social groups where values were prescribed and enforced (e.g. family and primary school). The adolescent experiences an increased freedom to select values; it is through this autonomy of value exploration that the adolescent eventually arrives at a personal system of values (56).

At the same time, the peer group, which typically holds values at variance with mainstream values, begins to play a major socializing role. Within the peer group, adolescents may create a subculture that embodies values which directly conflict with prevailing cultural values. The adolescent rituals which express these values (e.g. whatever the currently popular forms of music, hairstyle, or clothing may be) function as a critique of traditional authority and allow the adolescent to resolve conflicts created by the gap between the reality and ideal of school and work (24). Adolescents who can bridge this gap are more likely to identify closely with the formal values of school and work, rather than with the "subterranean" values of play (24).

Although popular cliches suggest otherwise, most adolescents agree with their parents on most issues (19, 29), and many adolescents adopt the work values, and even the careers, of their parents (48). Interestingly, when children and their parents have similar goals, there is more likely to be concordance between the goals of the adolescent and his or her friends as well (33, 51). In addition, many adolescents' values reflect older standards (10, 54). For example, a survey of high school students' values in the late 1970s found that in terms of work, girls ranked the goal of helping others as most important to them, whereas boys ranked high income and leadership as most important (54). However, adolescents with less traditional attitudes may actually have a more fully realized self-identity, since the choice of nontraditional beliefs often represents the consideration of a wider range of alternatives prior to selecting and committing oneself to a set of values (52).

For the same reasons that values mature during adolescence, moral reasoning also develops. Because they have achieved the level of formal operations in their thinking, and because this is a period of intense idealism and questioning, adolescents move beyond the initial egocentric reward or punishment type of moral thinking that characterizes childhood. Early adolescence tends to be characterized by conventional moral thinking, e.g. one conforms to the morals of peers or to the conventions of society. During later adolescence, one begins to search for more universal and ethical guidelines. Two basic moral issues emerge to dominate the decision making of young men and women. For men, the moral issue tends to be a concern for equality and fairness, and respecting the rights of others, whereas for women, the moral issue is one of caring, discerning and alleviating the troubles of the world (17). Ideally, a morality which blends both these concerns needs to be embraced by young men and women.

Temporal Orientation

During middle adolescence, the individual comprehends the future more fully and achieves the notion that one's life is a span of time with a beginning and an end. The adolescent comes to realize that his or her life is a personal possession (8). Along with this deepened appreciation of time and its personal nature, the adolescent receives messages from others that he or she is now expected to become oriented to the future, especially to the selection of an occupation (11). Because the future and the need to prepare for it take on new importance, the adolescent begins to see the present in a new light: present and future are more clearly linked, with future long-term outcomes being a function of previous behavior (11). The adolescent who previously was able to deal with the future largely in terms of fantasy now experiences it as real and cogent. There is a perceived sense of urgency of time as the previously distant "adult future" is suddenly looming ahead quite closely. The adolescent must either make a definite decision to move ahead into an occupation or to begin secondary preparation for an occupation in college.

Thus, it is accurate to say that for the adolescent, the future takes on gradual importance as a comprehensible, real and demanding time period. The present takes on new meaning as a determinant of the future. The present-dominated world of the child gives way to a new temporal orientation which emphasizes what one will become as time passes.

Meaningfulness of Activities

Along with the social expectations for entry into adult occupational roles, the adolescent should be achieving a sense of the meaning of productive and leisure activity, its personal significance and its place in the social order. The adolescent potentially develops a variety of meaningful occupations (e.g. driving and dating as leisure activities symbolizing adult maturity; hobbies as representations of a personal creative self; chores as a means of contributing to family well-being.) Further, the meaning of leisure for many adolescents may be that it is an opportunity to rehearse future lifestyles (24). Even television watching may share this meaning, as one's preference for types of shows may reflect beliefs in using skill, strategy, or relying on chance to get ahead in life (24).

However, the most pressing issue of adolescence becomes identifying a sense of meaning about work. Identifying with a worker (parent or acquaintance) is one of the most important steps one takes in achieving a sense of the meaning of work. If parents talk animatedly about their work and share some of its products with the adolescent, the meaning of work is likely to be different than if the parent returns from a hard and boring labor, exhausted and seeking solace and escape from the work day.

In addition to identifying with work as a meaningful activity via exposure to adult role models, the adolescent is exposed to a larger set of social conditions that influence the type of work he or she is likely to find significant and the general meaning of work that emerges out of the adolescent experience. For instance, during times of relative economic health, the adolescent may be more likely to view work in terms of its potential for contribution to society and its influence on people. During times of high unemployment and economic stress, adolescents tend to appreciate work more in terms of its immediate pay-off and its potential for a secure economic future.

The lack of worthwhile work for adolescents may be the single greatest predicament of adolescence (35). Adolescents need to do something meaningful, and the absence of work disrupts the balance of work, rest and play, denies the adolescent a feeling of worth, and distorts the meaning of work. Much of the discontent of youth stems from having little of importance to do; the resulting apathy comes from their insight that they are being denied access to involvements that would allow them to grow optimally (35). The family, too, can stifle the adolescent's opportunity to find meaning when the parents hold a monopoly on significant work.

In the end, whether an adolescent forms an image of work as a potentially fulfilling activity with obvious contributions to the welfare of society, as an opportunity for creative expression or use of personal skills, as a means of achieving status and worth along with financial security or, conversely, as a necessary evil for survival, likely to be boring and unconnected to any obvious good, depends on the adolescent's exposure to the world of work and to social values about human productivity, and on the general cultural values and economic conditions. Thus, one psychologist writes that, "without the hope of work that serves the healthy development of self and society, adolescent values curdle into cynicism and the young escape into speedy gratification through fantasy and drugs." (Ref 37, p A6).

Standards of Performance

As the adolescent faces the reality of long-term demands for performance in occupation

and as he or she searches for personal identity, standards of performance become increasingly of concern. They center on the quality and style of productive work and its ethicality. The adolescent develops a sense of pride in work and personal responsibility largely from experiences in the family (57). He or she achieves a growing sense of the importance of work both in terms of necessity as a part of the human condition and in terms of its reimbursability. Standards relating to doing things correctly, concern for the impact of one's efforts on others and such values as "giving an honest day's labor for an honest day's wages" emerge during this period. Experiences in high school such as collaborating on the production of a play or prom, sports, volunteering, and so forth, provide opportunities for the adolescent to comprehend the importance of working as a part of the team and giving one's all—standards that define how one should participate in both work and leisure social pursuits. The peer group, especially, is an important source of learning socially acceptable norms of behavior (31, 35, 48).

In addition to more general standards of performance, the adolescent internalizes particular standards related to a specific chosen occupation. This occurs as the adolescent comes to the final phases of occupational choice (e.g. if I want to be an accountant I will have to work hard and be exact in my work) and during the early phases of job training, whether it be vocational preparation or on-the-job training. Young persons in job training and apprenticeships are socialized into attitudes about what is important on the job. For instance, apprentices in steelwork on skyscrapers learn that the ability to give and take constant teasing (part of a process of assuring others whose life is often in one's hands that one is not the kind of person who carries a grudge) is critical (23). Beauticians learn to subordinate technical skills to a patron-centered attitude—thus, interpersonal dealings gain increasing importance over the technical aspects of their work (40). The "ethics" of allowing a patron to choose an unbecoming hairstyle is the kind of consideration that comes to be valued as part of a "professional beautician's standards of performance." In similar fashion, barbers' apprentices learn the importance of a careful job over giving many haircuts in the course of the day (58).

Occupational Goals

The most important aspect of adolescence for the achievement of a personal identity is the need to select an occupation (2). Common language expresses this importance in the recurring question of "what are you going to be when you grow up?" Whether by virtue of social press or personal desire, the adolescent comes to see the absolute importance of setting and achieving a goal of entering the world of adult productivity, either through paid labor or a homemaker role. Adolescence is also a time of looking forward to other adult roles which have an occupational component; the adolescent begins to consider marriage and parenthood, for instance, as goals for the future. The termination of adolescence means, in large part, the achievement of adult status through entry into adult occupational roles. Indeed, all of adolescence is a process of achieving the goals of adult status.

In sum, adolescence is a period of important value formation. The adolescent achieves an autonomous personal status as a self-regulated individual guided by values which specify the importance of the future and attaining goals, the meaning of adult work and leisure, and standards of performance which reflect larger ethical concerns as well as the situational demands of a particular occupation. Adolescence is truly a time of blooming of values. Because the task of acquiring a set of values is complex and because the sources of values in society are many and sometimes contradictory, the adolescent generally struggles with the process of value formation. The task is often one of tempering ideal values with the reality of life (24, 35). The adolescent who successfully achieves a first set of values acquires both a unique personal identity and a social identity which makes him or her acceptable to society at large and to a particular occupation or professional group.

INTERESTS

As with values and personal causation, interests undergo a major transformation during adolescence. Because adolescence is a period of substantial leisure time, developing the wisdom and skills to enjoy leisure is a critical task (24, 31).

One of the primary influences on interest change is the movement of the individual out of the family setting, where interests are often family-centered, into a peer group where new interests are espoused (31). In addition, interests change because the adolescent is recognized as being mature and capable of handling the responsibility associated with certain activities. Such diverse activities as social drinking, driving

a car, and using a gun for hunting represent the kind of newly available interests to the adolescent on the basis of increased social confidence in the maturity of the adolescent. Adolescent interests also represent a degree of experimentation with risk. The use of drugs and alcohol and speeding in automobiles in association with social recreation are examples of this. Finally, adolescents' interests become more of an expression of self-identity (12). Adolescents choose activities that say, in essence, I have control of my life; this is who I am and want to be. Leisure activities may also epitomize a life-style that is diametrically opposed to school and work. Thus, activities may be important for the chance to be hedonistic and spontaneous, and because they are exciting (24).

Discrimination and Pattern

In many ways the differentiation of interests in adolescence is a function of the particular peers of the adolescent (57). The rural adolescent who takes a job as a laborer or begins work on a farm after high school is likely to develop interests around hunting, four-wheel drive pickups, country-western music and the local fire rescue squad. The ivy league college student is more likely to be channeled into interest in intellectual games such as chess, cultural events, and participation in social-political activities. Both sets of interests represent a growing personal style, an orientation to socially accepted leisure and amateur pursuits, and a maturation of interests to show social and civic concern. Their pattern is in terms of the local milieu and its opportunities and established preferences.

Adolescent interests are particularly influenced by fads mediated and extolled by the adolescent peer group. For example, jogging is probably a more popular interest today than during the 1960s. Simply hanging around talking with peers becomes a major interest of adolescence (13). Sports in general are important interests for adolescents; traditionally this has been more so for men than women (13), although the pattern may be changing. Grooming and personal appearance are also major preoccupations during adolescence (13, 26), and often lead to an increase in magazine reading (48). Music plays an important role during adolescence. The themes of rock songs reflect problems and dreams of adolescents, and listening to music or playing an instrument gives adolescents a way to cope with their own feelings (48).

Potency

The issue of potency is especially critical in adolescence. The adolescent whose interests are based on adequate past experiences will be able to make more efficacious decisions. Interests based on vicarious experience, on passive observation, may be more fantasy-based than real (16). When the adolescent makes choices based on unrealistic interests, he or she may be in for a surprise when the interest is actualized in the choice. This is particularly consequential if the choice is for a job. The potency of interests in adolescence may be particularly problemmatical for two reasons. First, peer pressure may actually have more to do with interests than experience with, or satisfaction gained in, participation in an activity. Secondly, adolescents who are rich in information (via television, school, etc.) but poor in experience may develop interests which lack a sufficient basis in experience. Thus, the adolescent who develops a healthy set of interests is one who has had adequate opportunities to try out various activities and to experience like and dislike. Such an adolescent both understands what it is to find some occupation interesting and will develop a set of interests more clearly founded in action.

The Habituation Subsystem

Adolescence is a period of transformation in the roles and habits which regulate everyday behavior. The adolescent assumes an increasing variety of roles which are less circumscribed and externally regulated, and more complex, than were childhood family-centered roles. Because these roles are more complex, the individual emerges from adolescence with a more complex set of habits as well, able to regulate his or her own typical behavior and concomitantly freer of external sources of regulation.

ROLES

Some developmental theorists speak of an "adolescent role," characterized by marginal status (i.e. no longer a child, but not yet an adult) and ambiguous expectations (e.g. adults want the adolescent to grow up and assume adult tasks and responsibility, but do not feel comfortable giving the freedom that goes along with it). Adolescents are, nevertheless, engaged in a process of trying on many of the roles they will hold as adults. Role experimentation fills several needs for adolescents. It helps them to consoli-

date their identity (48), it allows them to satisfy some of their desire for status and independence, and it enables them to learn to deal with role expectations and to recognize their limits or capacities to meet the requirements for particular roles (35).

Role Expectations in Adolescence

The adolescent role is a kind of macro role which colors and influences the adolescent's other roles (e.g. roles as family member, student). Thus, while some roles continue from childhood into adolescence, the nature of those roles and expectations associated with them begin to change. The student role is exemplary in this regard. In childhood, the student role is largely a clear-cut status; the child is a student, and is expected to exist and function as a student. The adolescent in high school and college is still a student, but now the student role is related to becoming a worker. The role itself becomes transitional, and successful completion in order to enter work is increasingly emphasized. In similar fashion, the family role becomes transformed. Parents may see adolescents as becoming more responsible for taking care of themselves (e.g. buying their own clothes, cooking meals for themselves, maintaining their own car or the family car they primarily use). The adolescent may also be expected to contribute financially through part time work to his or her own maintenance or to the maintenance of the family. This transition within roles (i.e. increasing expectancy for productivity and responsibility within continuing roles) serves as a preparation for achieving adult roles which bear an even greater responsibility. That is, the student and family roles are changing so as to move the adolescent toward acquiring the homemaker and worker role.

The adolescent faces a dual task of internalizing new role expectations and beginning to negotiate around discrepancies in expectations. For instance, the same adolescent who is trusted and expected to carry on a part-time job may not be allowed to spend the money on a personal car. The adolescent who is allowed to earn money babysitting until 1:00 a.m. must return from a date before midnight. Adolescents perceive, sometimes correctly, injustice and inconsistency in such expectations and often rebel against fulfilling role expectations. While the rebelliousness of adolescence is usually perceived only in a negative light, it does give the adolescent an opportunity to negotiate role expectations and to begin to assert personal styles of role fulfillment in line with his or her own views of the role.

Internalization of Roles

In adolescence there are increasing opportunities to try on a variety of roles not available in childhood. High school provides an arena for more self-determining group activities, such as sports and student government, in which students can assume a variety of short-term roles. Dating allows the adolescent to explore aspects of roles that are associated with long-term relationships. The role of student remains important to most adolescents, although for some, not being with friends, racism or a lack of variety in classes may lead to dissatisfaction or truancy (29).

Probably the two most important roles for adolescents are the friendship role and worker role. For the adolescent, the peer group is a source of information about the world outside the family, and it is a testing ground for new ideas and behaviors (48).

The role of friend undergoes several changes during adolescence (14). Early adolescent friendships seem to focus on activity, rather than personality. That is, the adolescent chooses a friend on the basis of being able to "work" together, because someone is easygoing, cooperative or unselfish. In the next stage, the adolescent begins to seek friends who can be trusted. These friends serve as sources of guidance and vicarious experiences, and are sounding boards regarding how to act or to interpret one's own experiences. Finally, older adolescents begin to look less for someone to identify with and to choose friends more on the basis of their individuality and personal traits (14).

For young women, the female-female friendship may be particularly important to establishing a nontraditional identity (38). Adolescent girls still have few nontraditional role models, especially within their own families. Thus, the female who chooses a set of values that are less traditional may have difficulty finding support for her decision. It is in her friendships with other females, then, that she is most likely to find confirmation and encouragement for her unconventional goals (38).

The worker role is also important and valuable during adolescence, although the number of adolescents who work full time has decreased

dramatically since the turn of the century (48). Nevertheless, a great many adolescents work part time while they are going to school. Many adolescents babysit, work as waitresses or busboys, or hold other routine jobs (newspaper delivery, short-order cook, and so on) (29, 48). Such jobs, however, are generally unrelated to future vocational plans, and are done for spending money, not for any intrinsic meaning or satisfaction (29, 31). Apart from the money, though, other benefits do accrue to working adolescents. Through part-time jobs adolescents gain exposure to the work world, they develop skill in getting and keeping jobs, they learn to budget their time and money, and they can take some pride in their accomplishments (48). For adolescents who do not hold paying jobs, volunteer work can often serve as a means for finding a purpose in life and for exploring future vocations (31). In fact, volunteer work in some instances may be more rewarding than a paying job to the adolescent in terms of providing a sense of identity and worth. Volunteering can involve activities sponsored by scouting troops, community or church projects, being library assistants, teacher aides, candy stripers, supervising children, working in museums, zoos and parks, and so on (31).

Role Balance

At the same time that the adolescent has opportunities to enter new roles, he or she is experiencing increased demands for continuing roles in the family and school. For the first time the adolescent may experience role conflict, as he or she tries to handle a part-time job, high school or college studies, a relationship with another person, and involvement in school athletics. Balancing these demands frequently creates problems for adolescents, particularly in the roles that are less institutionalized (e.g. leisure). Thus, many adolescents express concern over having too little free time and knowing how to use their leisure effectively (26, 46).

HABITS

The adolescent faces the need to develop new habits for changing circumstances during adolescence and for the world of work. Habits also must take over much routine behavior which was formerly regulated by external factors. A major impact on the habits of the adolescent is the movement from grammar school to junior high. The student is no longer placed in a single classroom and led through the series of daily activities as part of the entire class (36). Instead, students have individual schedules and must be responsible for being in the right place at the right time. They have more autonomy over regulating their study habits. This is even further accentuated when the individual goes to college where fewer hours are spent in class while more time must be spent studying under one's own initiative. Study habits become a major factor in college success or failure.

Degree of Organization

The adolescent faces increased autonomy and responsibility for time use at school along with more leisure time which is at his or her personal discretion (31). Effective use of time and establishing a routine which allows one to perform the tasks required for school and other roles (including newly acquired roles) are habits which emerge during adolescence. The importance of a routine is clearly seen when looking at adolescents at risk for adjustment problems. For example, a study of eighth-grade boys whose fathers were absent from the family found that a factor which differentiated between well- and poorly-adjusted boys was participation in household tasks on a regular basis (30).

Social Appropriateness

The greatest demand on habit formation in adolescence is for habits relevant to the work role. The adolescent must learn basic habits of industry, the ability to put aside play and to use time and energy to do some productive activity (34). Habits of good workmanship, team behavior, promptness, and so on, are necessary for successful transition into the worker role. Persons who enter a homemaker role in place of, or along with, the worker role must have habits of daily living tasks in order to maintain the smooth functioning of the household. Most important for adolescents is the development of good work habits—i.e. planning work efficiently, organizing things and being dependable (41).

Adolescents are generally expected to do more around the house, and it is through household work that they have the opportunity to develop many work-related habits. Not surprisingly, the distribution of household chores is often influenced by sex (9). Girls generally spend more time in household tasks than boys, and their tasks are more likely to include housecleaning and food-related activities. Boys are more likely to do yard work, pet care or car maintenance. Generally, adolescents spend about an average of 1 hr daily in household tasks, unless the mother works fulltime (in which case, they are expected to help out more) (9).

The Performance Subsystem

As noted in the previous chapter, childhood is the time of most rapid development of skills. While most perceptual motor and many process skills have been developed in childhood, the adolescent continues to develop in these areas. A major growth of communication interaction skills occurs in adolescence. In addition, specific skills for various occupations are learned, especially toward the end of the adolescent period.

The musculoskeletal constituent of skills achieves its final development in adolescence. The major change is rapid growth of the long bones in association with puberty. Neurological changes during adolescence are minor compared to the tremendous development of the nervous system during childhood. A major change takes place in the symbolic constituent of skills as the adolescent reaches the stage of formal operations, becoming fully capable of abstract thought (27).

Changes in the school environment elicit the development of new skills. In senior high school and college, students are expected to become increasingly proficient in symbolic skills (36). The peer group life of college and high school and the changes in high school which bring the adolescent in contact with many teachers rather than with a single permanent teacher demand that the adolescent develop new interpersonal communication skills (36). The adolescent also has increased opportunity to learn cooperation and competition skills in team sports, and other extracurricular activities related to school.

As the adolescent enters actual preparation for work in professional college training, apprenticeship or training programs, the focus turns to development of specific skills for a given job. These specific skills are acquired during a formal preparatory phase (didactic or experiential) or during a job training phase, and during the early period of actual work—depending on the type of occupation.

OCCUPATIONAL CHOICE

As has been repeated throughout the previous discussions, adolescence is a time of upheaval and transformation. Values, personal causation and interests are changed, formulated, and refined; new roles and supporting habits are anticipated and developed; cognitive and interactional skills are honed. These changes prepare the adolescent for, and lead to, a choice of a future worker role.

The process of choosing an occupation dominates the adolescent period. It is a complicated process consisting of a series of periods and stages (18). Occupational choice actually begins with fantasy play in childhood. The second period of tentative occupational choices coincides largely with early and middle adolescence (ages 11–17). This period is characterized by three stages, which correspond to components of the volitional subsystem. The first stage is the interest stage; during this time the early adolescent makes choices based on interest—a sense of pleasure to be had in the chosen occupation. Following this are the capacity stage, when the adolescent takes into consideration his or her abilities and feelings of efficacy regarding these abilities, and then the value stage, during which the adolescent views and chooses an occupation according to internalized values. By age 17, the adolescent is in a transition stage looking toward college or work.

The realistic period begins in late adolescence and is characterized by three stages, the first of which is exploration. During exploration, the individual evaluates his or her alternatives. The choice is determined in the crystallization stage, and further delimited in the specification stage (e.g. deciding first to be a nurse, and then to be a nurse anesthesiologist).

Recent theorists have acknowledged that this process is not invariant, that it can proceed at different paces for different individuals, and that it may be repeated in adult life (18, 44, 53). In fact, because individuals and their self-concepts are continually evolving and changing with growth and experience, the process of occupational choice is continuous and dynamic (53). Through experiences in a variety of settings, identification of and with role models, role-playing activities, and expanded awareness of values, interests and capabilities, the adolescent engages in an ongoing process of trying to optimize his or her own goals with the demands, resources and constraints of the environment (53).

ENVIRONMENT AND OCCUPATIONAL CHOICE

Concomitant with the adolescent's own development, there are historical and socioeconomic changes in the larger environment that create demands for certain types of jobs, make others obsolete, and which make entry into the work world more or less likely for different social groups (6, 44). The entire process of occupational choice reflects the adolescent's history of interactions with the environment.

Although the family becomes less important, it is still a major environment during adolescence, and it affects occupational choice in a number of ways. Parents' attitudes toward their work is likely to affect the adolescent's ability to find meaning or purpose in work through the mechanism of role-modeling and imitation in the family (47). The modeling process is enhanced or impeded by certain parenting styles (55). For example, adolescents with "democratic" parents who provide explanations for their rules or requests tend to see their parents as positive role models (55). In addition, the more interaction there is between parent and adolescent, the more likelihood there is that the adolescent will use the parent as a role model. Interestingly, fathers who are seen as either positive *or* negative role models tend to have a significant effect on the occupational decisions and satisfactions of their sons. A negative role model can help the son achieve an occupational identity to a greater extent than a weak or nonexistent model (4). However, as the adolescent matures into early adulthood, a greater variety of role models becomes essential to occupational satisfaction (4).

Social class is also a powerful factor in career development, in terms of the careers that are thought possible and valued (48) and in terms of opportunities for experience and observation of a variety of role models.

School influence on the occupational choice process comes from association with peers, messages communicated through coursework, the adults who work in these schools, and the academic and nonacademic opportunities available to students. Interestingly, students in smaller schools have been found to participate in more activities, play more central roles in these activities than students in larger schools, and have more chances to develop their competence in more activities (3).

High schools shape and reinforce students' conceptions of the future roles open to them. In particular, they tend to reinforce narrow role stereotypes for girls (5). High school girls often reroute their mastery needs from academic channels into social channels. Unfortunately, avoidance of academic subjects, such as math and physics in high school, has repercussions in college when young women find their career options limited almost before they have even begun to seriously choose (5). In addition, because career choices are influenced by life experiences and most girls are not deliberately exposed to a variety of careers, their eventual choices are more likely than not to be traditional (29).

Teachers and other high school staff reinforce the sexual stereotypes encountered by girls. Most administrative positions in schools continue to be filled by men, most English teachers are women, and math and science teachers are often men. Textbooks communicate messages that women have played unimportant roles in historical events, and even subjects such as physical education prepare girls less adequately than boys for future work roles (5, 22).

The college environment continues to influence occupational choice, primarily through peer group influence and the climate of values on campus. Studies of college drop-outs have shown that these students often leave because their values differ from those of the campus mainstream (45). Further, students whose intended major substantially differs from the majors of most of their peers are likely to either change their field of study, or at least, become uncertain of their goals (7). Colleges also tend to have strong subcultural groups, such as fraternities and sororities, which serve to insulate their members from innovative forces and to foster conformity.

SUMMARY

Adolescence represents the interface of various social factors, such as extended schooling, with the individual at a time of intense personal change. As such, adolescence presents both opportunities and difficulties. The major transformation of the period is the movement from the roles of childhood to adult roles. Paramount in this process is the opportunity for the adolescent to be self-determining through occupational choice. The adolescent makes his or her entry into adulthood through assumption of the worker or homemaker role. When this achievement is a product of personal choice based on values, interests and a sense of personal causation, the adolescent has a strong foundation for success and satisfaction in adulthood.

References

1. Alissi AS: Concepts of adolescence. In Thornberg HD (ed): *Contemporary Adolescence: Readings*, ed 2. Monterey, Calif, Brooks/Cole, 1975.
2. Allport G: *Pattern and Growth in Personality*. New York, Holt, Rinehart, & Winston, 1961.
3. Barker RG, Gump PV: *Big School, Small School: High School Size and Student Behavior*. Stanford, Stanford University Press, 1964.
4. Bell AP: Role modeling of fathers in adolescence and young adulthood. In Conger JJ (ed): *Contemporary Issues in Adolescent Development*. New York, Harper Row, 1975.
5. Berkovitz, IH: Effects of secondary school experiences on adolescent female development. In Sugar M (ed): *Female Adolescent Development*. New York, Brunner/Mazel, 1979.
6. Blau PM, Gustad JW, Jessor R, Parnes HS, Wilcock RC: Occupational choice: a conceptual framework. In Peters HJ, Hansen JC (eds): *Vocational Guidance and Career Development*, ed 2. New York, MacMillan, 1971.
7. Brown RD: Manipulation of the environmental press in a college residence hall. In Moos RH, Insel PM (eds): *Issues in Social Ecology*. Palo Alto, Calif, National Press Books, 1974.
8. Buhler C: The integrating self. In Buhler C, Massarik F (eds): *The Course of Human Life*. New York, Springer, 1974.
9. Cogle FL, Tasker GE, Morton DG: Adolescent time use in household work. *Adolescence*, 27:451–455, 1982.
10. Conger JJ: A world they never knew: the family and social change. In Kraemer H (ed): *Youth and Culture: A Human-Developmental Approach*. Monterey, Calif, Brooks/Cole, 1974.
11. Cottle T, Klineberg S: *The Present of Things Future: Explorations of Time in Human Experience*. New York, Free Press, 1974.
12. Csikszentmihalyi M, Rochberg-Halton E: *The Meaning of Things*. Cambridge, Mass, Cambridge University Press, 1981.
13. Csikszentmihalyi M, Larson R, Prescott S: The ecology of adolescent activity and experience. *J Youth Adolesc* 6:281–294, 1977.
14. Douvan E, Adelson J: Adolescent friendships. In Conger JJ (ed): *Contemporary Issues in Adolescent Development*. New York, Harper Row, 1975.
15. Erikson EH: *Identity: Youth and Crisis*. New York, Norton, 1968.
16. Fidler G, Fidler J: Doing and becoming: the occupational therapy experience. In Kielhofner G (ed): *Health Through Occupation: Theory and Practice in Occupational Therapy*. Philadelphia, FA Davis, 1983.
17. Gilligan C: *In a Different Voice*. Boston, Harvard University Press, 1982.
18. Ginzberg E: Toward a theory of occupational choice. In Peters HJ, Hansen JC (eds): *Vocational Guidance and Career Development*, ed 2. New York, MacMillan, 1971.
19. Goodman E: Agreeable teen-agers. *The Washington Post*, April 3, 1984, p A-13.
20. Goodman P: *Growing Up Absurd: Problems of Youth in the Organized System*. New York, Ran-

dom House, 1960.

21. Hamburg BA: Early adolescence: a specific and stressful stage of the life cycle. In Coelho GV, Hamburg BA, Adams JE (eds): *Coping and Adaptation.* New York, Basic Books, 1974.

22. Harragan BL: *Games Mother Never Taught You: Corporate Gamesmanship for Women.* New York, Warner Books, 1977.

23. Hass J: Educational control among high steel ironworkers. In Geer B (ed): *Learning to Work.* Beverly Hills, Calif, Sage, 1972.

24. Hendry LB: *Growing Up and Going Out: Adolescents and Leisure.* Aberdeen, Aberdeen University Press, 1983.

25. Horner M: The motive to avoid success and changing aspirations of college women. In Conger JJ, (ed): *Contemporary Issues in Adolescent Development.* New York, Harper & Row, 1975.

26. House E, Durfee M, Bryan C: A survey of psychological and social concerns of rural adolescents. *Adolescence,* 1979, 14:361–376.

27. Jossyln I: *The Adolescent and His World.* New York, Family Service Association of America, 1952.

28. Keniston K: Youth: A "new" stage of life. In Kraemer H (ed): *Youth and Culture: A Human-Development Approach.* Monterey, Calif, Brooks/Cole, 1974.

29. Konopka G: *Young Girls: A Portrait of Adolescence.* Englewood Cliffs, NY, Prentice-Hall, 1976.

30. Kopf K: Family variables and school adjustment of eighth grade father-absent boys. *Fam Coord* 19:145–150, 1970.

31. Lambert GB, Rothschild BF, Altland R, Green LB: *Adolescence: Transition from Childhood to Maturity,* ed 2. Monterey, Calif, Brooks/Cole, 1978.

32. Lehr UM, Bonn R: Ecology of adolescents as assessed by the daily round method in an affluent society. In Thomas H, Endo T (eds): *The Adolescent and His Environment.* Basel, Karger, 1974.

33. Lesser GS, Kandel DB: Parental and peer influences on educational plans of adolescents. In Conger JJ (ed): *Contemporary Issues in Adolescent Development.* New York, Harper Row, 1975.

34. Maurer P: Antecedents of work behavior. *Am J Occup Ther* 25:295–297, 1971.

35. Mitchell JJ: *The Adolescent Predicament.* Toronto, Holt, Rinehart, & Winston, 1975.

36. Moor, CH: *From School to Work—Effective Counselling and Guidance.* Beverly Hills, Calif, Sage, 1976.

37. Morgan D. Growing up bored. *The Washington Post,* Dec. 29, 1981, pp A1, A6.

38. Morgan E: Toward a reformulation of the Eriksonian model of female identity development. *Adolescence,* 27:199–211, 1982.

39. Muuss RE: *Theories of Adolescence.* New York, Random House, 1975.

40. Notkin M: Situational learning in a school with clients. In Geer B (ed): *Learning to Work.* Beverly

Hills, Calif, Sage, 1972.

41. Oakland J: Measurement of personality correlates of academic achievement in high school students. *J Counsel Psychol* 16:452–457, 1969.

42. Offer D, Offer J: Three developmental routes through normal male adolescence. *Adolesc Psychiatry,* 4:121–141, 1975.

43. Ostro JM, Adelberg BZ: Community settings in the lives of adolescents: a research note. *J Commun Psychol* 4:401–402, 1976.

44. Perun, PJ, Del Vento Bielby D: Towards a model of female occupational behavior: a human development approach. *Psychol Woman Q* 6:234–252, 1981.

45. Pervin LA: Performance and satisfaction as a function of individual-environment fit. In Moos RH, Insel PM (eds): *Issues in Social Ecology.* Palo Alto, Calif, National Press Books, 1974.

46. Powell M. *The Psychology of Adolescence,* ed 2. Indianapolis, Bobbs-Merrill, 1971.

47. de Renne-Stephen, C: Imitation: a mechanism of play behavior. *Am J Occup Ther* 34:95–102, 1980.

48. Santrock JW: *Adolescence: An Introduction.* Dubuque, Iowa, Brown, 1981.

49. Sieg A: Why adolescence occurs. In Thornberg HD (ed): *Contemporary Adolescence: Readings,* ed 2. Monterey, Calif, Brooks/Cole, 1975.

50. Simmons R, Rosenberg R, Rosenberg M: Disturbance in the self-image at adolescence. In Conger JJ (ed): *Contemporary Issues in Adolescent Development.* New York, Harper Row, 1975.

51. Simpson RL: Parental influence, anticipatory socialization, and social mobility. In Conger JJ (ed): *Contemporary Issues in Adolescent Development.* New York, Harper Row, 1975.

52. Stein SL, Weston LC: College women's attitudes toward woman and identity achievement. *Adolescence,* 27:895–899, 1982.

53. Super DE: A theory of vocational development. In Peters HJ, Hansen JC (eds): *Vocational Guidance and Career Development,* ed 2. New York, MacMillan, 1971.

54. Tittle CK: *Careers and Family.* Beverly Hills, Calif, Sage, 1981.

55. Thomas DL, Gecas V, Weigert A, Rooney E: *Family Socialization and the Adolescent.* Lexington, Mass, Lexington Books, 1974.

56. Thornberg HD: Behavior and values: consistency and inconsistency. In Thornberg HD (ed): *Contemporary Adolescence: Readings,* ed 2. Monterey, Calif, Brooks/Cole, 1975.

57. Winch RF, Gordon MT: *Familial Structure and Function as Influence.* Lexington, Mass, Heath 1974.

58. Woods CM: Students without teachers: student culture at a barber school. In Geer B (ed): *Learning to Work.* Beverly Hills, Calif, Sage, 1972.

59. Wynne LC, Frader L: Female adolescence and the family: a historical view. In Sugar M (ed): *Female Adolescent Development.* New York, Brunner/Mazel, 1979.

CHAPTER 9

Early and Middle Adulthood

Roann Barris and Gary Kielhofner

AN OVERVIEW OF EARLY AND MIDDLE ADULTHOOD

The boundaries of adulthood are closely tied to one's working life. Chronologically, adulthood begins in one's early 20s—usually with the assumption of a first full time job—and ends with retirement, at around age 65 (30). Because a span of some 40 years is included in this stage, it is often more meaningful to distinguish between early and middle adulthood, recognizing that the tasks, goals and accomplishments of persons may undergo considerable change during this period. Some of these changes are externally recognizable, as the person passes through a series of steps, crises or transitions, such as settling down, starting a family, being promoted, or taking a new job (21, 25, 31); others are internal, as the individual sorts out the various meanings, goals and purposes that guide choice and self-evaluation in adult life. Table 9.1 summarizes the major themes of this chapter concerning adult development.

Historically, the phenomenon of adulthood itself is changing (18). Because the expected life span is continually increasing, the time frame for accomplishing major life tasks is also changing. People are raising families at older ages and retiring from work later. In addition, the historical events experienced by a particular cohort significantly affect the expectations and interpretations given to various activities (35). For example, work can never mean quite the same thing to a generation in which jobs are plentiful as it does to those who lived through the great depression.

Although adulthood is both a process and a changing phenomenon, we can still speak of some enduring and characteristic features of adult life. Perhaps the most salient is the centrality of work in adulthood. Work defines, shapes and structures the adult experience. Work provides, and is the means by which, adults carry out their responsibilities of caring for older and younger persons, and augmenting and passing on the knowledge, values and technology of society. Current conceptualizations of adult life tasks reflect this domination of work. These tasks include: developing an acceptable socioeconomic base; choosing and evaluating one's occupation or career in terms of a personal value system; assuming responsibility in occupational, social and civic groups; using leisure time in satisfying and creative ways; and fostering the growth of younger generations through teaching and mentoring relationships (29).

For the individual, these tasks are subsumed by the more encompassing and personal necessity of finding a balance between exploration, competence, and achievement in adult life. For many adults, the choice of a work role will represent the major path toward achievement in their lives, while leisure will become the chance to explore and be competent without having to worry about the stakes of failure. Others may not find the opportunity to achieve at work, and may look instead to their leisure, becoming amateur musicians, athletes, artists, and so on, in their spare time. In the past, this has been especially true of married women, who even when they worked outside the home, rarely had the chance to use work to satisfy their own needs to explore and master. Eventually, however, the ability to combine exploration, achievement and competence in one's life leads to the establishment of an occupational lifestyle.

The Volition Subsystem

The refinement of personal causation, interests and values and the ability to translate these into a meaningful choice of occupations reach their peak in adulthood. Adults have more freedom to make choices on the basis of their values than at any other stage of life. To be sure, such diverse factors as economic constraints, social discrimination, and obligations of parenthood or illness may impact upon these decisions, but for most people, adulthood is the time when one truly begins to live one's own life. As a result

Table 9.1.
Developmental phenomena in adult occupation

VOLITION

Within realistic constraints the possibilities of choice peak in adulthood
Self-reassessment may result in a transformation from concern with competence and achievement in early adulthood to a concern with value in middle adulthood; this may lead some adults to change work careers or drastically alter their lifestyles

Personal Causation

Adulthood is characterized by an increasing desire to achieve and work autonomously, generally accompanied by an increased sense of internal control
Early adulthood is a period of acquiring confidence in skills whereas middle adulthood is a time for self-assessment related to attainments
Persons in fields which require experience and judgment generally feel increased ability; in fields with rapidly changing technology, persons may feel threatened about their skills
Personal causation in women is more variable and is affected by their experience of working

Values

Young adults may be present oriented and at the same time hold values of getting ahead and experiencing success; in middle age persons may feel a time squeeze to attain their goals
Later goals may become more focused on humanitarian concerns and themes of legacy
Future orientation in adulthood is related to positive adjustment
Standards of adult performance have changed from a focus on industriousness and efficacy to self-fulfillment and pleasure
Sex-related work and family expectations are changing
Work is a major source of meaning for adults; leisure also serves as a source of meaning that complements work or may compensate for a lack of meaning at work

Interests

Interests are generally well established by adulthood, but their stability may be an artifact of cultural pressures against changing in adulthood
Adult interests are influenced by marriage, neighbors, organizations, sex, economic status, and other variables
While work is often a major arena for interest, not all adults find their work interesting and seek other avenues for interest
A major task of adulthood is carrying work-related interests into retirement

HABITUATION

Roles

Role shifts such as the beginning of parenthood, work transitions and participation in social organization occur throughout adulthood
Internalization of role expectations continues in adulthood with initiation into worker roles
Work roles characterize most adults, with many women now working out of the home while others are being recognized for their work role of housewife
Work roles may greatly influence leisure, friendship and other roles
Organizational and social roles peak in middle adulthood
Adults must divide time among many roles and may experience role conflicts

Habits

Habits must be efficient and allow routine performance in a variety of adult roles
External regulators give way to self-regulation with many jobs requiring flexible habits
Demands for synchronizing one's activities with partners, co-workers, children, and so on, also require highly organized habits
Habits of dress, work behavior and other behaviors are influenced by work and cultural expectations

PERFORMANCE

Skills

Physical changes in adulthood appear to have a minor, if any, impact on performance; the person's overall life-style may be more critical to continued performance than skill decrements
Throughout adulthood there are demands for new skills associated with work, parenthood, and so on; thus skill acquisition is ongoing
In some careers and jobs, skills may become obsolescent, contributing to the need for updating or learning new skills

adults tend to assess and reassess their own motives and choices. This reassessment reflects a transformation from an early concern with competence and achievement in work to a later concern with the significance and value of one's work and its potential to yield a sense of enjoyment. This transformation in volition, sometimes referred to as a mid-life crisis, may lead persons to reformulate the direction and goals of their lives, to change work careers, or to enact similarly drastic alterations in their occupational life-styles (5, 11, 15, 19, 21, 25, 29, 31).

In some ways adulthood brings into clearest focus what is meant by the urge to explore and master. We expect children and adolescents to grow and change because they are becoming adults. But adults themselves continue this process of becoming. Adults remain energized by a need to know about themselves, to explore their lives, their worth and meaning, and a need to achieve a degree of control over the circumstances and direction of their lives. For some adults this struggle results in a high level of well being; others do their best to hang on.

PERSONAL CAUSATION

Adulthood is characterized by an increasing desire to achieve and to work autonomously. For most people, this is accompanied by an increased sense of internal control and belief in one's competence (26).

Internal / External Control

The desire for more autonomy appears to be widespread in middle age, and not confined to a particular socioeconomic class or type of work. Older truck drivers, for instance, prefer to own their truck not so much to become entrepreneurs, but to achieve independence from supervision, to control their own working conditions and to be able to accommodate their work role with the rest of their life-style (23). The desire for more control also leads many older persons to enter managerial or teaching roles in which they supervise or prepare new members of their field.

Belief in Skill

One's belief in skill changes throughout adulthood. Early adulthood is generally a period of acquiring and refining skills for one's line of work; thus young workers see themselves as learning and increasing their skills and the efficacy of their abilities to manage the tasks of their work. While they may not feel fully competent, this feeling is judged in relation to still being a novice. By middle adulthood individuals have generally realized their peak performance and can assess how skillful they have become. The degree to which one believes in skill and its efficacy may be affected by a number of factors. In fields that require judgment and accumulated experience older workers may feel secure in their abilities. In rapidly changing fields they may be threatened by newly trained, younger personnel who may be closer to "state of the art" knowledge. One phenomena which has drastically affected persons' belief in skills has been the shift in available jobs from industry to human services and information technology. As assembly line jobs become scarcer, many persons may find that their skills are no longer efficacious and that they may need to acquire new abilities or face unemployment.

Expectancy of Success or Failure

In addition to one's belief in skill, the expectancy of success may undergo many changes over the adult years. The young adult may have dreams of success mixed with anxiety about how he or she will actually perform. As he or she learns the ropes, anticipatin of success is more reality oriented and the individual learns to read the markers of progress (i.e. promotions, salary increases, performance reviews, and more subtle feedback from colleagues and supervisors). In some positions one must either make the grade by moving through successive stages or levels of achievement or be considered a mediocre or failing worker, while in jobs which present more limited opportunities for laddering, there may be less need for concern over future progress (7).

Many individuals in middle age face a sense of panic related to the realization that one must either now achieve a certain status or accomplish a level of performance, or forego the dream of really "making it" in a career (25, 30). Thus, feelings of control may temporarily be overcome by the need to judge oneself by an external marker.

The Impact of Work and Other Factors on Personal Causation

While for most men, entry into adulthood means an opportunity to prove one's effectiveness in a job, the adult period may be more variable for women. Personal causation in women reflects this variability and is therefore less clearly understood.

Women have frequently been thought to be more externally oriented than men, and to be less motivated to achieve. This belief, however, may reflect social expectations for "proper" female behavior, as well as the assumption that achievement motivation can only be expressed in certain channels—e.g. success in the traditionally male work world. But, if one considers the possibility that achievement can be expressed either at home *or* in the work world, and either through one's own actions *or* through those of someone else, then it may be that for some women, being an efficient housekeeper, a gourmet cook or even married to a successful businessman is as much an expression of the urge to achieve and a source of feelings of personal efficacy as being a participant in the work world herself (30). On the other hand, more and more women out of choice and/or economic necessity are entering the work force and are taking on what were traditionally male careers. Women who work generally enjoy increased feelings of personal causation, although, in some cases, these feelings may decrease if the husband's occupational prestige outpaces their own (12).

While feelings of personal causation are generally dominated by one's relationship to work, other adult tasks and experiences such as rearing a family and maintaining a household and an economic base can be important challenges to, and sources of feelings of control, skillfulness and success. Young parents often find themselves facing great responsibilities with minimal training for parenting and may waver between feelings of success and being out of control as their children grow. Middle-aged parents tend to experience feelings of helplessness, often in response to their adolescent children's emerging independence and rebelliousness (22, 26).

Persons who find more limited opportunity to develop a sense of efficacy and success in their necessary life work may devote substantial time and energy to some amateur occupation or hobby in order to enhance their feelings of control and ability (28).

VALUES

During adulthood, values become increasingly important as a motivating force and a source of self-evaluation. Most adults have internalized a pattern of values reflective of the larger culture and can be relied on to self-regulate according to this value system. The occupational goals that are set in adulthood also strongly reflect social trends and one's socioeconomic status. For example, in the past, lower class adults have generally not aspired toward education beyond high school, unless it was clearly vocationally related (22). More recently, however, education has come to be increasingly valued by all members of society.

While personal values related to occupation tend to remain relatively stable throughout adulthood (30), a shift occurs from an early emphasis on standards of performance to the meaningfulness of activities in one's life. In addition, temporal orientation and goals also change substantially as the person ages and achieves or gives up certain objectives (22).

Temporal Orientation and Occupational Goals

Adults in western cultures are usually future oriented; view time as a commodity which can be sold, bought or wasted; feel tremendous pressure to fill time with activity, preferably work; and see time as linear, absolute and capable of being divided and compartmentalized (9, 16). The result of this orientation is an emphasis on plans, and the necessity for budgeting and allocating time. In short, adults are tremendously time conscious.

Young adults are highly present oriented, believing that now is the time to live and that the future holds unlimited opportunity (15). In fact, being future oriented during early adulthood often reflects "escapist" thinking as opposed to actual productivity (32). Maintaining a positive orientation to the present is critical to the formation and attainment of occupational goals in young adulthood. After spending adolescence in the arduous task of setting occupational goals and choosing a career, the young adult begins trying to fulfill these plans. The goals of early adulthood are thus focused on instrumental and material values, such as getting ahead at work, earning a satisfactory living, being able to support one's dependents, and being able to acquire the objects that signify success in contemporary society (22). Young adults are frequently expansive in their goals, and have high expectations of meeting them.

Because middle-aged workers begin to feel

that they have a limited amount of time left in which to achieve their goals, they often perceive a "time squeeze," a growing realization that only so much time is left to correct the course of one's life. After a period of an intense "last-ditch" effort to reach their goals, they often begin to focus more on their accomplishments of the past. Goals then become more focused on humanitarian concerns and on themes of legacy—what will I leave of myself to the future, how will I be remembered by my children (22).

As the person approaches old age the present again takes on growing importance along with the past (15). Attitudes toward the future are quite different among young and old people, reflecting a changed perspective on life in which one begins to think of time left to live (26). Possibly because of this changed outlook, future orientation seems to be related to positive adjustment in older adults. Being future oriented as one grows old enables one to make realistic plans and to continue to be productive into old age (22).

Although older adults are future oriented, the tempo of life which they experience appears to decelerate (22, 26). Older adults identify fewer stresses in a given period of time when compared with younger adults, and they exhibit more distance from events. As mastery becomes a striving to be in harmony with the environment, things that were once seemingly crucial become less significant or pressuring (29).

Performance Standards and Meaningfulness of Activity

In adulthood, the meaning of occupations and standards of performance are closely linked. This becomes particularly evident when considering some of the general shifts in values that have occurred in the past 20 or 30 years in this country. For example, in the 1950s, the chief adult aim of work was to make a good living and be successful in a traditional job. Standards accompanying such a goal might be efficiency, industriousness, a sense that work comes first in one's life, loyalty, and so on. In the 1970s, though, goals became more introspective and many Americans became preoccupied with self-fulfillment (34). This preoccupation led to more flexible performance standards, a belief that creativity and pleasure in work were more important than steadfast industriousness, and an attempt to balance the demands of work with the rest of one's life (34). Other standards that have changed and that have altered the meaning

of work are traditional sexual distinctions. The norm that only the man should provide an income has given way in many families which now expect and rely on both the husband's and wife's income to maintain their standard of living. In addition, more men now expect themselves to be actively involved in tasks of child rearing and homemaking, although many working women still perceive housework and child care to be their responsibilities (4, 33, 35). Other performance standards related to housework are also changing. Whereas in the past, women have maintained excessively high standards (possibly as a means of making their work more arousing) (4), women who now combine a paying occupation with housework may be less intent on spotless glasses and shiny floors.

Perhaps at no other time of life does the search for meaning in one's activities become as important as during adulthood. No other activity takes up as much of an adult's life as work; the type of meaning that work has for a person is therefore likely to pervade the individual's overall life-style.

For men, work is intimately bound to one's definition of self as being successful (22). Even for unemployed adults, work is a major source of identity or nonidentity. Characteristically, one of the first things we ask about someone we do not know is, "What do you do?" The answer, more often than not, is a statement of job title or function. People rarely introduce themselves as a conglomerate of roles—e.g. father, woodworker, bicyclist and engineer—but more often say simply, "I'm an engineer," leaving the rest to the imagination. Thus, although work may mean economic survival, a chance to achieve or a host of other things, above all it signifies one's identity.

Whether or not work has the same meaning for women is more complicated. Because women are not automatically expected to work, their reasons for choosing to do so influence its meaning in their lives (5). Women may work because their family needs a second income, because they need to get out of the house for a while or because of the intrinsic desire to have a career. However, even working women may still primarily identify themselves with their role of wife and mother, if they are married. On the other hand, for many women work may be an opportunity to achieve parity with men in an area dominated by males. Nevertheless, the woman seeking an identity in the modern world receives confusing signals from society.

Although to some extent the sociocultural importance of the work that one does influences its meaning (13), drudgery or unpleasant work can also be a source of identity and a satisfying experience. As workers develop social mechanisms for coping with the negative aspects of their job, the work environment can become an "occupational community" in which work and a positive self-identity become closely entwined (8).

The meaning of leisure is even more individualistic than the meaning of work (17). One reason that many adults offer for engaging in leisure is that it is a "welcome change from work" (10). Some people, for example, find in leisure the chance to engage in behaviors that are not used at work—to be creative if one has a routine job, or to be social, if one works alone. Other people, however, carry their work into their activities. Thus, an art teacher who makes jewelry when she's not teaching, or an engineer who builds model boats, may find the same meaning in their leisure that they find in their work.

Many playful activities have a further meaning of ritual in people's lives. Through ritual, people enter worlds that contrast with their everyday existence at the same time that they reaffirm their membership in their cultural group. For example, the monthly poker game for many American men signifies far more than just a change from work and an opportunity to socialize and play cards—it is also a sanctioned excursion into the world of adventure and risk (14).

The prevalent cultural view of leisure as something that is earned through one's work, but is less important and central to one's life than work (19), may be changing today, partly because of new social values emphasizing personal development and leisure as an arena for such development. In addition, in response to prevailing consumeristic life-styles, many persons are envisioning a change in which leisure becomes an important resource for fulfillment of personal needs as well as for contribution to society at large. However, such a culture does not currently exist, and many adults don't quite know what to do with their leisure or are uncomfortable in their use of leisure time.

INTERESTS

Most people have well-established interests by the time they reach adulthood. In both leisure and work these interests are more likely to be continuous throughout the life span than to change. This continuity, however, may partly be an artifact of having to do relatively similar things over a long period of time. Indeed, as the idea of midcareer change becomes more acceptable, more adults may find and acknowledge that their interests have changed over time.

A major task of adulthood concerning interests is to find ways of carrying work-related interests into retirement. Although some people at retirement completely transform their occupational life-style, for others, successful retirement is contingent upon being able to enact old interests in new ways (19).

Discrimination and Pattern

Adults' interests are formed by exposure to and participation in a variety of settings. In addition to work, most people find time to become involved in many community settings. Socializing with neighbors, joining civic organizations, adult education, and available cultural and natural resources influence the adult's interests.

Sex, age and socioeconomic status show some relationship to the discrimination of interests (17). Upper-middle class individuals more frequently participate in formal organizations, while lower-middle and lower class people often prefer manual hobbies and television. Women are more likely to be group members and to read, whereas men favor sports and fishing. Participator sports lose their interest for men as they become older, and many people in their 60s begin to prefer solitary activities such as gardening (17). Other popular activities among adults include visiting or being visited, and shopping.

Marriage also affects interests and use of leisure time. Newly-married couples frequently search for activities that can be done with another couple. Hence, small group activities such as playing bridge, or doubles in tennis, become popular among some adults.

Potency

If the pattern of interests does not show much overall change with age, the potency of these preferences and dislikes does increase over time (5). Probably this reflects two trends. First, at work, as one advances there is a tendency for the nature of the job to become more specialized. To succeed requires that one focus more attentively on a narrower body of work knowledge. At the same time, one must also give up mild interests for areas of work that have become less central to one's specialty. Second, because middle-aged workers feel pressured to make a last effort to gain promotions, they put more energy into work and have less left over for leisure (22). Having to use their leisure time more selectively means doing only those things that are truly enjoyed. Television, for example, is often the first leisure interest to be given up when adults are pressed for time (24).

Many adults entered their work because it embodied the opportunity to channel and develop personal interests (19). However, it is not a universal phenomenon that adults find their work interesting. White collar workers and professionals in general experience more interest in, and would be more likely to freely choose to spend extra time in, their work. For assembly line workers, though, the lack of connection between efforts and the final product, engagement in repetitive tasks which provide minimal challenge, and having little or no control over the working conditions often lead to disinterest in work (32).

The Habituation Subsystem

ROLES

While adolescence is marked by a predominance of ambiguously defined roles, adulthood is characterized by a variety of socially prescribed and individually chosen roles which structure the adult's daily life and provide a sense of identity and belonging to society. Apart from family roles, most of these roles are enacted in community settings that exist solely for the adult age-group (1).

Role shifts are highly characteristic of adulthood. The many transitions that occur include the initiation of parenthood, changes in work roles, transitions from work to homemaking or vice versa, joining civic and social organizations, and adopting major hobbies or amateur pursuits. Thus, the range of roles which adults expect to fill includes worker, homemaker, hobbyist or amateur, organization member, friend, and so on. Of all these, the work role is perhaps the most significant in this stage of life.

Perceived Incumbency

Most men and many women today have work roles. For men, expectations of entering the work force in adulthood are engrained at an early age. This early socialization leads them to be relatively career-oriented in both high school and college. It also leads them to define personal success in terms of having a job and, conversely, to attach a great deal of stigma to the condition of being unemployed.

Whereas being a housewife was once the only expectation of adult women, many women now choose to work as well, and their participation in the work force has increased strikingly in recent years. In addition, the role of housewife is increasingly being recognized as an occupational role in its own right (4). However, as an occupational role it is rather unusual, in that it is performed in a noneconomic setting without opportunities for advancement or for salary increase (4).

Many women first visualize themselves in a work role during middle age, when they no longer feel the need to subvert their own dreams to those of husbands or children (2). Some women, however, are unable to envision themselves as ever becoming a worker. The inability to perceive themselves in this role has created a syndrome known as the "displaced homemaker." These are women who assumed they would fulfill the homemaker role forever but, because of separation, divorce or widowhood, suddenly find themselves without economic and social support in their lives and needing to work, yet lacking any preparation for the worker role (6).

Many adults remain unemployed, especially those between the ages of 18 and 24, and 55 to 64. The older unemployed worker has an especially hard time finding a new job (30). Nevertheless, the work role is perceived by most adults to be a basic and normal condition of life.

The work role also influences other roles that are performed by the adult, especially friendship and leisure roles. For commuting men, the friendship role is particularly likely to be shaped by work. The adult male who commutes daily may actually share more confidences and decision-making with work friends than with his family (5). Similarly, workers who are periodically away from homes—such as professional athletes or salespersons—will develop strong friendship ties with colleagues. For persons who do not work, friends are likely to be limited to other people who also do not work.

The leisure role is influenced by work in terms of the amount of time available to leisure and when this time occurs, the meanings sought from leisure activities, and in terms of the types of leisure that may actually be engaged in. For example, housewives, whose free time usually falls in the afternoon, must choose leisure activities that are available at that time of day (3).

Or, certain forms of leisure may be expected as part of one's job. Large companies often sponsor teams for local league sports; playing on such a team may be a sign of loyalty to the company. Similarly, business persons reputedly complete major transactions on the golf course.

The leisure role takes several forms in adulthood. These forms are distinguished by the degree of intensity attached to them. Being a hobbyist is a typical leisure role characterized by enjoyment and enthusiasm. The amateur role, on the other hand, represents more of a middle ground between player and professional (28).

Participation in organizational and social roles reaches a peak in middle adulthood and then begins to decline in the early 60s (5). Service groups become quite popular for people between the ages of 35 and 55; however, there are fewer service groups for men than for women (5). Women's service groups tend to be church related whereas men's are more likely to be fraternal orders (5). Social roles are likely to be more important for women than for men because they are often an effective substitute for work or changing family roles (6). Volunteering is very popular with older women. Religious participant is another organizational role that many adults fill.

Internalization of Role Expectations

Many of the expectations that accompany adult roles are internalized in earlier stages of life. Playing house, children begin to assume the attitudes and behaviors of adult family member roles. In school, adolescents develop many of the habits and nonspecialized skills which they will later need in both work and leisure. But, at the same time, adult roles make new, unfamiliar demands and require corresponding socialization experiences.

Job initiation generally occurs in young adulthood and involves learning job-specific skills, forming new interpersonal relationships (7), reapportioning one's use of time to accommodate a new schedule and, frequently, developing a new image of oneself as a neophyte worker. Ultimately, the internalization of work role expectations involves a transformation in one's thinking as the individual becomes ideologically similar to others working in the same field (30)—a new resident begins to "feel" like a doctor, an accountant takes up bridge because his or her co-workers are bridge enthusiasts. This process is partly institutionalized, through vo-

cational preparation before actually taking a job, and on-the-job training and orientation programs for new employees.

Each work role potentially carries with it a range of expectations. Some persons internalize the highest expectations for full devotion and effort to the job; others internalize lower standards as their view of what they should do on the job. In addition, people vary in the degree to which they identify with work roles. The extent of role internalization is affected by the person's aspirations, the demands of other roles, the priority given to the worker role, and the tendency of the work setting to expect one or another level of performance in the role. For example, executives in one corporation may be expected to work longer hours than in another, or workers in a fast food chain might be expected to be more efficient than those in another. Thus, the press of the setting influences the kinds of expectations a worker comes to have of himself or herself. The level of performance of a person who previously held a position can often be a pressure for the level of expectations one internalizes; the phrase "a hard act to follow" refers to the expectations that have come to be associated with a position because of the previous role encumbant.

Internalization of work role expectations may be more problematic for women than it is for men. Women who enter the work world often continue to see themselves as first a homemaker, mother or wife, and only secondarily as a worker (22). Because they have less commitment to the work role, they may derive little satisfaction from their work and simultaneously underestimate the impact that future retirement will have on them (6).

Internalization of leisure roles also varies. Some adults strive to meet the standards of professionals who perform the same activity, and they acquire a level of expertise that, while not equalling the professional's, far exceeds that of the average person (28). The amateur role importantly differs from the player role in that the amateur is motivated to achieve, and not just to explore or become competent, and it differs from the professional role in that amateurs are not usually paid.

Role Balance

Most adults have to divide their time among three major roles—work, family and leisure. Because each of these roles can involve substantial investments of energy and time, a large number of people find inevitable conflicts in their use of time. These conflicts relate to age, sex and extent of role internalization.

Among working men and women, men are more likely than women to report conflicts between work and leisure (27), no doubt because of many women's lesser commitment to work. Older adults are less likely to report role conflicts than younger, again, possibly because of a lesser commitment. In addition, older adults have had time to develop a satisfying balance between leisure and work, whereas younger adults are probably more concerned with getting ahead and less concerned with the balance of activities in their lives.

While the amount of time spent in leisure does not necessarily relate to role conflict, incorporating a wide variety of leisure activities and engaging in activities of certain types do appear to contribute to conflicts in time use (27). Activities that need to be carried out away from the home and at certain prescheduled times are particular sources of conflict.

Women are more likely to experience conflicts between their leisure and family roles than men are (27). In part, this is because men frequently view many of their family tasks as leisure. Being only occasionally responsible for child care or meal preparation may allow these activities to be viewed as part of one's leisure rather than as daily chores.

The housewife may also experience role imbalance because the timing of the housewife role does not synchronize with the rest of the occupational world (4). The housewife's day begins earlier that most men's, and it often continues well into the evening, making it difficult to pursue certain forms of leisure. (3).

Despite conflicts in time use, having a combination of roles appears to be critical to well-being (2). A lack of arousal in one's life, from having too little to do, may be more of a problem than having too much (2).

HABITS

As the discussion of role balance implied, many habits of adulthood are necessarily concerned with the efficient allocation of time to various roles and tasks. The division of the week into time for work, play, rest, self-care, and family is to some extent contingent upon the norms of society. Because most American businesses operate between 9 and 5, most Americans

(or most male Americans) do not engage in leisure during these hours (24). However, due to the influx of women in the work force, the desire of men to be more involved with their families, increasing automation in the work world, and other trends, such practices as part time work, flextime, and job sharing are becoming more popular.

In addition to temporal organization, adult habits are influenced by social expectations in other ways. What constitutes appropriate food at a given meal, how often one bathes, how to dress for work, and so on, are all examples of cultural expectations that lead to the development of certain habits.

Organization and Balance

By adulthood, most external regulators (e.g. parents, school) of time use have been replaced with the need to autonomously regulate one's routine behavior. Different types of work may require vastly different structures. Some work requires a rather rigid adherence to schedules (e.g. factory workers) whereas other forms of work may require individuals to develop their own routines around changing workloads, seasonal variation and so forth (e.g. farmers, university professors). Marriage, purchasing a home and the advent of children also place demands on persons to change their routines, to synchronize activities with a partner, to be able to do additional tasks of home maintenance and caretaking of children and, generally, to meet the needs of one's family. Persons once accustomed to a routine organized around personal needs and desires find themselves having to orient their routines to a broader set of concerns.

A certain constancy underlies the organization of American adult life. Approximately 72 hours a week of the lives of most employed men and women and housewives are spent in sleeping, self-care and eating (24). Men, on the average, spend more time at work than women and usually have longer commutes to get to their jobs. Children have little impact on the amount of time men put in at work; however, they have an extensive impact on women's work time (24).

Spending more time at work means having less time for something else. For men, if work time increases, less time is spent on leisure. Women, however, compensate with reduced hours for sleeping, resting and visiting (24).

Women consistently put more hours into housework than men. Even women employed full time perform nearly 10 times as much housework as do men, frequently using the weekends to catch up (24).

The use of time is influenced conventionally by the day of the week. Saturday and Sunday even have a typical breakdown of activities for many persons, with Saturday being popular for housework, and Sunday a day to spend with the children (24).

Social Appropriateness

Work can have a far reaching effect on typical patterns of behavior. A person's style of dress, use of leisure time, performance of activities of daily living and a variety of other dimensions of habits can be influenced by work expectations, work schedule and other job-related factors. For instance, fast food employees typically wear a uniform to work, as do nurses, lab workers and certain professionals.

Whereas men become more conforming with age, adult women, interestingly, tend to increase in unconventionality as they get older (30). Nevertheless, most adults develop culturally prescribed habits which are slow to change. For instance, although clothing fashions have shown extreme variations in the past 30 years, the typical businessman still dresses for work in a suit and tie.

As the effects of women's liberation permeate society, many habits associated with sex roles are changing. Men are more routinely expected to develop habits relating to household management; women are more frequently developing habits associated with maintenance of cars and other machines.

Socially appropriate habits are not always productive—on the surface, at least. For example, approximately 10% of work time for most people is habitually spent in such nonproductive activities as taking breaks, socializing, or waiting for something (24). However, these seemingly unproductive uses of time may be necessary for "refueling" or for improving interpersonal relationships with co-workers.

The Performance Subsystem

SKILLS

One of the most common concerns of adults is the peaking and declining of their abilities. Whereas young adulthood is experienced by most as a time of acquiring new abilities for work and other areas of adult responsibility, middle and later adulthood is characterized by

some waning in capacity (19). However, although physical and cognitive abilities do peak either prior to or early in adulthood, the extent of decline in these abilities may not be as significant in adult performances as is the individual's life-style. A person's habits, including the use of time, eating and drinking patterns, routine amounts of exercise, and typical levels of stress have a major impact on various abilities as well as incidence of such diseases as heart attack and stroke which may impair skills (19, 29, 30).

Nevertheless, certain physical changes do occur and affect the occupational performance of adults. Over time, adults experience a decrease in energy and strength and may have to give up some more rigorous activities and take more time to perform others. Sensory perception also becomes less acute, causing many adults to require glasses, brighter lights for working and other adjustments (19).

However, the adult's response to decreased capacities may be even more important than any actual decline. Rather than withdrawing from or avoiding certain activities, many middle-aged adults find that engaging in physically or cognitively demanding activities is challenging and satisfying.

New skills are also acquired in adulthood, particularly at work. This sometimes occurs to the chagrin of young adults who have spent long periods of time in preparation for jobs and then find upon entering the work world that there is still much more to learn. Some of the skills that must be learned include performance of routine procedures for daily tasks and knowing how to use appropriate materials and equipment (20). A great deal of working knowledge and skills are learned informally, in the course of carrying out the job. These skills concern the ability to deal innovatively with unforeseen circumstances, to secure the cooperation of workers in other positions and to maintain an image of competence in one's own job (20).

Adults also find themselves newly responsible for a number of family-related tasks, including managing personal finances, home maintenance, caring for children, and communicating with a partner. These responsibilities often must be learned under "sink or swim" conditions. The abilities to find the information one needs, to learn new skills in the process of performing, and to problem solve in novel situations become more important than direct task performance capacities.

Although middle adulthood is often a time of confidence in one's mastery of skills necessary to a variety of roles, some occupations have a built-in obsolescence. Changing job technology may require the sudden learning of new skills (e.g. computer programming). Older athletes usually cannot compete against younger, and parents must learn how to communicate with adolescents and, later, adult children.

SUMMARY

Adulthood is popularly thought of as a period or state at which persons arrive and remain relatively unchanged until the next major phase of life, old age or later adulthood. However, throughout this chapter adulthood has been demonstrated to be a period of ongoing change and growth in the human system. While each individual's passage through adulthood is unique, there appears to be an early period of skill building, achievement orientation, and accomplishment followed by a period of self-examination and a search for meaning in work and other spheres of life. At the same time it must be recognized that adulthood is an ongoing phenomenon lived anew by each new generation and its own historical experiences.

References

1. Barker RG, Wright HF: *Midwest and Its Children.* Hamden, Conn, Archon, 1971 (1955).
2. Baruch G, Barnett R, Rivers C: A new start for women at midlife. *New York Times Sunday Magazine*, Dec. 7, 1980, pp 196–200.
3. Berk RA, Berk SF: *Labor and Leisure at Home.* Beverly Hills, Calif, Sage, 1979.
4. Bernard J: Between two worlds: The housewife. In Stewart PL, Cantor MG (eds): *Varieties of Work.* Beverly Hills, Calif, Sage, 1982.
5. Bischof LJ: *Adult Psychology*, ed 2. New York, Harper & Row, 1976.
6. Block MR, Davidson JL, Grambs JD: *Women Over Forty: Visions and Realities.* New York, Springer, 1981.
7. Brim, O.G, Jr: Adult socialization, In Clausen JA (ed): *Socialization and Society.* Boston, Little, Brown, 1968.
8. Bryant CD, Perkins KB: Containing work disaffection: the poultry processing worker. In Stewart PL, Cantor MG (eds): *Varieties of Work.* Beverly Hills, Calif, Sage, 1982.
9. Cottle TJ, Klineberg SL: *The Present of Things Future: Explorations of Time in Human Experience.* New York, Free Press, 1974.
10. Donald MN, Havighurst RJ: The meaning of leisure. *Soc Forces*, 37:355–360, 1959.
11. Farrell MP, Rosenberg SD: *Men at Midlife.* Boston, Auburn House, 1981.
12. Freudiger P: Life satisfaction among three categories of married women. *J Marriage Fam* 45:213–219, 1983.
13. Godbey G, Parker S: *Leisure Studies and Services: An Overview.* Philadelphia, Saunders, 1976.
14. Goodman W: The luck of the draw. *New York Times Sunday Magazine*, August 7, 1983, p 54.
15. Gould RL: The phases of adult life: a study in developmental psychology. *Am J Psych* 129:33–43, 1972.
16. Hall E: The Silent Language. Greenwich, Conn, Fawcett, 1959.
17. Havighurst RJ: The nature and values of meaningful free-time activity. In Kleemeier RW (ed): *Aging and Leisure.* New York, Arno, 1979.
18. Jordon D: Searching for adulthood in America. In Erikson EH (ed): *Adulthood.* New York, Norton, 1978.
19. Kimmel DC: *Adulthood and Aging*, ed 2. New York, Wiley, 1980.
20. Kusterer KC: *Know-How on the Job: The Important Working Knowledge of "Unskilled" Workers.* Boulder, Colo, Westview Press, 1978.
21. Levinson DJ: *The seasons of a man's life.* New York, Ballantine, 1978.
22. Lowenthal MF, Thurnher M, Chiriboga D, et al: *Four Stages of Life.* San Francisco, Jossey-Bass, 1975.
23. Peterson RA, Schmidman JT, Elifson KW: Entrepreneurship or autonomy? Truckers and cabbies. In Stewart PL, Cantor MG (eds): *Varieties of Work.* Beverly Hills, Calif, Sage, 1982.
24. Robinson JP: *How Americans Use Time: A Social-Psychological Analysis of Everyday Behavior.* New York, Praeger, 1977.
25. Sheehy G: *Passages: Predictable Crises of Adult Life.* New York, Bantam, 1978.
26. Schlossberg NK, Troll LE, Leibowitz Z: *Perspectives on Counseling Adults: Issues and Skills.* Monterey, Calif, Brooks/Cole, 1978.
27. Staines GL, O'Connor P: Conflicts among work, leisure, and family roles. *Monthly Labor Rev* 103:35–39, 1980.
28. Stebbins R: *Amateurs: On the Margin Between Work and Leisure.* Beverly Hills, Calif, Sage, 1979.
29. Stevenson JS: *Issues and Crises During Middlescence.* New York, Appleton-Century-Crofts, 1977.
30. Troll LE: *Early and Middle Adulthood.* Monterey, Calif, Brooks/Cole, 1975.
31. Vaillant GE: *Adaptation to Life.* Boston, Little, Brown, 1977.
32. Vroom V: *Work and Motivation.* New York, Wiley, 1964.
33. Wojciechowski D: I am a working mother . . . but who am I? *J Emp Counsel*, 19:106–112, 1982.
34. Yankelovich D: *New rules: Searching for Self-Fulfillment in a World Turned Upside Down.* New York, Random House, 1981.
35. Zimpel L: "The change in attitudes toward work." In *Work in America*, Report of a Special Task Force to the Secretary of Health, Education & Welfare. Boston, MIT Press, 1973.

CHAPTER 10

Later Adulthood

Joan C. Rogers and Teena L. Snow

The criterion used most frequently to define late adulthood is chronological age. In the past, age 65 was widely adopted as the criterion for mandatory retirement and for eligibility for social and health benfits and, hence, by implication, as the advent of old age. Recently, there has been a tendency to push "old age" back from 65 to 70 years.

Although chronological age may serve as a useful indicator of functional abilities in childhood, it tells us little about capabilities and potentials in later life. The rate and pattern of age-associated changes differs considerably from individual to individual and from system to system within the same individual. Furthermore, many of the decremental changes have little impact on overall functional performance.

Like middle age, old age is a relatively recent phenomenon. Whereas in 1900 only about half of the adults could expect to live to age 65; by 1976, 84% of the women and 70% of the men could anticipate reaching old age. Thus, old age has become accessible to a large segment of the American population rather than to only a minority. Even advanced old age is no longer rare. Whereas in 1900 less than 10% of adults lived to be 85; in 1976, 35% of the women and 16% of the men could anticipate reaching old age (71). These percentages highlight a salient characteristic of the aging population, namely, that it is predominantly female.

The period of old age often spans over 25 years. Hence, it may be longer than childhood and adolescence combined. Since the characteristics of older adults change over this period, gerontologists have sought to identify meaningful age groups. Age 75 has emerged as a significant indicator. On the average, the old-old (persons over 75) have more difficulty maintaining independent living, and thus need more social and health services than the young-old (those under 75).

Among the major challenges facing gerontological researchers is differentiating the effects of age and pathology. Although disease is not an inevitable accompaniment of old age, older adults are more vulnerable to debilitating conditions. Chronic conditions such as heart disease, cancer, stroke, arthritis, diabetes, and emphysema occur with increasing frequency in older individuals. Sorting out the effects of age from those of disease is critical for describing "normal" aging.

In addition to health, educational attainment is also significant for understanding aging. In general, people who are elderly today have not had the advantage of much schooling (72). Educational level is highly related to economic security. In addition, it impacts on a wide range of variables including type of occupation, health, longevity, and values.

This information about health, education, and income provides insight about the performance of different age groups. Developmental research employing cross-sectional designs, in which various age groups are compared, confound changes due to age and differences due to generational effects. It is likely that future generations of elderly will age in a manner that is very different from the current generation because of projected improvements in health and education.

This chapter deals primarily with the competent elderly, while Chapter 17 focuses on the frail elderly. Thus, this chapter describes what is known about normal aging from the perspective of the model of human occupation. The chapter reflects a composite of information drawn from multiple theories and studies, since the concepts that comprise the model have not as yet been investigated in a cohesive manner in the older population.

THE MODEL OF HUMAN OCCUPATION IN LATE ADULTHOOD

Performance Subsystem

Although age-related changes have been documented in all bodily functions, changes in the musculoskeletal and neurologic constituents of skills and in related cardiorespiratory functions have the most critical impact on occupational behavior in old age and, therefore, are briefly reviewed here. Recently, the inevitability of these decrements has been questioned. Many of these losses have been proposed as manifestations of disuse or misuse and of the older adult's acceptance of societal expectations for aging persons, rather than as necessary concomitants of the aging process. Future changes in behaviors and attitudes may well preclude or retard the development of what are today regarded as "normal" age-associated changes.

AGING AND PHYSICAL CHANGES

Musculoskeletal Constituent

Age-related changes in the musculoskeletal system are evidenced in the slowed movement, flexed posture, reduced height, and enlarged joints of many elderly individuals. Muscular activity diminishes in speed and strength. The number of active muscle fibers is reduced and the remaining muscle fibers contract less strongly. The arms and legs become flabby as muscular tissue atrophies and fatty tissue increases (25, 61).

Since cartilage erodes with extended use, the joints of older adults are generally less smooth, and thus less able to move through full range of motion. Connective tissue surrounding the joints becomes less elastic, making the joints less stable and less able to respond to quick changes in position (1, 61).

As aging progresses, bone mass decreases and the frailty of bone increases. Osteoporosis is a common occurrence in the aged, with women being more affected than men. Porous bones are easily broken and fractures of the vertebral column and at the neck of the long bones are common (67).

A thinning of the intervertebral disks contributes to a reduction in height. As the disks become dehydrated and less compressible, they are less able to absorb shock. The vertebral column becomes less flexible and more susceptible to injury. Back pain may become problematic. Postural alterations are typified by slight flexion of the hip and knees, varying degrees of kyphosis, and a forward tilting of the head and neck. In motion, these alignment difficulties are compensated for by the adoption of a wide stance gait (28, 61).

Neurologic Constituent

Structural changes within the nervous system include a loss of neurons, an increase in non-nervous tissue and lipofuscin, and decreased biochemical activity and cerebral blood flow. The efficiency of transmitting information from sensory receptors to the brain, within the brain and from the brain to the motor effectors is diminished (11, 29). Of greater functional significance are changes in the sensory receptors, particularly those receiving visual and auditory stimuli, since the output of the aging system is highly dependent on the quality of sensory intake.

Although sensory declines begin during the 40s and 50s, the changes are gradual, and they generally do not restrict activity until the 70s or 80s. The hearing loss that develops as a function of advanced age is called presbycusis. Presbycusis is a progressive and gradual hearing loss which may not be noticed until it becomes severe. It results in an inability to hear high frequency tones and a reduced ability to hear sounds in general. The major affect of presbycusis is on the consonants (high frequency tones) of human speech and, thus, speech may sound muffled and garbled. Speech is usually "misheard" rather than not heard at all (5, 17, 61).

Reduced visual functioning also shows a high correlation with age. The lens of the aging eye becomes rigid, opaque, and yellow; the size of the pupil decreases; and the eye muscles weaken. Structural changes are manifested in a decrease in visual acuity; presbyopia; a decreased ability to adapt to dark; an increased sensitivity to glare; a decreased ability to judge distances and color intensities, especially in the blue-green part of the spectrum; and a decreased ability to function in low light levels (5, 17, 61).

Receptors for gustatory, tactile, olfactory, vestibular, and kinesthetic stimuli also exhibit decrements. Reduced ability to perceive noxious stimuli, such as the smell or taste of spoiled foods, is of particular concern. Since the body's ability to respond to vestibular information becomes sluggish, the older adult's capability to recover balance is impaired, and the potential for falls is heightened (5, 17, 61).

Cardiorespiratory Processes

Cardiovascular and respiratory functions also undergo debilitating changes. The elasticity of the heart and blood vessels, the bronchial passages, and the chest walls is curtailed so that the ability to accommodate stress is reduced. Reductions in cardiac output and in vital capacity make it impossible for the body to perform at a youthful level. The efficiency of oxygen exchange diminishes and results in less oxygen profusion, in reduced nutrient delivery and in less efficient removal of carbon dioxide. The heart has to work harder to pump blood through the more rigid arteries, and the increase in peripheral resistance to blood flow contributes to rising blood pressure (34, 35, 56, 65).

SKILLED PERFORMANCE

The physical changes associated with aging may place the aging system at a disadvantage for interacting with the environment. Intake may be reduced and distorted. Output may be slowed and less accurate. However, the system acts as a coordinated whole, and it is a well documented fact that the impact of these bodily changes on the functional abilities of the individual may well be negligible.

Several factors account for the lack of correspondence between physical changes and functional declines. First, the habits of older adults enable them to do many tasks automatically. Less sensory information and thinking are needed to perform adequately. Experience outweighs the deficits. Second, older adults may compensate, consciously or unconsciously, for these changes. If visual acuity is reduced, one may wear glasses, increase the amount of light, and read large type print. The news may be heard rather than read. Slowness may become an adaptive mechanism, and the older adult may attend to things more carefully before responding. Overall, limitations on performance may be minimized or circumvented (5).

Perceptual Motor Skills

Among the most well documented findings in the gerontological literature is that it takes older persons longer to respond to stimuli than younger persons (75). Slowing occurs primarily in the premovement component, and involves the choice and shaping of movement rather than the overt action itself (8, 75). Although the delay in response time is negligible for most activities, it can become consequential in emergency situations where a rapid evasive response is needed.

In such situations the older adult may be unable to avoid an accident. Accidents are the sixth leading cause of death in persons over age 65 (72).

Process Skills

Older adults are less effective in solving laboratory problems than younger adults. They search for readymade solutions that are already present in their repertoires as opposed to formulating and testing new solutions. In obtaining information, they find it hard to distinguish relevant and irrelevant data and, hence, make many redundant inquires. The differences in problem-solving skills between younger and older persons may be more related to differential educational backgrounds than age. Laboratory experiments emphasize abstract thinking, which is highly related to educational level. Older adults find it easier to solve problems that are related to their past experiences than novel problems. In fact, when a problem can be managed with familiar strategies, older people may be more effective in problem solving than younger people. Little information is available on the relationship between problem solving inside and outside the laboratory (60).

Demming and Pressey (21) used test items reflecting everyday tasks, such as using a telephone directory, understanding common legal terms, and locating social services, to compare the performance of difference age groups. Both middle-aged and older adults performed better than the young adults. However, other (12, 31) studies employing practical problems have not been as optimistic. Younger subjects performed better because they used more efficient problem-solving strategies.

Problem-solving entails many component abilities, such as intelligence, capacity to learn and memory. Since these abilities are differentially affected by the aging process, the relationship between age and problem-solving capacity is complex. The "classic aging pattern" of intellectual function identified through intelligence tests exhibits decrements in psychomotor skills and little if any decline in verbal skills (9). The ramifications of age-related intellectual decrements on daily life are probably negligible because: the declines are small, there is little association between intelligence scores and the occupational tasks of adult life, and the life experiences of older adults can be used to bolster the decreased functions. In considering the relationship between age and intellectual capacity, health status must be taken into account. Birren (5) argued that observed decrements in the mental functioning of older individuals are closely linked to clinical or subclinical pathological conditions (5, 60).

Age-related changes in memory and learning may also impair the older adult's problem-solving potential. Memory deficits of late adulthood appear to reside in long-term rather than short-term memory (19). If the amount of material to be remembered is small and stays within the limits of short-term memory, memory differences between young and old people are unremarkable. If the memory task exceeds the management capabilities of short-term memory, older people remember less well than younger people. Older adults are also less able to retrieve items from long-term memory. Recognition of information is superior to recall (74). Overall, older adults can learn as well as younger persons, however, learning usually takes longer.

Communication/Interaction Skills

Communication skills enable the older adult to maintain contact with family, friends, caregivers, and service providers. It has been demonstrated that individuals can be identified as "old" by the quality of their speech (54). The aging voice is characterized by slurring, decreased volume, and imprecise consonants. Other facets of speech, including the selection of subjects for conversation, the length and initiation of conversation, and the ability to change topics, do not change appreciably with age (49). Similarly, the normal aged individual remains skilled in using facial expressions, hand gestures, and body language to enhance interactions and validate exchanges of information (49). Problems in communication are most apt to stem from auditory and visual impairments that impede the older person's ability to obtain information and hence to make appropriate responses.

Habituation Subsystem

The habits and roles comprising the habituation subsystem organize perceptual motor, process and communication/interaction skills into routines.

HABITS

The elderly have spent a lifetime developing habits to organize and streamline their daily lives. The aging human system is concerned with maintaining these habits, despite decreased energy reserves, so that tasks can be performed with a minimum expenditure of energy. At the same time, new habits must be developed to cover changing circumstances, such as widowhood or retirement, that often impose demands for new learning.

The learning of new habits may be handicapped by rigidity and interference. Habit rigidity involves resistance to change. With age, there does appear to be a tendency toward a lack of flexibility in intellectual and motor performance. Older adults are less inclined to modify their routine behavior even when the tactics employed are unsuccessful for task accomplishment. Current thinking on rigidity relates it more to cognitive than attitudinal factors. Limitations in obtaining and processing information make it difficult for older adults to adapt their response patterns and they persist in making ineffective responses (8).

Interference refers to the degree to which one's habits hinder new learning. Studies of older workers suggest that interference is maximal when the new job is highly similar to the old job, and minimal when retraining involves a task that is highly dissimilar (7). The fact that retraining takes longer for older than younger workers may be attributable to experience versus age, per se. People who are older have usually worked longer, and thus may have more old habits to overcome (7).

ROLE

In contrast to the role exits that occur at other life stages, the role exits of later life are often less voluntary and less pleasant. In other words, the older person has less control over them and they involve negative changes. For example, one may be forced to stop working because of mandatory retirement policies or failing health. Also, as a person ages the probability of losing one's spouse, adult children, or confidant through death increases. While the strain of role exits is cushioned at earlier life stages by the opportunities presented by new roles, the lost roles of old age may not be replaced. Since high social engagement is associated with life satisfaction, overall role loss may lead to discontent in old age. The adjustment process is complex, however, and concentration on role loss may obscure the strength derived from the quality of the remaining and substitute roles (6).

Perhaps the clearest expectations that society has for older adults is that they retire from work and find something useful to do. They are also expected to maintain financial and personal independence, and to exhibit social responsibility (4). Beyond these guidelines, society has few expectations. For this reason, the elderly are often spoken of as occupying a "roleless role."

Being in a roleless role has both advantages and disadvantages. On the negative side, the older population loses its ties to society, since it is through the fulfillment of socially valued role tasks that such attachments are formed. With the tapering off of work, parental and, sometimes, marital roles, social guidelines for time use are ambiguous. The lack of social regulation of behavior poses a potential threat to the identity of older adults. If satisfying replacements for lost or diminished roles are not found, the older adult is at high risk for boredom, loneliness, depression, substance abuse, and suicide.

On the positive side, older adults have gained considerable freedom to spend their time as they please. Normative guidelines for time use are minimal and they are free to explore role options that meet their needs and interests. The current generation of older adults is seeking to redevelop linkages to the social structure through a broad range of contributory roles, such as: continued paid employment; spouse, family, and friendship services; volunteerism; and education and leisure participation.

Work Role

The American experience with retirement is marked by several major trends. First, as a result of federal legislation enacted in 1978, people can now work longer. Congress abolished mandatory retirement for federal workers and raised retirement age to 70 in many work settings.

Coincident with the potential to increase work life, there is also a recognizable trend toward early retirement (66). While many of the present aged were forced to retire by mandatory retirement policies, many adults today are looking forward to retiring. These generational differences may be attributed to differences in attitudes toward leisure, as well as real differences in the financial feasibility of retirement.

Presently, both society and older adults are exploring work options for later maturity. One aspect of societal exploration is the introduction of a gradual withdrawal from work as opposed to an abrupt stoppage. A second pattern is the rehiring of older workers as consultants, as relief for workers on vacation and as additional help during peak production times. Job redesign, or adapting jobs to fit the older worker's abilities, is also being tried (30). On an individual basis, some older persons are retiring from one job and going to another (40).

Studies (4, 40) indicate that people continue to work past retirement age because of: a need for income, a desire to feel useful and to gain respect through contributory activity, the satisfaction derived from work, the need to have a significant activity around which to organize their lives, and the fear of being without a clear role.

Spouse, Family and Friendship Roles

Reduction or elimination of the work role is generally not simultaneously accompanied by disruptions in spouse, family and friendship roles. Thus, older adults may adjust their schedules by investing more heavily in these relationships. Marital satisfaction is apparently high in late life. The most rewarding aspects of marriage in late life are: companionship, the mutual expression of true feelings, economic security, being needed by the spouse, and the affectionate interaction. Different values and philosophies of life and a lack of mutual interests are the primary troublesome aspects (70).

Increased time during the postparental and postwork years may also be spent with adult children and grandchildren. Most older adults regard their relationships with their children as important and derive gratification from them. There is generally a reciprocal exchange between parents and children in the form of affection, gifts, money, and services (64). Social norms dictate that elderly parents should not interfere in the lives of their adult children. As frailty emerges, adult children may assume greater responsibility for the care of their aging parents. The young-old become the caregivers of the old-old.

Although the grandparent role carries no specific obligations, grandparents often act as surrogate parents, babysitters, supporters in times of crisis, housesitters, homemakers, teachers, confidants, and providers of income (23). The meaning of grandparenthood is variable. Commonly it is regarded as signifying biological renewal or continuity or emotional self-fulfillment. Less commonly, grandparents see themselves as being a resource to grandchildren and see their grandchildren as a means of vicarious achievement (47). Parents regard "good grandparents" as those who: do not interfere with parental upbringing and in the lives of their grandchildren, enjoy and love their grandchildren, set a good example, help when asked, are good listeners and provide discipline if needed (57).

Familial relationships are generally supplemented by relationships with age peers. The value of having a single confidant for safeguarding morale after retirement, widowhood, and decreased social participation has been demonstrated (42). Even though an extensive number of social relationships may not be needed, the person who has a number of friendships is more apt to find a replacement when a friend dies than the person who has none. Thus, the social interaction that is a part of other roles provides a valuable resource for promoting friendships.

The loss of one's spouse frequently occurs in old age and may severely disrupt the life of the remaining partner. Acute grief may last as long as 2 years and the incidence of mortality among the bereaved is high. Many roles may be simultaneously terminated with the death of a spouse—those of a friend, lover, confidant, homemaker, financial supporter, and comforter. Numerous other changes may be superimposed on the loss of a spouse. The remaining partner may have to learn to do or have done many things previously done by the spouse. Since women generally live longer than men, widowhood is more likely than is widowerhood.

The loss of pension benefits may precipitate a dramatic drop in style of living. Widows are the poorest segment of the American population with many getting by on an average income of less than $2000 a year (72). Widowers do better financially than widows since their pension benefits are not reduced or stopped if their wives die. Historically, the majority of American women have been homemakers and have not pursued full-time careers outside the home. As this pattern changes, some of the hardships of widowhood may be relieved.

Remarriage is a frequently overlooked transition of later life. Men are more likely to find a new mate than women. Although we generally assume that aged women would like to find a husband, one study found that the majority had no desire to remarry (41). Older men remarry for companionship and care, while women stress love and security (73).

Volunteer Role

A broad array of services is provided by older volunteers. For example, older persons have served as tutors for college students, drivers for handicapped persons, peer counselors, and providers of telephone reassurance for the homebound. Political activity, such as voter registration and lobbying, has also been attractive. Volunteerism allows older adults to continue to use their talents in a manner that benefits society. Men are prone to see volunteer work as a work substitute, while women perceive it as a vehicle for self-exression (51). Other reasons given for volunteer participation include contributing to the community, filling gaps in services, and increasing self-esteem and a sense of usefulness.

Student Role

A growing number of older persons are demonstrating that "no one is too old to learn" by assuming the student role. Older adults are attracted to courses aimed at: assisting them in coping with aging, increasing intellectual stimulation, improving communication skills, and enhancing performance for advocacy, citizenship and volunteer roles (53, 55). Educational institutions, churches, and libraries have developed special programs and incentives to attract older persons, thus increasing the opportunities to spend free time in learning. Older adults have also organized their own educational programs and have shared their talents by teaching other older adults.

Volition Subsystem

The volition subsystem directs the elderly person's choice of occupation and includes values, personal causation and interests.

VALUES

Values indicate what is desirable and meaningful in life and serve as central principles for mediating the way in which occupational goals are satisfied. Values have a pervasive influence on occupational choices in old age and are not linked to specific objects or situations.

Value Change and Stability

Research on value change in later maturity is contradictory. For example, evidence from several studies (58, 59) suggests that with age a shift from instrumental to terminal values occurs. Instrumental values, such as being ambitious, intellectual, capable, and responsible, become less important to older adults than terminal values such as a sense of accomplishment, freedom, equality, an exciting life, and a comfortable life. Evidence contradicting this switch in emphasis from instrumental to terminal values emerged from a study of three-generational families (3). Generational differences were observed on all instrumental values with the oldest generation reporting the highest scores. "A comfortable life" was the only terminal value on which differences were observed. This finding lends support to the consistency of terminal values across generations.

The significance attached to occupation by older adults is of particular interest. A decline in the importance of work and achievement with age is commonly regarded as appropriate for postretirement life. However, as age increases, work-related values have been shown to both increase (2, 77) and decrease (15, 27, 58). Antonucci et al. (3) hypothesized that work-related values may be retained by the older generation so that they can be transmitted to the younger generation.

Values and Adaptation

It is reasonable to anticipate some modification in values over the life span. Human development often involves a reappraisal of one's values to compliment changes in roles and physical and mental capabilities. Successful aging is an adaptive process that requires agreement between one's values, capabilities and activities.

Clark and Anderson (16) found that mental health in the elderly was correlated with the ability to redefine personal standards. Although elderly persons who were mentally healthy and mentally ill envisioned the same types of personal goals, the criteria against which they judged goal attainment varied substantially. Both groups desired independence, social acceptability, adequacy of personal resources, ability to cope with changes in the self, and having significant goals or meaning in later life. In seeking to fulfill these goals, the mentally ill appeared to be inclined toward competitiveness and ambition, whereas the mentally healthy were more relaxed and accepting in their attitudes. For example, concerning personal resources, the mentally healthy adopted a philosophy of conserving what they had, while the mentally ill persisted in striving to acquire new resources. Thus, healthy aging appears to be associated with a revision in the way in which values are satisfied.

Temporal Orientation

The ability to anticipate the future and to prepare for it can aid adaptation to shifting circumstances in later life. Futurity provides a guiding principle for structuring and interpreting life experiences and has been found to be an indicator of mental health in older adults (39, 43).

Although the elderly are commonly portrayed as living in the past, research has failed to confirm this notion. At all ages, people are most likely to be thinking about the present and least likely to be thinking about the past (13, 14, 26). The end of life is thus not accompanied by a change in conscious temporality.

Furthermore, older adults do not necessarily have a foreshortened view of the future. Kastenbaum (32) discerned that although the elderly are able to manipulate the future in the abstract, and hence to use time as an intellectual device for organizing experience, they are less able than younger people to project themselves into the future. Highly involved individuals have a more extensive future perspective than those lacking such involvement.

Valued Goals

Planfulness enables one to develop and work toward goals. Although the evidence (13, 68) suggests that planfulness declines with age, Cameron et al. (14) cautioned against interpreting this as a repudiation of the future. They noted that the elderly have less time to plan for than the young and that their need to plan may be lessened by the competence gained through years of experience. Having future goals and commitments has been related to the maintenance of morale in later life (62, 68).

PERSONAL CAUSATION

The passage from adulthood to old age is generally accompanied by multiple losses: loss of work, of social supports, of abilities. The accumulation of losses may place the elderly individual at risk for experiencing a diminished sense of competence and personal control. Sensing that they have little influence over these changes, older adults may become more externally oriented.

There is no clear evidence that aging and the accompanying changes in life situations negatively influence one's ideas of personal efficacy (10, 22, 69, 76). There is evidence to suggest that an internal control orientation is associated with a positive adjustment to old age and an external control orientation with maladjustment (37). Thus, from birth to death, the human organism strives to control the environment.

One aspect of personal causation is expectancy of success or failure. Level of aspiration refers to the level of performance a person expects to achieve on a particular task in view of past performance on that task. Compared to younger persons, older persons exhibit greater disparity in level of aspiration (36). They tend to both overestimate and underestimate their performance level. It is thought that overestimation may occur to protect self-esteem in the face of declining abilities, while underestimation may be motivated by a desire to avoid failure.

INTERESTS

Interests are valuable tools for use in structuring unobligated time because they serve to initiate and maintain involvement in activities. This premise was supported by a study in which participation in enjoyable activities was related to life satisfaction (52). Leisure participation patterns have been found to be a poor index of the interests of older adults. For example, considerable discrepancy has been observed between the actual and desired participation of older adults (45). While they were involved in activities that were solitary and less active, they wished to be involved in activities that were social and more active.

Activity participation is shaped by a person's preferences as well as by the actual and perceived availability of opportunities. Older adults report being constrained in their activity choices by factors such as: poor health; lack of transportation, facilities, money, leisure companions,

and skill; fear of crime; feeling too old to learn new activities; feeling that family and friends would not approve; and not getting a feeling of accomplishment from leisure participation (44, 46, 63). Thus, the constraints on leisure involvement from adulthood through later maturity may switch from work and family responsibilities to personal and social attitudes, personal capability, and availability of resources.

Output: Occupational Performance

Little research has been done to evaluate the influence of specific biologic and psychologic age-related changes on occupation. However, there is indication that tasks that were not formerly problematic become increasingly so for older individuals.

DAILY LIVING TASKS

Although most older persons continue to function independently in personal self-care and home management activities, functional dependency increases sharply with age because of chronic health problems. For example, in the 64–74 age category, about 52.6 persons per 1000 people require help in at least one self-care activity, while the rate for persons over age 85 climbs to 348.4 per 1000. Walking, going outside, and bathing are among the most difficult activities. For home management activities, the incidence per 1000 people increased slightly for each age group. The greatest needs were in shopping for personal items and doing routine household chores (24).

WORK

Productivity studies of workers of different ages have usually found that job performance remains stable through the 60s except where there is a time pressure. In considering these findings, it must be recalled that the older worker is a highly selected representative of the older age group and, compared to younger age peers, has the advantage of experience. It has also been observed that older workers tend to leave jobs that tax their declining abilities in speed, visual-motor coordination and short-term memory (5).

LEISURE

Compared to younger persons, older adults spend more time in activities of a sedentary and solitary nature, such as relaxation and reverie, and less time in activities that are more physically demanding and more social, such as dancing, going to the movies and participating in formal organizations (18, 20, 27, 33). In a longitudinal study conducted by Palmore (50), the elderly compensated for reductions in some activities by increasing their participation in others. This enabled them to maintain their overall level of activity. Other research (48) indicates that people tend to continue their participation in the same kinds of leisure activities as they grow old.

The Aging Human System and the Environment

Occupational behavior, the output of the human system, emerges from the interaction between the person and his or her surroundings. Lawton and Nahemow (38) suggest that behavior is adaptive if the competence of the older adult and the demands of the environment are matched. Adaptive behavior leads to positive affect. If there is an incongruence between personal competence and environmental demands, behavior is nonadaptive. If the older adult's competence is greater than the environmental (task's) challenge, the aging human system is deprived and underchallenged. On the other hand, if environmental demands exceed the older adult's ability to perform, he or she experiences overload and feels overwhelmed. In both situations, skill deficit and negative affect result.

Adaptation to aging is thus a process of maintaining a match between personal competence and environmental demands. According to the environmental docility hypothesis (38), as personal competence diminishes, the older adult becomes more vulnerable to the environment. For each person, there is an optimal level of environmental stimulation that will serve to maintain competence. The environment can be used to provide opportunities for action and interaction. High activity participation is associated with high morale and life satisfaction in later life (50).

SUMMARY

This chapter has dispelled the popular notion that late adulthood is marked only by decremental changes and discontent. The human potential for personal growth, achievement, and happiness continues throughout life. Table 10.1

Table 10.1.

Characteristics of occupational behavior in late adulthood

PERFORMANCE

Skills

Decreased efficiency of bodily functions
Maintainance of skills despite physical and psychological changes
Decremental changes may be due to pathology and disuse rather than age
Delays in response time may be critical in emergency situations
Maintenance of ability to learn new skills, although learning may take longer than at earlier ages

HABITUATION

Habits

Maintenance of old habits to facilitate the performance of daily living tasks
Development of new habits to adjust to age-related changes and to support new roles
Establishment and adaptation of habits may be more difficult than previously

Roles

Role losses associated with retirement, death of spouse, and relocation
Role continuity or gains associated with work options, kinship and friendship responsibilities, volunteerism, and educational and recreational pursuits.

VOLITION

Values

Reassessment of the ways in which values are satisfied
Inconclusive findings regarding the significance of instrumental values
Persistence of a primarily present orientation
Establishment of future goals and commitments

Personal Causation

Maintenance of need for personal control and drive to master the environment

Interests

Serve to structure unobligated time
Participation in solitary and sedentary pursuits is often accompanied by a desire to be involved in more social and more active activities
Leisure participation is constrained by personal and social factors

summarizes the characteristics of the occupational behavior of the aging human system. The integrated functioning of the performance, habituation, and volition subsystems enables most older adults to maintain competence in self-care, productive, and leisure activities, despite decreased efficiency in specific physical and mental functions. The aging human system requires environmental challenges to maintain its integrity and vitality.

References

1. Adrian MJ: Flexibility in the aging adult. In Smith EL, Serfass RC (eds): *Exercise and Aging: The Scientific Basis.* Hillside, NJ, Enslow, 1981.
2. Antonucci T: On the relationship between values and adjustment in old men. *Int J Aging Hum Dev* 5:57–69, 1974.
3. Antonucci T, Gillett N, Hoyer FW: Values and self-esteem in three generations of men and women. *J Gerontol* 34:415–422, 1979.
4. Atchley RC: *Social Forces in Later Life: An Introduction to Social Gerontology.* Belmont, Calif, Wadsworth, 1972.
5. Birren JE: *The Psychology of Aging.* Englewood Cliffs, NJ, Prentice-Hall, 1964.
6. Blau ZS: *Old Age in a Changing Society.* New York, New Viewpoints, 1973.
7. Botwinick J: *Cognitive Processes in Maturity and Old Age.* New York, Springer, 1967.
8. Botwinick J: *Aging and Behavior: A Comprehensive Integration of Research Findings.* New York, Springer, 1973.
9. Botwinick J: Intellectual abilities. In Birren JE, Schaie KW (eds): *Handbook of the Psychology of Aging.* New York, Van Nostrand Reinhold, 1977.
10. Bradley RH, Webb R: Age-related differences in locus of control orientation in three behavioral domains. *Hum Dev* 19:49–55, 1976.
11. Brody H, Vijayashanker N: Anatomical changes in the nervous system. In Finch C, Hayflick L (eds): *Handbook of the Biology of Aging.* New York, Van Nostrand Reinhold, 1977.
12. Burton A, Joel W: Adult norms for the Watson-Glaser tests of critical thinking. *J Psychol* 19:43–48, 1945.
13. Cameron P: The generation gap: time orientation. *Gerontologist,* 12:117–119, 1972.
14. Cameron P, Desai KG, Bahador D, Dremel G: Temporality across the life span. *Int J Aging Hum Dev* 8:229–259, 1977–1978.
15. Christenson JA: Generational value differences. *Gerontologist,* 17:367–374, 1977.
16. Clark M, Anderson BG: *Culture and Aging: An Anthropological Study of Older Americans.* Springfield, Ill, Charles C Thomas, 1967.
17. Corso JF: Sensory processes and effects in normal adults. *J Gerontol* 26:90–105, 1971.
18. Cowgill DO, Baulch N: The uses of leisure time by older people. *Gerontologist,* 2:47–50, 1962.
19. Craik FIM: Age differences in human memory. In Birren JE and Schaie KW (eds): *Handbook of the Psychology of Aging.* New York, Van Nostrand, 1977.
20. De Groot WL: *Analysis of Leisure Time Profiles of Selected Male Adults. Doctoral Dissertation,* Arizona State University. 1976.
21. Demming DR, Pressey SL: Tests indigenous to the adult and older years. *J Consult Psychol* 4:144–148, 1957.
22. Duke MP, Shaheen J, Nowicki S: The determination of locus of control in a geriatric population and a subsequent test of the social learning model for interpersonal distance. *J Psychol* 86:277–285, 1974.
23. Ebersole P, Hess P: *Toward Healthy Aging: Human Needs and Nursing Response.* St. Louis, Mosby, 1981.
24. Feller BA: *Americans needing help to function at home.* NCHS Advancedata. U.S. Department of Health and Human Services-Public Health Service, No. 92, September 14, 1983.
25. Fitts RH: Aging and skeletal muscle. In Smith EL, Serfass RC (eds): *Exercise and Aging: The Scientific Basis.* Hillside, NJ, Enslow, 1981.
26. Giambra LM: Daydreaming about the past: the time setting of spontaneous thought intrusions. *Gerontologist,* 17:35–38, 1977.
27. Gordon C, Gaitz CM, Scott J: Value priorities and leisure activities among middle aged and older Anglos. *Diseases of the Nervous System,* 63:13–26, 1973.
28. Gutman E: Muscle: In Finch C, Hayflick L (eds): *Handbook of the Biology of Aging.* New York, Van Nostrand Reinhold, 1977.
29. Hasselkus BR: Aging and the human nervous system. *Am J Occup Ther* 28:16–21, 1974.
30. Jacobson B: *Young Programs for Older Workers: Case Studies in Progressive Personal Policies.* New York, Van Nostrand Reinhold, 1980.
31. Jones HE, Conrad HS: The growth and decline of intelligence: a study of a homogeneous group between the ages of ten and sixty. *Genet Psychol Monogr* 13:223–298, 1933.
32. Kastenbaum R: Cognitive and personal futurity in later life. *J Individ Psychol* 19:216–222, 1963.
33. Keith PM: Life changes, leisure activities, and well-being among very old men and women. *Activ Adapt Aging* 1:67–75, 1980.
34. Klocke RA: Influence of aging on the lung. In Finch CE, Hayflick L (eds): *Handbook of the Biology of Aging.* New York, Van Nostrand and Reinhold, 1977.
35. Kohn RR: Heart and cardiovascular system. In Finch CE, Hayflick L (eds): *Handbook of the Biology of Aging.* New York, Van Nostrand Reinhold, 1977.
36. Krugman AD: A note on level-of-aspiration behavior and aging. *J Gerontol* 14:222–225, 1959.
37. Kuypers JA: Internal-external locus of control, ego functioning, and personality characteristics in old age. *Gerontologist,* 12:168–173, 1972.
38. Lawton MP, Nahemow LE: Ecology and the aging process. In Eisdorfer C, Lawton MP (eds): *The Psychology of Adult Development and aging.* Washington, DC, American Psychological Association, 1973.
39. Lehr U: Attitudes toward the future in old age. *Hum Dev* 10:230–238, 1967.
40. Lieberman L, Lieberman L: Second careers in arts and craft fairs. *Gerontologist,* 23:266–272, 1983.

41. Lopata HZ: *Widowhood in an American City.* Cambridge. Mass, Schenkman, 1973.
42. Lowenthal MF, Haven C: Interaction and adaptation: intimacy as a critical variable. *Am Sociol Rev* 33:20–30, 1968.
43. Lowenthal M, Thurnher M, Chiriboga D: *Four Stages of Life: A Comparative Study of men and Women Facing Transitions.* San Francisco, Jossey-Bass, 1975.
44. McAvoy LL: The leisure preferences, problems, and needs of the elderly. *J Leisure Res* 11:40–47, 1979.
45. McGuire F: The incongruence between actual and desired leisure involvement in advanced adulthood. *Activ Adapt Aging* 1:77–89, 1980.
46. McGuire F: Constraints on leisure involvement in the later years. *Activ Adapt Aging,* 3:17–24, 1983.
47. Neugarten B, Weinstein K: The changing American grandparent. In Neugarten B (ed): *Middle Age and Aging.* Chicago, University of Chicago Press, 1968.
48. Nystrom EP: Activity patterns and leisure concepts among the elderly. *Am J Occup Ther* 28:337–345, 1974.
49. Obler L, Albert M: Language and aging: a neurobehavioral analysis. In Beasley D, Daivs GA (eds): *Aging: Communication Processes and Disorders.* New York, Grune & Stratton, 1981.
50. Palmore E: The effects of aging on activities and attitudes. *Gerontologist,* 8:259–263, 1968.
51. Payne B, Whittington F: Older women: an examination of popular stereotypes and research evidence. *Soc Prob* 23:488–504, 1976.
52. Peppers LG: Patterns of leisure and adjustment to retirement. *Gerontologist,* 16:441–446, 1976.
53. Peterson DA: Participation in education by older people. *Educ Gerontol* 7:245–256, 1981.
54. Ptacek PH, Sander EK: Age recognition from voice. *J Speech Hear Res* 9:273–277, 1966.
55. Ralston PA: Educational needs and activities of older adults: their relationship to senior center programs. *Educ Gerontol* 7:231–244, 1981.
56. Reddan WG: Respiratory system and aging. In Smith EL, Serfass RC (eds): *Exercise and Aging: The Scientific Basis.* Hillside, NJ, Enslow 1981.
57. Robertson JF: Grandmotherhood: a study of role conception. *J Marriage Fam* 39:165–174, 1977.
58. Rokeach M: *The Nature of Human Values.* New York, Free Press, 1973.
59. Ryff CD, Baltes PB: Value transition and adult development in women. The instrumentality-terminality sequence hypothesis. *Dev Psychol* 12:567–568, 1976.
60. Salthouse TA: *Adult Cognition: An Experimental Psychology of Human Aging.* New York, Springer-Verlag, 1982.
61. Saxon SV, Etten MJ: *Physical Changes and Aging: A Guide for the Helping Professions.* New York, Tiresias Press, 1978.
62. Schonfield D: Future commitments and successful aging. I The random sample. *J Gerontol* 28:189–196, 1973.
63. Scott EO, Zoernick DA: Exploring leisure needs of the aged. *Leisurability,* 4:25–31, 1977.
64. Shanas E, Streib GF: *Social Structure and the Family: Generational Relations.* Englewood Cliffs, NJ, Prentice-Hall, 1963.
65. Shephard RJ: Cardiovascular limitations in the aged. In Smith EL, Serfass RC (eds): *Exercise and Aging: The Scientific Basis.* Hillside, NJ, Enslow, 1981.
66. Sheppard HL: Work and retirement. In Binstock RH, Shanas E (eds): *Handbook of Aging and the Social Sciences.* New York, Van Nostrand Reinhold, 1976.
67. Smith EL, Sempos CT, Purvis RW: Bone mass and strength decline with age. In Smith EL, Serfass RC (eds): *Exercise and Aging: The Scientific Basis.* Hillside, NJ, Enslow, 1981.
68. Spence DL: The role of futurity in aging adaptation. *Gerontologist,* 8:180–183, 1968.
69. Staats S: Internal versus external locus of control in three age groups. *Int J Aging Hum Dev* 5:7–10, 1974.
70. Stinnett N, Carter LM, Montgomery JE: Older persons' perceptions of their marriages. *J Marriage Fam* 34:665–670, 1972.
71. Treas J, Bengston V: The demography of mid- and late-life transitions. *Annals of the American Academy of Political and Social Science,* 464:11–21, 1982.
72. U.S. Department of Commerce. *Current Population Reports. Demographic Aspects of aging and the Older Population of the United States.* Washington, D.C., Bureau of the Census Special Studies Series P-23, No. 59, U.S. Government Printing Office, 1978.
73. Vinick B: Remarriage in old age. *Fam Coord* 27:359 363, 1978.
74. Walsh DA: Age differences in learning and memory. In Woodruff DS, Birren JE (eds): *Aging: Scientific Perspectives and Social Issues.* New York, Van Nostrand, 1975.
75. Welford AT: Motor performance. In Birren JE, Schaie KW (eds): *Handbook of the Psychology of Aging.* New York, Van Nostrand Reinhold, 1977.
76. Wolk S, Kurtz J: Positive adjustment and involvement during aging and expectancy for internal control. *J Consul Clin Psychol* 43:173–178, 1975.
77. Youmans EG: Age stratification and value orientations. *Int J Aging Hum Dev* 4:53–64, 1973.

SECTION 3

Generic Applications of the Model

Introduction

Earlier in the text it was pointed out that the model is intended as a tool to facilitate clinical thinking and problem solving. This section contains three chapters which address three types of clinical thinking and problem solving: treatment planning, occupational analysis and program development. Together the chapters can be conceptualized as offering a broad statement on the nature of clinical reasoning in which a therapist using the model engages.

The treatment planning chapter focuses specifically on the reasoning process which underlies questioning and decision making about the course of intervention for individual clients or patients. The occupational analysis chapter applies the model to the process of analyzing occupations for their inherent properties and therapeutic potential and the program development chapter outlines and demonstrates steps in the process of planning and evaluating an occupational therapy service based on the model. All three chapters are referred to as generic applications since they are potentially relevant to any client or patient group and to any type of setting or occupational therapy service.

The reader will necessarily want to translate the processes described in this section into his or her own situations of clinical reasoning. The corresponding exercises in the workbook provide structured opportunities to do so and should be especially helpful in operationalizing the concepts from this section.

CHAPTER 11

Treatment Planning*

Joan C. Rogers and Gary Kielhofner

Treatment planning is a problem-solving process in which the therapist selects relevant information about the patient and integrates it into a theory or explanation of each patient's unique occupational function or dysfunction (3, 8). This theory or explanation of the patient's status becomes the blueprint for therapy suggesting courses of action from which the therapist selects those best suited to the patient's strengths and weaknesses. Such treatment planning is not a rigid technical application of ameliorative procedures for discrete problems. Rather, it is a process of professional judgement which identifies right courses of action for a given individual. This chapter illustrates the use of the model of human occupation for treatment planning.

Patients come to occupational therapy when they, or others, perceive that they are not adequately performing their daily occupations or when there is reason to believe their performance is at risk of becoming unsatisfactory to themselves and/or others. Occupational behavior has been threatened or compromised by such factors as disease, trauma, abnormal development, age-related changes, imbalanced lifestyles, or environmental restrictions. The disruptions in occupational functioning characteristically are, or may become, severe and enduring. The therapist's role is to enable the patient to regain a former level of performance, maintain a current level, or achieve a more optimal one.

The occupational therapist must select appropriate therapeutic action for the patient (6). Correct therapeutic action emanates from an accurate and complete theory or explanation of the occupational dysfunction. To create an accurate explanation of occupational function and dysfunction, the therapist must determine and integrate both the positive and negative implications of different aspects of a patient's status. For example, a patient's limited active range of motion is a liability, but a patient's belief that he or she can overcome the disability is a potential asset. Both attributes are relevant to how the patient is likely to fare. The latter, belief in personal control, is a volitional trait. According to the model, volition governs the lower subsystems and it can lead to organization or disorganization of these lower subsystems. If the limited range of motion is correctable through active use of the joint, one can expect the patient's belief in control to lead to participation in occupations which will affect this remediation. This example draws upon only two aspects of a patient's status, but in clinical practice the therapist must identify and integrate a multitude of facts. The reasoning process is, therefore, much more complex. Use of the model gives the therapist more control over this process.

FIVE STEPS OF TREATMENT PLANNING

In the following sections we will illustrate the use of the model in five steps of treatment planning: (a) identifying clinical questions, (b) collecting data, (c) creating an explanation of the occupational function or dysfunction, (d) identifying and selecting from among treatment options, and (e) evaluating outcomes and adjusting therapy. This treatment planning process is illustrated in Fig. 11.1.

Identifying Questions for Clinical Assessment

From the model of human occupation one can identify five major questions which guide the process of collecting information on a patient's liabilities and assets. They are: (a) What is the volitional status of the patient?; (b) what is the habituation status of the patient?; (c) what is the performance status of the patient?; (d) what is the patient's history of performance?; and (e)

* Adapted from and reprinted with permission of The American Occupational Therapy Association, Inc., © 1983 *The American Journal of Occupational Therapy*, 9:601–616.

Identification of Clinical Questions to Guide Assessment
The therapist selects appropriate questions concerning occupational behavior strengths and weaknesses of a patient that will yield a holistic picture of the person's status

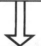

Collecting Assessment Data
The therapist gathers appropriate information on the patient through methods that are reliable and valid

Construction of an Explanation of the Occupational Function or Dysfunction
The therapist integrates data on the patient into a coherent theory of the person's status by drawing upon system principles concerning relationships between variables in the model

Identifying and Deciding Among Treatment Options
Treatment options are based on scientific data and past experience of the clinician. The therapist, having identified problems and strengths, and what could be done for a patient, makes a value judgment concerning what should be done

Evaluating Treatment Outcomes and Making Necessary Adjustments
After therapy is initiated the therapist determines whether goals are being approximated or met, looks for reasons why therapy may or may not be working and makes any necessary adjustments in treatment methods or goals

Figure 11.1. The treatment planning process.

what are elements in the environment supporting or constraining performance? Each of these questions can be further elaborated as will be illustrated next. The answers to these questions are integrated into an overall explanation of the patient's dynamic status in the second phase of treatment planning.

VOLITIONAL STATUS

Occupational therapy is an open system process in which patients influence their own well-being by their participation in occupations. Occupational behavior is ideally freely chosen by the individual. Before termination of occupational therapy, patients must show evidence that they will continue to choose to engage in adaptive patterns of occupational behavior or one can expect them to become disorganized and dysfunctional. By assessing volition the therapist determines how values, interests and personal causation influence the patient's choices for action, inaction or overaction. The components of each of these variables can be proposed as potential questions to assess all aspects of a person's volition (Table 11.1). This list of questions is fairly exhaustive for a thorough investigation of any patient's volition. For a particu-

Table 11.1.
Volitional questions for assessment

Personal causation

Does the person feel in control or does he/she feel controlled by external forces?
Can this person identify personal skills and liabilities?
Does this person feel his/her skills are relevant to his/her life situation and/or identify areas of needed skill development?
Does the person expect success or failure in various aspects of his/her life?
Are these views of personal causation realistic, given the person's actual abilities, environment, prognosis, and other assets and liabilities?

Values

What occupations, if any, have meaning for the person and why does he/she find them meaningful?
What standards of performance has this person internalized and how do they guide his/her action?
What is this person's relative orientation to past, present and future and what beliefs does he/she hold about how time should be used? Are they realistic and reflective of the culture at large and/or the person's subculture?
What goals does this person have?
Is the person's value system appropriate for his/her developmental level?

Interests

Can this person identify degrees of liking or disliking for various occupations?
What is the pattern of occupations this person enjoys? Is it reflective of a balanced life style?
Is this person's report of interest based on experience with the occupations and does his/her interest lead to participation in the activities?

lar patient, a therapist may identify from these questions those most important for clinical decision making. Thus it may be determined that for a chronic psychiatric patient, assessment should begin by focusing on what activities have some meaning to the patient; what activities provide the patient a basic sense of control; and what activities seem to evoke a sense of pleasure. Only later would it typically be possible for such a patient to be oriented to the future and establish realistic goals. For a depressed patient who has a pattern of exclusive work orientation, it may be most important to examine values about standards of performance and about how time should be used as well as leisure interest patterns. Thus priorities for assessment can be identified for different patients.

HABITUATION STATUS

While volitional assessment gives a picture of the patient's motivation for occupation, habituation is examined in order to determine possible sources of organization and disorganization of routine behavior. The questions indicated in Table 11.2 can guide assessment of habituation.

As with the volitional questions, the therapist will determine which aspects of habituation are most critical to examine first in assessing a given

patient. For an elderly person in a day care center, examination of availability of present roles to organize behavior might be most important, whereas for the coronary patient an examination of past role performance and possible role strain may be the initial focus.

PERFORMANCE STATUS

Evaluation of the person's performance is the aspect of assessment most fully developed in occupational therapy. It includes the assessment of a person's skills and of the underlying constituents of skills. Table 11.3 illustrates questions for evaluation of performance. These questions represent potential areas of patient assessment. The actual assessment of performance will depend on such factors as the patient's age and diagnosis. Once again, it is neither necessary nor feasible to evaluate all aspects of skills and skill constituents and the therapist must develop an approach to assessing performance that is comprehensive for the patient and his or her strengths and weaknesses.

ENVIRONMENTAL CONSTRAINTS AND SUPPORTS

Any assessment of a patient's functioning requires an understanding of the environments in

Table 11.2.
Habituation questions for assessment

Roles

What are the roles the person identifies as filling in the past, present and future?
What are the person's expectations of self for each current or anticipated role? Are they reasonable and commensurate with what others expect or would be likely to expect?
Does the person experience an overload or conflict of roles, or does he/she have too few roles to organize the use of time?

Habits

How organized is this individual's use of time? What is the nature of a typical day?
Does this person exhibit habits (e.g. promptness and attentiveness) necessary for role performance?
How flexible is this person? Can he/she adapt easily to changing circumstances?

Table 11.3.
Performance questions for assessment

Skills

Does the person demonstrate the ability to communicate and interact effectively with others in self-care, work and play activities?
Does the person have the ability to problem-solve, plan and organize personal behavior and the immediate environment in order to accomplish self-care, work and play tasks?
Does the person have the ability to receive and interpret sensory data and organize motor behavior in order to accomplish self care, work and play tasks?

Skill constituents

Are the person's symbolic processes intact? Does he or she have a cognitive limitation? Does the person show evidence of a poor internalization of rules to guide behavior? Is he or she aware of the properties of objects, persons and events and the expectations and possibilities for action they convey?
Does the person have an intact nervous system? Is there evidence of damage to, or developmental delay in the nervous system? Are there problems of sensory processing and integration?
Does the person have an intact musculoskeletal system? Does the person have functional strength and range of motion? Is there any disturbance of muscular, skeletal and joint integrity?

---

which the person has performed, is performing and will be performing in the future. Occupational behavior is interaction with the environment and an individual's occupational function or dysfunction is always influenced by the environment. Unless the environment for performance is considered, a therapist may underestimate or overestimate a person's actual ability to function. For example, a person who demonstrates independence in cooking in a clinic with appropriate level cabinets and working spaces may be unable to function in his or her own kitchen at home where architectural barriers prevent it. Or, a mentally retarded adult who appears unable to communicate effectively in a clinic may be able to manage effective exchanges with those in the residential facility where he or she lives. Assessment of the environment in-

volves such questions as those illustrated in Table 11.4.

HISTORY OF PERFORMANCE

Historical data are a source of information about how the patient arrived at the current condition; where he or she is likely to be headed; what past strengths or limitations will augment or constrain future success; and what kind of life-style he or she has led and will be attempting to reinstate, overcome or adjust. It allows a determination of the strength of certain values, goals, interests, and convictions about self. For example, the history could reveal lifelong values about work, a long-standing feeling of incompetence or a recurrent pattern of making poor choices because of a value conflict.

Table 11.4.
Environmental questions for assessment

What is the physical and social press for performance in this person's environment? That is, what performance demands are made by objects, tasks and other persons in the environment? Do these provide an appropriate level of challenge for the person? Are these demands relevant to the person's needs and goals?
What values will be held up as standards to judge the person's competence?
What supports exist or may be needed in the environment to maintain this person's competence in spite of limitations?
Does the environment foster or deprive the person of a sense of internal control?
Does the person have opportunities to practice new roles and habits in a variety of contexts?

Means of Collecting Assessment Data

To answer questions for clinical assessment the therapist selects an appropriate battery of assessment tools. Several factors such as time constraints, the person's capacity to respond to types of data collection procedures, and the importance of some data over others for treatment determine what assessments are chosen. In addition, the therapist is often constrained by what assessments are available for use and the degree to which scientific properties of these assessments have been developed and demonstrated. Ideally, the therapist should use assessment procedures that have been shown to yield results that are consistent, stable and valid for the intended purpose. In addition to formalized assessment procedures, therapists employ informal observations and conversations with patients and clients and integrate information from them into their pool of assessment data.

Constructing an Explanation of Occupational Dysfunction or Function

Once data have been gathered on relevant questions concerning various aspects of the person's status, they must be integrated into an explanation of the occupational function or dysfunction of the patient. Persons entering treatment will generally be in a state of occupational dysfunction, but this is not always the case. Some patients may require support to maintain or enhance a state of occupational functioning which is threatened by such factors as disease, environmental factors or a change in roles.

Developing an explanation of the patient's occupational function or dysfunction is facilitated by the model of human occupation because: (a) the model indicates relevant variables on which to gather information; (b) the model specifies relationships between these variables by indicating their place and function within subsystems and the hierarchical relationships of subsystems; (c) the model indicates the relationship between inner states of the person (i.e. status of subsystem components) and the environment and the influence of this relationship on the open system cycle; (d) the model provides a map of changes expected at different developmental levels; and (e) the model posits a continuum of occupational function and dysfunction from which a determination of the patient's level of performance can be made.

EXPLAINING SYSTEM DYNAMICS

By examining the information collected in light of the model and the proposed relationships of variables on which data are collected, a coherent explanation of the dynamics of the open system cycle can be generated. In a study of clinical assessment (4, 5), patients were rated on a continuum of function and dysfunction. The clinical reasoning used in this study illustrates how one integrates data on several variables to generate an explanation of a patient's occupational dysfunction. For example, stated goals were compared to skill level to determine whether each patient had sufficient skills to support his or her goals. Goals were also compared to a person's anticipation of future roles to examine whether the individual had a sense of intermediate roles necessary for goal attainment. If a person's goals were to enter a career for which he or she had no scholastic preparation, the therapist examined whether the person anticipated entering the student role in the future. Patients' reports of their past, present and future roles were used to determine how consistent their patterns of role enactment were and whether they supported or allowed enactment of interests and values. Through this type of data comparison the therapist arrived at an overall assessment of the degree of organization or disorganization in the person. If there was a pattern of consistency and congruency, the organization was rated higher. That is, if a patient's goals, interests and roles were consistent with his or her skill level, such a patient was considered more organized than a patient with more skills, but with a discrepancy between those skills and stated goals and interests. A patient's dysfunction was thus explained in dynamic terms as a lack of congruence or harmony between different subsystems variables as opposed to discrete deficits in various areas.

Generating explanations which take into consideration dynamic conditions between aspects of a patient and between the patient and the environment obviously requires conceptual problem solving on the part of the therapist. The model can be helpful to the therapist in this regard since it provides a framework for comparing and contrasting information and for constructing an explanation of function or dysfunction.

After constructing an overall explanation of the patient's status, the therapist can, by matching the patient's profile to the functional continuum proposed in Chapter 5, determine the patient's approximate level of function or dysfunction. This can be useful in deciding placement with groups or determining the treatment needs of the person since it allows identification of the degree of organization or disorganization in the person's occupational behavior.

GOING BEYOND THE MEDICAL DIAGNOSIS

It is important to recognize that the open system cycle of a patient cannot be adequately delineated from knowledge provided by the medical diagosis. Rather, the medical diagnosis is used in conjunction with other data gathered on the subsystems, on the environment and from the occupational history. The following example will demonstrate this and also illuminate how the process of identifying the open system cycle is undertaken.

Consider two patients with a diagnosis of hemiparesis secondary to a cerebrovascular accident. The diagnosis tells us an individual will have a weakness on one side of the body which affects ambulation, and upper extremity strength and coordination. What is not known from this information is the specific occupational behavior which is interrupted by this dis-

ability. If the patient is a retired individual living in a rural setting with a supportive extended family who occupies himself with entertaining grandchildren, doing small chores around the farm, fishing in the nearby pond and spending long hours playing checkers and talking with other elderly neighbors on his front porch, the implications of the hemiparesis might be quite different than if the individual is a 55-year-old, single, female dance instructor living in a high-rise apartment in mid-Manhattan, whose major recreation is travel. While the status of the two persons may be similar in respect to some basic functional abilities, each faces a very different set of needs in order to adjust to the disability. In the case of the first patient the open system cycle will likely be characterized by a reduction in performance. The patient may have difficulty in performing self-care and limited mobility. In the context of the patient's occupational roles as a retired grandfather with a strong friendship network, the constraints imposed at the performance level may be expected to be moderate. The patient may need family assistance in daily living tasks and to be able to continue his habits of playing with the grandchildren, fishing and visiting with friends. He will most likely continue to operationalize his values and interests. While he will experience some loss of control, he may adjust his values to allow family to assist him. For a period of time his level of occupational function might be at the competency level as he learns new habits such as walking with a walker or cane and dressing himself with adapted equipment. He should be able to return to achievement, filling the life roles he had prior to the onset of the stroke.

The second patient, on the other hand, may have a more severe disruption of the open system cycle. The constraints imposed on performance by the stroke will prevent her from continuing the same kind of involvement in dance instruction, it will likely make her role of an independent homemaker in a large urban setting untenable, and it will interfere with her recreation of travel. Because the constraints imposed by performance for her are more dramatic than for the previous patient, it is likely that this patient will feel more out of control, will perceive herself as separated from meaningful activities in her life and from pursuit of her interests. The result could be occupational dysfunction leading to helplessness.

As data are gathered on these patients, one's expectations are either confirmed, refuted or elaborated. For instance, one might find contrary to expectations that the dancer is able to draw upon her strong history of independence to begin to explore new options for her life-style. Thus, one might discover that she is actually beginning a process of occupational functioning at the exploratory level.

It is also expected that patients' occupational dysfunction and function will change over the course of therapy. As functional movement returns, as depression subsides, or as the patient learns new adaptive skills the constraints imposed by the performance subsystem will be lessened. Patients may begin to move from learning skills to integrating them into habits, thus moving from the exploratory to competence level of occupational functioning.

RECOGNIZING THE MULTIFACTORIAL NATURE OF DISABILITY

The most important aspect of constructing an explanation of dysfunction is that it provides an appreciation for the multifactorial nature of disability and subsequent adaptation requirements. For example, we might observe in the clinic that a patient cannot dress herself. Ostensibly this is because she has contractures in her upper extremities. Thus, we attribute the cause, in part, to the musculoskeletal constituent of skill. In addition, we might also find she does not dress herself because of a memory problem and attribute the problem also to the symbolic constituent of skill. We might also find that, in concert with contractures and the memory problem, she is unable to reach her clothes from a wheelchair. In this case, the dressing dysfunction is also produced by a combination of limitations in the performance subsystem and environmental constraints. Further assessment of the volition and habituation subsystems of this woman may reveal yet other contributing factors to the dressing dysfunction. We might discover that she is not motivated to dress herself because she has lost her homemaking role as a result of the disability and that the disability also interferes with her hobby of needlework. For this woman dressing has always been part of a routine which prepared her to go about her lifework, taking care of her home and participating in her leisure pursuits. Now she literally has nothing for which to dress. This woman has lost access to things she values and finds pleasurable and she feels she has lost personal control over her life. The

volitional factors not only account for the reasons why she is unmotivated to dress but reveal the potential for further disorganization. At this point it becomes evident that a whole complex of factors may contribute to why this woman is not dressing herself. If we are to expect her not only to be able to dress herself when therapy is terminated, but also to carry on this activity as part of her daily routine, then therapy must attend to other aspects of her occupational dysfunction.

As illustrated in this example, to construct a theory of the patient's function or dysfunction, one engages in a process of examining alternative interpretations of the dysfunction. The evidence supporting or opposing each alternative is weighed. Through this process the explanation of the individual patient is polished and repolished. In this way, the therapist arrives at a cohesive conception of the patient and, having grasped the whole, goes back and reinterprets the parts in the light of this gestalt understanding. Once a holistic picture of the patient has been devised, treatment planning moves from explanation to decision making.

Identifying and Deciding Among Treatment Options

Having proposed an explanation of the patient's occupational status, the therapist then begins to explore the actions that could be taken to enhance occupational role performance. The intent is to generate a list of the treatment options available for both problems and assets presented by the patient. The aim, at this stage of treatment planning, is to foster an awareness of the range and kind of treatment possibilities. In effect, the therapist uses the explanation of the patient's occupational function or dysfunction to construct a theory of practice for the particular patient.

CONSIDERATIONS OF TREATMENT EFFECTIVENESS

The therapist's consideration of what could be done, includes a review of the relative effectiveness of treatment approaches relevant to problems and strengths the patient exhibits. One considers for a particular treatment option what results can be expected, and how long it will take to achieve them. Any hazards associated with the various treatments or with no treatment, are evaluated in the light of the potential benefits.

Decision making concerning the appropriate action can approach certitude, if the deleterious effects of a disorder without treatment are known, and if there is substantial evidence of how these effects can be altered by a particular treatment. For most occupational therapy approaches or procedures, however, the scientific evidence is not definitive. In the absence of scientific knowledge about the effectiveness of treatment options, clinicians rely on knowledge gleaned from their own clinical experience or from the experience of others. Thus, each time a therapist treats a patient, a clinical experiment is performed, in which the objective is to replicate a successful outcome of a past experiment (2). As a first step in reproducing the experiment, the therapist mentally reviews previous patients whose occupational status resembled the patient at hand. Although no two patients are exactly alike, the therapist assembles subgroups of patients who are most similar to the patient under study (9). Treatment is selected for the new patient by analyzing and comparing the therapeutic actions and outcomes of the patients in the reference group.

Organizing information about treatment effectiveness is facilitated if the therapist has a conceptual framework for clinical decision making. The model serves as such an organizational framework for comparing past patients. For example, a therapist may know that arthritic patients with homemaker roles tend to do best with a given type of adaptive equipment and that they routinely have to learn a specific set of skills for energy conservation and problem solving.

The model also serves as a framework for considering differential outcomes of therapy. For example, it may be observed that one patient did better at learning cooking skills than another because she had a deeper interest in cooking and the latter's values tended to fall outside the homemaker role and to relate more to her volunteer role. Thus, explanations for positive and negative outcomes of therapy can be generated.

ETHICAL DECISION MAKING

The final task of selecting among treatment options involves an ethical question of what *ought* to be done to enhance the person's occupational competence. Simply because a treatment or a goal appears technically feasible for the patient, does not mean that it should be selected.

Assessment of the patient's performance and habituation subsystems generally provides the evidence of problems which can be addressed. For example, therapists may discover that various patients have poor grip strength, poor visual-motor integration, a cognitive deficit, imbalanced use of time, or extreme anxiety interfering with task performance. From identification of these problems the therapist could reasonably initiate the following kinds of treatment: activities to increase muscle strength of the upper extremity, visual-motor integration tasks, cognitive retraining procedures, planning for time use, and training in stress management techniques.

While these modalities are potentially appropriate for the corresponding problem, the therapist must decide whether and how each ought to be implemented for the patient. To make this decision two sources of information are critical: (*a*) information on the patient's volition, and (*b*) information on the patient's social and task environment. That is, to decide what ought to be done for a given patient, a therapist cannot be limited to knowledge of performance deficits. The therapist must also know to what personally meaningful and socially valued ends the patient would be willing to direct performance. For instance, one should know that a child who has visual-motor problems wants, above all, to play ball with his peers and that his parents are concerned over his school performance. One should know that a woman, who lost her dominant upper extremity secondary to sarcoma, is an artist who makes her living painting watercolors. Without such information the therapist cannot be assured that treatment is directed toward those objects which the patient finds personally relevant and that modalities employed as therapy relate to those personally meaningful goals.

It may mean that the child's therapy must include consideration of his desire to play ball (a developmentally appropriate activity) and that his parents may need training to understand the importance of his play as a source of self-esteem to increase his confidence for school work. It may mean that the woman will be more anxious to transfer motor skill to her nondominant hand in order to resume painting than she will be to engage in prosthetic training and that both will have to be pursued in therapy. The ethical aspects of clinical decision-making are thus two-fold. First, the therapist must be careful not to impose personal values on patients, thereby negating patients' dignity and right to determine their own values and objectives. Secondly, the therapist must select a course of action that is aimed at eliciting the patient's own volition (i.e. the patient's personal choice to engage in meaningful action) so that therapy will be more efficacious. Thus, ethics apply both to the objectives of therapy and to choosing the most efficacious means in therapy. Since occupational therapy is a process that absolutely depends on the patient's own participation and action, the efficacy of therapy is closely tied to an understanding of the patient's volition.

The impact of considering volition in the ethical choice of the most efficacious therapy is aptly illustrated in the following example that a student therapist provided of a patient she was treating. This man, Charlie, experienced a cerebrovascular accident (CVA) 4 months before his planned retirement from running a family business. He had recently purchased a new boat and fishing equipment in order to pursue an interest for which he had little time during the years as a worker. The patient was engaged in what was routine for stroke victims in the setting: he was placed on a skate board to range the affected upper extremity and offered a deltoid assist. However, Charlie was extremely unmotivated, he would not range his arm unless constantly cajoled by the therapist and he tended to be sullen and tearful. He also complained that he saw no reason or end to the process of using the skate board. The therapist's response to the situation is aptly described in her own words:

I went home and thought about Charlie. He wasn't intrinsically motivated to push that skateboard, he didn't want to use the deltoid aid. He hated therapy. At that point, I did too.

It was not so much the fact that he had a CVA but what else was going on and what it all meant for Charlie. What was his life like before the stroke? What was the status of his volition subsystem? Did his interest lead him to playful behaviors and allow recreation or was he too concerned about work time for recreation? My mind flooded with related questions. During our next skateboard session we discussed these matters.

It turned out that there was much more to

his CVA than left sided hemiparesis and hemianopsia. There was Charlie and his life. We talked about his work and what it means to him, his recovery, and his future "at the end of the ramp."

It seemed that his past roles had no relationship to his interests. He never wanted to be a salesman but his father's death led him to feel responsible to the family business. Therefore, Charlie took over and became a dedicated businessman to the point of totally devoting himself to his work. His concern now centered around his forced early retirement and around how he was going to spend his time. Because of his hemiparesis he was also afraid his wife would have to take care of him.

We planned alternate ways of maintaining the business and how it could be handed over to someone. Charlie was unsure about his life after retirement, as all his energy has always been absorbed in work. He wanted to pursue his leisure interests to fill the void left by retirement, but now he felt that his stroke would render him incapable of this. How could he ever think of driving his new boat or casting his fishing rod? He had no other strong interests.

It was time to toss the skateboard and deal with what really mattered to Charlie. The next day his wife brought in his new fishing rod. We attached graded sized fish (weights) to the leader line and practiced casting and reeling using the affected extremity as an assist originally and later to cast the rod. We spent time developing grasp and prehension patterns by practicing "cleaning fish" using a leather strip which would later be used as a strop to sharpen his knife blade. I never had to count his repetitions again. Charlie later developed the coordination to tie his own lures and leader lines. His outlook and prognosis improved with each passing day. Therapy was what it needed to be. It was something to take home. It had value (7).

As the example illustrates what is in the best interest of the patient and what will work best as a mode of therapy cannot be decided on an *a priori* basis by the therapist. One cannot know for all patients with the same medical diagnosis that a given regimen of therapy will always be the most efficacious. There is a temptation to do this, but the pitfall is that a conflict between what the therapist thinks is best and what holds meaning for the patient may be at odds. If the therapist's idea prevails over the patient's there is the very real possibility that potential for recovery or enhancing a patient's ability is ignored or prevented. This is where the ethical nature of the clinical decision becomes most evident. It is not just that the therapist must respect the rights of the patient for choice, but also that the positive outcome of therapy depends on the degree to which the patient can choose the course of action or come to see the wisdom of a particular course of action. There are, of course, times when a therapist must disagree with a patient's own goals and attempt to provide information so that the patient has a more realistic view or, at least, has a clearer sense of the consequence of a particular course of action.

In addition to respecting the particular views and concerns of the patient, the therapist is also placed in a moral position of mediating to the patient reasonable expectations of the social environment. The therapist becomes a socializing agent bringing societal demands to bear on an individual. This occurs when, for instance, an adolescent patient is expected to engage in self-care and to participate in chores in a halfway house. While this is often a difficult position for the therapist since it involves a coercive element, it should also be recognized that the message that one is expected to perform is also an expression of societal confidence in the person's ability to perform and of the value society places on that performance. Thus it can be an affirmation of the person's basic worth and dignity and his or her belonging to society as a contributing member. Expectations for performance must, therefore, be reasonable and reflect culturally valued means and ends.

The importance of making the patient's own concerns and values the guiding principle in clinical decision-making is best recognized by considering what therapy is. It is the patient and not the therapist who is the agent of change. As open systems, patients organize or reorganize themselves through engagement in occupation. The choice to effectively occupy oneself comes from a sense of personal freedom. The patient ultimately must will the action which is undertaken as part of the clinical process or else true change cannot result. This is equally true of the child who must actively pursue needed sensory input in play and of the adult who must identify goals for future performance.

In cases where a patient might not initially be able to choose a course of action deemed necessary for therapy, the therapist must be careful so that the ultimate freedom of the patient to

choose is always the guiding principle. For instance, a severely depressed individual may, if not influenced by a therapist, choose to do nothing, continue to feel sad and helpless and remain in a chronic cycle of maladaptation. The goal of the patient's participation in activity would be for such patients to begin to discover pleasure in action, to feel some control over their own bodies and emotions, and over their immediate environment. When these volitional elements are nurtured in therapy, patients are brought to a point where they can begin to more fully take over their own volitional processes in therapy.

It almost goes without saying that this is a delicate and complex decision-making process. The methods used to answer ethical questions differ from those used in science. While scientific questions are answered by accumulating data and testing hypotheses, ethical questions are resolved by coming to grips with values and making value judgments [1]. To empower the patient to act as his or her own moral agent, the therapist provides the patient with the knowledge needed to participate effectively in decision making. The therapist presents the possible options for treatment, projects the outcomes of each option, explains how the outcomes are achieved, and outlines a time sequence for goal attainment. The selection of treatment becomes more difficult as the merits of one action over other actions become more ambiguous. The therapist makes known his or her preferences for the patient's treatment as well as the rationale for this decision. The patient and/or a family member or guardian† ends the deliberation by making a choice. Once the course of action has been determined, the therapist supports or confirms the decision. The therapist strives to bolster the patient's belief that he or she can carry out the treatment and achieve the goals. The treatment process ends, therefore, in persuasive rhetoric by which the therapist seeks to influence patients to fully engage in occupations which appear in their best interests.

Evaluating the Outcome of Clinical Action

While the therapist may identify goals and means for therapy through careful evaluation

---

† When patients are unable, because of their age or disabilities, to act alone as their own moral agents, family or legal guardians may act with them or on their behalf to make such decisions.

and obtain a patient's willingness to embark on a course of action for therapy, there is no final assurance that any selected action will be efficacious. This can only be assessed by determining whether the outcomes are those desired by the patient and therapist. Ongoing assessment allows both the patient and the therapist to determine whether therapy is working.

In some cases it will be found that desired outcomes are attained. A patient who has been doing woodworking to increase upper extremity strength will show gains. Another patient will have attained the needed confidence to problem-solve independently. Still another will have learned to use a prosthetic device to perform simple tasks. When goals have been attained, the therapist and patient may together set new goals and choose new, more demanding, tasks for the patient to perform in order to reach those goals.

In some cases it will be found that desired outcomes are not attained. It may be determined that the original objectives were not realistic or it may be determined that the therapeutic means chosen were not optimal for goal attainment. Depending on the mutual decision of the therapist and patient, new goals and/or new means may be chosen.

In order to facilitate reasoning that underlies these kinds of decisions the therapist returns to the explanation of the patient's occupational function or dysfunction and enters the new information. Consideration of these data may lead to a new explanation for an existing problem, or it may lead to the recognition that a person's status has changed from occupational dysfunction to occupational function, or from one level of dysfunction or function to another level. When the explanation is altered to take into consideration the new information, the therapist is enabled to decide new alternatives for therapy and bring them to the patient.

References

1. Brody H: *Ethical Decisions in Medicine.* Boston, Little, Brown, 1981.
2. Feinstein AR: Scientific methodology in clinical medicine III. The evaluation of therapeutic response. *Ann Intern Med* 61:944–966, 1964.
3. Line J: Case method as a scientific form of clinical thinking. *Am J Occup Ther* 23:308–313, 1969.
4. Oakley F, Reichler R: Pilot study of a battery assessing psychosocial function. Paper presented at the *American Occupational Therapy Association Annual Conference*, Portland, Oreg. 1983.
5. Oakley F, Kielhofner G, Barris R: A Study of a battery assessing psychosocial function. *Am J Occup Ther* (in press).
6. Pellegrino E, Thomasma DC: *A philosophical basis of medical practice.* New York, Oxford University Press, 1981.
7. Plummer T: Untitled, unpublished paper. Virginia Commonwealth University, 1983.
8. Rogers JC: Eleanor Clarke Slagle lectureship—1983; Clinical reasoning: the ethics, science, and art. *Am J Occup Ther* 37:601–616, 1983.
9. Schon DA: *The reflective practitioner: how professionals think in action.* New York, Basic Books, 1983.

CHAPTER 12

Occupational Analysis*

Sally Hobbs Cubie

The study of occupations is essential for occupational therapists because the use of occupation as a therapeutic agent is the foundation of practice (1, 4, 7, 9). Historically, therapists have studied the qualities of occupations which evoke such diverse desired behaviors as cooperative social interaction and increased range of motion. Various formats for this kind of activity analysis are currently in use (2, 3, 5, 6, 8). Some emphasize detailed analysis of specific behaviors (5), while others explore patterns of behavior and behavioral contexts (2). This chapter builds upon the approaches of these analyses, and proposes an occupational analysis method based on the model of human occupation.

The model emphasizes the mutual ongoing influence of person and environment upon each other. Consequently, occupational analysis must deal with the following issues; in general, what kind of environmental press occurs within this occupation? How can this occupation, as it is usually performed, activate or support adaptive behavior for the person? What types of output are generated? How can this occupation be presented so that desired roles, habit patterns and skills can be learned?

The occupational analysis method is proposed as a two-part process. The first part is a descriptive study of how occupations correspond to the human open system—as environments for performance, and as potential activators of values, personal causation, interests, roles, habits, and skills. This analysis of *inherent qualities* in occupations overlaps with a second process of examining occupations as *potential therapeutic media*. This clinical occupational analysis explores how occupations can engage a client group in exploration, competence and achievement levels of behavior.

Occupational analysis aims toward developing a science of occupation. Clinical occupational analysis aims at clarifying the practical relationship between occupations and therapeutic goals. The two processes are presented in separate sections of this chapter and can be undertaken separately. However, they are designed to complement and reinforce each other.

Table 12.1 illustrates guiding questions for occupational analysis, and Table 12.2 presents questions for clinical occupational analysis. The occupation of meal preparation will be analyzed throughout this chapter to illustrate both processes.†

OCCUPATIONAL ANALYSIS: THE STUDY OF OCCUPATIONS

Just as occupational behavior is examined in terms of the environment, volition, habituation, performance, and output, so must occupations themselves be explored in relation to these variables. Those who use occupation to encourage adaptive behavior must study the qualities of occupation which engage the will, organize behavior and foster skills. Occupational analysis examines five areas: the environment created by the occupation, the motivation it can elicit, the ways it organizes behavior, the skills it uses, and the kinds of output it generates. Each of these analyses are explored in the following discussions.

Environmental Analysis: What Press is Created by Objects, Tasks, Social Groups, and Culture in This Occupation?

As noted in Chapter 4, the environment can be understood as a hierarchy composed of objects, tasks, social groups or organizations, and

---

* Howard University occupational therapy students have worked with this information at various stages of its development. Their experiences and suggestions have been very valuable to the author, and are much appreciated.

† Sequential steps for occupational analysis and appropriate forms for undertaking these steps are provided in the workbook. The reader will find it helpful to work back and forth between the chapter and the workbook.

culture. A particular occupation can also be studied in terms of the environment it creates. The environmental press within an occupation can be understood by answering several questions: What objects are used in the occupation, and how available, complex, flexible, and meaningful are they? What are characteristics of the task (complexity, rigidity, degree of playfulness, temporal requirements, social nature)? What social groups and/or organizations use this occupation? And, finally, what cultural attitudes pertain to and/or can be communicated in this occupation?

The answers to these questions provide information about the environmental qualities which are part of an occupation. The following brief environmental analysis of meal preparation illustrates the kind of perspective generated by this analysis.

Table 12.1.
Occupational analysis: the study of occupations

1. *Environmental analysis:* what press is created by objects, tasks, social groups, and culture in this occupation?

2. *Volitional analysis:* how does this occupation activate personal causation, values and interests?

3. *Habituation analysis:* how does this occupation organize behavior into habits and roles?

4. *Performance analysis:* in the performance of this occupation, how are perceptual-motor, process and interpersonal skills used?

5. *Output analysis:* how is this occupation used in work, play and/or daily living tasks?

ENVIRONMENTAL ANALYSIS OF MEAL PREPARATION

Cooking and serving a meal includes preparation, consumption, and clean-up; it may be a simple meal for one or a dinner for many people.

Objects. The required objects include food; places for storing food; and utensils for measuring, mixing, cutting, cooking, serving, and cleaning up. These objects are generally available in a wide cost range, and can be as simple as an iron skillet or as complex as a computerized microwave oven. They can be used for many different processes, and are therefore flexible. A primary symbolic connotation of these objects is caregiving and nurturance.

Task. A task sequence for meal preparation will include some of the following steps: choosing a menu, buying groceries, planning cooking time, following recipes, cooking the meal, serving it, dining, and cleaning up. The task can be very simple, as when a fast-food meal is selected, purchased, consumed, and disposed of; or it may be very complex, as when a large family holiday meal is prepared. The task can be approached in either a rigid or a flexible manner (e.g. following a recipe exactly, or substituting available ingredients). Meal preparation can be very playful (cooking hot dogs over a campfire) or serious (a religious group supper acknowledging world hunger). Temporal requirements for meal preparation tend to be explicit and closely linked with cultural patterns. Economically advantaged Americans expect to eat three substantial meals a day. This is turn poses temporal requirements for preparation and clean up. Cooking may be a public task as when preparing food for guests or it may be private. It may be done cooperatively; and it can be competitive, as in a "best desserts" contest.

Table 12.2.
Clinical occupational analysis: the use of occupations in therapy

Level of occupational function	Needs of the patient or client population	Occupational analysis
Exploration	What skills must they learn? What skill constituents must be enhanced?	What arrangements (of object, task, social group, and cultural context) will provide a safe environment to encourage skill learning and enhancement of skill constituents?
Competence	What work, play and daily living task routines do they require, given their developmental level, disability and expected environment?	How can the occupation be practiced as part of their daily routines?
Achievement	What roles must they perform in their everyday lives?	How can the occupation be used in performance of these roles?

Social Group/Organization. The social environments for meal preparation range from the solitary individual, through the family and groups of friends, to large public settings.

The activity is basic to the family social unit, as an organizing and socializing process for all family members, whether they share in tasks of preparation and clean-up, or only in enjoyment of the food. Restaurants employ many people in food preparation, and create public environments for dining. Large organizations often hold dinners and banquets to celebrate special events or to entertain members.

Culture. The preparation and consumption of food is central to any culture; the way it is carried out comunicates important qualities of a culture or cultural subgroup. Reliance on fast-foods and convenience foods suggests that higher values are placed on work and leisure than on nurturance of self and others, for example. Frequent ceremonial gatherings for food (church suppers, business lunches) reconfirm the importance of memberships and traditional values for participants. Soup kitchens provide a setting where homeless people can share meals together, and a degree of community can be forged.

From the previous analysis one can see that the preparation and consumption of meals is a highly adaptable and flexible activity. Therefore, great variation in the press from this activity is possible. Occupational therapy requires adaptable environments for individual learning. An occupation such as this which has many possible variations of object, task, social group, and culture is likely to be much more useful than one which can only be presented in limited ways. Certain occupations allow this flexibility in environmental variables without extensive investments in materials, or unusual adaptations which would make the activity irrelevant to everyday life. Occupations which can generate various levels of arousal and can be easily practiced in a variety of settings will generally be greater resources for therapists than those which are limited in the dimensions of object, task, social group, and/or culture.

Volitional Analysis: How Does This Occupation Activate Personal Causation, Values and Interests?

An understanding of the volitional aspects of occupation allows a therapist to incorporate opportunities for personal choice (through interests, values and the sense of personal causation) into the treatment process.

The personal causation dimension of an occupation can be examined by asking the following questions: what opportunities does it provide for exploring personal effectiveness? Does it emphasize internal or external control? Is it relevant to skills used in everyday life? Can participants anticipate outcomes and identify success reliably?

The potential for enacting values in an occupation is assessed by several questions: what kinds of objectives can participants meet? What are inherent standards of performance? How does it encourage awareness of past, present and/or future? What values about time use does it reflect? The interest dimension of an occupation can be assessed by asking whether it involves enough variety to have wide appeal and to encourage discrimination; if it is likely to have been part of past experiences; and whether it can be frequently chosen and enacted in many environments.

VOLITIONAL ANALYSIS OF MEAL PREPARATION

Personal Causation. Meal preparation gives many opportunities for experiencing personal effectiveness, because personal choice of foods and recipes and actual preparation determines the outcome almost entirely. It develops and maintains skills which are crucial to everyday life. Most outcomes can be reliably predicted as long as recipes are chosen which are suitable to the skill level of the cook.

Values. Meal preparation encourages awareness of the past in cultural links with favorite foods (e.g. cookies after school and grandmother's lasagne recipe). The use of seasonal foods encourages awareness of the present. Future objectives concerning diet (nutrition and weight) can be met using this occupation. The importance of nurturing is reflected in food preparation. Cooks are expected to prepare meals that look and taste good, and are in keeping with budget and dietary needs.

Interests. Taste preferences, social preferences (frequent or infrequent entertaining) and simple or complex daily routines (fastfood or gourmet meals) can find expression in this occupation, giving a wide range for choice and discrimination. It is likely to have some interest for most people because it is an inevitable part of daily life. It can be enacted in a very wide variety of environments.

The previous volitional analysis illustrates that meal preparation and consumption has motivational potential. It allows many opportunities for personal choice. It embodies many kinds of values. And it offers expression to a wide range of preferences. Motivation is crucial to all other aspects of occupational behavior. Therefore, occupations which allow a wide range of choices will be particularly useful in a variety of individual treatment plans. Highly motivating occupations are those which are clearly linked to establishing mastery in culturally valued routines of work, play and daily living tasks. Of course, there are individual differences in motivational appeal of activities, and treatment planning will ideally use the widest possible range of activities both within and outside of the clinic. However, occupations having a high potential for motivating a large number of people provide the most flexible foundation for a therapeutic program.

Habituation Analysis: How Does this Occupation Organize Behavior Into Habits and Roles?

Performance of occupations is the core of occupational role behavior; therefore it is useful to explore how an occupation may be used in various roles, and how habit patterns are organized within the occupation. These two aspects of habituation analysis—role relevance of the occupation, and habits required to organize the performance of the occupation, are briefly illustrated in the following analysis of meal preparation.

HABITUATION ANALYSIS OF MEAL PREPARATION

Roles. Preparing and consuming meals is behavior relevant to many roles. For example, care givers and family members may have responsibility for all aspects of meal preparation. Workers may be cooks, chefs, home economists, or caterers. Friends share recipes, cook for ill or bereaved friends, have dinner cooperatives, and invite each other to formal and informal meals. Students may study clinical nutrition or other food-oriented professions. Volunteers teach others to cook, work in soup kitchens and bring in meals for others. Hobbyists may engage in gourmet cooking or other special interests such as breadmaking or regional foods.

Habits. Habit systems—meal planning, shopping, cooking, dining, and cleaning up—organize behavior in meal preparation and consumption. Components of meal planning include reading recipes and making choices based on financial limits, nutritional needs, food preferences, and time available for shopping and preparation. Shopping involves making lists, purchasing groceries and storing them at home. Cooking requires habits of cleanliness and orderly arrangement and use of cooking space and utensils. Habit components in dining include pleasant table manners and serving food. Clean up involves clearing the table, cleaning dishes and the kitchen, and storing leftovers. The person who has mastered these habit structures has the basic repertoire for integrating meal preparation into many different roles.

Meal preparation is an important component of a wide variety of roles. Since meals must be prepared and consumed in some fashion every day in all settings, opportunities for practice are plentiful, and the development of habit structures for the activity are a routine part of daily life. Activities like this which are practiced naturally and frequently in the community environment have obvious benefits for the therapeutic program over those for which practice opportunities are rare. If habit pattens are to be learned and subsequently incorporated into role behaviors they must be practicable under ordinary conditions of life.

Performance Analysis: In the Performance of This Occupation, How Are Perceptual-Motor, Process, and Interpersonal Skills Used?

Most activities use, or can use when adapted, a great range of skills and skill components. Therapeutic use of the activity requires knowledge of which skills are emphasized, so that the activity can be easily graded, and people can practice those phases of the activity most relevant to their needs.

Skill analysis requires identification of the perceptual-motor, process and interpersonal skills that are necessary to perform occupations. The following analysis of skills used in meal preparation shows that perceptual-motor, process and interpersonal skills are used throughout the activity.

PERFORMANCE ANALYSIS OF MEAL PREPARATION

Perceptual-Motor Skills. Meal planning involves checking to see what is available before shopping. Then one must get to a shopping area; reach for, grasp and lift groceries; discriminate among foods and brands; and put items into storage areas. Cooking requires measuring, mixing, cutting, and baking. Dining involves using a fork, knife and spoon for serving and eating. For clean up, carrying dishes to the sink and washing, drying and putting away food and dishes is required.

Process Skills. Meal planning involves deciding what foods will balance preferences, nutrition requirements and budget needs. One must also decide where to shop, which brands to buy and where to store food at home. To cook one must measure, monitor oven temperature and time various processes. When dining, one follows etiquette requirements for the particular setting. To clean up, one chooses the most efficient sequence for cleaning dishes and putting food and dishes away.

Communication/Interaction Skills. Meal planning may involve discussion of food preferences, nutrition needs and costs. Shopping can require conversation with other shoppers, making transactions with clerks and asking for assistance. Cooking may include discussing who will do what work in a shared project. Dining with others involves social conversation.

Occupations are clearly most useful for therapeutic programs when they require a wide range of skills for performance. Some occupations may rely heavily on one skill area, but can be linked with other activities to increase opportunities for skill development. While the clinical conditions of clients or patients will predispose a program toward emphasis on one set of skills over another (e.g. psychiatry settings using interpersonal skills and physical dysfunction settings concentrating on perceptual-motor skills), a program should generally provide balanced opportunities for development of all three major skill components.

Output Analysis: How is This Occupation a Part of Work, Play and/or Daily Living Tasks?

A final aspect of occupational analysis is determining the kind of output an occupation generates. It is vital to look at how the occupation is used in work, play and daily living tasks because output will be the key to self-transformation via the open-system cycle.

OUTPUT ANALYSIS OF MEAL PREPARATION

Work. Many people are employed in restaurants, cafeterias, by catering firms, and in other food service settings. In addition, meal preparation can be seen as part of the work of a caregiver's role, and of the student whose work is the study of food services.

Play. Many parties are planned around the food that will be served at them. Skill in meal preparation can lead to increased entertaining during leisure time. Meal preparation as a hobby offers a wide range of interests to develop, from picnic foods to special pastries. Good meals are very enjoyable; they can build community between people in a way that transcends self-maintenance.

Daily Living Tasks. Meal preparation is an essential component of self-maintenance. Food is also a large expense in most household budgets, so skill in money management is closely related to meal preparation.

A balance among work, play and daily living tasks is essential to adaptive occupational behavior. The occupations included in a treatment program should allow the development of balance in these areas. A program using only crafts and games will not provide the best learning environment for people whose work and self-care output has been dysfunctional. And a program emphasizing daily living skills alone does not address essential occupational issues of work and play behavior. Programs should use occupations which contribute to a balance among these three areas of output.

The Value of Analyzing Occupations

Analyzing an occupation in terms of environment, volition, habituation, production, and output has several useful results. One gains awareness of how an occupation may motivate individuals, how it can organize skills and habits into role behavior, and how it can contribute to a balance among work, play and daily living tasks. In addition, some preliminary conclusions can be drawn about the usefulness of occupations for treatment. Occupations which analysis shows to be flexible, easily practiced and relevant to various roles are likely to provide a sound foundation for therapeutic programs.‡

Analysis of environmental, volitional, habituation, performance, and output aspects of an occupation is primarily a method for study aimed at developing a science of occupation. The essential purpose is to build a knowledge base about the qualities of occupations. How occupations are related to therapeutic goals is the second step in occupational analysis.

CLINICAL ANALYSIS OF OCCUPATIONS

Therapists designing treatment programs face two important questions about occupation: what are the occupational needs of the client or patient group, and how can an occupation be graded to meet those needs? The occupational analysis process just discussed provides background for these questions, but does not address them directly. Clinical occupational analysis examines how an occupation can engage a client group in exploration, competence and achievement learning. Table 12.2 outlines guiding questions for this type of analysis. Clinical analysis is part of treatment planning for any individual and will be most useful when developing a program, or making plans for changing or updating treatment media in a setting.

Occupations and Exploratory Learning: What Arrangements of Object, Task, Social Group, and Cultural Context Will Encourage Skill Learning?

Skills are learned when an environment permits exploration and discovery. Occupations can be presented so that exploratory learning of various skills is facilitated. Different arrangements of objects, tasks and social/cultural factors can make the same occupation useful for different purposes. For example, a therapist will present woodworking in one way to develop motor skills, and in another way to develop social interaction skills. In both cases the craft will be organized to encourage exploratory learning, but the different needs of client groups dictate different arrangements of the occupational environment.

Table 12.3 illustrates an example of clinical

---

‡ Following the forms for occupational analysis, the workbook provides forms for summarizing the content and therapeutic relevance of occupations.

analysis for exploratory learning; the hypothetical client population in this example needs to develop *basic group interaction skills*. Meal preparation is graded so that this learning is likely to occur. In this case three sequential types of groups are identified. As clients acquire skills at each level, they can move on to the next level. The match between levels of skill and the demands and supports of the environment assure a safe setting to nurture exploration.

In any program, typical client roles will determine which skills will be emphasized and which occupations will be used frequently for treatment. For example, one clinic might have a large population of caregivers and workers, many of whom have suffered recent loss of perceptual-motor skills due to peripheral nerve injuries, cardiovascular accident or degenerative neuromuscular diseases. Clinical occupational analyses for this population would focus on such activities as meal preparation, mobility and money management, which are necessary for these roles, and would emphasize task components which require frequent and gradeable use of perceptual-motor skills.

Occupations and Competence Learning: How Can the Occupation Be Practiced as Part of Daily Routines?

Occupations contribute to competence learning when they can be practiced in work, play and daily living task routines. Therefore, a clinically useful occupational analysis should describe practice routines for an occupation and how it can be incorporated into occupational behavior on a regular basis. Again, characteristics of particular client groups must be considered.

Table 12.4 shows how meal preparation can be planned as a habitual part of work, play and/or self-care routines for people who have access to kitchens and grocery stores. In this example, competent performance of the occupation itself is the aim of treatment, so the occupation is graded with emphasis upon mastering the basic habit patterns within the occupation: meal-planning, shopping, cooking, dining, and clean up.

Habitual performance of specific skills is the aim of treatment. The analysis can be modified to emphasize a particular relevant skill. For example, if therapy is aimed at acquiring habits of group interaction, the practice routines described in Table 12.4 could be undertaken in

Table 12.3.
Clinical analysis for exploratory learning: basic group interaction skills using meal preparation

Skill sequence	Occupational environment
Parallel group: individuals work and play in the presence of others, with mutual stimulation and minimal sharing of tasks	Therapist plans a picnic meal and buys groceries. Each group member makes his or her own sandwich, chooses fruit and packs bag with food and dishes
Associative group: individuals are involved in short-term tasks requiring some sharing or interaction. Interaction is task oriented and may be cooperative or competitive	Therapist plans picnic meal, buys groceries and assigns tasks to group members. One member makes sandwiches, another packs fruit, another packs dishes, and a fourth is responsible for clean up
Interactive group: members decide on relatively long-term activities, carry them through to completion and meet esteem needs of others	Therapist provides several picnic menus and necessary group leadership. Members choose menus, make shopping list, shop, and prepare food. Group members also decide who will be responsible for each task

Table 12.4.
Clinical analysis for competence learning: meal preparation in work, play, and daily living task routines

DAILY LIVING TASK: PRACTICE ROUTINES

1. Plan breakfasts for one person for a week; purchase groceries; prepare and serve the meals; and clean up afterwards
2. Plan lunches for one person for a week, being sure the menus require a variety of cooking techniques (baking, frying, sautéeing, and so on); prepare and serve the meals; and clean up
3. Plan suppers for two or more people for a week; purchase groceries from more than one store if necessary; cook some food ahead and freeze; serve; and clean up

LEISURE: PRACTICE ROUTINES

1. Buy fast food meals from different restaurants for several days; analyze which are the "best buy" in terms of cost, nutrition and serving time
2. Plan and carry out (cooperatively) a picnic meal for several people; include some cooked foods
3. Plan and carry out a dinner party for a group of friends

WORK: PRACTICE ROUTINES

1. Prepare three cakes for a fund-raising sale, keeping track of costs, time requirements and profits
2. Prepare cookies for a fund-raising sale every day for a week; vary the kinds prepared in response to customer demand; keep records as above
3. Prepare a catered meal to the general specifications of a client; keep records as above

groups; if competence in one-handed activities is desired, the same or similar activities can be practiced using necessary adaptive techniques.

As the person performs in work, play and daily living task routines, habit patterns are developed. It is very important to grade occupations for habit acquisition, just as they are graded for skill learning.

Occupations and Achievement Learning: How Can the Occupation Be Used in Role Performance?

The final component of clinical occupational analysis is assessing how an occupation encourages role performance (the achievement level of occupational function). The occupation can be examined in terms of the conditions it provides for trial enactment of a role, with realistic standards of performance. Table 12.5 demonstrates analysis of meal preparation for the role of caregiver. First, standards for meal preparation expected of caregivers are delineated. These expectancies will be modified in individual cases by factors such as developmental needs, type of disability, individual preferences, and so on. However, there are general expectancies of persons functioning in the caregiver role, which also serve as standards by which performance is measured and feedback given. Clients approaching the achievement level of function must come to terms with these standards. Therefore, performance standards for particular occupations and roles must be identified.

Second, a graded sequence for trial enactment of the role, using the occupation, is identified. Again, this sequence can be modified to meet the needs of different individuals during treatment planning.

APPLICATIONS OF OCCUPATIONAL ANALYSIS

Occupational therapists " ... design activity experiences that offer the client opportunities for effective action. Those activities are purposeful in that they assist and build upon the individual's abilities and lead to the achievement of personal goals" (Ref 1, p 805). Underlying these individual applications of therapeutic occupations is knowledge of the therapeutic potential of an occupation. This knowledge is heightened through use of occupational analysis. It does not take the place of individual decisions for each client. It does, however, provide an outline of general considerations which can be refined for the individual client, and it requires clear statements about the relationship between occupations and the behaviors they evoke, which can encourage further study.

Clinical programs based on the model of human occupation encourage person-environment interaction through occupation; these interactions elicit competence in skill, habit and role behaviors. Occupations used for treatment in the clinical programs must have qualities which encourage this kind of learning. These qualities can be discovered and explored through occupational analysis. As research generates increasing knowledge about the nature of occupation, the analysis process will be further refined. This method is presented as one way of continuing a long journey.

Table 12.5.
Clinical analysis for achievement learning: the caregiver role using meal preparation

STANDARDS OF PERFORMANCE

1. Prepare daily meals for self and others which meet:
    a. Nutritional requirements
    b. Budget limits
    c. Taste preferences
    d. Time constraints
2. Nurture others by preparing food for:
    a. personal celebrations (e.g. birthday parties)
    b. ceremonial occasions (e.g. graduation or reunions)
    c. community gatherings (e.g. Labor Day picnics, covered dish suppers)
3. Maintain clean and safe kitchen

TRIAL ENACTMENT

Stage 1. planning

Identify nutrition, taste and budget requirements of family or friends; plan a week of menus and make shopping lists. Include one celebration in addition to regular meals

Stage 2. implementing

Prepare and serve the meals planned for the week; experiment with ways to save time and to serve food attractively

Stage 3. feedback

Ask others about their satisfaction with meals; assess nutrition, budget, time, cleanliness, kitchen safety factors; make new plans based on feedback

References

1. American Occupational Therapy Association. Purposeful activities: a position paper. *Am J Occup Ther* 37:805–806, 1983.
2. Cynkin S: *Occupational Therapy: Toward Health Through Activities.* Boston, Little, Brown, 1979.
3. Hopkins HL, Smith HD, Tiffany EG: Therapeutic application of activity. In Hopkins HL, and Smith HD (eds): *Willard and Spackman's Occupational Therapy,* ed 6. Philadelphia, Lippincott, 1983.
4. Kielhofer G: Occupation. In Hopkins HL, and Smith HD (eds): *Willard and Spackman's Occupational Therapy,* ed 6. Philadelphia, Lippincott, 1983.
5. Pedretti LW: *Occupational Therapy: Practice Skills for Physical Dysfunction.* St. Louis, Mosby, 1981.
6. Reed K: *Models of Practice in Occupational Therapy.* Baltimore, Williams & Wilkins, 1984.
7. Rogers JC: Why study human occupation? *Am J Occup Ther* 38:47–49, 1984.
8. Trombly CA, Scott AD: *Occupational Therapy for Physical Dysfunction.* Baltimore, Williams & Wilkins, 1977.
9. Wiemer R: Traditional and nontraditional practice arenas. In *Occupational Therapy: 2001 A.D.* Rockville, Md, The American Occupational Therapy Association, 1979.

CHAPTER 13

Program Development

Sally Hobbs Cubie, Kathy L. Kaplan and Gary Kielhofner

Program development is important for existing programs as well as new ones, and for individuals in private practice as well as employees of large organizations. Coherent plans for delivery of occupational therapy services make treatment purposes and methods explicit to patients and clients, to other professionals, and to providers themselves. An accessible program plan allows a clear picture of treatment goals, creates relevant expectations about the nature of occupational therapy services, and provides standards against which therapists, professional peers and providers can measure the effectiveness of services.

Questions about occupational therapy programs often reflect confusion about the exact role of occupational therapy. If a patient needs to increase range of motion, why can't a physical therapist or a nurse provide the exercises? If clients need diversional leisure activity, shouldn't the recreational therapist, or a group of community volunteers, lead the activity? Isn't the occupational therapist really doing bits and pieces of things that are done better, cheaper or more comprehensively by a variety of other professionals and nonprofessionals?

Program development is particularly relevant to occupational therapy because of increasing demands for accountability. Competition in the health care arena, stimulated by budget cuts and a surplus of professional groups, means that occupational therapists need to justify their position in the system (3). By articulating an organized plan, based on facts and grounded in theory, occupational therapists can more effectively secure their place in health care. This means, however, that occupational therapy program plans must clearly identify occupational therapy's contribution to a particular health care system or population. This amounts to being able to point to special problems or aspects of problems which occupational therapists are well suited to address; being able to articulate an understanding of those problems, their dy-

namics and implications for the persons being served; and being able to explain and justify a course of action for remediation which has identified measurable outcomes.

THE MODEL AS A FRAMEWORK FOR PROGRAM DEVELOPMENT

This chapter will illustrate how the model of human occupation can be used as a theoretical framework for developing an occupational therapy program with clearly identified occupational therapy problems, processes and goals. Using the model as a framework for program development means that the patient or client group will be analyzed in terms of this framework, program goals and implementation methods will be consistent with it, and program effectiveness will be measured by standards inherent in the model.

This chapter proposes a general outline for program development based on the model of human occupation, and demonstrates how this approach was applied in two different programs: a preventive community program for inner-city adolescents, and an adult inpatient and outpatient physical medicine program. These two groups also represent two different types of program development: developing a new program and articulating and improving an existing successful program.

Program Orientation Under the Model

The model provides an orientation to occupational function and dysfunction as the domain and expertise of occupational therapy. Whatever diagnostic categories or types of delivery systems are involved, occupational therapy programs based on this model will focus on problems of occupational dysfunction, with the aim of enabling clients or patients to enter into an adaptive cycle of occupational behavior in their native environments. This generic focus can be further elaborated as criteria for program development.

CRITERION ONE: ORIENTATION TO OCCUPATIONAL FUNCTIONING

A program based on the model has as its ultimate goal returning clients or patients to optimal occupational functioning. This means that persons who leave the program should be enabled to engage in a balanced routine of work, play and daily living tasks appropriate for their environments, their disabilities and their developmental levels. Treatment goals are always oriented to this ultimate objective. Thus, for example, muscle strengthening, increasing problem-solving abilities, clarifying values, and providing adaptive equipment, are all seen as intermediate steps toward enabling the individual to return to or enter occupational roles. Additionally, programs will recognize and address multiple factors beyond performance deficits which impair occupational functioning. Knowledge of holistic factors which enhance occupational functioning is as essential to program development as is awareness of dysfunctions which limit performance.

CRITERION TWO: OCCUPATIONAL DYSFUNCTION AS THE PROBLEM FOCUS

Occupational therapy programs can be developed for a wide range of clients and patients with diagnoses ranging from mental disorders, to physical disabilities, developmental delays, and terminal diseases. In addition, they may be developed to prevent the occurrence of dysfunction in an at-risk population. In many settings models of delivery tend to focus on the patient's pathological state or disease and, consequently, on reducing identified pathology. Occupational therapy programs can be complementary to such models. However their focus is on actual or potential disorganization in the human system and in the fit between the system and the environment that are factors in occupational dysfunctions. By identifying occupational dysfunction as the target problem area of the occupational therapy program, the boundaries of occupational therapy are more clearly identified. Thus, problems of emotional disturbance, limited range of motion, skill deficits and the like are attended to by the occupational therapy program within the context of occupational performance. The occupational therapy program should identify how various pathological states impair occupational functioning and include a plan for assessing the degree of occupational dysfunction.

CRITERION THREE: OCCUPATION AS THE REMEDIATIVE STRATEGY OF OCCUPATIONAL THERAPY

Occupational therapy is defined as a process of facilitating engagement of patients and clients in directed occupations. Recognizing the open systems nature of the person, occupation or output is identified as part of the open system cycle that maintains and changes the system. Thus occupation is the remediative or change strategy of occupational therapy. Ancillary interventions such as splinting or counseling are part of the occupational therapy process only in so far as they facilitate and direct the client or patient's participation in occupations.

CRITERION FOUR: OCCUPATIONAL BEHAVIOR AS ENVIRONMENTAL BEHAVIOR

According to the model, occupational behavior is behavior directed at and influenced by the environment. The occupational therapy program has two environmental implications. First, it recognizes that patients and clients function within their own environments with specific sets of demands and characteristics. Knowledge of an individual's environment is critical for evaluating ability to function and for setting program goals. Second, occupational therapy is, itself, an environment in which patients and clients are enabled to function. Whether the client engages in occupations in a therapeutic workshop or in some guided community activity, therapy always consists of participation in a planned environment.

The Process of Program Development

Program development can be broken down into three steps: (*a*) identifying characteristics of the patient/client population, (*b*) identifying characteristics of the treatment program, and (*c*) evaluating effectiveness of the program. These steps are to a degree sequential; however, in ongoing program development therapists may move back and forth between them. Figure 13.1 outlines these steps in detail; they are discussed

I. **Identify characteristics of the patient/client population**

    A. Describe actual and potential performance deficits for this group

        1. Major pathological conditions, or conditions for which the population is at risk
        2. Causes (stress, disease, trauma, developmental delay, other)
        3. Occupational performance areas of skill deficit
            a. Perceptual-motor skills
            b. Process skills
            c. Communication/interaction skills

    B. Identify typical occupational behavior and environmental characteristics

        1. Roles
        2. Values, interests, sense of personal causation
        3. Habit patterns
        4. Skills needed and used in everyday life
        5. Environment: objects, tasks, social groups, cultural values

    C. Describe nature of occupational dysfunction (actual and/or potential)

        1. Level of dysfunction (inefficacy, incompetence, helplessness)
        2. Type of dysfunction: problems in role, habit and skill performance
        3. Contribution of environment and typical behavior patterns to dysfunction
        4. Probable length of time needed to reverse the occupational dysfunction

II. **Identify characteristics of the treatment program**

    A. Qualities of the treatment setting affecting the program (staff, space, money, time, relationship of occupational therapy to the total program)

    B. General program goals

        1. Volition
        2. Habituation
        3. Performance
        4. Environmental interaction

    C. Therapeutic procedures

        1. Program content and sequence
        2. Evaluations and occupations used

III. **Program evaluation**

    A. Quality assurance

    B. Outcome and effectiveness studies

Figure 13.1.   Steps in program development.

in the following sections and illustrated in two examples of program development.*

STEP ONE: IDENTIFY CHARACTERISTICS OF THE PATIENT/CLIENT POPULATION

Program development must begin with a clear identification of the patients or clients to be served. The program serves as a general context within which individual treatment plans are

---

* The outline for program development is provided in the Workbook, with space for notes and planning.

generated and implemented. It also serves to identify needed resources, personnel, and processes for affecting desired changes in patients or clients. The identification of patient or client characteristics involves three interrelated processes: (a) identifying performance deficits, (b) identifying typical occupational behavior and environmental characteristics, and (c) describing the nature of typical occupational dysfunctions.

Performance Deficits

Persons come to occupational therapy programs because of a reduction in or interference with their occupational performance, or because they are potentially at risk for maladaptive performance. Disease, trauma, stress and other factors interfere with persons' abilities to perform. The occupational therapy program must reflect a thorough understanding of performance deficits and their implications. For example, a program serving cardiac patients must incorporate an understanding of the nature of myocardial infarction, its implications for activity and the risks involved, and the nature and implications of medical interventions. Similarly a program for depressed clients must reflect an understanding of affective states, their possible causes, their impact on performance, the nature of medical interventions, and the necessary risks and preventive measures related to suicidal patients. Preventive programs must be grounded in a knowledge of epidemiology, risk factors and potential areas of dysfunction. Thus, the occupational therapy program must be founded on a thorough knowledge of the factors limiting performance. In addition, the contributions of others on the interdisciplinary team remediating the total adaptation problems must be clearly understood.

Occupational Behavior and Environmental Characteristics

While clients and patients come to occupational therapy because of performance deficits, they have patterns of occupational behavior and environments to which they seek to return or which they seek to enter. Thus the program must identify the life roles and daily routines which are typical of the patients or clients, and their characteristic values, interests, and feelings of personal causation.

The cultural background, values and interests a client brings into the treatment setting will profoundly affect what can be achieved within the program. It is also necessary to know something about important reference groups for clients in the program. Attitudes of these social groups toward disability, chronic illness, acute illnesses, and health can influence expectations about recovery and adjustment to permanent disability.

Clients may come from families where there is much chronic illness; therefore they may expect little improvement in their own condition. They may live in an ethnic community in a large city, where everyone is known to each other and much community support is available; or they may live in an affluent but highly transient

suburban neighborhood which places very high values on work achievement and financial success, with few valued relationships outside of the immediate family. They may come from a subcultural group which emphasizes stoic endurance in the face of misfortune, and so may deny the very real burdens imposed by their dysfunction.

In addition to values about health and illness, clients reflect their community experience in other values and interests. For example, spinal cord injury patients coming from a cultural background emphasizing sports achievement and physical strength will need a different program emphasis than will clients with similar injuries, whose friends and family value intellectual achievement. For the first group, it may be essential that the program allows enactment of competitive, aggressive behaviors such as winning games; for the second, individual performance in educational pursuits may be more highly motivating.

Occupational Dysfunctions

Once both performance deficits and occupational characteristics of the target population have been identified, expected occupational dysfunctions can be delineated. Performance deficits interact with occupational characteristics to determine the occupational dysfunction. For example, hand injuries may differentially affect white and blue collar workers so that one group will lose their work roles while others will only have to make adjustments in their work roles.

Identifying the occupational dysfunction involves determining typical levels of dysfunction (inefficacy, incompetence or helplessness) represented in the population. It also entails describing typical disruptions of volition, habituation and performance as well as their impact on the open system cycle. This amounts to a needs assessment which determines target areas for intervention and the types of goals which will be set. It also includes identifying any contribution of the environment and typical behavior patterns to the onset or exacerbation of the performance deficit. For example, the absence of leisure activities among cardiac patients, or the erratic work records of emotionally disturbed persons may be occupational dysfunctions which preceded and contributed to the onset of a performance deficit.

Identifying the occupational dysfunction also gives some indication of the amount of time which may be required for the dysfunction to be

remediated. If the dysfunction is at the inefficacy level and is precipitated by a temporary
performance deficit, a relatively short course of
readaptation can be anticipated. If the dysfunction is at the helplessness level, is precipitated
by a major and permanent loss in performance
and will involve reorganization of life roles,
habits, values, interests and personal causation,
then an extended course of recovery is likely. It
is important to determine whether or not the
program can serve the client or patient throughout the course of recovery. If it cannot, identification of prior and postdischarge resources
along with the appropriate referral will be
needed to assure continuation of support for
occupational functioning.

STEP TWO: IDENTIFY CHARACTERISTICS OF THE TREATMENT PROGRAM

The first step in program development
amounts to a needs assessment in which client
characteristics and requirements for change are
analyzed. The second step in program development is a delineation of how the program will
respond to these characteristics, problems and
needs. It involves three processes: (a) description of the treatment setting, (b) delineation of
general program goals, and (c) identification of
therapeutic procedures.

Qualities of the Treatment Setting

It is useful to review issues of staff, space,
money, and time prior to defining general program goals and identifying therapeutic procedures. These factors may serve as constraints
on subsequent plans, or they may represent
strengths upon which the program can build.
The general relationship of occupational therapy to the total program should also be examined at this point, so that services are not dupli-
cated unnecessarily, and so that the occupational therapy program complements existing
services rather than being isolated from them.

Program Goals

The overall objective of all occupational therapy programs is to enhance the occupational
functioning of clients and patients. Stating program goals amounts to proposing the steps for
accomplishing this overall purpose. Two important aspects of this task are making sure that

all relevant goals are identified, and determining
that the goals identified can be addressed in
some fashion within the constraints of the setting in which the program will take place. A
helpful method for assuring that all relevant
goals are met is to systematically review components of the model. Thus, for example, goals
for volition, habituation, performance, and environmental interaction should be delineated.

Therapeutic Procedures

Once goals have been identified for a program,
it is necessary to specify how these goals will be
addressed in the program: what are the therapeutic activities and aids that will be part of the
program's service package? These procedures
will be affected by the setting's budget and personnel resources, and by the interface of occupational therapy service with other services in
the setting. For example, if a program goal of
increasing client work skills is identified, the
therapeutic service may be a simulated work
program in an inpatient setting with adequate
resources, or a community volunteer program
for clients in a day care setting.

The selection of therapeutic procedures and
equipment should also be relevant to occupational behavior in the home environment. Programs for physically disabled clients from low
income facilities which emphasize use of expensive equipment may not achieve any carryover
beyond the inpatient setting. Training in skills
should be relevant to the environments in which
clients will live, or they will be inadequately
prepared for resuming functional occupational
roles once they leave the treatment setting.

The core of therapeutic procedures will be the
involvement of patients or clients in directed
occupations. As noted earlier, other procedures
and equipment should be supportive of this process. Identification of treatment procedures
should also delineate how occupational therapy
will serve as a physical and cultural milieu to
enhance performance.

STEP THREE: PROGRAM EVALUATION

The final step of program development is
evaluation of processes and outcomes. When
program goals and procedures have been identified clearly, program evaluation can be conceptualized and implemented. Basically there are
two types of program evaluation: quality assurance and determination of program effectiveness.

Quality Assurance

Quality assurance studies determine whether specified procedures are being implemented where they are needed. Quality assurance is a problem-solving approach to assessing and improving health care delivery (14). By capitalizing on the subjective judgements of health care professionals, an objective approach is used to identify and resolve common problems. The five-step procedure allows for improving productivity, cost containment, and clinical outcomes (9). The comparison between the expected, optimal outcomes and the actual achievable goals in a given facility documents the quality of care.

Outcome and Effectiveness Studies

Outcome studies are examinations of whether stated program goals are being met. They may also involve studies of whether different therapeutic procedures are more or less effective in achieving these goals (4, 12).

Program evaluation is essential to effective development of a program. Documenting goal accomplishment and efficacy of services increases the viability of the occupational therapy program for maximal funding and continuation. It also allows the program staff to respond to demands for accountability. If goals are not being met or if certain procedures are found to be more effective than others, then there is a data base to justify change.

SUMMARY

The previous section outlined a process of program development using the model of human occupation as a conceptual framework. The process of program development is seen as critical to defining and justifying occupational therapy services and as essential to the quality of occupational therapy services and their relevance to the client or patient population. In the following section two cases of program development are presented to illustrate the process in developing a new program and changing an existing program.

A PREVENTIVE COMMUNITY PROGRAM FOR ADOLESCENTS

An increasingly important area of health care is health promotion and disease prevention (13). As Johnson and Deuschle (7) have noted, "The broad implementation of preventive services . . . is easier said than done in a culture which gives overwhelming priority to the management of firmly established disease." However, such services are being recognized as cost effective in all areas of health care. Jackson and Pellegrino (6) suggest that "The essential question is no longer whether or not a preventive health care system can supplant a curative one; rather, it is how can a new health delivery system accommodate both types of services and multiple types of health care deliveries." Thus it is useful to examine how a preventive program in occupational therapy can be developed.

Step One: Identifying Characteristics of the Patient/Client Population

The clients in this program are inner-city adolescents ages 12 through 21, who attend an after-school outreach program jointly sponsored by the city government and private foundations.

PERFORMANCE DEFICITS

This client group is at risk for experiencing substance abuse, unwanted pregnancies, and homicides. These problems have substantial links with environmental stress. The following performance deficits may occur among these clients:

Perceptual-Motor Skills

Undiagnosed perceptual-motor dysfunction may contribute to delinquent school behavior and related social disorders. Perceptual-motor dysfunction may also result from substance abuse.

Process Skills

The ability to set and achieve long-term goals may be impaired or affected by environmental limitations; problem-solving skills may be poorly developed.

Communication/Interaction Skills

Friendships may encourage destructive behavior patterns (such as drug abuse); family relationships may be only minimally supportive due to poverty and deprivation throughout the family system.

OCCUPATIONAL BEHAVIOR AND ENVIRONMENTAL FACTORS

These clients are developmentally at the stage of engaging in occupational choice (1), making the gradual transition from the role of student to the role of worker. They are doing so in an environment in which there is very high unemployment.

Roles

In general, these clients occupy the primary roles of student, family member and friend. In some instances, they also are volunteers, religious participants and workers. Those who have small children may also be caregivers and home maintainers.

Values, Interests, and Sense of Personal Causation

These clients share the predominant values of the larger culture—money, success and physical attractiveness. In addition, they may value education as a means to these goals. Their interests are wide-ranging, but actual experience with a variety of interests is often limited. Their sense of personal causation may be impaired due to the very great discrepancy between what the culture advertises and what is presently possible for them.

Habit Patterns

Their adaptive habit patterns center around school attendance, friendships, after-school employment, and family responsibilities, such as caring for younger brothers and sisters. Maladaptive habit patterns may include extensive television watching and late and frequent parties involving drug and alcohol abuse.

Skills

Their skills include perceptual-motor abilities gained from school and extracurricular sports such as karate or running; cognitive skills which center around school performance and problem solving for "street survival"; and interpersonal skills which are demonstrated in friendships with peers, maintaining family ties and developing mentor relationships with adults (teachers and counselors).

Environment

The immediate environment of objects, tasks, and social groups is pervaded by the realities of poverty. Most money is spent on necessities of life—food, clothing, housing, and transportation. Tasks also center around these self-maintenance necessities, with leisure being sought in inexpensive informal gatherings such as parties at someone's house.

Important social groups are peer groups from school and after-school activities, and family. Cultural values influencing clients in this age group range from the conservative religious and social views of some older family members to the more consumer-oriented images of television, movies and advertising.

OCCUPATIONAL DYSFUNCTION

Many young people in this client group are functioning at the level of inefficacy, or are at the risk of doing so. They may demonstrate marginal management of the roles of student, worker and family member. Their skill repertoires are limited. There is often a sense of frustration, inadequacy and lack of trust in the future.

The primary occupational dysfunction seen in this group is disruption of the occupational choice process. Drug abuse may alter basic capacity for skilled performance; early pregnancy and parenthood can create time demands that seriously interfere with school and work; and violent encounters are often directly life threatening. Aside from these problems, many of these young people see a discrepancy between cultural values of monetary and career success and easy access to expensive goods, and the high unemployment and general environmental deprivation around them. This conflict can result in confusion about how to set goals and achieve them, and about identifying pathways to successful work experience.

Step Two: Characteristics of the Treatment Program

The occupational therapy treatment program will be a new program designed to augment an existing multidisciplinary program.

QUALITIES OF THE TREATMENT SETTING

The treatment setting is a partially renovated three-story building in the neighborhood in which most of the clients live. Staff includes employment counselors, teachers and tutors, health care workers, a family planning coordinator, and numerous volunteers. A combination of private and public funds support the program. Increased funding from the private sector is being sought. Clients attend the center in the afternoon and early evening. The staff welcomes participation by additional professionals. Occupational therapy services will be provided by faculty and students in a nearby university occupational therapy program under a training grant, and so will not bring the program additional salary expenses. The occupational therapy program will augment the existing program emphasis on education and employment.

GENERAL PROGRAM GOALS

An overall program goal for this client group is promoting competence in the occupational choice process, thus preventing future occupational dysfunction. Objectives supporting this goal include the following.

1. *Volition.* Identify interests and values relevant to work roles; set goals for work experience.

2. *Habituation.* Develop activity patterns that balance current role requirements (student, family member, friend) with exploratory learning about work. Develop a balance among work, leisure and self-care activities.

3. *Performance.* Explore perceptual-motor, cognitive and interpersonal skills related to getting and keeping a job. If necessary, develop skills useful in leisure activities and daily living tasks.

4. *Environmental Interaction.* Identify and use objects, tasks and social groups in the school and community to further occupational goals.

THERAPEUTIC PROCEDURES

Fortunately, the program which is already in effect at the center is well designed and managed, and is oriented toward similar goals. The occupational therapy program will focus on a combination of assessment, education and practical experience; it will aim at developing client awareness of the occupational choice process, and providing opportunities for exploratory, competence and achievement learning.

Program Content and Sequence

The program is based on three levels of learning, each of which is related to the occupational choice process:

1. *Discovering Occupational Assets and Preferences.* Exploratory learning about values and interests can occur during experiences with available occupations, and during prevocational training. Clients can begin to identify skills that they enjoy using, and which can be transferred to possible career choices.

2. *Learning Time Management.* Competence in using time so that work, leisure and daily living tasks are carried out is an important step toward assuming the worker role.

Clients will learn to schedule time involving their experiences at the center, in the community and at school.

3. *Making an Occupational Choice.* Achievement of the worker role ultimately depends upon the ability to meet personal goals and social requirements. Practice in identifying goals, and trial enactment of the worker role at the center and in the community will provide opportunities for feedback and revising priorities in the process of role acquisition.

Evaluations and Occupations Used

Evaluations that will be administered and discussed with the clients include the Adolescent Role Assessment (1), the Interest Check List (8), the Bay Area Functional Performance Evaluation (2), the Activity Configuration (15), the Role Checklist, and others (such as the Purdue Pegboard (10), sensory-integrative evaluations and developmental screening of infants and children as needed).

Certain structured activities are already available at the center, varying somewhat with the availability of volunteers to provide instruction. With the addition of occupational therapy services, clients may be able to participate in a wide range of activities in the center, including clerical tasks, small crafts, exercise groups, carpentry, and others. In addition, the occupations clients pursue outside of the center will be points of reference in the occupational therapy process.

Step Three: Program Evaluation

Some evaluation will be ongoing in the form of feedback to clients; if a client could identify only a few interests early in the program, and can describe a variety of them after participation in classes, this is useful information for the client and for the program. The ability to manage time will be monitored throughout the program, as will the setting and achieving of valued goals. Client performance and self-report on the interest check list, the activity configuration, variations of the role check list, and other assessments will indicate progress, or lack of it, toward program goals, and will suggest areas of the program requiring further development.

Two additional forms of program evaluation may be used. The first is ongoing evaluation based on feedback from the clients concerning the value and efficacy of occupational therapy services. Clients can routinely fill out questionnaires concerning how they perceive occupational therapy and what, if any, benefits they see coming from it.

Additionally the program can be evaluated through a research design in which participants and control subjects from the same neighborhood are evaluated initially and after a period of participation in the project. Measures of change can be focused on the occupational therapy program goals (e.g. measure of occupational choice development). This research can provide evidence of whether or not the program helps clients make the desired changes.

DEVELOPING AN OCCUPATIONAL THERAPY PROGRAM FOR PATIENTS WITH RHEUMATOID ARTHRITIS[†]

This example demonstrates the application of the model in the development of a program for individuals with rheumatoid arthritis. The program is located in a large urban research facility, and persons served through the program are seen on an inpatient and outpatient basis. Previous to the development of the present program the focus was biomechanically oriented. However, the chief occupational therapist and the therapist in charge of the program had begun to incorporate such activities as time management into treatment and were searching for a conceptual schema which would define the program as occupational therapy's legitimate domain. The model of human occupation provided a coherent framework within which program goals and treatment outcomes could be articulated in terms of occupational behavior. This case example presents the program after it had been reformulated in terms of the model.

Step One: Identifying Characteristics of the Patient Population

The patients in this program are primarily local, middle-aged women who have a medical diagnosis of rheumatoid arthritis. They have been referred by their family physician to this research hospital for help in managing the disease.

PERFORMANCE DEFICITS

This group of individuals is identified by their common medical diagnosis. Although the severity and extent of the disease varies, typical performance deficits include:

---

† Much gratitude is expressed to Cynthia Smith, O.T.R., Chief of Occupational Therapy at the National Institutes of Health, Bethesda, Maryland, for providing information about their program development.

1. *Perceptual-Motor Skills.* Musculoskeletal problems of diminished strength, dexterity and range of motion interfere with performance of daily living tasks.

2. *Process Skills.* Changes in motor capacity, the experience of pain and fatigue, and the needs for following joint protection principles place new demands on the process skills of these individuals. Some manage to be adequate problem-solvers while others are often frustrated by their inability to plan around and solve problems which arise in connection with their symptoms and the necessity of joint protection.

3. *Communication/Interaction Skills.* Due to diminished energy, pain and restricted movements, resultant patterns of performance affect interpersonal relationships. Family and friends may encourage pathological dependence or support healthy interdependence. The patient may not be comfortable asking for help or working out interdependent arrangements.

OCCUPATIONAL BEHAVIOR AND ENVIRONMENTAL CHARACTERISTICS

Most of the patients referred to this facility tend to be 35- to 60-yr-old married, suburban housewives with families. They are generally middle class persons and some have past work careers. Their occupational traits can be characterized as follows.

Roles

In general, these persons occupy primary roles in family member, caretaker and home maintainer. In addition they are involved as friends, religious participants, volunteers, and as organizational members. Some have interrupted a worker role either to raise children or because of the disease process.

Values, Interests, and the Sense of Personal Causation

In general, these persons value child care and family involvement, responsible household management and community and religious involvement. Their interests center around their roles in the home and community, shopping and leisure sports and crafts. Prior to the disease most have been active in a variety of these interests. Their sense of personal causation derives primarily from their various role involvements, an especially from family-related roles. Some persons with past work careers derived a sense of personal causation from that involvement. For some others, hobbies and other leisure pursuits provide a sense of efficacy.

Habit Patterns

These persons, prior to the onset of the arthritis, were well organized and efficient homemakers. Their habits of time use revolved around family duties and participation with family, friends and neighbors in leisure activities.

Skills

For the most part, prior to the onset of rheumatoid arthritis, these individuals had the skills to pursue their goals and interests related to child care and household management. Some had special skills they learned as part of occupational preparation in college or on the job.

Environment

The environment of objects, tasks and social groups is characteristic of residents in middle class communities. Money is budgeted for family needs and wants and community contribution. Tasks center around routine cooking, cleaning and caretaking as well as pursuit of leisure interests and social gatherings for family and friends. However, the disease process can profoundly affect how the environment is experienced. Many common objects such as stairs and small kitchen utensils become difficult to manage for patients with this disease. Family and social values pertaining to independence and dependence strongly influence how well patients are able to make the adjustments necessary to effectively cope with their physical limitations.

OCCUPATIONAL DYSFUNCTION

Various levels of dysfunction can be seen depending on the severity of the disease and its impact on the daily life of the person. In general, routine tasks of living take longer to perform because frequent rests are required. In addition, patients need to deal with the unpredictable quality of the disease; they may feel relatively healthy one day and too ill to carry out their planned activities the next day.

Most patients have difficulty maintaining their primary roles, setting priorities on what they most value, and delegating tasks. They are required to give up their previous standards of independence because they are dependent upon support in order to function. Loss of goals, values and interests may occur because of the necessarily altered time frame and reduced ability to perform valued activities. Habits are disrupted for most persons. Skills are not only interfered with by the disability, but the person may also lack the process skills necessary for adapting to the disease process.

Step Two: Characteristics of the Treatment Program

QUALITIES OF THE TREATMENT SETTING

There is a room with a table and storage for equipment and supplies which is used for the occupational therapy component of the arthritis program. There are separate areas for the other members of the interdisciplinary team: the physical therapist helps the patient to maintain joint range by using hotpacks and other techniques; the physican monitors the patient's prescribed arthritic medication, and the social worker provides family support and group therapy. Transportation is provided to the research facility if the patient has no access to it. This is an especially important feature of the program, as many patients may feel too ill to come to the facility on their own for appointments. The patient makes separate appointments with each part of the program as needs are determined. They attend occupational therapy weekly, for 1- to 1½-hr sessions for about 7 weeks. Each patient is seen by the same occupational therapist to provide continuity of care.

GENERAL PROGRAM GOALS

Overall, the program goal for the patient population is to increase awareness of, and adjustment to, the effects of rheumatoid arthritis on the individual's occupational behavior. Objectives supporting this goal include the following:

1. *Volition*. Identify and develop interests and goals which are compatible with values and physical abilities; maintain sense of personal causation through planning and problem solving.

2. *Habituation*. Set priorities about how time is spent; incorporate habits of rest, joint protection and energy conservation, and make realistic decisions regarding enactment of current and future roles.

3. *Performance*. Maintain or increase range of motion, strength and coordination for performance of self-care, household and play tasks; assess for aids which would support adaptive behaviors; develop interactional/communication skills which enable the pa-

tient to negotiate for support and interdependence; and develop necessary planning and problem-solving skills.

4. *Environment.* Identify objects in the home and community resources which need adaptation for effective use.

THERAPEUTIC PROCEDURES

The occupational therapy program is part of an interdisciplinary program of evaluation and treatment for rheumatoid arthritis in a research setting. The occupational therapy component focuses on the impact of a medical diagnosis on the person's occupational behavior. Based on a needs assessment, each individual participates in selected evaluations and treatment procedures designed to augment adaptive occupational behavior.

Program Content and Sequence

The program involves individual and group sessions and homework assignments which are outlined in a workbook (5). Areas of treatment include:

1. Discussion of assessment results and discrepencies among any of the subsystems. Priorities must be set to achieve satisfaction in occupational behavior.

2. Practice of energy conservation and joint protection; practice of relaxation and other methods to decrease pain and fatigue.

3. Education and practice of principles of activity analysis and problem solving, so the patient need not rely on an occupational therapist when dealing with, and avoiding, crises due to exacerbations of the disease.

4. Practice of communication skills necessary for educating family and others about disease and negotiating new role relationships, as necessary.

5. Provision of assistive devices and environmental adaptations to increase ability to function as independently as possible.

Evaluations and Occupations Used

The following evaluations may be used for assessment of patients in the program: range of motion, sensation, fine motor coordination, and upper extremity strength evaluations; an arthritis hand assessment; an activity questionnaire; an activities of daily living checklist; the Role Checklist; an occupational therapy functional screening tool; the Rotter Internal/External Scale (11); a modified interest checklist; and a home evaluation. (Most of these assessments are contained in the Instrument Library at the back of this text.)

The main occupations used in the program center around the educational character of the program. Patients attend presentations and discussions and they engage in clinic activities aimed at using the information provided. Additionally, homework assignments are given in which patients carry out activities at home and report back to the group.

Step Three: Program Evaluation

This research facility expects and supports program evaluation. An outcome and follow-up study are being conducted to assess the efficacy of the program. Preliminary analysis of data indicates positive trends.

CONCLUSION

The two previous discussions indicate how the program development process outlined in the beginning of this chapter can be implemented. As the cases illustrate, using the process allows the therapist to articulate specific patient or client needs in a framework unique to occupational therapy; to specify program goals, parameters and processes; and to provide justification for the services, so that program goals can be altered or achieved.

The organized approach to planning and articulating a program outlined in this chapter is considered an essential part of all occupational therapy services. It is central to developing new programs, improving existing programs and assessing the need for future programs.

References

1. Black M: The Adolescent Role Assessment. In Hemphill BJ (ed): *The Evaluative Process in Psychiatric Occupational Therapy.* Thorofare, NJ, Slack, 1982.
2. Bloomer J, Williams S: *Bay Area Functional Performance Evaluation.* Palo Alto, Calif, Consulting Psychologists Press, 1979.
3. Christiansen C: Research: an economic imperative. *Occup Ther J Res* 3:195–198, 1983.
4. Cook TD, Reichart CS: (eds): *Qualitative and Quantitative Methods in Evaluation Research.* Beverly Hills, Calif, Sage, 1979.
5. Furst G: *Rehabilitation Through Learning: Energy Conservation and Joint Protection: A Workbook for Persons with Rheumatoid Arthritis.* Bethesda, Md, National Institutes of Health, U.S. Department of Health and Human Services, 1982.
6. Jackson L, Pellegrino ED: Introduction: change agents in a changing system. *Prev Med* 6:379–385, 1977.
7. Johnson KG: Deuschle KW: Strategies for prevention using allied health professionals. *Prev Med* 6:386–390, 1977.
8. Matsutsuyu J: The interest check list. *Am J Occup Ther* 22:323–328, 1969.

9. Ostrow P, Williamson J, Joe B: *A Quality Assurance Primer*. Rockville, Md, American Occupational Therapy Association, Inc., 1983.
10. *Purdue Pegboard*. Chicago, Science Research Associates, Inc., 1968.
11. Rotter JB: Generalized expectations for internal versus external control reinforcement. *Psych Monogr* 80:1–28, 1966.
12. Schulberg H, Shelton A, Baker F: *Program Evaluation in the Health Fields*. New York, Human Sciences Press, 1969.
13. U.S. Department of Health, Education, and Welfare: Public Health Service. *Healthy People: The Surgeon General's Report on Health Promotion and Disease Prevention*. Washington, D.C., Superintendent of Documents, 1977.
14. Williamson J, Ostrow P, Braswell H: *Health Accounting for Quality Assurance: A Manual for Assessing and Improving the Outcomes of Care*. Rockville, Md, American Occupational Therapy Association, Inc., 1981.
15. *Willard and Spackman's Occupational Therapy*, ed 5. Hopkins HL, Smith HD (eds): Philadelphia, Lippincott, 1978, p 157.

SECTION 4

Specific Applications of the Model

Introduction

The chapters in this section discuss applications of the model to treatment and intervention with specific target populations. Most of the chapters are divided into subsections which address an even more sharply defined group than the chapter as a whole. As noted earlier, the categories of discussion in this section reflect both conventional ways in which patient and client groups are categorized and the areas in which applications of the model are most fully developed. This section does not present an exhaustive coverage of relevant applications and is intended to be exemplary, inviting other applications.

The format of each chapter or chapter section is a review of relevant literature leading up to a description of the dynamics of occupational dysfunction potentially reflected in the particular group of persons being discussed, followed by recommendations for assessment and intervention. General discussions of these topics are both summarized and elaborated in the tables which accompany them. Instruments which are merely identified by name in the tables will be found in the Instrument Library in the Appendix at the end of this text. The various treatment strategies which are identified in the tables represent a potential (and not exhaustive) list of approaches from which the therapist selects, and builds upon, to develop a coherent approach to intervention. Cases at the end of each section illustrate how these strategies are used in the context of developing and implementing a coherent treatment plan. In many places specific treatment techniques are mentioned but not elaborated when more thorough discussions of these techniques are available elsewhere. The purpose of the chapters is not to elucidate the details of various treatment strategies or techniques but rather to show their integration into the total picture of intervention.

The treatment planning exercise in the workbook provides an opportunity and structure for the reader to make applications of the concepts in these sections to specific patients of interest.

CHAPTER 14

Physical Disabilities*

Gary Kielhofner, Jayne Shepherd, Cynthia A. Stabenow, Nancy Bledsoe, Gloria Furst, Jana Green, Betty Herlong Harlan, Carol Lee McLellan, and Joan Owens

Occupational therapists offer services to persons with a wide variety of physical disabilities.† Their problems result from trauma and diseases which may disrupt the musculoskeletal, neurological and symbolic constituents of skills. In order to treat such persons, occupational therapists must have extensive knowledge and expertise concerning the nature of the medical problem, the related precautions and the functional implications. Further, the therapist must employ a number of therapeutic regimes and techniques aimed at preventing deformity and functional loss and maximizing mental, sensory and motor capacities. In order to extend limited capacity, therapists also prescribe and provide training in the use of adapted equipment, and assess and recommend modifications of physical environments. The knowledge and expertise for these contributions to the rehabilitation of physically disabled persons is well developed and documented in occupational therapy literature.

The aim of this chapter is to demonstrate how these physical disability approaches and practices can be integrated within the model of human occupation to yield a holistic approach to treatment of the occupational dysfunctions of physically disabled persons. We begin with a discussion of how the model of human occupation orients the occupational therapist to problems of the physically disabled person in general. Subsequent discussions illustrate applications of the model to persons with chronic progressive disease (illustrated through arthritis and multiple sclerosis), spinal cord injury, coronary disease, brain damage (including both traumatic injury and cerebrovascular accident), and cancer, as well as persons seen in acute care.

OCCUPATIONAL DYSFUNCTION IN THE PHYSICALLY DISABLED PERSON

The impact which disease, trauma and residual limitations have on persons is a complex and individually unique matter. All persons with physical disabilities face some threat to, or interference with, their ability to continue to function within their occupational roles. Persons who experience sudden and permanent change in their physical status, must often reconstruct everyday life and life plans (82). Those with chronic illness face ongoing problems and challenges for maintaining their daily lives over an extended period of time—usually their lifetimes (75). Some manage to adjust and maintain occupational life-styles while others have more difficulty adjusting. Pathological states alone do not account for differences in individual outcomes (127). These differences may be explained by a number of environmental and personal variables. The model of human occupation provides a means of identifying, describing and synthesizing these variables. Consequently, it can serve as a framework for understanding an individual's unique reaction to, and needs after, the onset of physical disability and for developing treatment plans.

---

* The first three authors had responsibility for the overall content and organization of the chapter. Nancy Bledsoe made primary contributions to the acute care section, Gloria Furst to the chronic progressive disease section, Jana Green to the cancer section, Betty Harlan to the brain damage section, Carol McLellan to the coronary disease care section, and Joan Owens to the spinal cord injury section.

† This Chapter deals only with physical disabilities in adulthood and adolescence. Chapter 16 will address physical dysfunction in pediatrics.

Impact of Physical Disability on the Hierarchy of Subsystems and the Open System Cycle

Physical disabilities are disturbances to the performance subsystem that resonate throughout the system constraining the higher habituation and volition subsystems. This first general discussion will overview the impact of disability on the status of the three subsystems, on the environment and on the maladaptive cycles that may follow.

PERFORMANCE

Physical disabilities are, by definition, disturbances to the neurological and/or musculoskeletal constituents of skills. There may also be associated symbolic disturbances. In all cases the organization of skills in the performance subsystem is disrupted. Since the performance subsystem produces output, a person's occupational behavior is interrupted, limited or jeopardized as a result of the physical disability.

HABITUATION

Physical disabilities disrupt and place new demands on the habits and roles which regulate patterns of routine behavior. Whenever a person is faced with physical limitations, habits and roles will have to be reorganized to accommodate them (52, 84, 117).

Habits

Since habits build upon skills in the performance subsystem, disruption to those skills means that habits will become disorganized. For example, getting bathed and dressed in the morning after a disability is not only a matter of having lost performance capacities, but also of the loss of viable automatic routines. In addition, new habits related to the need to accommodate to or manage the disability are often required (e.g. bowel and bladder care, joint protection, energy conservation needs, requirements for rest).

As a consequence of all these changes the task of organizing the entire day may become overwhelming. Accommodations and trade-offs must take place. Certain behaviors may be eliminated from the person's routine or the person may have to delegate some tasks to family members or an attendant in order to have time for other more valued activities. Thus, physically disabled persons may have to change much of their manner of accomplishing daily routines.

Habits are disturbed not only by the loss of skills, but also by the inactivity imposed by the disability and hospitalization. When habits are not practiced they degenerate. The learning of new habits may also be impeded if opportunities for practicing them are not provided during rehabilitation (97).

Roles

In the same way that performance limitations interfere with habits they may also disrupt or terminate role performance (123). Depending on the performance demands of a particular role, it may be impossible for an individual to maintain or return to it. If a person is to retain a role, major modifications in the expectations for the role may be required. In other cases, persons may have to find new ways to enact roles. A person may desire to continue being a worker, but be unable to engage in the old line of work necessitating a new occupational choice.

Persons forced to undergo loss of roles or changes in roles may experience a loss of the identity that the roles provide (123). Decreased self-esteem may occur as they take on roles believed to be less important or as they lose roles (112).

Another major impact of disability may be placement of the individual in the sick role and later in the invalid role (123). The sick role is characterized by demands for the patient to comply with medical regimes and to assume a passive and dependent relationship with medical personnel. The sick role is, however, counterproductive in a rehabilitative setting where it is critical that the individual take responsibility for his or her own course of recovery and for adapting to permanent or progressive limitations. The invalid role may occur after rehabilitation if an individual internalizes a view of self as incapable and resorts to passive and dependent behavior. Often the reactions of strangers, family and friends can serve to reinforce the invalid role. This occurs when others unnecessarily lower their expectations of the disabled person, become overly protective or helpful, or consider the disabled person to be inferior or handicapped beyond his or her actual limitations.

VOLITION

Volitional elements are critical determinants of the physically disabled person's maintenance of, or return to, occupational functioning. They also influence the patient's choices relative to participation in the rehabilitation process. For example, the individual who recognizes the need to adjust values and goals will more readily identify personal rehabilitation goals and will be enabled to more fully adjust to the disability (36).

Personal Causation

Physical disability confronts the individual with experiences that challenge and contradict a view of self as competent (127). All physical disabilities in some measure reduce a person's ability to perform. Pain, fatigue and loss of sensory, cognitive and/or motor capacities impose limitations and interruptions of function that can erode the individual's belief in skill (123).

The fact that disease and trauma are visited upon one with little or no hope of escaping its consequences engenders feelings of being externally controlled. The loss of function accompanied by necessary dependence on medical personnel and family or friends exacerbate such feelings. Disability also imposes new requirements for performance such as the need to learn and to use adaptive equipment. The physically disabled person must also learn new communication and interaction skills. In sum, physical disability creates conditions in which old skills are lost and new skills are required, thereby threatening an individual's belief in the efficacy of skills.

Concerns and fears about future success and failure also arise. The potential for success in the future may be uncertain because the disease process is variable. Or, if the interruption of function is acute and drastic it may be difficult or impossible for individuals to imagine any possibility for success in the future, short of denying the permanence of the disability.

Values

Physical disabilities can impose a discontinuity between what persons can do and what they value or believe they should do. This discrepancy may result in an invalidation of some values, in lowered self-esteem or in alienation from values (128).

Physical disability may make the future seem uncertain and interrupt the continuity of past and present (82). Not only does the physical disability often prevent an individual from using time as in the past, but the demands of the disease process and its management or treatment may also impose new conflicting values for time use. Persons may be torn between their belief that time should be used productively and the medically dictated necessities of rest, reduced stress and the like.

The individual's valued goals may be partially or totally invalidated by the disability. Orientation to future goals gives meaning and direction to present activities. When they are disrupted, much of the purpose for present efforts may be lost. Without a sense of who or what they are becoming, persons may be unable to find reasons for struggling with the problems imposed by physical disability (66, 86, 87).

Discomfort, performance limitations and the necessity of precautions and adaptations may negatively impact the ambience and spirit of activities, making it difficult for a person to experience the same sense of meaning in them. Further, persons may be prevented from participating in activities that formerly had meaning for them.

Interests

Interests are affected in ways very similar to values. Premorbid interests represent an individual's avenues for pleasure and satisfaction. Disability may interfere with the pleasure in action or with the ability to engage in pleasurable occupations.

Willingness to engage in occupations as part of therapy may be both a function of the interest the person has for the activity and the general anticipation the person has for being able to return to participation in pleasurable and satisfying occupations. For the disabled person the future may seem a bland and undesirable existence without the potentials for enjoyment and investment that existed in the past.

ENVIRONMENT

The environment is one of the most critical variables affecting occupational behavior of the physically disabled person after the onset of the physical disability. Each of the four environmental levels impact on the human system and thus influence what occupational behavior is possible, valued and facilitated.

Objects

Man-made objects in the environment are naturally geared for able bodied individuals in their size, shape, weight, and mechanical functions. Physical disability often makes it impossible or contraindicated for persons to handle objects of everyday life. Many physically disabled persons must also learn to use new objects which extend or substitute for motor function, replace lost senses or provide protection to the body. The patient is also confronted during treatment and rehabilitation with new, albeit usually temporary, objects which must be accommodated to and used as part of a rehabilitation process. The symbolic value to the patients of many of these objects may determine how they react to them. Some patients may retain use of objects which are less functional than substitutes but which signify some value for them. Other objects may be rejected because they are unfamiliar or because in a patient's perception they accentuate his or her handicap.

The summative experiences of inability to manage familiar objects, the need to accommodate to new objects and their significances for rehabilitation and ultimate adjustment to the physical world can create for the physically disabled person an intensely arousing situation with considerable press for change. Patients can, under such conditions, be easily over-stressed and can experience a sense of discontinuity with the artifactual world which constitutes part of their sense of reality.

Tasks

Physical disability may force an individual to relinquish or alter the manner of performing tasks and to take on new tasks. The physically disabled person may also find that he or she must relinquish some tasks to others.

The temporal nature of tasks may be changed because more time is necessary for performance or because they must be performed when others can assist. Disability and necessary adaptive equipment may mean that tasks that were more flexible in the past must now be performed more rigidly. Finally, the need for assistance and the increased noticeability of the disabled person in public may make many previously private tasks more public after disability. Thus, for the physically disabled person the world of tasks that is "out there" and that was taken for granted in the course of normal life becomes radically altered.

Social Groups

Following the onset of physical disability, individuals may find themselves interacting with new groups, losing access to past groups and having to negotiate and change relationships within continuing groups. In many ways the social environment in which the individual exists may be fundamentally changed.

Much of the individual's success in maintaining or rebuilding of personal abilities, habits and roles will be dependent on others, and their willingness and ability to shift responsibilities and roles and to accommodate to necessary adaptations. The group which is ordinarily most significant for, and most altered by, the person's physical disability is the family (84). Outside the family unit the physically disabled person may experience a shrinking social world. The work environment along with other social groups may not be accessible. Groups which were permeable in the past may no longer be because of physical barriers or social attitudes in the group. At the same time the physically disabled person may find in other disabled persons a new and important reference grouping giving support and even political strength (118).

Another important dimension of the changing social environment for disabled persons is their tenure of stay in a medical, rehabilitation and/or extended care institution. While medical personnel view these institutions as agents of therapy and support, they are also, for the disabled person, new and often complex social groups to which they must adapt (62). Physically disabled persons may also have to interact with new governmental and bureaucratic groups related to receiving financial support, vocational training or other public services.

Culture

Cultural prejudices may make it difficult for the disabled person to achieve a satisfying and productive occupational life-style. American culture tends to place a high premium on physical beauty and able-bodied self-reliance and vigor. The physically disabled person can thus easily be devalued. Some disabled persons themselves have carried these prejudices and must reconcile them to their own disabled status.

Disabled persons may be viewed in this culture as persons who cannot contribute to society. There tends to be in American culture an all-or-none value system that places individuals either in the category of tax-paying independent citizens or as public dependents. This is reflected, for instance, in laws which do not allow for physically disabled persons to supplement their public assistance incomes through as much work as is feasible for them.

The Maladaptive Cycle of Occupational Dysfunction

The previous discussions briefly illustrated how the effects of physical disabilities can resonate throughout the human system. By interfering with the output of the system, physical disabilities also negatively impact the open system cycle and may lead to a maladaptive cycle of occupational dysfunction. Whether the occupational dysfunction is at the inefficacy, incompetence or helplessness level depends on the severity of the disability and the impact it has on the habituation and volition subsystems. Aside from the degree of performance incapacitation, if the disability interferes with major roles and values, the occupational dysfunction is likely to be more severe. The return to adaptive cycle of occupational function will thus require changes and reorganization in all subsystems.

Occupational Therapy with the Physically Disabled Person

The occupational therapist aids the reorganization of all subsystems by engaging the disabled person in occupations and by modifying the environment to facilitate function. Traditional occupational therapy approaches focus primarily on the performance subsystem. These practices are necessary to incorporate into the total therapeutic program. The model helps conceptualize what additional strategies of treatment are useful and also how the traditional performance-oriented procedures fit into the total picture. Thus, from the perspective of the model, the evaluations and treatments of current practice become an integral part of the approach to treating the occupational dysfunction holistically. The following discussions will illuminate those strategies of practice which might be less familiar and about which less has been written in occupational therapy. Less detail is given to the knowledge necessary for addressing performance in order to avoid redundancy with other sources.

CHRONIC PROGRESSIVE DISEASES

The person with chronic progressive illness faces, above all, the task of trying to maintain a life which has some level of productivity and satisfaction in the face of ongoing and changing impediments posed by the disease process. The problems generated by multiple sclerosis (MS) and rheumatoid arthritis (RA) are representative of chronic progressive illness and will thus be used in this section as examples to demonstrate application of the model of human occupation. These two diseases can be considered to have the following characteristics in common: onset in early adulthood; a possibly chronic, degenerative course characterized by unpredictable periods of exacerbation and remission; unknown etiology and cure; fatigue of emotional and physical origin; and progressively decreasing physical abilities (14, 49, 73).

Transient and permanent changes in perceptual motor functioning and physical appearance are common to many chronic illnesses. Persons suffering from a chronic disease, like those who are well, must manage their personal, social and occupational activities but with the additional prolonged and often unpredictable impact of a disease and medical regimen. Two characteristics common to all chronic illnesses are their negative impact on multiple areas of functioning and the long-term nature of demands for adjusting to the disease and its functional implications (108, 115).

Impact of Chronic Disease on the Human Open Systems

The person with progressive chronic disease may develop a pattern of occupational dysfunction secondary to the physical limitations in the performance subsystem which resonate through habituation and volition and disrupt the open system cycle. To facilitate occupational functioning in persons with chronic progressive diseases it is important for the occupational therapist to identify how all components of the human open system may be affected.

PERFORMANCE SUBSYSTEM: IMPACT OF CHRONIC DISEASE ON SKILLS AND THEIR CONSTITUENTS

As MS is a central nervous system (CNS) disease, skills can be affected by such CNS symptoms as blurred or double vision, ataxia, muscle weakness, spasticity, sensory losses, incontinence and fatigue. Remissions and exacerbations may be present for years with increasing disability or a person may follow a continuous downhill course (8). In RA, motor skills are affected primarily by fatigue, by joint pain and inflammation, by muscle weakness and atrophy, and by progressive joint destruction resulting in deformity, contractures or subluxation, and limited strength and range of motion (74). In both of these chronic diseases, exacerbations of symptoms can possibly be accelerated by tension and overfatigue.

Perceptual motor disturbances interfere with the ability to carry out skilled performance in self-care, work and leisure. Therefore, process skills become increasingly important as physical abilities decrease. To compensate for physical limitations, the person must be able to problem-solve, use adaptive equipment and plan for and anticipate difficulties. Because of medication side effects and the disease process, persons may also have difficulty directing or managing daily activities due to cognitive problems which tend to interfere with such things as problem solving (80). In all chronic disease, emotional and personality reactions to the disease can interfere with information processing, judgement and other process skills.

If speech or hearing is affected in the person with MS, communication skills may be particularily handicapped. As more occupational behaviors become difficult or impossible to accomplish alone or at all, adaptation depends on the ability to appropriately communicate and interact with others in the environment. Persons able to fulfill only parts of a task would need to get help with other parts or be forced to give up the entire activity. Yet, the person with RA or MS may not appear to be in pain or show visible signs of deformity. Requests for help must be carefully communicated lest they be met with resistance by a family member, co-worker or friend who knew that a short time ago the person *could* do the activity independently.

HABITUATION

The chronically disabled person faces the problem of maintaining an occupational lifestyle in the face of long-term, progressive disability. As limitations vary the person must make adjustments in habits and roles.

Habits

Remissions and exacerbations that include decrease in physical functioning make organization of habits extremely difficult. Because physical abilities are so variable and unpredictable, chronically disabled persons must be flexible in their habit patterns. New habits must also be learned which allow performance within the limitations of disability. For example, habits of appropriate rest and distribution of energy become important not only for performance, but to avoid potentially unnecessary disability such as joint damage in RA (27).

Roles

As chronic disease interferes with skills it also threatens occupational roles. In addition, the chronically disabled person often must maintain a continuing role related to management of the disease symptoms and compliance with medical procedures. This role may include such expectations as rest and joint protection, combined with routine visits to treatment facilities. This role can interfere with occupational roles.

As physical abilities fluctuate with remissions and exacerbations of the disease, persons with MS and RA may acquire and give up various occupational roles making role balance unstable. A worker may become a volunteer if full-time employment is no longer possible; a caregiver may have to relinquish this role for a while, and so forth. Such role changes can be extremely stressful.

In the early stages particularly, joint pain in RA, weakness in MS and fatigue in both MS and RA are not visible to others, but can severely limit participation in occupational activities (95, 121). These particular symptoms may be interpreted by friends, family and co-workers as signs of laziness or malingering (95). The result can be conflicts between others' expectations and what one can actually do in the role, adding to role stress and conflict. If friends, co-workers and family expect invalid behavior, the patient may perceive and internalize the invalid role.

In later stages of chronic disability, persons may be forced to give up or change roles. A loss of identity and increased self-esteem may occur as persons take on roles they believe to be less important or as they lose roles (112).

Because of the perceived obligations and stress of keeping up productive roles of work and homemaking, other roles such as participation in an organization, amateur roles or friendship roles may fall by the wayside. Because the disease process is gradual and progressive, this may take place slowly over time and the chronically disabled person experiences decreasing life satisfaction and a shrinking sense of personal identity (118).

VOLITION

While the most obvious effects of chronic disease are the interference with performance abilities and routines of daily living, there may also be devastating effects on a person's feeling of personal causation, values and interests. When volition is undermined by chronic disease the handicap imposed on the individual is accentuated. Further, since the disease process is progressive and results in irremediable losses of function, ultimate adaptation of the chronically disabled person depends on adaptive volitional changes and choices.

Personal Causation

The onset of chronic disease is accompanied by pain, fatigue and a reduced ability for performance—all of which may rob one of belief in internal control. As persons increasingly feel externally controlled they may develop undue dependence on medical services and family members and at the same time fail to develop necessary adaptive skills. Such patients may be reluctant to participate in rehabilitation activities which require effort and further confront them with their limitations.

Because of exacerbations and remissions it is difficult for the individual to develop a clear and realistic view of abilities. The prognosis for decreased abilities over time makes it difficult for persons to continue an expectation for success in the future. Persons with MS and RA may, during periods of exacerbation, become unduly discouraged by problems which arise.

Because of the gradual onset and symptom variability associated with MS and RA, some persons may fail to recognize or may deny limitations and necessary precautions, failing to appropriately limit or alter activity and exacerbating their own symptoms. The person with chronic progressive disease must achieve a fine balance between necessary hope for the future and unrealistic expectations. There is often little tangible information from experience or medical knowledge that can assure the individual of what

the future may hold. Thus, it is important for the person to develop a belief in ability to cope with functional losses and suffering, to problem solve and to negotiate with others over management of necessary life tasks (18).

Values

The interference of chronic progressive disease in everyday occupation greatly affects values. In the face of an uncertain disease course with likely periods of exacerbation and remission, persons with chronic diseases cannot easily anticipate what the future will hold and what goals are feasible. They also may find that the disease process may interfere with their own standards for performance, making it necessary to compromise them and sometimes experiencing loss of self-esteem as they are unable to meet their own standards. For example, one arthritic woman, whose role as the spouse of a successful businessman included routine entertainment of her husband's business associates, highly valued her ability as a gourmet cook and expert hostess. However, she found that her routine of shopping for produce, preparing a complex meal, dressing and decorating the home for guests was no longer feasible because the pain was so great by the time guests arrived that she could not enjoy the evening. Though she valued all components of the routine, she had to make difficult choices as to which aspects could be dropped or modified.

As orientation to the future and to goals is affected and as the person is unable to perform up to personal standards, there may be a loss of meaning in activity. For example, one man who found meaning in his hard work as he sought a promotion, was no longer able to find the same meaning in his work after diagnosis of RA, as he knew the disease may prevent the promotion no matter how hard he worked.

Interests

The impact of chronic disease on pleasure or satisfaction in occupation is often great. The disease may prevent the individual from participation in some interests. For example, persons with RA may have to give up activities involving excessive physical stress to joints such as bowling or piano playing. A person with MS may no longer participate in running because of blurred vision or foot drop. In other cases the fatigue, pain and reduced performance in occupations may make them less enjoyable so that the individual begins to lose interest and reduce participation in these activities. The potency of interests may also be affected as the person requires more time for work, daily living tasks and rest, leaving less time for pursuing interests.

ENVIRONMENT

The physical environment may pose many problems for the chronically disabled person as architectural barriers and other features interfere with the performance of work, play and daily living tasks. The variability and progressive nature of chronic disease also mean that new problems in the physical environment will arise from time to time requiring attention.

The social and cultural environment plays a major role in the ability of the chronically disabled person to achieve satisfactory occupational functioning. Attitudes and behaviors of family members, rehabilitation and medical personnel, and others will influence how the individual views his or her disability and how roles are maintained and altered. A great deal of stress may be placed on family members who must accommodate to changing limitations in the disabled person (114).

OCCUPATIONAL FUNCTION AND DYSFUNCTION IN CHRONIC PROGRESSIVE DISABILITY

The impact of chronic disease on personal causation, interests and values can lead to a breakdown of morale in the individual. When the future seems bleak with goals uncertain or obliterated, pleasure in activity diminished, and meaning and purpose in life eroded, it is difficult for the individual to make adaptive choices to engage in occupation. Maintaining a satisfying and productive life through positive choices is a major task for the chronically disabled person. The strength of past success, a belief in ability to cope with problems and strong personal values are strengths upon which many persons draw in order to adapt to disability, but they become extremely vulnerable under the stress and pressure of chronic progressive disease. These factors all may converge to produce various levels of occupational dysfunction. Inefficacy may accompany each period of symptom exacerbation. Repeated negative experiences and forced retreat from life roles and daily habits

may bring a person to the levels of incompetence or helplessness.

Assessment

The person with chronic progressive disease potentially faces a number of problems in each subsystem as the effects of the disease process resonate throughout the system. Additionally, the environment is an important variable in successful or maladaptive occupational behavior. Thus, assessment of the individual with chronic progressive disease should provide the clinician data on the status of all subsystems, the open system cycle and the environment of the person. Table 14.1 indicates potential problems in the person's occupational status and related evaluation procedures for each component.

Treatment

Chronic progressive diseases threaten and gradually cause irremediable damage to the performance subsystem. One role of the treatment process is to prevent increasing limitations and symptom exacerbations and to maximize function within the inevitable constraints imposed by the disease process. Treatment may also facilitate recovery of function after surgical procedures, as in the case of an arthroplasty.

Treatment goals for chronically disabled persons also include: (a) maintaining and altering habit structures to prevent symptom exacerbation and maximize functional capacity within daily routines, (b) enabling balanced performance in roles and while taking into consideration fluctuations in performance ability and gradual decreases in capacity, and (c) maintaining a realistic sense of personal causation and participation in valued and interesting daily activities.

Particular strategies of treatment for each system variable are noted in Table 14.1. These strategies represent a collection of treatment approaches potentially relevant to the chronically disabled person. Their configuration and integration into a particular patient's total treatment plan depends on the stage of the disease process, the level of function or dysfunction and the type of delivery system in which the service takes place.

Intervention with disabled persons can be categorized into four main areas. The first includes fabrication of splints and introduction of adaptive equipment (76). The second is identifying

Table 14.1.

Occupational status, recommended assessments and treatment considerations for persons with chronic progressive diseases

Occupational status	Recommended assessments	Treatment considerations
VOLITION		
Personal causation		
Unpredictable and decreasing skills can lead to feelings of external control and loss of belief in efficacy of skills. Uncertain disease course make expectancy of success difficult	Occupational History (OH) Activity Questionnaire (AQ) Occupational Therapy Functional Screening Tool (OTFST) Internal/External Scale	Provide realistic guidelines for independent decision making in choice and execution of activities in treatment and at home. Reinforce positive feedback from environmental interaction, using structured craft, and vocational and other activities for positive experience
Values		
Inability to participate in past occupational activities and unpredictable future may cause temporal disorientation, mismatch between abilities, and meaningful activities, occupational goals and personal standards, as well as loss of self-esteem from inability to participate in valued activities	OH, AQ, OTFST Values portion of Role Checklist	Assist in refocussing values and goals in line with current and potential abilities. Reinforce the need for flexible future planning providing clinic or home experience
Interests		
Disease process may make past interests no longer viable, may interfere with pleasure and spontaneity of interests, reducing potency and narrowing interest pattern	OH, AQ, OTFST Interest Checklist (modified)	Exploration of new interests related to daily living tasks, work and play in treatment and on free time at home or elsewhere. Opportunities to adapt/modify participation in continued interests. Generation of a wider range of interests so that activity is feasible during exacerbations
HABITUATION		
Roles		
Inability to participate and inconsistency of participation in occupational roles results in confusion regarding perceived incumbancy and internalization of expectations for performance	OH, AQ, OTFST Role Checklist	Identify skill and abilities for valued roles, ways and means of partial role participation and suggestions for participation in new or previously less important roles
Invisible symptoms such as fatigue, pain, sensory loss, etc., can result in a discrepancy between the patient's and other's expectations for role performance		Patient and family education to clarify realities of illness and help reduce patient/ other expectation discrepancy. Explore and plan for role options if discrepancy diminishes

Table 14.1—*Continued*

Occupational status	Recommended assessments	Treatment considerations
Habits		
Limitations imposed by disease require restructuring of daily habits to allow performance. New habits related to disease management may be required. Variability in symptoms and performance ability make stability in habits difficult	OTFST, AQ, OH	Recognition of need to change or develop habits should be emphasized and programs (outpatient if possible) should be designed to monitor development of necessary habits which emphasize time management, energy conservation and a balance of time use

PERFORMANCE

Occupational status	Recommended assessments	Treatment considerations
Skills		
Perceptual and/or motor skills are affected inconsistently, progressively and unpredictably by the specific neuromuscular (MS) and musculoskeletal (RA) symptoms, and by disease and/or emotionally generated fatigue	Passive and active range of motion, sensory evaluation, eye hand/fine hand coordination, and activities of daily living assessment (52, 114) (in RA and MS)	Use of neurodevelopmental and biomechanical treatment approaches (114) as would be determined by assessment results and priorities guided by the patient's values and interests
	Arthritis hand assessment (in RA)	Teach proper precautions, body mechanics and energy conservation and provide opportunities to practice these skills
Pain, fatigue, muscle weakness, and progressive joint destruction reduce ability to perform daily activities (in RA)	Functional status index (in RA) Occupational therapy evaluation for persons with MS Jebson-Taylor Test of Hand Function (in RA and MS) Klein-Bell Activities of Daily Living Scale (in RA and MS)	Provide splints, adaptive equipment and recommendations to reduce deformity and to facilitate environmental adaptation
Process and communication/ interaction skills become increasingly more important as physical skills decline	Informal observation of problem solving and planning abilities	Emphasis should be on developing the ability to evaluate personal situations and apply problem-solving skills. It will also be important to learn how and when to ask for help from others

ENVIRONMENT

Occupational status	Recommended assessments	Treatment considerations
Architectural barriers hinder or prohibit daily activities and disrupt routines	OH Home evaluation appropriate for particular situations	Evaluation and recommendations for modification of home, work, hospital, school environment(s), and for personal assistive devices
Attitudes and behavior of others can have positive or negative effects on adaptation		Provide education and recommendations for family, co-worker and patient regarding coping with this problem and/or refer to counselor

necessary modification of the physical and social environment. This includes family intervention to increase support and realistic expectations for the disabled person's performance. The third is a combination of education, counseling and training. Education is necessary to inform the patient of the disease and necessary precautions and compensations. Counseling involves such processes as values clarification, identification of discrepancies between values and physical abilities, goal setting, mutual evaluation of performance, and time management planning. Training involves such factors as enabling persons to use adaptive equipment, to enact joint protection and energy conservation measures, and to communicate effectively with others (76). The goal of these efforts is to affect change in volition and habituation subsystems. Such change may take a significant amount of time. For example, habit development is a process of gradual internalization of behaviors which initially requires conscious planning and organization. One program designed to teach habits of energy conservation and joint protection to adults with RA required 6 weeks (with 1½-hour sessions/week to achieve initial changes in habit patterns (39).

The fourth aspect of therapy is the engagement of persons in various occupations. These may be designed to achieve physical goals such as increasing range of motion, strength, coordination and endurance (76). They may also serve as opportunities for persons to practice skills and habits for self-care, work or leisure. Finally, participation in occupations provides a setting where problems may be discovered and overcome through adapting activities or performances; where confidence is increased through success, or through ability to compensate for problems or to cope with limitations or failures; and where new interests and values are discovered or enacted.

Delivery of such services may occur in a variety of formats. Persons with chronic progressive disease may have periods of hospitalization coupled with longstanding outpatient therapy or home-bound services. The occupational therapy clinic or workshop may be a setting for remedial activities and exploration and modification of various activities. Outpatient groups may be a particularly efficacious way to engage persons in time management and other problem-solving activities as they allow group support and opportunity to practice what is learned or planned

in the home environment (39). Services rendered in the home have the advantage of allowing the therapist to monitor performance in the actual environment to more directly impact environmental modifications.

ARTHRITIS CASE: SALLY

Sally is 37 years old and has seropositive rheumatoid arthritis (RA). Since her diagnosis 5 years ago she has undergone the standard medical approach to her disease. She progressed through aspirin therapy to nonsteroidal antiinflammatory medications and, finally, began gold therapy 2 years after the original diagnosis. Side effects of skin rash and proteinuria forced her to discontinue the gold therapy after 6 months. A combination of aspirin (Ecotrin), indomethacin (Indocin) and hydroxychloroquine (Plaquenil) was used after the gold therapy but they failed to stop the erosive progression of the disease and Sally was subsequently placed on D-penicillamine medication.‡ A rash developed with the use of this medication and it had to be discontinued. Sally's first referral to occupational therapy, in concert with a referral to a research-rehabilitation facility, was after this course of medication and 5 years after the original diagnosis. Her chief complaints were pain and swelling in both wrists, metacarpophalangeal (MCP) joints and proximal interphalangeal (PIP) joints, knees, ankles, and feet. Because of anemia and weight loss secondary to the chronic nature of her disease she was also referred to a nutrition clinic. Her medications at the time of the occupational therapy referral included a second trial of the Plaquenil, piroxicam (Feldene) and Ecotrin. Consideration was being given, by the rheumatologists, to a course of experimental medications or plasmapheresis because of the progressive nature of her rheumatoid arthritis and the failure of the usual medicine regimen to successfully place the disease in remission.

Evaluation

Sally's evaluation included an occupational therapy assessment to document active and passive range of motion in both upper extremities, a hand assessment, activities of daily living evaluation, the Occupational History,

---

‡ This course of medication is indicated when rheumatoid arthritis is unchecked by a more conservative medication regime. This medication has the ability to place the disease in remission for many arthritis patients.

the Interest Checklist (modified), the Activity Questionnaire and an informal interview concerning her values. Sally finished the paper and pencil assessments on her own time, demonstrating openness and interest in the evaluation process.

UPPER EXTREMITY FINDINGS

Sally had limitations in active range of motion for elbow extension (−10°) bilaterally and loss of finger tip to proximal palmar crease measured in centimeters (Table 14.2). Grip strength could not be measured on the dynamometer but measurements using the standard mercury sphygmomanometer were the following: right, 40 mm Hg, and left, 35 mm Hg, as averaged over three trials. Grip strength measurements were limited by synovitis and pain in MCP joints and PIP joints in both hands. These results indicate a severe loss of grip strength.

On the activities of daily living assessment all activities involving strong grip were difficult for Sally to do. Dressing activities such as buttoning and the use of zippers; self-care activities such as teeth brushing, showering and haircare; and household activities, especially cooking, were difficult due to her loss of grip strength, joint pain and fatigue.

OCCUPATIONAL HISTORY

Sally is a trained and credentialed secondary educator who interrupted her career after 1 year of work to become a full-time homemaker, raising her two sons who are now in their early teens. She had planned to return to teaching after the children were grown. Sally appeared to enter the homemaker role primarily out of sense of obligation to raise her children full time. While she had no complaints about the homemaker role, it did not seem that she had found it highly satisfying or important for her self-esteem. Concurrently, with her homemaker role and previous to the onset of arthritis, she was an active

Table 14.2.
Sally: distance from finger tip to proximal palmar crease

	cm		cm
Right index	4.0	Left index	3.0
Right middle	4.0	Left middle	4.0
Right ring	3.0	Left ring	2.5
Right little	1.0	Left little	2.0

volunteer in her church, running an education program for senior citizens. Volunteer work appeared quite satisfying and important to her. With the onset of arthritis, she relinquished the volunteer role and concentrated her efforts on the homemaker and patient roles (i.e. compliance with treatment and with rest practices for the arthritis were quite demanding of her time). Sally acknowledged that her children will be gone from home in the foreseeable future and that she would need to find a new major occupational role. She had some vague ideas about returning to teaching as a substitute teacher, but seemed both apprehensive and uncertain about her future.

Sally indicated in the occupational history interview that the arthritis interferred with many of her routines and posed problems for undertaking new activities. She admitted running into problems in her daily activities which she could not easily solve and was anxious to learn more about methods of preventing pain and joint deterioration. She also expressed a desire to achieve more enjoyment from her daily schedule.

INTEREST CHECKLIST

The modified interest checklist used for Sally assesses past, present and desired future interests. Of 80 items Sally indicated 11 past strong interests in the past 10 years. In the year previous to the evaluation she had maintained a strong interest in only two of those areas, singing and mending. Many past strong interests which involved both a physical and social component had been dropped. Interests with stressful physical components such as bowling will likely have to be permanently dropped. She had only acquired one new interest, swimming, which she did as "therapy" for her arthritis. However, she indicated a wide range of activities in which she wished to participate in the future.

ROLE CHECKLIST

Sally's perceived role incumbency as she reported it on the Role Checklist is indicated on Table 14.3. Sally had been able to maintain continuous friend, family, home maintainer and religious participant roles. Both the student and worker roles were not part of her current life and she did not indicate them for the future. The volunteer role was interrupted but she planned to return to this role.

Table 14.3.
Sally's Role Checklist responses

Role	Past	Present	Future
Student	X		
Worker	X		
Volunteer	X		X
Caregiver	X	X	X
Home maintainer	X	X	X
Friend	X	X	X
Family member	X	X	X
Religious participant	X	X	X
Hobbyist/amateur			
Participant in an organization			

VALUES

The pattern of values which emerged from the interview was that Sally gave a very high priority to fulfilling external expectations and demands of others while she placed much less emphasis on personal satisfaction, and self-development. The discrepancies between these two areas were substantial, indicating a possible imbalance of values.

ACTIVITY QUESTIONNAIRE

On the activity questionnaire, Sally reported and answered eight questions about her activities over 2 consecutive days. Table 14.4 summarizes Sally's day in terms of the percent of waking hours she spent in relation to various system components. Overall, her day appears deficient in activities providing a feeling of value, personal causation and interest. She rated only about a third of the activities in her day as related to major life roles. She had several long periods of rest, but does not routinely rest during activities. Finally, she experienced a moderate amount of difficulty in daily activities.

Occupational Status

Sally's occupational status is summarized in Table 14.5. She is an articulate and intelligent young woman who is attempting to cope with a progressively debilitating and painful disease process. Her arthritic condition gave her moderate daily pain, limited range of motion and reduced her strength and fine motor abilities.

Her daily routine reflected a lack of oppor-

Table 14.4.
Sally's Activity Questionnaire results

System components	Percent waking hours	
	Initial	Discharge
VOLITION		
Personal causation		
How well done		
Very poorly	0	0
Poorly	19	0
Average	79	83
Well	1	16
Interests		
Time in recreation and leisure	22	32
Enjoyment of activities		
Not at all	3	0
Very little	21	0
Some	51	61
A lot	24	39
Values		
Meaningfulness of activities		
Not meaningful	8	0
Slightly meaningful	6	0
Meaningful	69	76
Very meaningful	16	23
Value of activities to others		
Not at all	5	0
Very little	3	0
Some	35	95
A lot	56	5
HABITUATION		
Roles		
Role related activities	30	44
Habits		
Rest during activities	1	22
PERFORMANCE		
Skills		
Level of difficulty		
Very difficult	5	0
Difficult	6	0
Slightly difficult	41	40
Not difficult	46	59

tunities for exercising feelings of competence and enjoyment. She maintained some roles, but relinquished an important volunteer role to which she hoped to return.

Table 14.5.
Sally's occupational status, treatment goals and intervention

Occupational status	Treatment goals and intervention
VOLITION	
Personal causation	
Failure to recognize current strengths	Facilitate positive feedback through support in therapy and opportunities to review accomplishments
Lack of occupations that provide a sense of efficacy	Increase feeling of efficacy through acquisition of process skills necessary to increase performance and minimize symptomatology
Values	
Value discrepancy	Achieve value balance through values clarification
Future goals unclear	Explore options for future roles
Interests	
Good past interest pattern—loss of major interests due to disability	Explore possible reactivation of some past interests and generate new interests through exploration with activities in therapy and at home
Low level of enjoyment in some daily activities	Incorporate interesting activity into the daily schedule through planning and time management
HABITUATION	
Role	
Good maintenance of several life roles	Support role performance through enhancing necessary skills and time use
Loss of the volunteer role	Begin occupational choice for a new role by exploring values and interests
Habits	
Routine is deficit in providing meaning, interest and feelings of personal causation	Develop a routine with more time for enjoyable and efficacious activity through time management
PERFORMANCE	
Skills	
Reduced motor capacity (strength, range of motion, fine motor coordination)	Protect joints, minimize pain through joint protection training, splints and adaptive equipment. Enhance process skills to compensate for motor loss through practicing problem solving related to joint protection, work simplification in activities related to homemaking role
Difficulty with process skills related to performance problems and pain	

Sally's values were imbalanced, reflecting a strong external orientation and related neglect of self-development and enjoyment. She also had no clear goals for herself in the future. She had lost most of her strong interests due to the interference of arthritis. Sally appeared to be attempting to keep the arthritis from interfering with her perceived homemaker obligations and to keep control over the arthritic process. In so doing she had not fulfilled her urge to explore and master. Her consequent occupational dysfunction was at the inefficacy level.

Treatment Goals and Strategies

The overall objective of treatment was to move Sally to an exploratory and later competence level of occupational functioning where she could begin to investigate and implement ways of changing her occupational lifestyle. Specific objectives of treatment are noted in Table 14.5. Sally's treatment program included instruction in an active range-of-motion program for both upper extremities. In the outpatient occupational therapy program contrast baths, coban wrapping and intrinsic stretching exercises were introduced in an attempt to increase finger tip to proximal palmar crease motion in both hands. Sally was fit with polyform custom-made wrist splints to decrease the pain and increase the stability of both wrists during activities of daily living. She was cautioned to check for an increase in MCP joint synovitis due to the rigid immobilization of both wrists in the splints. Sally was also given two resting hand splints for rest periods or night time use to maintain hand and wrist alignment. In the occupational therapy clinic, Sally had the opportunity to try various adaptive devices that would allow her to continue to be independent in spite of the loss of hand strength and range of motion. A jar opener, vegetable peeler, key holder, long-handled shoe horn, mit to hold soap, and wooden push/pull stick for the oven rack all were devices Sally needed. In addition, Dycem (a blue tacky plastic) and black foam cylinders were useful to increase grip strength and accommodate loss of hand range of motion. Sally put the black foam cylinders around her toothbrush, hairbrush, kitchen utensils, and cleaning equipment. Pieces of the Dycem were wrapped around juice or milk cartons and other cooking and bathroom supplies to help Sally hold onto these items. Sally was encouraged to problem solve when she encountered limitations or pain.

Sally's treatment also included enrollment in a joint protection and energy conservation program which provided information on the disease process and offered opportunities to learn problem-solving techniques and activity analysis skills and to modify interests so that they could still be pursued. Further, all the results of the evaluation (with emphasis on her assets and competence) were shaped with and validated by Sally and she collaborated with the therapist in values clarification and goal setting, and planning time use in her daily schedule. She also had opportunities to explore potential interests through engaging in activities in occupational therapy where she could discuss problems and receive suggestions for modifications from the therapist.

Outcomes

After a period of 6 months of outpatient occupational therapy, a number of notable changes occurred. Sally seriously responded to the feedback concerning her imbalance of values, and her lack of enjoyment or feelings of competence. She was able to identify that in many ways she was quite competent in managing her arthritic condition and still maintaining major life roles. She engaged earnestly in values clarification and, at her own request, retook the Life Goals Inventory 3 months later; her scores showed a marked decrease in discrepancies between value areas.

Sally also identified that teaching had never been a career of strong interest or value for her, but that she had gotten into teaching because of family pressures and lack of a clear occupational choice on her own part. She recognized that her true interests were in the areas of science and health care and began exploring opportunities for education and volunteer work related to medical technology.

Sally learned about analyzing and planning her activities to conserve energy and protect her joints and was able to practice her new skills at home and discuss the changes with her therapist. Training in the use of splints and adaptive equipment helped protect joints and facilitate otherwise painful or difficult activities. These changes are reflected in Sally's activity questionnaire results 3 months after her initial evaluation at discharge (Table 14.4). Sally increased the interest, value and feelings of competence in her day. She was able to increase both leisure time and time related to major life roles. Overall, Sally shows evidence of having successfully moved through exploration and competency levels in therapy. She is now performing at an achievement level with less difficulty and more life satisfaction and continues to explore possibilities for future roles.

MULTIPLE SCLEROSIS CASE: BETTY

Betty is 33 years old and was diagnosed as having multiple sclerosis 3 years ago. Symptoms of weakness and pain in her back and lower extremities, blurred vision, decreased rectal tone, and some slurring of speech occurred intermittently for 5 years prior to the diagnosis.

Betty was admitted to a rehabilitation center after spending a 4-month period in exacerbation of the disease. During the exacerbation, Betty had decreased endurance and ascending muscle weakness with difficulty breathing, dysphagia and optic neuritis. She was not walking or propelling a wheelchair. Prior to her admission, she had been hospitalized for 1 month in acute care on bedrest while receiving corticosteroid therapy. This was her first referral to occupational therapy.

Evaluation

Betty was assessed in the occupational therapy clinic. Assessments included: manual muscle testing (MMT), range of motion evaluation (ROM), sensory testing, self-care and homemaking evaluation, the Minnesota Rate of Manipulation Test (MRMT), the Occupational History, the Interest Checklist, the Role Checklist, an unstructured interview to determine values and goals, an unstructured interview to determine her activity pattern before hospitalization, a home evaluation 2 weeks prior to discharge, and a driving evaluation.

UPPER EXTREMITY-PERCEPTUAL MOTOR STATUS

Betty is right-handed. Her bilateral active range of motion was within normal limits. The MMT at admission revealed proximal upper extremity and trunk weakness with the left side being more affected (Table 14.6). Betty utilized neck and trunk compensation to accomplish shoulder abduction and flexion. No ataxia was noted in upper extremity movements. Betty had a slightly exaggerated thoracic curve and protracted shoulders which are counterproductive to efficient breathing.

Betty had fair coordination; she was able to button small buttons, pick up objects 1 inch in diameter and had definite, legible handwriting. The MRMT was given to Betty to assess her hand dexterity to determine feasibility of vocational goals. She could not endure a testing session of 60 minutes, as she became short of breath and complained of low back pain and heaviness in her arms. Therefore, the test was given in two 30-minute sessions. During bilateral testing, she could not maintain her balance and fell to the left side and onto the testing board. Betty's scores (summarized in Table 14.7) indicated she was not likely to be able to maintain any worker role demanding dexterity and endurance.

Betty's bilateral upper extremity sensation for light touch, pain and temperature was

Table 14.6.
Betty's upper extremity strength on admission[a]

Muscles	Left	Right (dominant)
Neck		
Flexors	G	G
Extensors	N	N
Rotators	G−	G−
Trunk		
Flexors	F	F+
Extensors	F	F+
Lateral flexors	G−	G
Shoulder		
Flexors	F	F+
Extensors	F	F+
Abductors	F−	F
Adductors	N	N
Rotators	G−	N
Elbow		
Flexors	G	G
Extensors	G	G
Pronators/supinators	N	N
Wrist		
Flexors	N	N
Extensors	G	N
Gross Grasp[b]	32 lb	61 lb

[a] Muscle grades (G, good; N, normal; and F, fair) in this table are based on Trombly C: *Occupational Therapy for Physical Dysfunction*, ed. 2. Baltimore, Williams & Wilkins, 1983, p 174.
[b] Norms for Betty's age and sex: 53–60 pounds.

Table 14.7.
Betty's performance on the Minnesota Rate of Manipulation Test

Subtests	Percentile for age and sex
Placing	0
Turning	60
Displacing	60
One-hand turning and placing	2
Two-hand turning and placing	0

intact, as was her proprioception and stereognosis. Her 2-point discrimination was impaired at ½ inch and diminished at 1½ inch on the dorsal and volar surfaces of both upper extremities. She complained of paresthesia in both hands.

SELF-CARE AND HOMEMAKING SKILLS

At admission, Betty was dependent in lower extremity dressing, bathing, transfers, and mobility. Betty dressed her upper extremities but was unable to maintain her balance or bend at the waist to reach her lower extremities to get her clothes over or on her feet. She took sponge baths at home and hadn't been in the shower for over 1½ years. She required minimal assistance for transfers from the wheelchair to the bed, commode, straight back chair, and car. Betty could propel her wheelchair 200 feet on a level surface with two or three rest stops to catch her breath.

For the past 5 months, Betty has made two or three meals for her family and has relied on her children or parents to do most homemaking tasks. She confessed she was unsure of how to approach these tasks from a wheelchair. During a basic kitchen performance test, Betty was unable to maneuver her wheelchair around the kitchen to get items in or out of the cabinets, stove or refrigerator unless given 10 or 15 minutes for each item. She exhibited difficulty with problem solving and planning when asked to plan a simple meal and write down the necessary steps.

OCCUPATIONAL HISTORY

Betty completed high school, was married and had a baby within a year. She worked as a cashier for 6 months in a supermarket before quitting when her daughter was born. She disliked working with the public on a daily basis. For 2 years, her main job was being a homemaker and mother; a second child was born 2 years after the first. After divorcing an alcoholic, indigent husband, she returned to work as a secretary in an architectural firm. She filed papers, did some typing and bookkeeping, and acted as a receptionist for 8 years. Betty resigned from this job 3 years ago when her multiple sclerosis had progressed and she was unable to fulfill her job responsibilities. Two years prior to her resignation, she had numerous absences due to fatigue, muscle weakness and low back pain. Betty stated in retrospect that she had enjoyed the job and liked the moderate contact with other people, but always felt guilty about not being with her children during the day.

VALUED GOALS

When asked what she valued the most in her life, Betty named five things and ranked them in the following order of importance: children and family, independence, financial security, being useful to others, and walking. Betty expected her rehabilitation to enable her to operationalize these values. Nevertheless, she was unable to identify her specific goals for 6 months, 1 year or 5 years in the future.

ROLE CHECKLIST

Betty identified family member as her only continuous role for the past, present and future. Her daughter is now 14 years old and her son 12 years old. She has been completely out of touch with her husband for 12 years and has depended on the support of her parents to assist in child rearing. When questioned if she wasn't a caregiver to her children, she responded, "No, I'm inadequate and unable to do those responsibilities, my parents are their caregivers." She rated the roles of caregiver, home maintainer and family member as very valuable and as the roles she wanted to fulfill in the future. Betty's biggest concern was being a burden to her children when they were coming to an age where they needed more independence. Her comments indicate a perception of being in an invalid role.

Betty identified the following roles as disrupted: worker, caregiver, home maintainer and friend. She felt she had lost a few friends due to her decreased mobility and to her friends' misconceptions about her capabilities. Betty missed the lack of social contact with others besides her family. She realistically identified being a homemaker as her major role in the future.

INTERESTS

Betty identified eight strong interests on the 80-item modified interest checklist. Most interests centered around socialization or sports. In the past year, she has participated in only one area, watching television. She identified a need to develop new interests.

RECENT ACTIVITY PATTERN

Prior to her hospitalization, Betty spent 70% of her waking day in bed watching television or talking to family members on the phone. The other major portion of the day was spent talking with or directing her children. She had no set schedule for meals or self-care activities. Household chores were completed sporadically by the children or her parents. When she had more energy, she would get up and spend an hour or two folding clothes or straightening the house, but afterwards would be exhausted for the next 2 or 3 days.

HOME EVALUATION

Two weeks prior to her discharge, a home visit was made. Betty and the therapist went to her house and were met there by her parents who participated in the review of the possible home modifications. Betty lives in a one-floor, ranch style home. Neither of two entrances to the home was wheelchair accessible, but a ramp and sidewalk could be constructed at the front entrance to make it accessible to Betty. The home was small and crowded with excess furniture. After rearranging the furniture, all the rooms were wheelchair accessible except the utility room and the bathroom. Neither of these rooms could be modified for improved accessibility. But a system of transfers onto a chair and the commode was practiced and was feasible so that Betty could use the bathroom independently.

Betty's father and mother were impressed with the improvement therapy had brought in her transfers and mobility throughout the house. They added suggestions for possible home modifications. Both parents were extremely supportive and praised Betty for her new physical capabilities. Her father planned to make necessary home modifications with the help of Betty's two brothers who lived nearby. Both of Betty's children were accepting of their mother's illness and did household chores with few complaints. Family members admitted that their willingness to help Betty may at times have made her overly dependent and agreed to facilitate her maximal functioning with the future.

Treatment Goals and Strategies

Betty was an inpatient and came to therapy twice a day for an hour and a half. She came in a wheelchair or on a stretcher if she was fatigued from sitting. The objective of treatment was to move Betty from her helplessness level of occupational dysfunction to an exploratory and later competency level of occupational functioning with an aim toward achievement in chosen roles. Specific intervention strategies related to her occupational status are summarized in Table 14.8.

Intervention was developed in conjunction with physical therapy and nursing, and modified weekly according to Betty's endurance level and increased strength. Therapies and self-care activities were scheduled hourly with half-hour rest periods between major activities.

Treatment began by educating Betty about multiple sclerosis: the symptoms, possible precursors to exacerbations and how future planning needed to be flexible. Throughout the hospitalization, Betty's children and parents were also educated about these things by the therapist. Prior to relearning any self-care or homemaking skills, work simplification techniques were taught, reviewed and then practiced within the hospital routine and occupational therapy sessions. Adaptive aids such as a reacher, dressing stick and long-handled bath sponge were given to Betty to increase independence.

During self-care and homemaking tasks, Betty learned how to plan her actions ahead of time with efficiency. Hypothetical problem situations were given to Betty in a graded sequence of simple to complex, with Betty trying many solutions and then choosing the most efficient and comfortable solution for her. She identified when it was acceptable to ask for help from her children or parents to complete tasks.

For 2 weeks, Betty kept an hourly time log of her activities in the hospital and on the weekends when she went home on pass. She also reported her level of fatigue for each hour. Prior to each weekend pass, Betty developed a schedule with the therapist and then compared the schedule with her actual activity. By doing this, Betty learned the value of future planning and of flexibility according to her strength and endurance.

Numerous value clarification activities and goal-setting sessions were conducted with Betty. She decided to set daily, weekly and monthly goals and learned to prioritize them. Treatment stressed the exploration of various, meaningful activities to identify new interests while at the same time increasing upper extremity strength and coordination and improving trunk balance. For example, Betty chose to learn macrame. She learned the basic knots while sitting at a table and then was able to macrame with her arms up in the air, with the same macrame secured to a stationary object. As her strength and endurance improved, weights were put on her wrists, time spent doing macrame was increased and the wheelchair seat belt and armrests were removed. Later she sat on the edge of a mat while doing the activity.

Table 14.8.
Betty's occupational status, treatment goals and intervention

Occupational status	Treatment goals and intervention
VOLITION	
Personal causation	
Feels out of control and expects failure after experiencing an exacerbation	Identify what she can control at home and in hospital and give choices in treatment
Lacks occupation to generate a sense of efficacy	Clarify strengths and provide opportunities for success and positive feedback
Is unable to recognize her strengths	Compare expectations with actual outcome of activity and periodically review accomplishments
Values	
Has clear values but is not incorporating them into daily activity and not all are realistic	Engage in values clarification and prioritization to determine which values should be pursued
Is unclear about short- and long-term goals	Involve in goal-setting daily, weekly and monthly, with revision as needed
Interests	
Lacks participation in interests	Assist to reactivate past, realistic interests
	Provide opportunities to explore new activities and interests
Maintains old interest pattern of which most interests are unrealistic	Incorporate interesting activity in therapy for physical problems
Recognizes need to develop new interests	Involve in daily scheduling to balance work and play
HABITUATION	
Roles	
Has lost worker, caregiver, home maintainer, and friend roles	Assist in prioritizing importance of certain roles given their feasibility and her values and interests
	Provide assertiveness training to enable her to negotiate role relationships
Is currently in an invalid role	Provide practice of role behavior from wheelchair level
	Assist her to incorporate role behaviors into daily schedule at hospital and at home during weekend passes
Habits	
Inconsistent routine	Collaborate in developing a routine schedule according to physical capabilities
Inefficient organization of behavior	Provide instruction and practice of time management techniques
Imbalanced work and play	Involve in routine with time for work, play, rest, and with flexibility

Table 14.8—*Continued*

Occupational status	Treatment goals and intervention
PERFORMANCE	
Skills	
Reduced motor capacity (i.e. strength, endurance, sitting balance, and bilateral coordination)	Use of graded activities providing exercises with frequent rest periods
	Record endurance for an activity and compare daily
	Provide adaptive equipment and practice skills in clinic and as part of routine
Dependence in self care, homemaking and mobility	Provide opportunities to learn problem solving and organizational skills in relation to homemaker role and practice work simplification techniques and body mechanics
Difficulty with process skills (i.e. organization and problem solving in daily performance)	Provide driver's training with adapted hand controls
ENVIRONMENT	
Supportive family whose members can be overly helpful	Educate family and Betty on her disease and her capabilities, and her needs to perform meaningful activity
	Support her accepting new responsibilities and asserting her need to perform her roles with minimal assistance
Physical environment is wheelchair inaccessible and disorganized	Identify environmental barriers, problem solve with Betty and provide recommendations
	Assist Betty in reorganizing furniture, cabinets and placement of household items for greater efficiency

Prescription of bathroom equipment and wheelchair evaluations and recommendations were also done. Betty was instructed in body mechanics, time management, assertiveness behavior, wheelchair maintenance, and accessibility requirements. She was encouraged to participate in community leisure activities and with occupational therapy she shopped using a wheelchair grocery cart. She also received driving instruction.

Outcome

After a period of 2 months in occupational therapy, Betty had recognized and accepted her strengths and weaknesses and stated her long-term goal was to be an independent homemaker and caregiver. She recognized her former degree of withdrawal from her role as a homemaker and her social isolation as both unnecessary and counterproductive for her own life satisfaction. She no longer felt helpless; she was in "control" of her life, feeling competent and was indeed in a state of occupational functioning, able to return to and achieve in her homemaker and mother roles.

At discharge, Betty's sitting tolerance had increased to 12 hours a day and she complained very little of back pain. She improved in sitting balance so she could do bilateral activity for 30 minutes with no rest periods and only two or three readjustments to her posture. She improved a full muscle grade in her shoulders and trunk and was independent in self-care, advanced homemaking and wheelchair management. Betty could propel her wheelchair up and down ramps, on flat level surfaces and over rough terrain; she balanced her wheelchair on the rear wheels to ascend a curb and was able to maneuver the chair around objects and through small hallways. She could push her wheelchair for 30 minutes with two rest periods of a minute each. Betty completed adaptive driving training, was able to drive using hand controls and was able to put her own wheelchair in and out of her car. She identified this accomplishment as her "ticket to freedom," but was concerned about financing the hand control adaptations.

Betty practiced work simplification techniques 80% of the time during four ½-hour observations. She was able to correct her actions and state alternative ways to perform an action. Previous to discharge, she planned her weekends at home independently and was flexible with her actual activity. Betty no longer required her parents' assistance on weekends and she managed the cooking and cleaning and her own self-care independently with minimal help from her children. One weekend, she stayed in the house by herself while the children were at camp. During this time, she invited two friends over to play cards.

After discharge, Betty was referred to a vocational counselor at the Department of Rehabilitation Services. Her stated goal of independent homemaking was recognized by the department as a vocation and it financed the recommended home modifications and the hand controls for her car. Betty continues to identify her family as supportive and as allowing her to perform the homemaker and mother roles as she wishes.

Betty continues to write out weekly schedules and goals and states she is less fatigued by her activities. She is socializing again with her old friends and neighbors and has joined a bimonthly bridge club. Betty continues to macrame and has given many of her projects as gifts and was "even paid for a macramed pocketbook." Though Betty will have more exacerbations and remissions and loss of skills, she identifies realistic goals and feels "more prepared and optimistic about the future."

SPINAL CORD INJURY

Damage to the spinal cord can be caused by injury from trauma such as automobile or diving accidents, gunshot or knife wounds, and falls. Spinal cord damage may also be caused by vascular accidents, by degenerative diseases such as amyotrophic lateral sclerosis or spondylytic osteoarthritis, or by back or spinal surgery. For the patient who has sustained spinal cord injury (SCI), the results are far reaching and all subsystems may be negatively impacted.

Occupational Function After Spinal Cord Injury

The devastation of physical capacity is only part of the total impact of the cord injury and only one factor in successful adaptation. The cord-injured person generally experiences disorganization in the habituation and volition subsystems which threaten the occupational lifestyle. Coping with the physical losses is complicated by losses of control over the course of life,

of interest and meaning in everyday activity, of identity, and of familiar routines. Thus, cord-injured persons must reconstruct for themselves a new sense of being and becoming (82). How this takes place depends both on the extent of performance deficits and the premorbid traits and developmental level of the cord-injured person.

PERFORMANCE

SCI leaves a sudden and severe loss to neurological and musculoskeletal skill constituents of the performance subsystem. Depending upon the injury to the spinal cord, the disability may include lower extremity paralysis (paraplegia); loss of trunk stability, mobility and bowel and bladder functions, and upper extremity paralysis (quadriplegia) (125). Because symbolic constituents are predicated on normal movement and sensation, they will be largely invalidated as the person is faced with the need to acquire new basic rules for body awareness, moving, sensing, and accomplishing tasks.

Skills

Loss of both sensation and voluntary muscle movement precipitates the need to develop new perceptual motor skills. Residual innervated muscles must be strengthened as much as possible and remaining movement may be used to accomplish tasks previously carried out by other movements. For example, paraplegics will use upper extremities for wheelchair mobility and some quadriplegics may use tenodesis action for grasp.

Loss of sensation requires that visual scanning and activity monitoring skills must substitute to avoid decubiti or damage from heat or physical insult (114). Other residuals of the SCI, such as loss of bowel and bladder function, require such skills as self-catheterization, the use of condoms, leg bags and other equipment, and being aware of preventive measures to avoid urinary tract infections and autonomic dysreflexia (114).

For the quadriplegic, implications of relearning daily living, work and play tasks are greater, although both paraplegics and quadriplegics face a major task of relearning skills of daily life. Cord-injured persons with higher lesions may function only with assistance and, to some degree, will have to learn such basic skills as sitting, transferring, dressing, and using adapted equipment.

Communication and interaction skills are both affected by and become more important as a result of the disability. The status of being paralyzed and the reactions to it create impediments to successful communication and interaction. In addition, being in a wheelchair and losing control over upper extremities impairs the ability to communicate through posture and gestures (82). Yet, oral and graphic communication skills are extremely important to the spinal cord-injured person. For example, quadriplegic persons must be able to direct their own care with precise communication.

HABITUATION

Predisability roles and habits are impacted by the residuals of SCI. For the cord-injured person there is a sudden and drastic alteration of daily routines and life roles. Everyday roles and tasks take on a whole new ambience and character; they must be done in new ways, in a different time frame and often with the assistance of others.

Habits

Spinal cord injury radically alters the most basic dimensions of routine performance space and time (82). For example, the cord-injured person must learn to organize behavior around the constraints of where he or she can freely go in a wheelchair and how long it will take.

Habits of the cord-injured person must accommodate a more limited number of daily activities than in the premorbid habit structure. Temporal constraints may require decisions to perform more valued activities while others are performed by an attendant family member or other person. Temporal constraints are further imposed by the necessity of new self-care habits such as bowel and bladder care. Habits must often be flexible since dependence on others and the greater impact of some contingencies (e.g. bad weather, crowded public places, unavailability of facilities accessible to a wheelchair) may require spontaneous modification of routines.

Roles

Cord-injured individuals experience a disruption of their normal occupational roles during hospitalization and rehabilitation (118). Residual limitations may prevent or radically alter role performance after discharge. Many cord-injured persons who are young and whose work

and leisure roles involved robust physical activity, must undergo extreme role change. It may be especially difficult for them to imagine themselves in, and eventually choose roles which do not demand, the same level of physical activity. Such new roles may require skills that the person did not possess premorbidly, intensifying the difficulties of entering productive and leisure roles after cord injury. Peer reference groups which were a source of friendship and organizational roles may have a high degree of demands for physical performance. Consequently, the cord-injured individual may have to find new peer groups or a new basis on which to maintain contacts with old friends and colleagues. Family roles may also be greatly altered. For example, the cord-injured person who previously was a head of a family may become the most physically dependent member.

Reconstitution of roles after SCI may take quite some time because of the tremendous demands placed on persons for changes in identity and skills. For example, cord-injured persons may take several years to return to a worker role although they are physically capable much earlier (26).

VOLITION

The loss of function after SCI is dramatic and permanent. To return to occupational functioning, the cord-injured person must make a series of difficult decisions leading to life-style changes. The interests, values and sense of personal causation which can guide adaptive decision making will be different in some aspects than those which characterized the person premorbidly. Thus, volitional change is essential to adapting to SCI.

Values

SCI interferes with an individual's participation in meaningful life occupations and pursuit of valued goals. For many persons whose activity and goals included substantial physical ability, the injury can have an overwhelming negative impact. Identification with premorbid values centering on physical beauty and prowess may become a source of self-devaluation for the cord-injured person who can no longer live up to these values (85). Because premorbid reference groups often held such values the cord-injured person may be faced with either rejecting group values or devaluing self.

For the newly hospitalized SCI patient, temporal orientation is dominated by the here-and-now reality of a paralyzed body and the routines accompanying its care. A sense of discontinuity with the predisability past may be felt since former abilities can no longer be taken for granted (82). The sense of progression toward an ideal image of self is interrupted, future expectancies and future planning may diminish. The cord-injured person may be hampered in setting occupational goals because of uncertainty over the future (26). Others may have problems identifying effective strategies to pursue their long-term goals.

Interests

After spinal cord injury a general decrease of interest and participation in, and a decline in enjoyment of, occupations may occur (86). The greatest decreases in interest enactment from predisability levels center on activities involving manual dexterity, physical exertion and mobility outside the home (86).

Personal Causation

SCI represents devastating loss of control. The cord-injured patient soon after injury is fully aware and confronted with varying degrees of paralysis, immobility and dependence upon others for even the most basic of bodily functions. Early phases of recovery amount to sensory deprivation in which patients may not even have control over what is available in their perceptual fields.

SCI severs the individual from former taken-for-granted capabilities and results in feedback related primarily to limitations (82). The cord-injured person is faced with a sequence of situations in which his or her inability or difficulty in task performance becomes manifest. There is the realization that one cannot move or receive sensations from parts of the body. There is confrontation with everyday self-care tasks and tasks in rehabilitation which can demand monumental efforts for small results and which require help and supervision. Beyond rehabilitation, the cord-injured person faces a physical and social world that is not designed to accommodate his or her limitations. Each phase along the way the person's sense of control and efficacy may be threatened.

A decrease in positive expectations for the future and a lack of control over the present may result in passivity, dependence and inability

to set goals. Former skills that gave a sense of ability to the person may be impossible or irrelevant to the hospital setting.

In the early stages after SCI, a modicum of hope for recovery may be necessary (24). Hope for recovery is directed at the only kind of existence the patient can imagine—i.e. a future like the past. Until the patient has a sense of remaining skills and some experience in developing and using new skills, no alternative and comprehensible future can be grasped (82).

ENVIRONMENT

The cord-injured person experiences an abrupt and permanent withdrawal from the everyday world of things and people. Upon reintroduction to the community, he or she finds out that the world that is "out there" is vastly altered. Immediately after injury, the environment is narrowed to include primarily the circular bed or Stryker frame, a portion of the hospital room and medical personnel. Being totally immobilized and paralyzed, the cord-injured patient, especially the quadriplegic, finds that he or she is in an environment over which there is no personal control (123). The new social surround of the hospital may also be one which treats the cord-injured person as a depersonalized object (122).

In the rehabilitation phase the environment of the cord-injured person expands. First encounters with the new problems that the disability imposes are presented through both organized and casual interactions with tasks and persons. Tasks presented in therapy are a source of information about how the environment can be explored and mastered through remaining capacities. Rehabilitation personnel, peer patients and others in the setting also become a source of experimentation with personal identity and with interaction from the new social position of being a paralyzed person (26, 82).

The cord-injured person is removed from role partners and role audiences (94). Prolonged hospitalization may also cause role strain within the patient's family and other predisability role settings. The family may be a vital influence on the successful reintegration of the cord-injured individual into occupational roles. Family members can support adaptation of the cord-injured person if they value and are willing to support enactment of alternative occupational roles. Positive family adjustment is influenced by the flexibility of role partners, the strength of relationships within the family before and after the injury (122), the economic needs of the family (102), and the shared values related to occupational roles (118).

Assessment and Treatment

To facilitate occupational functioning of the cord-injured individual, the therapist evaluates and intervenes in all subsystems. Relevant assessments and treatment considerations related to potential problems in the occupational status of the spinal cord-injured person are noted in Table 14.9.

Evaluation and treatment of the performance subsystem will include such factors as upper extremity strength and range of motion, endurance, coordinated use of residual musculature, sitting balance, and mobility (125). These basic abilities must be integrated into indirect or direct responsibility for self-care management (i.e. bowel and bladder care, dressing, feeding, hygiene, skin care) and other desired areas of competence. These are enhanced through the provision of adaptive aids and splints, wheelchair prescription, automobile adaptations and modifications of the home and work environment. Additional skill training includes opportunities to practice planning, problem solving, and communication/interaction skills. Simulation and role playing may provide nonthreatening circumstances for the development of such skills (89).

By learning about the patient's past goals and roles, the therapist can determine along with the patient which of these are still viable, what modifications might need to be made and what new choices may be required. Activity-centered exploration in the clinic provides a concrete means of discovering what role behavior and valued activity is still viable or can be maintained if modified. Beyond this, patients must begin in therapy the task of altering their values, interests and personal causation. This process will likely extend over several years after the cord injury so the goal of therapy is to successfully initiate the process and give the patient confidence in self and hope in the future.

Four types of personal value change are generally necessary: (a) enlargement of scope of values, (b) subordination of values concerning the physical self to values pertaining to personality and other nonphysical factors, (c) realization that the effects of the disability do not involve all characteristics of the self and self-

worth, and (d) transformation of comparative values to asset values by learning to appreciate one's inherent worth and relinquishing unnecessary self-comparison with standards, norms and others (28, 127). Values clarification coupled with concrete goal setting should be included in the rehabilitation process to facilitate effective goal formulation and follow through (87).

The cord-injured person should have opportunities to reconstitute a sense of personal causation and develop new interests or find ways to enact old interests. Treatment should stress personal control over life circumstances by maximizing patient choice and control over the goals and content of therapy and by focusing on personal coping problem solving and communication as successful ways of overcoming physical limitations. When issues of control focus too much on physical ability, the cord-injured person may develop a sense of failure and inability and lose sight of other means of retaining control.

Identification of the roles to which patients desire to return and focusing treatment to maximize the required skills is an important part of therapy. In some cases patients may have to make new occupational choices for entry into a number of new roles to replace lost roles. Exploration of potential work, amateur, leisure, family, organizational, and other roles should be initiated in therapy.

Ultimately, the skills which are acquired in therapy must be organized into habit patterns which relate to the patient's chosen life roles and environmental circumstances. Routines of daily living should be planned and practiced during rehabilitation and carried over to the home. Without opportunities to practice routines and prepare for the course of a routine day, the discharged cord-injured person may have unrealistic expectations and an inability either to accomplish what is desired or to fill the day with appropriate activity.

When possible, treatment goals for all subsystems should be included in each activity. For example, a cord-injured patient engaged in some purposeful activity to strengthen remaining upper extremity function might also be exploring a new activity which could become an interest and which generates belief in ability.

Treatment goals during rehabilitation should take into account the long-term life plan of the patient (100) and the potential function of treatment goals in restructuring a life-style that is meaningful to the patient. By definition, this

Table 14.9.
Occupational status, recommended assessments and treatment considerations for the spinal cord injured person

Occupational status	Recommended assessments	Treatment considerations
	VOLITION	
Personal causation		
Feelings of external control due to loss of sensory and motor functions, isolation, loss of control over routines and interpersonal interactions	Occupational Therapy Functional Screening Tool (OTFST) Occupational History (OH) Occupational Questionnaire (OQ) Activity Questionnaire (AQ)	Maximize opportunities for control over immediate environment through adapted equipment and controls Acknowledge right to, and provide opportunities for, personal decision making and control related to aspects of treatment
Confrontations with loss of skills in most areas of performance	Internal/External Scale	Identify remaining skills. Explore opportunities to adapt existing sensory and motor capacities to optimize performance and success. Stress problem-solving and communication skills as a means of control
Loss of control over decisions because of personal limitations	Informal interview concerning past and anticipated capacities	
Retention of hope for total recovery coupled with difficulty grasping the reality of permanent limitations of skills		Acknowledge areas where patient desires control and incorporate into treatment as much as possible Emphasize remaining and potential abilities and their efficacy
Values		
Premorbid values may be a source of current self-devaluation	OTFST, OH, OQ, AQ	Examine value pattern and identify possible discrepancies between values and capacities. Engage in value examination and clarification emphasizing need for value changes including enlargement of scope of values, subordination of values related to physical prowess and developing or maintaining values related to remaining capacities and roles
Temporal orientation to past and future disrupted	Time Reference Inventory	Support continuity with past by acknowledging past values and identities as still being part of the self while focusing on transformations toward the future

Table 14.9.—_Continued_

Occupational status	Recommended assessments	Treatment considerations
Goals are negatively impacted and may no longer be viable	Expectancy Questionnaire	Support transition to future orientation by examining goals to determine viability, needs for goal changes and intermediate goals necessary for long-term goal attainment
Interests		
Potency of interests lost through discrepancy between demands of interest participation and performance	OTFST, OH, OQ Interest Checklist (modified)	Provide opportunities to explore new interests and to adapt and continue old interests
HABITUATION		
Roles		
Disability initially removes persons from occupational roles and places in a sick role which can become an invalid role	OTFST, OH, AQ Role Checklist	Identify important occupational roles and provide opportunities to practice relevant behaviors
May be discrepancies between past role expectancies and performances and present abilities invalidating or vastly altering roles		Engage in occupational choice and planning for entry into new roles Examine possible modifications of role performance to allow maintenance of roles after discharge
Habits		
Predisability habits invalidated by sensory and motor losses. Time and space dimensions of routine performance are vastly altered	OTFST, OH, OQ, AQ Informal interview to determine present time use in rehabilitation setting and at home on passes	Examine with patient needs for time use to accomodate desired daily activities. Plan for times when assistance is needed. Set priorities for activities and develop a schedule to accomodate it
Self-maintenance and disability management require new routine behaviors		Provide opportunities to practice habits
PEFORMANCE		
Skills		
Insult to neurological constituent produces major loss of perceptual-motor skills. Sensation and movement are lost and may include all four extremities depending on level and completeness of the lesion	Active and passive range of motion evaluation, manual muscle test, sensory evaluation, fine motor coordination evaluation, wheelchair mobility evaluation, driving evaluation, evaluation for orthotics, and prevocational, work	Evaluation and treatment concerns may vary with the timing of intervention. They will generally include the following: Provision of graded, valued and interesting activities to maintain and maximize range of motion, strength,

Table 14.9.—*Continued*

Occupational status	Recommended assessments	Treatment considerations
Perceptual motor limitations place new demands on process and communication/interaction skills	endurance/tolerance and/or homemaking evaluations (52, 114)	endurance and coordination in innervated muscles while increasing sitting balance and tolerance, and while developing relevant leisure and/or other skills
		Retraining in self-care, homemaking, and driving according to patient's capacities and future goals and roles
	Informal observation of problem solving and planning skills	
		Provide activies to maximize communication skills and verbal expression using adaptive aids if needed
	Information observation of communication interaction skills	
		Educate in precautions, in the need to visually compensate for loss of sensation and in wheelchair maintenance and accessability requirements
		Provide opportunities to learn wheelchair mobility in different types of physical settings
ENVIRONMENT		
Abrupt withdrawal from everyday environment	OQ Home evaluation (preferably visitation)	Allow personalization of environment through presence of personal objects and control over some tasks (the latter may simply include decision-making responsibility for when tasks will occur)
Discrepancy between the demands of tasks, objects, roles, and values and remaining capacity	Discussions with family and/or relevant persons in posthospitalization environment	Gradually introduce and prescribe new objects to maximize control and efficacy in environment
		Provide instruction to family concerning patient needs and abilities. Provide information to patient concerning special transportation, support groups and other community resources
		Introduce to graded tasks which have relevance to predisability environment

Table 14.9.—Continued

Occupational status	Recommended assessments	Treatment considerations
		Allow opportunities to take roles in groups and to practice and maintain continuity with predisability roles
		Maintain a value climate which emphasizes values consistent with limitations of capacities

connotes a cooperative process or co-management involving patient and occupational therapist (127). Many rehabilitation facilities have adopted the principle of a team approach which includes the cord-injured person as a full member of the team, with input into the decision making and problem solving required in planning the course of rehabilitation. This approach gives control to patients and encourages the exercise of process skills.

Ultimately, treatment involves transition into an exploration of the environment outside the hospital. Beyond physical modifications in the home, the cord-injured patient may need to plan and practice for community mobility, use of community stores and other resources for leisure and daily living needs. Since the return to work is a process that may take a long period of time (26), in therapy exploration of possibilities is begun and the patient is given opportunity to plan intermediate roles such as homemaking, return to school or training for a new job. If return to work is a possibility and a goal of the patient, then consideration of the work environment and planning and problem solving for adaptations may become part of therapy.

SPINAL CORD INJURY CASE: ALEX

Alex is 30 years old and lives in a moderate sized midwestern city. He was diagnosed as having transverse spinal cord syndrome C_7 complete after sustaining a fracture and posterior displacement of C_7 and a bilateral comminuted fracture of C_{6-7}. The accident occurred when he dove into shallow water in a local creek. Alex stayed in acute care for 4 weeks in Gardner Wells tongs and then was transferred to a rehabilitation unit in a halo vest. His condition was complicated by sacral pressure sores, a urinary tract infection and orthostatic hypotension. He was first referred to occupational therapy in the rehabilitation unit.

Evaluation

Alex was initially assessed mostly at bedside due to his high fevers and unstable blood pressure. Assessments included: manual muscle testing (MMT), range of motion evaluation (ROM), sensory testing, self-care evaluation, the Occupational History, the Interest Checklist, the Life Goals Inventory, the Role Checklist, an interview to determine his activity pattern in the hospital and a predischarge home evaluation.

UPPER EXTREMITY, PERCEPTUAL MOTOR STATUS

Alex is right handed with bilateral upper extremity passive range of motion within normal limits. The MMT at admission and 2 months later after the halo vest was removed is summarized in Table 14.10. At the time of the first testing, neither hand had a measurable grip. The right upper extremity was more functional than the left and Alex was able to pick up objects 2 inches in diameter, operate a call bell, and use a built-up pen to write legibly although his performance was slow, shakey and inaccurate. He demonstrated difficulty working with all fine motor tasks.

Sensation was intact at and above the C_7 dermatone. Light touch, proprioception and stereognosis were intact bilaterally. Sharp/dull sense was intact in the right and impaired in the left upper extremity at the C_8 dermatome. Alex complained of a dull aching pain throughout the left upper extremity. His endurance for activity was low; e.g. he could do an upper extremity activity for only 5 minutes before needing a rest or tilting back due to dizziness.

INITIAL SKILLS IN SELF-CARE

At admission, Alex was dependent in all aspects of self-care and mobility. After the initial evaluation, adaptive aids were given to Alex and with practice he could perform some of his self-care. When given built-up utensils,

Table 14.10.
Alex's upper extremity muscle examination at admission and 2 months later[a]

Left		Muscle	Innervation	Right	
Testing				Testing	
1st	2nd			1st	2nd
SHOULDER GIRDLE					
N	N	Anterior deltoid	C_{5-6}	N	N
N	N	Middle deltoid	C_{5-6}	N	N
N	N	Posterior deltoid	C_{5-6}	N	N
—	G	Upper trapezius	C_{2-4}	—	N
—	G	Middle trapezius	C_{2-5}	—	N
—	G	Lower trapezius	C_{2-4}	—	N
—	G	Serratus anterior	C_{6-7}	—	G
—	N	Rhomboids	C_{5-6}	—	N
G−	G	Pectoralis major-sternal	C_7-T_1	G	G
G−	G	Pectoralis major-clavicular	C_{5-7}	G	N
—	G	Latissimus dorsi	C_{7-8}	—	N
G−	G	Internal rotators	C_5-T_1	G	N
G−	G	External rotators	C_{5-6}	G	N
ELBOW					
F	G−	Biceps	C_{5-6}	G	N
F	G−	Brachioradialis	C_{5-6}	G	N
F	F+	Triceps	C_{7-8}	G	N
F−	F+	Supinators	C_{5-6}	G−	G
F	F+	Pronators	C_{7-8}	G−	G
WRIST					
0	T	Flexor carpi ulnaris	C_8	G−	G
T	P	Flexor carpi radialis	C_{7-8}	G−	G
T	P	Palmaris longus	C_{7-8}	G−	G
P	F−	Extensor carpi radialis longus	C_{6-7}	G−	G
P	F−	Extensor carpi radialis brevis	C_{6-7}	G	N
P	P+	Extensor carpi ulnaris	C_{7-8}	G−	G
HAND					
T	T	Lumbricales	C_8-T_1	F−	F+
T	P−	Flexor digitorum profundus	C_8-T_1	F	F+
T	P−	Flexor digitorum superficialis	C_8-T_1	F	F+
T	P	Extensor digitorum communis	C_{7-8}	F	F+
0	0	Dorsal interossei	C_8-T_1	P	P+
0	0	Palmar interossei	C_8-T_1	P	P+
0	T	Abductor pollicus longus	C_{7-8}	P	F−
0	0	Abductor pollicus brevis	C_8-T_1	P	F−
0	0	Adductor pollicus	C_8-T_1	P	P+
0	0	Flexor pollicus longus	C_8-T_1	P	P+
0	0	Flexor pollicus brevis	C_8-T_1	P	P+
0	0	Opponens pollicus	C_8-T_1	P−	P+
0	T	Extensor pollicus longus	C_{7-8}	P	F
0	T	Extensor pollicus brevis	C_{7-8}	P	F

[a] Muscle grades (N, normal; G, good; F, fair; P, poor; T, trace; 0, zero) in this table are based on Trombly C: *Occupational Therapy for Physical Dysfunction*, ed 2. Baltimore, Williams & Wilkins, 1983, p 174; the format of the table is based on Wilson DJ, McKenzie MW, Barber LM: *Spinal Cord Injury: A Treatment Guide for Occupational Therapists*. Thorofare, NJ, Charles B. Slack, 1974.

Alex fed himself with his right hand, but was unable to complete an entire meal due to poor endurance. After set-up, Alex independently washed his face and upper extemities and brushed his teeth with a built-up toothbrush. He was totally dependent for dressing, bathing lower extremities and bowel and bladder control. He required maximal assistance from one or two people to transfer with a sliding board, and required moderate to maximal assistance in bed mobility, rolling side-to-side and sitting up from supine. He could propel his wheelchair 150 feet on flat surfaces, but propulsion was difficult. Alex's sitting balance was poor; he could not sit upright more than 2 seconds without losing his balance due to his halo vest and decreased trunk musculature strength and innervation. His ability to interact and communicate was limited due to his poor fine motor coordination (e.g. he could not dial a phone or manipulate money). He also did not initiate conversation and answered questions in one- or two-word phrases.

OCCUPATIONAL HISTORY

Alex completed the 10th grade and dropped out of school "to start earning money." At this time, he worked on a maintenance crew for the city and on road construction. In the interim, Alex became involved in drug abuse and eventually turned to a substance abuse unit for help. Following rehabilitation, he entered a federally funded work-training program where he worked with handicapped persons as a counselor. Alex enjoyed this tremendously and stated his occupational goal was to be a rehabilitation counselor. Due to a cut in federal funding, Alex's job as a counselor was eliminated. Alex then attended school for plumbing and worked as an apprentice for 6 months. He became disillusioned with his coworkers and the tediousness of the jobs. At the time of his injury, he was employed as a stock clerk for a large supermarket.

Alex acknowledged that his future occupation was questionable. He felt there was no other satisfying job besides counseling the handicapped, but he recognized his limited education as a deterrent to fulfilling this dream. However, he was willing to obtain short-term job training. He indicated in the interview that he has had difficulty keeping a job for more than 9 months or a year, but could state no reason why.

ROLE CHECKLIST

Prior to his accident Alex lived with his wife and their 3-year-old son and two children from her previous marriage. They were ex-pecting another child within the month. Alex identified family member and friend as his only continuous roles for the past, present and future. He recognized that these roles would be different than in the past. He stated his family role has changed from being a provider and caregiver to his child and wife to being cared for or dependent on others. He rated the role of caregiver and family member as very valuable, and was concerned about his son's reactions to the halo vest and the wheelchair and about his own ability to care for a new baby.

Alex identified the following roles as disrupted: caregiver, worker, home maintainer, church member, and hobbyist. Each of these he rated as very valuable roles. He was anxious and uncertain about his ability to fulfill these roles in the future and was apprehensive about others' reactions to his appearance. Both the student and volunteer roles were not part of his present life, but he indicated they may be roles for the future. After completing the Role Checklist, Alex stated the role he missed the most was as an independent caregiver to himself.

INTEREST CHECKLIST

Of 80 items in the modified interest checklist, Alex indicated strong interests in 10 areas, most of them being sports or involving physical components. In the past month, he maintained a strong interest in only two items—listening to popular music and watching television. For the future, Alex expected to participate in all his strong interests and stated that he would do so as soon as he "walks out of here."

LIFE GOALS INVENTORY

The pattern which emerged from the Life Goals Inventory was high emphasis on love and family, pleasure, social values, and avoidance of hardships. The last was probably related to his questions and concerns about his injury. He placed less emphasis on the areas of accepting limitations, submissiveness and self-development.

This inventory indicated incongruencies among values and a discrepancy between his values and his physical capabilities and what must typically occur in the rehabilitation of a cord-injured person (i.e. accept limitations and develop new and different skills).

CURRENT ACTIVITY PATTERN

Alex reported the typical day at the hospital as being controlled by others. If the staff were running late, so was he. He was dependent on others for his self-care, transfers and being pushed to therapies. He attended occupational therapy and physical therapy twice a day and recreational therapy once a day. A Spinal Cord Support Group was held twice a week and Alex participated in this sporadically. He ate his breakfast in his room and had lunch and dinner in the dining room with 24 other patients. This schedule was varied if his skin was too red, if his blood pressure dropped, if he spiked a fever, or if he had a bowel accident.

Throughout the day, Alex had little or no time to himself. Visitors came but they never visited at a regular time. They would come during therapy, lunch, catheterizations, bathing or postural drainage time.

HOME ENVIRONMENT

Two months prior to discharge, Alex had made good progress in his self-care skills, transfers, mobility, and fine motor manipulation skills. A home evaluation was done at this time as Alex was approaching his expected level of independence. Alex and his therapist left the hospital for 2 hours and written recommendations for modifications were given to Alex after the home visit was completed. Alex lived in an apartment complex in a two-bedroom apartment with his wife, her brother, her two children, and their 3-year-old son and their second child born during Alex's treatment, now 2 months old. The entrance to the apartment was wheelchair accessible but the bedrooms and bath were inaccessible as they are upstairs (14 steps). At the time of discharge, Alex planned to live in the living room, sleep on the couch, have a bedside commode, and wash in the kitchen sink. There was no way to divide the small crowded living room to give Alex some privacy.

Alex's relationship with his wife was increasingly difficult. Prior to his injury, they had difficulty getting along and coping with their extremely active 3-year-old son. Throughout his hospitalization, their relationship had been stormy with frequent disagreements and periods of not talking with each other. Both expressed feelings of depression about their "lost" partner.

During the home evaluation, Alex and his wife had difficulty controlling their son and resorted to spanking or hitting him when he misbehaved. However, Alex's son interacted with him naturally—he asked questions, sat on his lap, got items for him and kissed him. Alex also held his 2-month-old son and played peek-a-boo with him.

Alex's family was supportive and expected Alex to do as much for himself as possible. His parents and younger brother and a married sister live nearby and participated in therapies in order to be trained in Alex's care. His parents offered their house as an alternative living situation for Alex if things did not work out with his wife. They lived in an inaccessible house with the bedrooms and bathroom upstairs. The parents and Alex's 20-year-old brother lived there and all three worked during the day.

Treatment Goals and Strategies

Alex was an inpatient coming to therapy twice a day for a total of an hour and a half. The initial objective of treatment was to move Alex from his helplessness level of occupational dysfunction to an exploratory and later competency level of occupational functioning where he could learn to cope with his injury and acquire the necessary organization to achieve in chosen life roles. Specific treatment goals and intervention for the full course of his occupational therapy are summarized in Table 14.11.

As in most rehabilitation centers, treatment was based on a team approach. This was especially crucial for occupational therapy treatment as many skills and self-care habits needed to be discussed and integrated with nursing care, and physical and recreational therapy needed to be complimentary to occupational therapy goals.

The first phase of treatment for Alex included educating him about his medical status and care and learning how to direct his own care while he was in a halo vest and dependent on others. Through collaboration, a workable time schedule for daily routine care and leisure time was developed, and Alex was responsible for adhering to the schedule. Once the halo vest was removed, Alex moved from directing his care to performing his own care as he acquired the needed skills.

Treatment included the use of purposeful activity to increase upper extremity strength and fine motor coordination, and to improve problem-solving skills. For example, Alex chose to make a toy wooden truck for his new son. He used the bilateral sander with weights, a paint brush, hammer and nails, glue and a wax dobber while constructing his truck. He had to problem solve how to stabilize and position himself and the wood, how to use the tools, how to sequence the construction steps, and how to maneuver his wheelchair to get needed items and clean up.

Treatment also included the fabrication of

Table 14.11.
Alex's Occupational status, treatment goals and intervention

Occupational status	Treatment goals and intervention
VOLITION	

Personal causation

Constraints of performance imposed by the injury	Educate about his medical needs and status and typical outcome for C_7 quadriplegic
No control over scheduling and carrying out his care	Make responsible to direct and later perform care
No feeling of control and fear of failure in the future	Provide positive, exploratory activities in self-care to improve sense of efficacy
	Engage in joint monthly review of accomplishments
	Rearrange environment so Alex is able to use phone and appliances in his hospital room

Values

Value discrepancy and incongruency with physical limitations	Engage in values clarification and exploration to achieve balance and congruency
High commitment to family roles and to attaining maximal independence	Use family-related activities and involvement of family in treatment
	Stress independent function within realistic limits
Unclear future goals	Set future long- and short-term goals

Interests

| Interests incompatible with limitations | Explore old interests and methods of adaptation to limitations and incorporate interests into treatment sessions |
| No participation in interests | Explore new interests |

| **HABITUATION** | |

Roles

Loss of all past roles—entry into an invalid role of being dependent and helpless	Progressive re-entry into productive roles through graded responsibility beginning with directing his care and continuing through living in the hospital apartment
Desire for future participation in family, caregiver, homemaker and worker roles	Practice roles of child caregiver and homemaker
	Explore interests and capabilities in possible work roles

Habits

Controlled by hospital routine which is inconsistent depending on the availability of caregivers	Develop time schedule for self-care and leisure routine in hospital and when discharged
Unaware of importance of habits for own care	Educate in the need for, and practice new habits of, bowel and bladder and skin care, and preventative measures
Premorbid difficulty in maintaining habits	Evaluate and prioritize which routines could be done by others for sake of time
	Give expectation to attend therapies regularly and promptly and dressed appropriately

Table 14.11.—Continued

Occupational status	Treatment goals and intervention
PERFORMANCE	

Skills

Occupational status	Treatment goals and intervention
Decreased upper extremity strength, endurance and coordination	Maintain range of motion and increase upper extremity strength and coordination for functional activities through progressive resistive exercises and repetetive meaningful activity
Low physical endurance and stamina	Provide graded activities for increasing sitting tolerance and time in activity
Dependency in bed mobility, transfers, dressing, bathing, driving, toileting	Driving evaluation and training and independent placement of wheelchair in car
Poor sitting balance	Provide adaptive equipment and splints
Good verbal comprehension and fair communication/interaction skills	Develop homemaking and self-care skills
Difficulty with planning and organizing	Give practice in writing, typing and telephone skills
	Enhance process skills through problem solving related to organization of time, self-care, work simplification and generalization to new situations
ENVIRONMENT	
Supportive nuclear family	Provide family with support and education of Alex's ability
Unstable relationship with wife who is assuming role of caregiver to Alex	Support Alex in negotiations to change roles and reintegrate self into family
Inaccessible housing leading to unnecessary dependence	Recommend a change in living situation; giving Alex responsibility to make phone calls to look at, and obtain, accessible housing
Lack of personal equipment	
Architectural barriers may interfere with mobility	Recommend and obtain wheelchair and personal bathroom equipment
	Practice wheelchair mobility within the community and educate Alex about accessibility requirements and preferences

a left dorsal cock-up splint to maintain his wrist in neutral position which made it more functional as an assist. Adaptive equipment was also given to Alex and he was trained in how to use it. Adaptive equipment included: a reacher, a long-handled sponge, a long and short transfer board, a digital stimulator, a button hook, a zipper pull, an adaptive can holder/dispenser, a transfer belt, Futuro cuffs, and wheelchair gloves.

Alex's treatment stressed exploration of various activities to identify new interests, values clarification and patient-therapist goal setting. Short-term goal setting was done for each week and long-term goals were reviewed monthly and modified if needed. Results of all evaluations were discussed with Alex to help with values clarification and goal setting. Numerous practice sessions were used to assist Alex in re-entering his roles as a father and homemaker. Role playing how to diaper a baby, how to discipline a child, and how to react to emergency situations was used, followed by an hour in therapy where Alex was responsible for the care of his own two children. These sessions occurred in a private environment and began with using a doll for diapering and dressing. During the first three sessions with his own children, the therapist stayed with Alex, made suggestions, modeled appropriate disciplinary action and provided immediate feedback to Alex. Later, Alex cared for the children himself, first in the hospital setting and then when he went home for the weekend. Alex also practiced homemaking tasks such as cooking, cleaning and laundry. He went out in the community for grocery shopping, going to the store and using a local public transportation system for the handicapped.

Outcomes

After a period of 5 months in occupational therapy, Alex improved in all areas of occupational functioning. He moved from a state of occupational dysfunction (helplessness) to a functional state with a feeling of competency. At the time of his discharge, Alex's feelings of efficacy had changed dramatically.

Physically, Alex improved in upper extremity muscle strength and coordination, graphic communication, sitting balance, wheelchair mobility, maintenance and management, bed mobility, and transfers. Range of motion in both upper extremities was maintained and he improved in muscle grade in all innervated muscle groups. He had a gross grip of 20 pounds in the right hand, and 3 pounds in the left hand. His right hand was more functional than the left and with his right hand he was able to write legibly, accurately and at a good rate with no assistive device; he typed 60 words in 10 minutes; and he manipulated objects ⅛ inch in diameter, money and letters. The left upper extremity was being used as an assist but was beginning to develop claw hand with slight edema at the metacarpal joints on the volar surface of the hand. Intrinsic wasting was evident in both hands.

Alex lived in the hospital apartment for 1 week prior to discharge home. He did all self-care independently except for use of a digital stimulator and spotting for tub transfers since the bathroom was not set up to his advantage. He dressed, cooked, cleaned, made his bed, did laundry, took his medicines, and kept his own schedule independently. Occasionally he would slip back into the dependency role by conning others to do things for him that he was capable of doing. When questioned about this, he would state he gets tired of doing everything for himself and likes others to pay attention to him. This issue was discussed with Alex and his family, and they prioritized when assistance could be given if wanted by both parties involved. The family was also given a self-care checklist describing when Alex needed assistance in certain activities.

Alex received feedback concerning his imbalance of values and his incongruency of values and interests with his physical capacities. Although Alex continued to maintain hope for more improvement and thought he may walk again, he clarified his values and developed some realistic long-term goals. He expressed a desire to obtain vocational training and to work with handicapped persons. Following discharge, Alex went to another facility for vocational training and 3 months later began work for Goodwill Industries as a cashier and assisting in supervision of handicapped workers.

In addition to working he is currently pursuing interests as a sports spectator and participating in woodworking and swimming. He is on the waiting list for an apartment designed for the handicapped and hopes to move to more accessible quarters within a few months. During his admission, Alex studied for, and successfully passed, the test for a learner's permit for driving. He completed his behind-the-wheel training at the vocational center and is able to drive with hand controls.

Alex reports feeling more competent in his capabilities and feels he has some active goals to pursue. Even though his marriage ended in divorce and he moved in with his parents, he continues to visit his children and have them over to his parents' home while he babysits. He has met new friends and has renewed friendships which are extremely important to him. Although his medical condition with frequent urinary tract infections has hospitalized him sporadically, he continues to state that he feels in control of his life and is doing what he wants to do.

CORONARY DISEASE

Coronary disease is the leading cause of death in the United States. For survivors it can be severely debilitating. Occupational life-style is a major risk factor in the occurrence of a myocardial infarction (MI) and is of even more importance for survival after the MI (90).

A large body of research outlines a behavior pattern that makes a person more susceptible to cardiac disease, specifically MI. This coronary disease-prone behavior pattern, labeled type A, consists of a complex of personality traits including free-floating anxiety, excessive competitive drive, aggressiveness, impatience, a sense of temporal urgency, and over-arousal by too challenging an environment (38, 42, 67, 91, 93, 98). Not all type A individuals manifest all of these maladaptive characteristics. Nontype A individuals may also possess a few characteristics typical of coronary disease-prone individuals.

While life-style modifications should take

place *before* and to prevent coronary disease, most persons come to the attention of therapists only after the occurrence of a MI. This section discusses both the pre- and postmorbid factors affecting the disease process. Treatment implications after the onset of coronary disease which are discussed here are also relevant to prevention.

Occupational Dysfunction Before and After Coronary Disease

The overall profile of the coronary disease-prone individual reflects disorganization and stress throughout the system which are related to factors in the social environment. The system is "wound up too tight" and eventually breaks down in the form of coronary disease (38, 54)§. Postcardiac patients face a dual challenge. First, such persons must adjust to initial or lasting limitations on activity. Secondly, coronary disease-prone traits that remain must be modified in order to decrease the risk of further coronary morbidity or mortality.

VOLITION

Coronary disease-prone individuals can be characterized volitionally as overachievers. They are driven by an excessive valuation of accomplishment and by an inability to realistically admit limitations or to experience satisfaction from success.

Values

The coronary disease-prone individual's orientation to time is characterized by a sense of urgency. The passage of time is perceived to be too rapid for the accomplishment of desired activities resulting in a ceaseless striving. This temporal urgency results in a chronic and excessive discharge of catecholamines and various

---

§ The purpose of this chapter is to describe occupational life-style problems which may precede and follow coronary disease. A variety of other risk factors such as smoking and diet are important in the etiology and prognosis of coronary disease. While the therapist working in the areas of coronary disease should be aware of these risk factors, they are not described here because of the purpose and focus of the chapter. Also, the chapter is not intended to suggest that all persons who manifest coronary prone life-styles will be victims of coronary disease or that every person who has suffered coronary disease has all or any of the premorbid traits described here.

hormones which encourages the development of coronary artery disease (32, 38).

Coronary disease-prone persons tend to be oriented to task accomplishment and to external recognition as opposed to the intrinsic worth of the tasks they perform. All sense of self-worth is based on success in competition and productivity. The high value placed on completion often leads to a rigid set of standards for performance which paradoxically can decrease efficiency. This individual will continue along the same path even when more creative solutions might reframe the nature of the task or problem and reduce the stress it poses.

In group tasks, these individuals stress task performance, recognition, and power over interpersonal satisfaction and congenial collaboration. Obsessive acquisition of objects and accomplishments along with competition as a central value enter into all aspects of performance and interaction with others. The coronary disease-prone individual thus finds it difficult to relax, to relate to others, or to derive satisfaction in activity (38, 56, 93).

Cardiac patients may continue the same value system after an MI or they might react to the close encounter with death by reflecting and reevaluating their life goals and values. Fear, denial and a general resistance to change may hamper the process of reviewing and changing their value systems. The cardiac patient may be caught in a dilemma of fearing the consequences of retaining past values, but at the same time feeling unable to relinquish them. The person may deny the disease and risk or may accept an invalid identity and withdraw from all activity (78, 104, 107).

Personal Causation

The values of coronary disease-prone individuals emphasize control and mastery, yet these persons often experience themselves as being in jeopardy of losing control. They may perceive greater demands in the environment than are really present and thereby widen the gap between their own perceived abilities and environmental challenges (67, 98). Fear of loss of control or mastery is the major source of stress for the coronary disease-prone individual (42).

These persons often enter into jobs for which their educational or training background is less than adequate, increasing their concern over their own skills. Interpersonal stresses, inability to perform up to personal standards and perceived environmental demands prevent coronary disease-prone individuals from developing belief in their skills and in the efficacy of these skills. Their orientation to the future is dominated by concerns over possible failure (30, 119).

After coronary disease, the cardiac patient may have increased feelings of loss of control and lowered sense of ability, perceiving self as pemanently disabled when such a view is not physiologically justified. They may become incapacitated by fear of another heart attack and disengage from most activity (1, 46, 104). On the other hand, cardiac patients may be unwilling to accept realistic precautions for activity and stress.

Interests

Coronary disease-prone individuals typically experience little pleasure or satisfaction in daily life (55). They are often exclusively involved in work-related activities and have little or no leisure, social and daily living interests. Whether problem solving at work or playing on the golf course, such persons are so fixed on competition and achievement that they cannot enjoy activity and are likely to experience a high degree of frustration.

After a heart attack, patients may resume interests too early against medical advice; they may return to the same pattern of narrowed interests or interest-deficit activity; or they may accept a view of themselves as invalids unable to engage in any activities.

HABITUATION

Both pre- and postmorbidly, individuals with coronary disease exhibit routines of behavior which are stress producing. Both roles and habits reflect rigidity of behavior, a lack of balance between serious and playful activity, and a futile attempt to fit excessive amounts of activity into daily routines.

Roles

Coronary disease-prone individuals characteristically exhibit an imbalance of roles manifest in almost exclusive orientation to the worker role and competitive avocational pursuits while familial, organizational and leisure roles are neglected (54). These individuals also experience stress over conflicting role demands and over role expectations which they typically perceive as being greater than they are. These

persons may also experience stress related to status inconsistency (e.g. being in a role that typically requires more education than they possess). The coronary disease-prone individual may be attracted to occupational roles that encourage and reinforce the coronary-prone behavior pattern (109, 119).

Instead of experiencing their roles as a link to others in the social system, coronary disease-prone individuals tend to feel isolated. They often exhibit strained relationships with peers and superiors, feeling unappreciated for all their efforts (16, 56). Coronary disease-prone males often are unfulfilled in the traditional family roles (1). Sometimes marriage to a woman with higher educational status can exacerbate status inconsistency felt in work roles (30).

After an MI, entry into the cardiac or invalid role is a problem for patients who accept a view of themselves as permanently impaired and whose families, employers and others reinforce such an impression. On the other hand, persons may deny both the limitations they must face and the maladaptive aspects of former role stress.

Habits

The habit structure of coronary disease-prone individuals reflects the volitional sense of temporal urgency, competition and excessive achievement. These persons are likely to work longer hours than others and to carry work-related tasks with them from the workplace. They will persist in stressful work situations despite feelings of overwork. These persons also may attempt to carry out more than one job activity at a time, often shifting back and forth from one task to another (16, 55, 111, 119).

There is typically an imbalance of habits manifest in little time for leisure, family and home-related activities. Even when engaged in leisure the approach may be inflexible. For example, such people characteristically plan their weekends and vacations hour by hour (54, 55). Inflexibility in habits is also manifest in work where such individuals will persist in efforts that are not efficacious or necessary. Overall, the habits of coronary disease-prone individuals are a source of stress for them. Being overly hurried and rigid in their approach to daily behaviors, they seek to maintain control but, paradoxically, become less efficient (38, 54).

After the MI, patients may deny risks involved and attempt to reinstate former patterns lacking restful, meaningful leisure activities increasing risk for further coronary problems. On the other hand they may develop a fear of activity and habits of over-restricting activity and somatic preoccupation (47).

PERFORMANCE: SKILLS

The coronary disease-prone individual speaks emphatically with an air of certainty, increases the tempo of conversation, and may cause the other participants to feel hurried. The coronary disease-prone person gestures with tense, energetic movements. Often, both extensor and flexor muscles are contracted creating movements with an abrupt quality. This person will often motorize by tapping feet or playing with a pencil. Different from nervous fidgeting, these movements are more repetitive and constant in their form and more assertive in style (54).

Coronary disease-prone individuals can be poor observers, failing to register the necessary details of their physical and social environment. They may differ from others in processing stimuli, experiencing their day in a hypervigilant, overscanning, perceptual mode which may be associated with greater physical stresses and different patterns of sympathetic nervous system response (54, 124).

The coronary disease-prone person fights a "time barrier" in skilled performances and is unable to accept inevitable delays and to give up when problems cannot realistically be overcome. He or she pushes harder and does not give up when fatigued. Inadequate problem solving and planning skills may increase the coronary disease-prone individual's feeling of stress, tension and job demands. Preoccupation with competition and task performance increases feelings of stress and tension that can interfere with problem solving (54, 109).

The coronary disease-prone individual typically has difficulty communicating thoughts and feelings to others, is uncomfortable in interpersonal relationships and may have difficulties with authority figures in the work environment (16). Often social relationships are limited to other coronary disease-prone individuals. Excessive competitiveness among these persons often results in tense competitive interaction even in social gatherings (38).

After MI, the cardiac patient may experience varying degrees of limitation of motor performance. The amount and duration of limitations depends on the type and severity of the disease process. In severely complicated post-MI or postsurgery patients, as well as in patients with chronic cardiomyopathy, long-term hypertension, valve disease, or myocardial ischemia, complications may continue for the person's lifetime and cause permanent functional limitations.

There can be interpersonal stress and conflict with the spouse after an MI (103). Previous communication/interaction problems continue and can be a source of interference with recovery as such persons are resistant to communicating feelings and thoughts about the self and may not readily participate in needed self-examination and future planning (53). Process skills may be even further impeded by some patient's concerns that activity will bring on a heart attack. Other patients may be unwilling to learn necessary problem-solving skills for making adjustments in life-style.

ENVIRONMENT

Coronary disease-prone individuals overidentify with values of achievement and competition in the culture. However, the existence of a strong cultural focus on competition over cooperation or satisfaction in performance cannot be underestimated as a factor contributing to coronary disease-prone behavior. Coronary disease-prone individuals strive for jobs that involve greater challenges and higher demands. In turn, these jobs and organizations tend to press for performances that characterize coronary-prone individuals. Thus, the person and the environment mutually reinforce coronary disease-prone behavior patterns (109, 119).

After the occurrence of an MI, the attitudes of family and those in the workplace are important to convey to the individual a realistic set of expectations for return of function. Family members fearing the consequences of another heart attack may become overprotective and may take over the person's previous family obligations. In some cases, the spouse may replace the person as the family wage-earner. The individual with the MI may thus experience a reduction of status within the social system (104, 107, 116).

Assessment and Treatment

Assessment and treatment of the cardiac patient involves identification and modification of premorbid coronary disease-prone behaviors and traits along with identification and implementation of an appropriate activity program to restore endurance. The overall goals of treatment are to restore physical abilities, generate needed new skills and achieve a balanced and satisfying life-style. Both of these foci are critical for restoration of functional ability and for longevity (78). Assessment procedures and treatment considerations are noted in Table 14.12.

Generally, occupational therapy treatment includes graded participation in purposeful activities which increase cardiac capacity, and reduce anxiety and cardiac stress (114). The particular nature of the program and related precautions depends on the patient's diagnosis, cardiac damage and type of surgery.

The occupational therapist may also provide training in skills of stress management and relaxation (109, 110) which allow the patient to more fully cope with tension and stress. However, it is also critical for the patient to alter volitional and habituation factors that create stress. The use of crafts and leisure-related activities may provide the patient an opportunity to try out and learn more flexible and creative approaches to problem solving and provide the patient with an opportunity to develop more balanced values. Engaging patients in time management sessions aimed at developing more flexible habits of work and play, and reestablishing a balance of life roles can help assure avoidance of return to a coronary disease-prone life-style. Identification of interest patterns and providing persons opportunity to explore new interests or to operationalize old interests is very important. Varied and interesting daily activity is a strong predictor of longevity among cardiac patients. Leisure interests involving physical activity can further reduce the patient's coronary risk (15, 37, 51).

Enactment of interests under supervision of an occupational therapist can help prevent cardiac invalidism. Supervised monitoring of progressive activity reduces fear about the risk of activity, provides immediate feedback regarding one's ability to perform interesting, relaxing activity and can enable the patient to explore and gain pleasure in performing daily occupations in a less stressful manner. With supervised monitoring and work simplification techniques, the cardiac patient can practice previous and new role-related and leisure-related activities gaining competence and confidence while gaining strength and endurance.

Enabling patients to identify maladaptive values which are sources of stress is essential. The importance of quality of life over sheer productivity should be stressed. Patients should have opportunities to identify and to value their own inner qualities and resources rather than to base their judgment of worth solely on their number of accomplishments (46). Also, patients should have opportunities to plan for ways in the future they can seek moderate achievement in concert with leisure, family participation and pursuit of satisfying avocational occupations. In therapy the importance of occupation for its intrinsic worth should be stressed and reinforced through participation in activities.

Since patients may be resistive to such programs it is important that occupational therapy receive endorsement by other team members, that the risk factors associated with former lifestyles be stressed by the physician and that the program overall be nonthreatening and exploratory. The use of inpatient and outpatient groups may be useful so that patients can practice collaborative interpersonal skills and provide mutual support.

Finally, the importance of family and work environments for either nurturing or preventing adaptive behavior cannot be overlooked. Family discussion can identify misimpressions concerning patient's abilities and needs for future activity, elicit support for a more balanced life-style, and avoid overprotectiveness (37, 51, 72). Involvement of the family in treatment can help facilitate communication and support for therapy and its carry-over into the home. Assessment of the physical and social aspects of the workplace may be in order, along with modification of aspects of the job and negotiation of clearly stated reasonable expectations for performance. This can serve to alleviate both the employer's and the patient's concerns about adequate job performance. If the coronary problem precipitates retirement, then retirement planning and practice of retirement skills and habits is an important focus.

The life-style changes described here are often difficult to make and may require substantial follow-through by therapy after the initial hospitalization. This is especially true if the cardiac patients are denying the illness and their maladaptive habits. However, given the high risk of further disability and death, such changes are critical for the patient.

CORONARY CARE CASE: MR. JEFFRY

Mr. Jeffry was admitted to the hospital having experienced angina, followed by a myocardial infarction (MI). Sixty years old, he is the owner of a successful small-town

Table 14.12.
Occupational status of the pre- and postmorbid coronary-disease care patient; recommended assessments and treatment considerations

Occupational status	Recommended assessments	Treatment considerations
VOLITION		
Personal causation		
Very high need for achievement premorbidly, coupled with temporal urgency may lead to sense of being out of control. Has a tendency to seek jobs for which skills may be marginally efficacious and thus feels tremendous stress	Occupational Therapy Functional Screening Tool (OTFST) Occupational History (OH) Occupational Questionnaire (OQ) Activity Questionnaire (AQ) Internal/External Scale	Identify reasonable levels of achievement, areas of probable success in the future with the aim of increasing sense of control through more realistic self-assessment and standards for self-assessment
Postmorbidly may have heightened feelings of being out of control and assume a helpless position or have unrealistic view of control and take on contraindicated stressful activities		Engage in graded activities that illustrate tolerance for activity and the unrealistic nature of fears or denial
Values		
Premorbidly, person may have a distorted sense of time characterized by urgency, fear of loss of control over time, and need to fill all time with productive activity. There is a tendency to place too much value on achievement and too little on interpersonal relations. Goals may be overly ambitious and unrealistic	OTFST, OH, OQ, AQ Values portion of Role Checklist Expectancy Questionnaire	Values clarification focusing on a shift from overemphasis on "doing" values to values of "being" and "relating" and values pertaining to leisure Goal setting which stresses accomplishment of quality of life along with achievement
After heart attack the person may be moved to reflect on and alter values or may obsessively continue past value pattern		Examination of standards of performance to identify and modify unnecessarily high and rigid standards
Interests		
Premorbidly lacks variety of interests; most interests are centered on work activity. Tends to engage in interests for competition instead of pleasure	OTFST, OH, OQ, AQ Interest Checklist (modified)	Provide opportunities to enact or discover interests. Emphasize pleasure in activity as opposed to competition and achievement

Table 14.12.—Continued

Occupational status	Recommended assessments	Treatment considerations
HABITUATION		

Roles

Premorbidly roles may reflect a lack of role balance. May have a tendency to enter high stress roles or roles with requirements for training or education beyond what the person has. Obsession with worker role is often evident with neglect of family and other nonwork roles. Work role may lack feelings of colleagiality and include poor supervisor relationships	OTFST, OH, AQ Role Checklist	Emphasize importance of role balance and provide opportunities to plan for and begin to practice and enact role-relevant behavior Examine work role, and sources of work role stress, considering options for reducing stress
There is a tendency for the patient to enter into an invalid role or to return to former maladaptive role patterns		Counteract tendency toward invalid role through graded activity and expectations for performance

Habits

Premorbid habits demonstrate compulsivity and excessive pressure from competition and time. Unrealistic persistance and attempts to do several tasks at a time characterize habits; may have no leisure habits for relaxation	OTFST OH,OQ, AQ	Explore and plan a habit structure which maximizes pleasure and control in daily activity and avoids stress, imbalance of work over recreation, and overestimation of what can be done in a given amount of time
Postmorbid habits may reflect denial and return to contraindicated levels of stress or fear and consequent inactivity		Train in habits of stress management and provide opportunities to practice these habits

| **PERFORMANCE** | | |

Skills

Premorbidly exhibits tense movement patterns and poor observation skills coupled with sense of urgency, poor problem solving and difficulties in interpersonal relationships	OTFST, OH Clinical observation Monitored work evaluation Appropriate formal/informal evaluation of daily living skills	Teach relaxation skills and proper body mechanics. Provide opportunities to learn more flexible problem-solving. Provide training in communication/interaction skills, role playing and group activities
Premorbidly, coronary status may limit activity temporarily or permanently		Provide graded program of increasing activity while monitoring cardiac status. Teach work and activity simplification and energy conservation skills Provide oppportunities to practice self-care and other tasks incorporating simplification techniques Provide any needed adaptive equipment

Table 14.12.—Continued

Occupational status	Recommended assessments	Treatment considerations
ENVIRONMENT		
Environments chosen are often characterized by high stress. Family environment may lack cohesiveness. Hospital environment can contribute to passiveness	OH	Serve as a liaison to family and work to facilitate negotiation of role performance. Examine ways of reducing stress in work environment. Provide an exploratory and activity oriented environment. Plan with the patient and family a home activity program

business, is married and has one son. He has several coronary disease risk factors, including cigarette smoking, diabetes mellitus and a family history of coronary problems (a twin brother died of a heart attack a few years ago). An additional risk factor is his coronary disease-prone life-style. He has extreme involvement in his work coupled with a lack of restful, leisure activity. Mr. Jeffry confided that he often escaped a stressful relationship with his wife by spending long hours at his job. He also complained of a general inability to relax. Mr. Jeffry experienced a second MI in the hospital. Cardiac nursing and counseling staff attributed the second MI to his aggravated state after a recent visit by his spouse. His prognosis was poor; he has a total occlusion of the left anterior descending (LAD) coronary artery, a mild disease of the distal circumflex system and status post two myocardial infarctions.

Assessment and Treatment

During Mr. Jeffry's hospital stay, he agreed to participate in a cardiac rehabilitation program that included a series of seminars developed by the occupational therapist. Mr. Jeffry was assessed with the Interest Check List, Occupational Questionnaire and the Occupational History. At this particular hospital, the occupational therapy program complimented the physical therapy cardiac program which provided graded activity exercise and monitoring of cardiac capacity. Mr. Jeffry's occupational status and treatment goals and strategies are summarized in Table 14.13.

INTERESTS

According to the Interest Check List, Mr. Jeffry has no present interests in the activities of daily living, manual arts, cultural/educa-

tional and physical sports categories. The only activities which he pursued before hospitalization were card games, visiting and shopping. He listed popular music, television and reading as future possible interests.

OCCUPATIONAL HISTORY

Mr. Jeffry started and has managed a successful auto-parts business for the past 30 years. He reports enjoying his work environment although he admits aspects of it are very stressful. This includes management responsibilities and paperwork, and physical labor. He stated that he enjoyed working with his 12 employees and considers many of them personal friends. This is in contrast to a strained relationship with his wife.

OCCUPATIONAL QUESTIONNAIRE

His roles as friend and employer appeared functional but his ability to perform adequately as husband and father were questionable. His interests were minimal and his personal causation were low in his personal relationship with his wife, as he felt controlled by her, allowing her to dominate and control him. Mr. Jeffry's values centered around work with a high desire for business success. He appears to have a low valuation of leisure activities as he has never taken the time to develop and pursue interesting and valued leisure activities.

His reported routine indicated an excessive amount of time devoted to work-related activities, allowing little time for leisure (Table 14.14). When he is not working, his time is taken up with daily living tasks about the house that he perceives as obligatory. These further prevent him from having time to recreate.

Mr. Jeffry's poor medical prognosis made

Table 14.13.
Mr. Jeffry's occupational status and treatment goals and strategies

Occupational status	Treatment goals and strategies
VOLITION	
Personal causation	
Felt some competence at work	Clarify standards by which he judges self at work
Felt very out of control in his relationship with his wife	Assertiveness training
Values	
Strong emphasis on work with devaluation of leisure and family-related activities	Examine values related to work, family and leisure as well as the value of the latter two for survival
Interests	
Narrow interest pattern centered on work. Participation in noninteresting activities	Explore areas of renewed and new interests and emphasize importance of leisure activities
HABITUATION	
Roles	
Stressful spouse role along with imbalanced focus on work role also producing stress	Examine role imbalance and methods of achieving a better integration of roles
Potential for entry into invalid role	Avoid invalid role through focusing on future activity
Habits	
Rigid imbalance of work and play	Time and stress management training to emphasize a better use of time for relaxation and leisure
Long hours and need for physical labor provide contraindicated levels for stress	
PERFORMANCE	
Skills	
Coronary damage places constraints on physical output	Teach energy conservation through simplification
Appears to have good work-related skills but lacks skills for leisure and relaxation	Teach relaxation skills, and explore ways to learn leisure skills

him a candidate to develop cardiac invalid traits. In addition, because Mr. Jeffry highly valued his work role and spent the majority of time at work he expected difficulty adjusting to a need for decreased stress in the worker role.

Treatment

Given the brevity of his hospitalization and the unavailability of outpatient therapy, the focus of occupational therapy treatment was to assist Mr. Jeffry to recognize and learn how to deal with daily and personal stresses and to recognize the importance of including more rest and recreational activities in his daily schedule. The goal was to begin Mr. Jeffry in the direction of life-style change which he would continue on his own after discharge. This was addressed in a series of seminars in which he and other coronary patients participated.

Table 14.14.
Percentage of time Mr. Jeffry spent in occupations pre- and postmyocardial infarction

	Pre-myocardial infarction	Post-myocardial infarction (1 year)
Types of occupations		
Work	42	29
Daily living tasks	29	18
Rest	21	39
Recreation	8	14
Competence in occupation		
Done very well	0	15
Done well	77	62
Done about average	23	23
Done poorly or very poorly	0	0
Value in occupation		
Extremely important	35	38
Important	35	62
Take it or leave it	30	0
Interest in occupation		
Like very much	28	40
Like	54	56
Neither like nor dislike	18	4

The seminars consisted of training in work simplification techniques that would specifically provide patients with physical methods of performing daily living activities with less energy thereby accomplishing more with less physical effort; time management techniques that would enable patients to organize their time by becoming more aware of personal goals and by planning activities through prioritizing; leisure counseling techniques to encourage patients to incorporate more leisure activities in their daily life; and stress management and assertiveness training to improve the cardiac patients' ability to handle daily stresses, interpersonal and otherwise.

Outcome

Mr. Jeffry was contacted a year after his myocardial infarctions. He was doing markedly well, had remained in business and was involved in marital counseling with his wife. When asked what he was doing differently than before his heart attack, Mr. Jeffry stated that he "handles stressful events differently and takes life slower." He also stated that he

had a realistic appraisal of his condition and had modified his life-style appropriately. Mr. Jeffry also agreed to complete a second Occupational Questionnaire. Data from the two questionnaires are compared in Table 14.14. The percentage of time in work activities and daily living activities have decreased. Now, Mr. Jeffry spends more time engaged in rest and recreational activities than prior to his myocardial infarction.

Mr. Jeffry's feelings of control over his environment have changed in that he now spends more time engaged in activities that he feels he does very well. Specifically, these activities that he marked as "very well" were work activities. This may reflect an adjustment in his work-related standards of performance. Mr. Jeffry related that since his myocardial infarction he has achieved a long sought after goal—making a million dollars. He felt that this was partly due to the fact that he was not as rigidly concerned with being in control and was now a "chance-taker." In addition, he said that he is handling stressful events differently and is now more relaxed in his business dealings.

Mr. Jeffry's work-related activities continue to be extremely important to him as they were before his myocardial infarction. Notably, there has been an increase in the amount of time he spends in activities that he finds important and a decrease in the amount of time spent in activities that he could take or leave. Since his myocardial infarction, Mr. Jeffry has also come to see the significance or value of spending time in all types of activities—rest, recreation, daily living, and work.

An increase has occurred in the amount of time Mr. Jeffry spent in activities he likes very much along with a decrease of those he neither likes or dislikes (Table 14.14). This change seems to have occurred because Mr. Jeffry does not spend as much time in daily living activities he previously felt obliged to perform. He now spends more time in rest and recreational type activities that he finds interesting. Mr. Jeffry stated that he attributes his successful recovery in large part to including more leisure-related activities and dealing with stressful events in a more relaxed manner.

THE BRAIN-DAMAGED ADULT

The acute brain-damaged adult is one of the most challenging patients seen by the occupational therapist. Such patients experience dysruptions in all subsystems and in the open system cycle. These dysruptions are often quite severe. Damage to the brain can be caused by a blow from an external source resulting in an open or closed head injury, craniotomy, anoxia, hemorrhage, tumor, infections, thrombosis, or an emboli (50). In this section traumatic head injury and cerebral vascular accidents will be addressed together as types of acute brain damage. However, since the traumatically head-injured person is typically a young adult and the cerebrovascular accident (CVA) patient is frequently over fifty (52, 77) their likely developmental differences must be kept in mind. Additionally, cerebrovascular accidents and head traumas may present widely differing clinical pictures, courses of recovery and ultimate performance limitations. Therefore, performance subsystem disturbances are discussed here only in a general way. The reader is referred to more specific and detailed treatments in this topic, many of which are referenced in this section.

Phases of Recovery from Brain Injury

Brain damage typically results in a course of recovery that can be conceived of as involving three stages (106). The acute phase encompasses the time when the patients are comatose, semi-comatose, or beginning to show generalized, but inconsistent, responses. The rehabilitation phase begins when the patient demonstrates that he or she is aware of the environment and can be a more active participant in treatment. The final, community or outpatient phase refers to the person's preparation for, and return to, home or some other residential situation. Table 14.15 summarizes the occupational status, recommended assessments and treatment considerations for the brain-damaged person in each phase.

The Acute Phase

Brain damage represents an insult to the central governing biological organ in the human body. Depending on the nature and location of the damage, a variety of conditions may be present initially; they often involve a near-complete shutdown of the system.

PERFORMANCE

The brain-damaged person in the acute phase of recovery may have fluctuating mild-to-severe deficits in one or all of the perceptual motor and symbolic areas of the performance subsystem

(69). The brain-injured victim may exhibit abnormal postural reflexes and abnormal tone which dominate all motor control. This abnormal muscle tone as well as limitations in strength and range of motion, and apraxia or ataxia may interfere with patterned, selective and/or coordinated movements (7). In the head trauma patient, bilateral upper and lower extremity function may be affected while in the CVA patient, usually only one side of the body may be affected (41).

In intensive care, motor function may be limited by the life-support machines, monitors and preventative devices (restraints, splints, pillows, casts) that are attached to the patient (92). Oral motor and swallowing functions may be affected and the patient may be fed through hyperal or nasogastric tube feedings (59).

Responses to sensory stimulation may be absent, impaired, delayed, inconsistent, or exaggerated (58). Brain-injured persons may or may not increase their rate of breathing, open their eyes, or vocalize in response to deep pain or speech (71). Responses to auditory, visual, olfactory, tactile, kinesthetic, gustatory, and vestibular stimulation will vary from patient to patient but, in general, responses are inconsistent in this acute stage (77).

In this phase, alertness, the ability to attend to a task, and the fatigue level of the brain-injured person will constantly affect performance. Confusion, disorientation, lack of attention, and inconsistent response to one-word commands typify the general mental status of the patient. Patients may respond more readily to familiar persons such as friends and family than to their therapists or nurses (48).

HABITUATION AND VOLITION

For the brain-injured patient whose behavior does not appear to be under volitional control, volition and habituation may appear to be irrelevant. Severe dysruptions of the performance subsystem does impose constraints on these two subsystems so that their role in the patient's functioning is not immediately apparent. However, past volition and habituation traits represent the ways in which the brain has been processing information and may represent the types of environmental stimuli which could enhance the patient's present ability to process sensory information. Typically, the environment of the intensive care unit or hospital room presents the patient with an array of foreign sensory stimuli.

Table 14.15.

Occupational status, recommended assessments and treatment considerations for persons with brain damage

Occupational status	Recommended assessments	Treatment considerations
	Key: **(A)** = acute phase **(R)** = rehabilitation phase **(C)** = community phase **(ALL)** = all three phases	

VOLITION

Personal causation

An overwhelming sense of being out of control occurs due to confusion, sensory deficits, cognitive and motor deficits, and loss of control over emotions. Uncertainty of functional return and outcomes may also produce feelings of inefficacy. Denial of deficits can lead to an inappropriate belief in skills	**(A)** Family interview Occupational History (OH) **(R, C)** Activity Questionnaire (AQ) Internal/External Scale Occupational Therapy Functioning Screening Tool (OTFST)	**(A)** Give the opportunity to explore body in space and act purposefully. Educate and reassure patient of concerns; provide reality orientation and sensory stimulation with meaningful activities **(ALL)** Provide support and realistic guidelines for independent decision making in choice and execution of activities in treatment, home and community Assist patient to identify strengths and weaknesses, current and potential future capabilities

Values

Inability to participate in past valued occupational activity due to functional limitations. Uncertainty of functional return and outcomes may cause temporal disorientation (especially to the future), lack of motivation, lowered expectations and standards. Mismatch between abilities and meaningful activities and occupational goals may be present. Self-esteem may be threatened or lost when unable to operationalize old standards and goals	**(R, C)** OH, AQ, OTFST **(A)** Family interview **(R, C)** Values portion of Role Checklist Expectancy Questionnaire	**(A)** Sensory stimulation that is meaningful to the patient **(R, C)** Assist in setting realistic goals and values according to current functioning and interests Values clarification and prioritization of goals can assist in future planning. Incorporate values and goals into treatment rationale to motivate and build self-esteem

Interests

Motor, cognitive or perceptual deficits may make past interests no longer viable. Spontaneity and pleasure in interests may be reduced	**(A)** Family interview **(R, C)** Interest Checklist (modified)	**(A)** Stimulation programs centered on past interests **(ALL)** Exploration of old and new interests related to daily living tasks, work and play. Incorporation of interests into treatment to improve motor, cognitive, perceptual and social functioning. Assist in ways to continue interests in hospital and home

Table 14.15.—*Continued*

Occupational status	Recommended assessments	Treatment considerations
	HABITUATION	

Roles

| Inability to participate in occupational roles results in a feeling of helplessness or a loss of interest on role re-entry. Roles may be interrupted or terminated leading to an invalid role exacerbating functional limitations | **(R, C)** OH, AQ, OTFST
(A) Family interview
(ALL) Occupational History
(R, C) Role Checklist | **(ALL)** Identify skills needed and current abilities available for valued roles. Provide opportunities to practice old, new or partial roles in the hospital, at home and in the community. Provide suggestions and feedback for role re-entry |
| Invisible cognitive and perceptual deficits can result in a discrepancy of patient's/others' expectations for role performance | | Patient and family education to clarify capabilities and limitations to help reduce any expectation discrepancy |

Habits

| Limitations imposed by injury require restructuring of daily habits to allow performance. Inability to adapt to changes, habit rigidity, and/or perseveration may be evident. Cognitive, motor and perceptual deficits may interfere with execution of daily routines. May become disorganized and inadequate in performing daily habits in a timely fashion if faced with a new, unstructured situation | **(R, C)** OH, AQ, OTFST | **(A)** Incorporate elements of past routines into sensory stimulation
(R, C) Help patient and family recognize the need for a routine and habits to cope with limitations imposed by brain injury. Initially a structured routine should be developed and treatment organized with meaningful tasks, on a time schedule and with expectations clearly stated
Structure should decrease gradually with more patient responsibility for initiation
Instruct in time management and assist with development of a routine for home |

| | **PERFORMANCE** | |

Skills

| Perceptual and motor deficits may affect upper extremity function, head and trunk control, sitting and standing tolerance, ambulation, communication, and self-care capabilities. Return of function or outcome is uncertain | **(R, C)** OH, OTFST
(ALL) Range of motion evaluation, manual muscle testing, and sensory evaluation (52, 114)
Motor function assessment (12)
Appropriate tests of motor coordination
Appropriate perceptual motor testing | **(ALL)** Use of various treatment approaches (neurodevelopmental, biomechanical, rehabilitative, cognitive) (114) would be determined by assessment results, and priorities and treatment activities would be guided by the patient's values and interests |
| Daily living tasks, work and play skills may also be limited due to cognitive deficits. Memory, judgement, prob- | | **(ALL)** Preventative and corrective splinting, positioning |

Table 14.15.—*Continued*

Occupational status	Recommended assessments	Treatment considerations
lem-solving and decision-making skills can be impaired, thus limiting independence in self-care and mobility	Appropriate assessment of cognitive functioning Appropriate activities of daily living evaluation	and casting may be provided along with instruction and practice of graded self-care skills and mobility skills (bed, wheelchair, automobile) leading to maximum independence in activities of daily living. Provide adaptive equipment and recommendations to facilitate independence in the hospital and in the community Stimulate higher cognitive functioning through challenging, meaningful activities such as crafts, homemaking, functional community tasks and games while increasing attention, concentration, memory and problem solving skills **(R, C)** Provide opportunities to interact appropriately with others and develop verbal and graphic communication skills. Prevocational training if appropriate
Communication/interaction skills may become more important as physical skills are limited but they also may be affected, thus increasing isolation and frustration	Appropriate evaluation of social skills	

ENVIRONMENT

(A, R) Foreign environment of ICU and hospital and personnel is confusing, frightening, unfamiliar, and overstimulating	General observation Appropriate home and work evaluations	**(ALL)** Provide safe, reassuring, comforting, structured environment. Gradually, decrease structure to approximate expected discharge environment. Speak in calm voice and model behavior for other staff members; educate staff on program goals and workable techniques
(C) Architectural barriers can hinder or prohibit daily activities and disrupt routines		Evaluation and recommendations for modifications of home, work, hospital, school environment, and personal assistive devices
(ALL) Attitudes and behavior of others can have positive or negative effects on adaptation		Provide education and recommendations for family, co-worker and patient regarding coping with this problem and/or refer to counselor

As they impact on an already disorganized system, processing of sensory data may be impeded. Stimuli that are volitionally relevant or part of the patient's life routine may have the potential to trigger more effective sensory processing as well as volitional activity.

An example is a 21-year-old male who suffered a head injury. He had been an active singer and had frequently sung with his brother and sister. They began singing to him after he had been comatose and in decerebrate posturing for about 3 weeks. A calendar and family photos were also placed at his bedside. He became responsive within the next 2 weeks; several weeks later he was able to recall the songs, the calendar and photos and even conversations which he heard during the semicomatose state. The presence of these familiar stimuli appeared to facilitate his recovery.

ASSESSMENT AND TREATMENT DURING THE ACUTE STAGE

During the acute phase, the therapist makes the important initial contact with the patient and family. This is frequently in the alien environment of intensive care. The first concern is whether the patient is stable so that there will be no undesirable autonomic nervous system reactions from therapeutic stimulation. A primary reason for becoming involved with patients at this phase is that an optimally arousing environment and contact with a patient has the potential to facilitate the patient's responsiveness and to prevent sensory deprivation.

It is also important at this stage to make contact with family members and assist them in their interactions with the nonresponsive patient (88). Families welcome this instruction and sometimes they are the therapist's only source of information about the patient's unique values and interests. Families need reassurance that they can interact with their loved one in a meaningful way, not just as an unresponsive person connected to tubes and machines.

Assessment of performance at this stage includes such factors as upper extremity passive and active range of motion, pain, tone, strength, control, function, and sensation for deep pain and light touch. Abnormal reflexes and associated reactions (7, 114); abnormal posturing (decerebrate and decorticate); contractures; heterotrophic ossification, defensiveness and sensory (i.e. tactile, auditory, olfactory and visual) responses should be evaluated and documented.

Any fluctuations in responses due to change in the patient's position or time of day should be noted. Evaluation of primitive oral motor reflexes, a gross evaluation for dysphagia (126) and the observation of facial muscle use may also be used to assess oral feeding potential (11). Therapists should test visual tracking, and note if there is a possible field deficit. The patient's responses to one-step commands should be observed, allowing enough time to observe any delayed response. During this acute stage and during all stages, it is helpful to assess the patient's cognition by using Rancho Los Amigos Hospital's Levels of Cognitive Functioning which is arranged hierarchically, levels I–VIII (48). These levels describe a wide range of behaviors that can be assessed by observing the patient. Therefore, the comatose or uncooperative patient can be assessed.

During evaluation and treatment of the brain-injured patient, the therapist should always talk to the patient and explain what he or she is doing and why, even if the patient is comatose or semicomatose.

Volition and habituation assessment is aimed at determining the patient's past interests, feelings of ability, roles, and familiar routines. Information gathered from family and friends about the person's interests, preferences, important roles, and routines can guide the therapist in appropriate selection of visual, auditory and tactile information which is familiar and meaningful to the patient. For example, tapes of favorite music might be more meaningful than the extraneous auditory information from a TV or a radio.

Since the acute phase is when the patient first begins to become aware of and respond to the environment, treatment should provide the patient opportunity to explore his or her body and environment, to determine personal capacities and to learn what has occurred to his body, family and environment. At this phase, the patient needs an environment which is safe, reassuring and comforting.

A multisensory, organized stimulation program should be instigated during the acute phase (71). Meaningful objects from the patient's past may help to increase his or her responses to sensory input. Brief, multiple daily sessions may be preferable as they do not overload or bombard the already confused and disorganized patient. All hospital personnel and visitors should be encouraged to touch the patient while talking to him, and to participate in some aspects of treatment (71).

The Rehabilitation Phase

After a patient has regained consciousness and is able to begin volitional activity, the rehabilitation phase begins. Performance constraints affecting both emotional states and symbolic abilities may still impair some habitual and volitional functions.

PERFORMANCE

In the rehabilitation phase, the brain-injured patient's performance subsystem will vary and may change dramatically from the acute phase. Initially, the patient's ability to process information may be severely affected. He or she may be confused, responding to questions or requests inappropriately or incoherently. The patient may be uncooperative and agitated. Short-term and long-term recall, attention span, concentration level, and ability to follow directions may be diminished. The patient may have impaired judgment, organizational ability, problem solving, abstract reasoning and insight, thereby requiring constant supervision. Language, reading, spelling, math, sequencing, and comprehension skills may be affected as well (7, 48, 50, 69).

In the rehabilitation phase, patients are relearning how to manage their bodies and adapt to such changes as paralysis, sensory loss, spasticity, or residual deformities from the insult (e.g. lacerations, fractures, contractures, atrophy, orofacial changes, surgery scars). All the motor problems from the acute stage may exist in this phase and may inhibit the patient's bed mobility, sitting and standing tolerance, functional upper extremity use, transfers, mobility, dressing, feeding, hygiene, and communication skills. Depending on the severity of the motor involvement, the patient may remain dependent on others for all aspects of his or her care in the early rehabilitation phase (7). As the patient progresses, and motor functioning and self-care skills improve, the patient may gain the ability to perform skills with minimal assistance or independence.

Perceptual motor problems may be multiple in the brain-injured person as central nervous system pathways have been disrupted. If these problems exist and continue to persist, the patient's ability to be independent in activities of daily living may be hindered (6, 70, 99, 120). Depending on the location and extent of the lesion site or brain damage, perceptual motor and visual perceptual skills may be affected mildly or severely. Common problems may include apraxia, unilateral neglect, impaired constructional abilities, visual spatial deficits and poor tactile discrimination (7, 50, 61, 70, 99). These and other related percepual motor problems frequently result in difficulty with wheelchair mobility, transfers, dressing, and other self-care skills (83, 84, 120).

HABITUATION

The person who has regained consciousness may still be disoriented to time and space (106). Or, he or she may be in an agitated and confused state also characterized by an inability to identify and relate to any routine (106). Some special problems, such as amnesia, may affect the patient's recollection or perception of his or her roles.

Removal from familiar surroundings and routines and from everyday life roles adds to this. As the process of recovery continues, a variety of problems may interfere with habits and roles and make acquisition of necessary alterations in routines difficult (65).

Habits

Following brain damage, persons may show an inability to flexibly adapt to changes in the environment (84). This habit rigidity may be either a reflection of the insecurity experienced because of symptoms from the brain damage or a direct manifestation of their cognitive and perceptual motor deficits resulting from the brain damage. Rigidity in habits may be manifest in difficulty with changed time schedules, changes in the social environment, and changes in methods of performing familiar activities (84). Such rigidity may be an impediment to learning necessary adaptations in routines because of performance deficits. Rigidity can also be manifested in perseveration in which the patient continues in some meaningless behavior until someone intervenes.

Brain damage may directly impair the ability to enact once familiar routines. Ideomotor apraxia, for example, is the inability to conduct ordinary behaviors that were once part of such daily routines as self-care (50, 84).

Roles

Brain damage and subsequent loss of abilities immediately remove the individual from participation in life roles. The extreme disability and disorientation that can accompany brain damage casts the individual into a helpless and passive role. Motivational difficulties and aphasia may make it difficult for the patient to begin assuming a more active and responsive role and some patients appear to have lost interest in their former roles.

The family of the brain-injured person must accomodate and take over role obligations that formerly belonged to the person. Further, because of family members' confusion and anxiety over the patient's tremendous loss of function, personality changes, and so on, they may have difficulty maintaining appropriate role expectations as the person recovers. For example when a former preacher who had a stroke with moderate global aphasia began to swear and speak lewdly, his wife would run and hide. She would not talk to him after these episodes, forbade his church members to come visit him and often had him in his room in isolation from others, even though this patient was not responsible for what he was saying and was going through the normal agitated stage of cognitive functioning. Whenever there is a brain injury, families and friends should be educated about the behavioral and personality changes they may see, and how they personally should handle this behavior. Family expectations may be unrealistic and could impede the patient's return to old or to new roles.

VOLITION

As the patient regains consciousness volitional processes must again take over. However, damage to the neurological structure underlying symbolic processes results in a number of symptoms which can interfere with normal volitional activity. Notably, some patients appear to lose their urge to explore and master. This lack of motivation may be the result of organic factors in combination with the overwhelming sense of loss and the monumental efforts required to struggle against the symptoms of the brain damage (84).

Personal Causation

Distortion of sensory information, confusion, pain, loss of control over emotions, and related anxiety can produce an overwhelming sense of being out of control (106). The conditions in the environment can easily produce a state of over-arousal exacerbating these feelings. After brain injury the person may display a flat affect and

decreased motivation and initiative to act (68, 84). Managing the external environment can have a positive effect on reducing confusion and anxiety and giving the patient opportunity to feel increasingly in control.

Later, as the initial symptoms subside and the patient has a more realistic grasp of self and the environment, realization of limitations such as paralysis and sensory loss can produce feelings of inefficacy. The uncertainty of how much physical return may exist can leave the individual ambivalent about the possibility of success or failure in the future. Confusion and other altered sensory, motor and effective experiences may generate a fear of insanity (106).

Belief in skill can also be affected by cognitive and perceptual deficits. For example, a patient may deny hemiplegia due to perceptual deficits and psychological reaction to the pain or loss (84). Thus, belief in skill may initially be characterized by confusion over, or a lack of, recognition of skills or their absence.

Values

Certain personality changes associated with brain damage may affect an individual's standards of performance. Persons may exhibit a reduced level of expectations and may exhibit these lowered standards through shoddy peformance; this problem may begin because of organic disturbances, but it is exacerbated by the lack of activity and the impact of the illness on self-confidence (84).

Brain damage may also impair the individual's ability to abstract and thus to be oriented to the future (84). Future orientation may also be negatively impacted when persons face the uncertainty of physical outcomes and when future plans and goals have been interrupted because of the loss of perceptual motor and symbolic capacities.

Interests

After brain damage, the ability to concentrate and to filter sensory information may be impaired (84), negatively impacting an individual's ability to pursue interests. Perceptual motor and cognitive losses may limit the ability to participate in interests.

At the same time, interests can be an important key to remotivating the patient. Because of the struggle involved in recovery from brain damage, the presence of tasks that are interesting and not overarousing are important (84). Sensory stimuli that are related to past interests may be more readily recognized and responded to by the patient.

VOLITION AND RECOVERY

While both the amount of initial loss of ability and recovery are affected by the nature and extent of brain damage, the motivational state of the patient is a major factor in the recovery process (84). Some patients may simply give up because of frustration or the inertia created by confusion and inability. On the other hand, volitional elements can be the key to establishing a pattern of occupational behavior that enhances recovery. The following case illustrates the role of volition in the rehabilitation phase.

John was a 34-year-old dentist in the army who incurred a head injury in a skiing accident. He had significant damage to motor, sensory and speech areas of his cerebral hemisphere and also sustained brachial plexus injury. His problems included a severe hemiparesis of the right side of the body, decreased sensation, motor apraxia of speech and mild slowing of congnitive processing. Two months after the accident he had spontaneous recovery of most motor aspects, but he did not have the coordination to use his right hand for activities requiring finer motions such as writing. He could walk brief distances with a cane, but tired quickly. He was very self-conscious of his speech and problem-solving ability.

Initially he decided to concentrate on pursuing goals of returning to function as a dentist since this was his greatest area of concern. He engaged in playful bilateral activities such as tossing a ball with the therapist and progressed to whittling and woodcarving—activities he had to do as a dental student. He progressed to being able to do dental procedures on a dental plate model, but realized his fatigue level would prevent him from returning to the direct practice of dentistry.

He began to interview patients who were being prepped for oral surgery and simultaneously explored other ways that he might use his dental background. Eventually he applied to a dental radiology program and was being retained by the army.

In his case, volitional factors were important because he was able to engage in activities relevant to his values and interests which at the same time had therapeutic value for the return of perceptual motor skills. Further, by exploring the area that was important to him he was able to discover both his strengths and limitations and to adjust long-term goals.

ASSESSMENT AND TREATMENT DURING THE REHABILITATION STAGE

It is during the rehabilitative phase that the brain-injured patient explores his world and begins to develop competence in handling a "new" self. Information is gathered which will assist the therapist in enhancing the patient's maximal participation in therapy. The motor, sensory, perceptual, cognitive and behavioral skills of the patient must be evaluated and treated. Initially, the patient may be unable to tolerate standardized evaluations and the therapist will need to use the same gross evaluations and observations used in the acute phase. As the patient's attention span and concentration level progresses, more standardized evaluations can be used (34). The therapist may obtain information directly from the patient on interests, values, personal causation, role, and habits from the premorbid life-style. Possible evaluations are noted in Table 14.15. Consideration of how these might fit with the patient's present condition and likely outcomes will guide the therapist's choices of therapeutic activity.

With the brain-injured person, it is necessary to structure evaluation and treatment sessions so the best performance can be elicited. The environment should be calming to the patient, distraction free yet stimulating. Variables in the environment, time of day, difficulty of stimuli, nonphysical or physical responses required, medications, evaluator, and level of awareness and behavior of the patient, can invalidate assessments (11) and must be considered when planning treatment. A calm voice, giving slow simple commands and the use of gestures and repetition of instructions should be used by the therapist. The therapist can also serve as a role model to family members and assist them in learning how to interact with the patient. Opportunities to meet with persons with similar disabilities can help both the family and patient maintain positive attitudes towards rehabilitation.

Treatment in this phase allows the patient to experiment with new skills, roles and habits. The treatment program should begin with very concrete, familiar and functional tasks that are meaningful to the patient (83). Numerous facilitation techniques (12, 17, 35, 114), compensation techniques for perceptual, cognitive, sensory, and motor deficits; and cognitive retraining (10, 21, 22, 23) may be incorporated into treatment. Splinting, serial casting (13, 25, 63), slings (105), and adaptive devices may be needed to improve motor or self-care skills, so that habits and routines can be incorporated into treatment and be relearned by the brain-injured adult.

Routines and habits should be emphasized during the rehabilitation phase. As much as possible, treatment routines should be matched to patterns of behavior to which the patient will return after discharge. Patients may need written schedules or routines posted to help them remember, and organize their habits. The treatment program should encourage variety as well as repetition in order to develop adaptive skills, habits and routines. The environment should also provide opportunities for the patient to be in a variety of settings that approximate community settings.

The therapist may start with one or two activities during a treatment session. This can usually be increased to at least four 15-minute sessions which incorporate several areas, such as self-care or life skills, communication tasks, cognitive skills, social abilities, upper extremity function, perceptual motor tasks, games/sports, and a leisure activity. After going through the treatment schedule with the patient and family, the patient should be allowed to choose the order, duration and variety of the activities. This gives a sense of control, independence and the freedom for the necessary repetition a patient needs to regain skills and habits. The schedule should be expanded and changed as the patient's tolerance increases and as he or she needs less structure.

Prior to entering the community phase, treatment should emphasize the teaching of safety precautions in the home, community, at work, and when using transportation, cooking, or engaging in leisure activities (9). The brain-injured adult needs instruction on how to handle emergency situations if judgment, and problem-solving abilities remain impaired. Community outings, work simulation and driving evaluation (60, 64), if appropriate, should be incorporated into the treatment process as the focus shifts from the rehabilitation to the community phase.

Therapeutic leaves for the weekend should be utilized prior to discharge into the community. These leaves can prepare the patient and his family for discharge and can determine if other areas of treatment should be addressed. A home visit could be done at this time to assess not only the physical but also environmental expectations. An on-the-job evaluation may be necessary if the patient is returning to work. This would assist the therapist in assessing actual performance skills, work habits and routines needed by the patient, and incorporating these into treatment. Also, architectural barriers or the expectations of the employer may need to be discussed and modified.

Community Phase

Depending on the nature of the brain damage, the course of recovery and the delivery system, the rehabilitation phase may begin months after the head trauma or CVA or it may occur relatively soon and overlap with the recovery of skills (57). What is most critical in the community phase is the return of the patient to a daily living environment that may pose either supports or obstacles to optimal occupational functioning.

PERFORMANCE

Upon leaving the hospital, the brain-injured individual is reintroduced to old tasks and objects. During this initial period of reentry, inabilities may become more obvious. For example, a former homemaker returning to the home may encounter difficulties maneuvering in a wheelchair or with a walker because of architectural barriers. The absence of someone to assist or cue, or oversolicitousness by family members, may lead to decreased independence in self-care, mobility, social, or cognitive skills. Families become more aware of processing difficulties as the brain-injured person may not understand their instructions or the reasoning for doing certain tasks, or is unable to remember or generalize learned skills such as bathing, dressing, wheelchair mobility, transfers, or homemaking from the hospital setting.

The brain-injured individual may not be able to perform the skills he or she learned in the hospital if there is decreased structure, predictability, and familiarity in the home or community setting (71). The patient may have difficulty initiating, organizing and completing a task or applying feedback from others. Skills learned during the last phases of rehabilitation such as money management, safety, work skills and habits, and job seeking skills (if appropriate) may not generalize to a different environment.

After returning home, one brain-injured person stated he felt as if he was in a foreign, yet somewhat familiar world. Little things such as where the sheets were kept, how his room was arranged, how his younger sisters competed for attention, how his mother prepared dinner and how his family watched every move he made were confusing and disconcerting to him. He felt as if he was a "Martian from outer space" for the first 4 or 5 months he was home.

HABITUATION

The successful reintegration of the brain-injured person to routines and roles, depends largely on the transition from hospital to home or other setting. Reintroduction to routines of daily behavior and to various occupational roles may be slow and require much understanding and patience from those in relevant social systems.

Habits

During the rehabilitation phase, habits are largely imposed by the hospital schedule and physical plant. Upon return home the individual may face difficulties in routines because the lack of structure of the different physical setting. Because of the needs of the household, there may be different temporal demands for performance so that the habits learned in the hospital may be inadequate. Persons may have difficulty organizing their day and using time meaningfully and efficiently.

Roles

Reintegration into the family role is a primary task for the head-injured person in this phase. Success in resuming role responsibilities within the family may have an impact on a person's adaptation to other roles. Residual limitations, personality changes and other factors may make it difficult for the family to facilitate role reentry. However, a supportive family milieu can have a major impact on the continued adaptation of the person (84).

The worker role and other roles in social organizations may be interrupted or terminated by the brain injury. Persons may be forced to retire early, to alter their vocational plans or careers, or to begin almost anew in achieving occupational roles. When brain damage and residual disability are severe, role participation may be extremely limited. An invalid role which exacerbates functional limitations may be taken on by the individual and reinforced by others. During this phase, families as well as the brain-injured person may be unsure of what role he or she is in now that he or she has returned home.

VOLITION

Leaving the hospital or other facility can have a variety of effects on an individual's volition. Much depends on the degree of impairment and on the attitudes of those in the social surroundings.

Additionally the person may be faced with a number of important occupational choices. If retirement has been forced by the disability, then the person must find leisure or volunteer alternatives to structure time use. If ability to perform at work is impaired, modifications in the work setting and in work responsibilities may be necessary.

Personal Causation

Return to the community can be threatening if the individual encounters overarousing task demands, architectural barriers and requirements to perform with less structure and assistance. Facing old objects and tasks that can no longer be adequately handled, seeing one's roles assumed by others and attempting to maintain old routines or standards without success may negatively impact personal causation. Fears of failure can become exacerbated if obstacles are encountered which cannot be overcome.

Values and Interests

In similar fashion, the values and interests of an individual may be threatened when the person is faced with inability to operationalize old standards or goals or to participate in old interests. On the other hand return to familiar surroundings may enhance pleasure and satisfaction and the individual may feel more capable of returning to activities he or she valued and found pleasurable.

ASSESSMENT AND TREATMENT DURING THE COMMUNITY PHASE

Too often patients may never achieve success at the community phase of treatment. The patient becomes caught in the maladaptive cycle, obsessing over losses. The community phase is a critical area for occupational therapy to assist patients in developing confidence in their personal causation, obtaining a sense of achievement, new appropriate values and goals, and pursuing opportunities for acquiring societal worth (81). Community treatment could occur in home health care, adult day care settings and outpatient programs.

The therapist should ascertain in assessment whether the person is involved in interests in the home and community and if he or she is working toward valued goals and anticipating success.

The current status of performance skills must be carefully evaluated to determine not only what the patient is capable of but also what is he actually doing at home, at work and in the community. Families need to be given concrete examples of the patient's actual capabilities and should be encouraged to identify problem areas from their standpoint. Often brain-injured persons continue to have difficulty remembering how, what, where, and when they are to do certain tasks. They need to utilize certain memory aids such as lists, calendars and schedules to assist them in successfully completing occupational tasks and organizing their time (71).

In the community phase the person assumes a more autonomous role in treatment. The patient explores his effectiveness in the environment, begins to experience success in the real world and adapts to failures as he looks to the future. At this phase the person should return to mastering the environment at the achievement level. Meaningful activities at this phase would be participating in an interest, or day care group, returning to school, volunteering or working half-days.

HEAD INJURY CASE: JESSY

Jessy is a 22-year-old white female who was injured in a single car automobile accident resulting in a grade IV closed head injury¶ with right occipital scalp lacerations, left intracerebral hemmorhage, right hemiparalysis, left 7th nerve palsy, aphasia and multiple contractures. Jessy was comatose for 4 weeks and semicomatose confused for 7 weeks while in an acute care hospital. During the acute

---

¶ A grade IV closed head injury refers to the patient's initial status in the emergency room and means that she needed full cardiorespiratory support and exhibited no signs of brain function.

phase, Jessy had a ventriculostomy, central hypertension, pneumonia, recurrent urinary tract infections, and bouts of agitation. She was referred to occupational therapy 7 days after the accident.

Jessy was initially assessed in the intensive care unit (ICU) and was later seen in the occupational therapy clinic and at bedside during the acute phase. After 11 weeks in acute care, Jessy was medically stable and was transferred to a rehabilitation center. In rehabilitation, Jessy was assessed in the occupational therapy clinic. Assessments throughout the three phases included observations, informal testing and later formal tests of motor, cognitive, perceptual, self-care and social skills, as well as evaluations of habits, roles, goals, interests, and values.

Performance Subsystem Assessment: Acute and Rehabilitation Phase

ACUTE PHASE

Initially, Jessy was nonresponsive to sensory stimuli except for pain. As she became semicomatose, Jessy responded favorably to visual, auditory and tactile stimulation, but cried to kinesthetic stimulation. She was unable to follow one-step commands and remained in decorticate posturing with marked spasticity and contractures of all extremities which severely limited any voluntary, controlled movement. She made no attempt to speak; she only cried.

In the ICU, Jessy was on numerous monitors, had an IV, a Foley catheter and was fed nasogastrically. Throughout the acute phase, in the ICU and in a private room, Jessy was restrained as she often thrashed her body around and would fall out of bed. Jessy was dependent on others for all aspects of her care including feeding, bathing, toileting, dressing, communication, bed mobility, and transfers. She was unable to sit up for more than 5 minutes without going into a pattern of total extension and sliding out of the chair.

In the later stages of the acute phase, she could attend to a task for 2–3 minutes. She was able to follow one-step verbal directions 50% of the time and began to use facial and other physical gestures to communicate.

REHABILITATION PHASE

Perceptual Motor Skills

Jessy is right-handed and at admission was severely limited in active and passive range of motion of both upper extremities. The right upper extremity (UE) was frozen at the shoulder, internally rotated and adducted, fully flexed at the elbow, with three quarters wrist and finger flexion (see Table 14.16 for specifics). There was no active movement and pain occurred during movement of all joints of this UE. The left UE was also limited in range of motion with apraxia. Jessy often dropped items, was unable to write with her left hand and could not button large buttons. Jessy's left gross grip was 10 pounds and her sensation for light touch, pain, temperature, proprioception, and stereognosis was intact. Jessy's right UE sensation for pain and temperature and deep pressure was intact; she had impaired proprioception, light touch and stereognosis.

Jessy had multiple lower extemity contractures and spasticity which inhibited sitting. She sat with her legs adducted, her left hip and knee at −30° extension and −35° dorsiflexion of both feet. She could roll side-to-side in bed utilizing the bedrails but could not sit up from supine. Jessy required maximal assistance for a stand-pivot or sliding board transfer. She was paralyzed on the left side of her face and was unable to imitate lip or tongue movements on the left, and she drooled constantly. Perceptually, Jessy had no difficulty with body image or scheme, figure ground, position in space, or spatial relations.

Communication/Interaction and Process Skills.

Initially, Jessy was alert when attending, but became agitated and frustrated after 10 minutes of activity. She exhibited the confused-agitated, confused-inappropriate, and confused-appropriate levels of cognitive functioning (48). By gesturing, shaking or nodding her head, or by pointing to objects, letters, words, or pictures, Jessy demonstrated cognitive awareness to her environment and this increased daily. She was oriented to person, place, year, city, state, and President and could follow simple two-step commands 2 out of 5 times. She could immediately recall three out of four objects shown to her, but her remote memory was impaired; she could not state her address, her mother's full name, or her brothers' names, or what she ate for breakfast. Jessy was able to place objects, pictures, the days of the week, and the letters of her name in the correct sequence. She identified objects as same or different according to size, shape and functioning. Jessy pointed to items needed to brush her teeth, but could not put the items in the correct order in which the task is done.

In the early rehabilitation phase, Jessy was agitated and would be constantly moving or would be crying with her hand on her forehead. She had a low frustration tolerance, would give up on difficult tasks and would not initiate interaction with others. As Jessy improved and was able to speak (with dysarthria), she began to interact with others but would be manipulative by acting helpless or childlike. For the first 3 to 4 months of her rehabilitation phase, she carried stuffed animals and pictures of rock stars with her, became embarrassed easily, giggled inappropriately, and interrupted other's conversations or tasks. She had difficulty expressing her frustrations in other ways beside crying, pouting or yelling. Jessy demonstrated questionable judgment, poor problem solving and difficulty making decisions for herself, yet resented being "bossed around." When things bothered her emotionally, she would develop migraine headaches and would go to bed for a day or two.

Self Care

With a scoop dish and a built-up spoon, Jessy was able to feed herself with moderate cueing so she would not drop the spoon or cup. Jessy assisted with bathing, toothbrushing and dressing but required maximal assistance for these tasks as flexion contractures, spasticity, incoordination, poor balance, and poor memory limited her. Early in rehabilitation, the Foley catheter was removed and Jessy had frequent incontinency. She was unable to propel her own wheelchair.

Habituation Subsystem Assessment: Acute and Rehabilitation Phase

During the acute phase information concerning Jessy's roles and routines was provided by her parents and friends. After Jessy's confusion had cleared in the rehabilitation phase she was administered the Occupational History, Role Checklist and an informal activity configuration interview.

OCCUPATIONAL HISTORY

Jessy completed high school and was a senior in college, majoring in chemistry at the time of the accident. During college, she worked part-time for 3 years in a fast-food restaurant as a waitress. Jessy had previously worked as a babysitter, a salesclerk and a housekeeper to earn money. Jessy stated she liked all of the above jobs as they helped her to have spending money and she liked working

Table 14.16.
Jessy's upper extremity range of motion initially in the rehabilitation phase[a]

| LEFT | | | RIGHT | |
Active range of motion	Passive range of motion		Active range of motion	Passive range of motion
		SHOULDER		
0–90°	0–120°	Flexion		0–5°
0–10°	0–30°	Extension		0–7°
0–60°	0–90°	Abduction		0–10°
0–40°	0–60°	Internal rotation: arm in abduction		0°
0–30°	0–50°	External rotation. Arm in abduction		0°
		ELBOW AND FOREARM		
−10–100°	−5–120°	Flexion		(−)90–140°
0–50°	0–80°	Supination		0°
0–80°	0–90°	Pronation		0–45°
		WRIST		
		Flexion		(−)10–40°
		Extension		(−)10°
		Ulnar deviation		0–15°
		Radial deviation		0–10°
		THUMB		
		MP flexion		(−)15–30°
		IP flexion		(−)10–50°
		Abduction		25°
		Opposition		Touch finger tip digit No. 2
		INDEX FINGER	No active range throughout upper extremity	
		MP flexion		(−)10–80°
		PIP extension		(−)5–95°
		DIP flexion		(−)5–80°
		LONG FINGER		
		MP flexion		(−)7–83°
		PIP flexion		(−)30–95°
		DIP flexion		(−)5–70°
		RING FINGER		
		MP flexion		(−)10–80°
		PIP flexion		(−)5–90°
		DIP flexion		(−)5–77°
		LITTLE FINGER		
		MP flexion		(−)5–90°
		PIP flexion		(−)10–100°
		DIP flexion		(−)5–75°

(Left Active range of motion and Left Passive range of motion from WRIST downward: Within Normal Limits)

[a] The abbreviations used are: MP, metacarpaphalangeal joint; IP, interphalangeal joint; PIP, proximal interphalangeal joint; and DIP, distal interphalangeal joint.

with people. Jessy stated that her occupational goal for the future was to be a chemist, working in a university laboratory doing research. She saw her accident as delaying this goal but not obliterating it.

Jessy is the oldest of three children and before entering college she often spent time babysitting her 9-year-old brother. Jessy lived with her brothers and mother and stepfather until 2 years ago when she moved out of the house. Prior to her accident, she lived on campus in an apartment with her boyfriend (against her parents wishes) and they shared financial costs and household chores. Besides working in a fast-food restaurant, Jessy volunteered at the local humane society, worked on the school newspaper and maintained a high B average.

ROLE CHECKLIST

Table 14.17 summarizes Jessy's past, present and expected roles for the future. Since the accident, Jessy had been placed in a dependent role and stated she had no control over her previous role tasks. Her parents controlled her finances, visitors, mail, and phone calls whenever they could. Since her parents lived 2½ hours away from the rehabilitation center, they did not participate directly in her progress in rehabilitation, but as her court appointed legal guardians, they made many decisions for Jessy.

Table 14.17.
Jessy's Role Checklist responses

Role	Past	Present	Future
Student	X	X (in rehabilitation)	
Worker	X		X
Volunteer	X		X
Caregiver	X		X
Home maintainer	X		X
Friend	X	X	X
Family member	X	X	X
Religious participant			
Hobbyist amateur	X		X
Participant in organization	X		X

ACTIVITY CONFIGURATION

Jessy was interviewed informally to determine her activity pattern before the accident and in the hospital. Prior to the accident, Jessy was extremely active. Her typical day included getting up at 6, studying, going to classes or work, volunteering, or working on the school paper. She had no set times for meals or household chores, and she saw her boyfriend erratically as he also had a part time job.

In the rehabilitation phase, Jessy's day was initially structured by the hospital routine. She was awakened at 6, and was bathed, dressed and given breakfast. For 8 hours, she attended therapies. She had ½ hour of freetime during the day, but evenings were generally free except for 45 minutes of self-care activities before bedtime.

Volition Assessment: Acute and Rehabilitation Phase

ACUTE PHASE

Family members and friends were also interviewed briefly during the acute phase to determine Jessy's interests and valued activities. It was determined that she enjoyed and valued rock music, animals and nature.

REHABILITATION PHASE

When Jessy became able to respond to interview questions and structured evaluations she was interviewed concerning values and feelings of personal causation and administered the Interest Checklist.

VALUES

When asked what she valued the most in life, Jessy named four things and ranked them in the following order: independence; being with her boyfriend; having pets; and living away from home. Jessy stated that her goal in 6 months was to walk independently and be able to wash and dress herself and have a weekend pass to her apartment. Jessy expected her other goals to be achieved soon after she was independent in self-care and ambulation.

PERSONAL CAUSATION

Jessy repeatedly complained of her lack of control over her life. She felt as if she had lost her last 2 years of independence from her family and had been put back into a child's role. In acute care and in rehabilitation, Jessy would try to take control of situations, but would give up after one attempt, especially if communication was a problem. Due to the accident, Jessy no longer saw herself as an independent, capable woman. Instead, she saw herself as inferior, dependent on others and incapable of making decisions.

INTERESTS

Jessy identified 10 strong interests on the 80-item modified checklist. Interests clustered around crafts, nature, cooking, and socialization. Initially, Jessy participated in none of these areas, but 4 months into her rehabilitation, she became an active participant in five of her identified interest areas.

Treatment Goals and Strategies

Jessy was an inpatient in both the acute and rehabilitation phases. Initially she was seen for treatment for 10–15 minutes, 2 to 4 times a day. As her attention span and concentration level increased in the rehabilitation phase, she came to therapy twice a day for 1½-hour sessions. Treatment sessions were initially held in a room where distractions were eliminated as much as possible. Activities were varied every 20 minutes. Slowly, Jessy progressed to moving into the kitchen and then finally into the occupational therapy clinic when she had learned to tune out distractions and focus on tasks. The objective of treatment in both these phases was to move Jessy from her helplessness level of occupational functioning to an exploratory and later competency level of occupational functioning. In the community phase, Jessy was seen as an outpatient 3 times a week for an 1½ hours. Later in this phase, she went to a vocational training center, stayed in a dormitory and had occupational therapy twice a week. The objective of treatment was to build on Jessy's competency level of occupational functioning and to move her into an achievement level of occupational functioning. Table 14.18 summarizes Jessy's occupational status and occupational therapy treatment strategies.

ACUTE PHASE

Most of the time was spent in sensory stimulation, reality orientation and preventive and corrective splinting and positioning. Jessy had bilateral elbow extension splints, bilateral footdrop splints, a knee abductor splint, and a right hand cone splint. During this phase, the nurses and family members were taught how to stimulate Jessy most effectively and how to position her to elicit normal posturing and responses. Stimulation programs using rock music, animals and nature objects and pictures were developed according to Jessy's interests as stated by her friends and family. When possible, her restraints were removed or she was sat in a chair during treatment sessions.

Near the end of the acute phase, Jessy made some progress in self-care skills and in her attention span. A swallowing and feeding program was initiated and Jessy learned to feed herself with adaptive equipment and supervision. Other self-care skills were tried during this phase as they were habits that were natural or familiar to Jessy. A picture communication chart was used with Jessy. Matching and sorting tasks were given to Jessy and she began to demonstrate to hospital staff how alert she could be.

REHABILITATION PHASE

Throughout the 6 months that Jessy remained in the rehabilitation phase, intervention strategies were developed in conjunction with physical therapy, nursing, psychology, and recreational therapy. Goals were reviewed and modified weekly (if needed) according to Jessy's improvements and her personal goals.

Preventative and corrective splinting, range of motion (ROM), and facilitation techniques for normal posturing and movement and reduced pain were still a major part of Jessy's treatment. Through ROM, and serial casting techniques, Jessy's right UE became less contracted with reduced spasticity and slight voluntary movement. Voluntary movement was facilitated using Bobath techniques and functional activities, such as dressing, rolling cookie dough and sanding a project. As Jessy's right UE became more functional with movement throughout, her splints were used only at night and were later discarded.

Through trial and error, a seating arrangement was developed so Jessy could tolerate sitting for an hour or more. A wooden wedge seat insert, seat belt, plexiglass lapboard and footstraps were added to her wheelchair. She was instructed on wheelchair mobility and 2 months later, after building up the strength and endurance of her left UE, she was independent in propelling her wheelchair on flat surfaces.

During the early months of rehabilitation, Jessy was constantly (night and day) restricted in her movement by splints, straps, casts, and her inability to propel her wheelchair or ambulate. Treatment time was set

Table 14.18.
Jessy's occupational status, treatment goals and intervention

Occupational status	Treatment goals and intervention

Key: **(A)**   = Acute phase
(B)   = Rehabilitation phase
(C)   = Community phase
(ALL) = All three phases

VOLITION

Personal causation

(A, R) Lack of occupation to feel a sense of efficacy

(ALL) Stimulate with meaningful tasks, objects, music and pictures to perform purposeful responses

(R, C) Review lists of accomplishments and have a picture booklet of new things she is doing

(ALL) Lacks control and unable to make decisions

(R) Identify what she can control; give choice in treatments

(R, C) Facilitate decision-making skills, weighing pros and cons

(R, C) Assertiveness training

Values

(R, C) Unrealistic goals for cognitive and physical status

(R, C) Practice realistic goal setting (daily, weekly, monthly, yearly)

(R, C) Exploration and practice of skills needed for goals and self-evaluation of current skills

(ALL) Identified values but no incorporation into daily activity

(A) Incorporate values into sensory stimulation program

(R, C) Exploration and redirection of vocational and avocational goals

(R, C) Values clarification, prioritization, and review of actual activity

Interests

Premorbid life-style of participation in many interest areas

(ALL) Use previous interests for stimulation program and include in treatment sessions

(ALL) Lack of participation in interest areas

(ALL) Reactivate past interests in hospital and community

(ALL) Explore old and new interests and problem solve how to do them with current physical and cognitive status

HABITUATION

Roles

(ALL) Loss of worker, volunteer, caregiver, home maintainer, hobbyist, organizational participant roles

(R, C) Practice role behaviors, gradually increasing responsibilities

(C) Assist in planning reentry into roles and give feedback

(ALL) Loss of age-appropriate family role

(R) Practice age appropriate behavior through role playing and analysis of actual situations with feedback

(ALL) Instruct family on patient's capabilities and need to be treated as an adult

Table 14.18.—Continued

Occupational status	Treatment goals and intervention
(C) Change from helplessness role to achievement with supervision	(C) Support in role transitions providing corrective feedback as needed

Habits

(A) Inconsistent routine	(A, R) Develop structured schedule for activity
(R, C) Inefficient organization of time	(A, R) Structure treatment and organize meaningful tasks with clear expectations
	(R, C) Practice time management techniques
	(R, C) Decrease structure with more self-initiation of routine habits leading to prevocational readiness
	(R, C) Develop mnemonic aids to assist with routine (checklist, charts, notes, daily planner, etc.)

PERFORMANCE

Skills

(A, R) Reduced motor capacity (range of motion, strength, balance, coordination, motor planning, control, oral motor skills)	(A, R) Preventive and corrective splinting, positioning and casting
	(A, R) Facilitate normal oral motor function, movement and positioning through meaningful activity
	(R) Graded activities to increase strength and endurance
(A, R) Dependence in self-care skills (feeding, communication, dressing, hygiene, transfers, homemaking) and mobility skills	(A, R) Instruct and practice daily: self-care and mobility skills with gradual increase in independence and decrease in supervision
	(R, C) Practice skills in community (grocery store, restaurant, shopping mall, riding a bus, etc.)
	(C) Driver training
(ALL) Impaired memory and cognitive functioning affecting vocational status	(A, R) Stimulate higher cognitive functioning through optimally arousing tasks
	(R, C) Increase attention, concentration, and problem solving through graded functional tasks, crafts, homemaking, and prevocational tasks
	(R, C) Instruct in, and practice use of, mnemonic aids
(A, R) Inappropriate social behavior	(ALL) Encourage age-appropriate behavior, social interaction through modeling, role playing and feedback, using tape recordings, videotape and a social skills group

ENVIRONMENT

(A, R) Overstimulating, distracting and confining intensive care unit, hospital room and occupational therapy clinic	(A) Remove restraints and loud noises as possible and treat in quiet environment
	(A, R) Progress from an isolated, nondistractable environment to a more stimulating, everyday environment for treatment

Table 14.18.—Continued

Occupational status	Treatment goals and intervention
(ALL) Overprotective family	**(ALL)** Educate family on Jessy's capabilities, limitations and needs to perform meaningful, valued and age-appropriate tasks
	(R) Provide home program
	(ALL) Support Jessy in assuming new roles and being assertive
Accessible home environment (as reported by family and patient)	**(R, C)** Weekend passes and warning of possible hazards and need for emergency plans

aside daily, where all restrictions were removed and Jessy explored moving her body on the mat, on the bed or in front of the mirror.

Writing, typing and spelling on a letter communication board was used while Jessy was still nonverbal. This was not always successful as she confused or forgot letters. But, some information about her values, interests and goals were obtained from this method. One day, a month into rehabilitation, Jessy was asked what she wanted to cook. She spelled out sugar cookies. When she was given a sugar cookie mix, she became horrified. She had been a gourmet cook and would not think of using a mix! Her desire to bake cookies from scratch was respected and although she struggled with cognitive problems which made gourmet cooking difficult, her motivation to cook according to her own standards counterbalanced the difficulties.

Oral motor facilitation techniques were used successfully; Jessy was eventually able to imitate tongue and lip movements and to control her drooling. She was especially fond of popsicles. After 1½ months of rehabilitation, Jessy's oral motor skills improved and she began talking, though the left side of her face remained paralyzed. Her speech was slow at first, and dysarthric but intelligible. She revealed how frustrated she had been without speech: "I felt trapped inside my own body!"

Her right UE was nonfunctional; time was spent increasing the ROM, coordination and strength of the left UE. As Jessy's ataxia decreased, she was able to write legibly though inaccurately. Previous interests were incorporated into activities to increase coordination such as cross-stitching, cutting out pictures of rock stars, meal preparation and leatherwork. These activities were also used to increase decision making, problem solving, sequencing, memory, attending, and frustration tolerance. Eventually, Jessy's right UE became coordinated so she could write and use it in bilateral activities.

Throughout the rehabilitation phase, Jessy improved in cognitive functioning. Tasks were graded in difficulty and were gradually reduced in structure as Jessy improved. Cognitive skills were developed through self-care, homemaking, craft, functional, and prevocational activities. Through daily repetition, instruction and memory aids, Jessy learned to independently dress, bathe, style her hair, brush her teeth, and shave her legs. She initially required stand-by assistance for all transfers as she often lost her balance when standing.

Jessy progressed from living with a roommate to modified independent living and finally staying in the hospital's apartment prior to discharge. Progressively, Jessy was made responsible for more of her own care, and learned to develop workable habits. Her responsibilities included: bedmaking, laundry, room organization and clean-up, making and keeping her own appointments, taking her own medicine and, later, cooking one meal a day. Mnemonic aids were developed to assist Jessy with her memory problems.

Since Jessy continued to identify independence as a valued goal, she collaborated with the therapist to develop a list of her previous responsibilities. A budget system was worked out and Jessy had to "pay weekly bills" to different people for the following things: rent, food, electricity, water and sewage, phone, therapies, entertainment, clothes, toiletries, medical, transportation, and savings. At the time of discharge, Jessy was writing checks correctly and balancing her checkbook, but frequently forgot payments unless reminded or sent an overdue bill.

Other functional tasks done with Jessy to increase cognitive skills and to prepare her for the community phase included using a phone book, the newspaper, a library, a dictionary, an encyclopedia, a time clock, and a vending machine; filling out a job application, doing word problems and mathematics; using abbreviations; filing; reading maps; giving directions; writing letters and reading bus schedules. At the time of discharge from the rehabilitation phase, she performed these skills with 80–100% accuracy according to her concentration level. Jessy had difficulty with selective attention and became flustered and emotional in emergency situations or when confronted by others.

Throughout therapy, problem-solving and decision-making skills were practiced. Explanations of how things are done and weighing the pros and cons of decisions were discussed. In the last 3 weeks of her hospitalization, Jessy planned her own schedule, setting up her own therapies, bedtime, self-care schedule and leisure time.

Assertiveness training and socially appropriate behavior were practiced in a variety of settings with corrective feedback given. Jessy learned to initiate conversations and tasks, participated in community outings, and became friends with numerous patients and staff members. She often advocated for other patients and encouraged them to get out of the hospital and to forget their disability. Though Jessy wanted total control of her life at home, she had to accept that her memory and problem-solving deficits and her needed stand-by assistance for transfers and ambulation limited her independence. Prior to discharge, Jessy went on numerous weekend passes and her family was given a list of things Jessy could do independently so they would let her, and expect her, to do them. A schedule and home program was developed and reviewed with Jessy and her family.

COMMUNITY PHASE

Assessment

Jessy returned to live at home with her parents and brothers and went to outpatient occupational therapy to continue to increase her right UE function and occupational functioning. Upon re-evaluation it was found that her right UE remained as functional as in rehabilitation and had improved in ROM and in speed on the Minnesota Rate of Manipulation Test.

The Role Checklist was given again and it was evident that Jessy had not followed through with enrolling in a community college class or volunteering at the local humane society. She was having difficulty structuring her day, but was able to generalize skills and habits of self-care, homemaking, simple problem solving, and decision making. Jessy had reacquainted herself with some girl friends and had gone to the movies and out to eat with them. She had pursued her leisure interest of cross-stitching and frequently played games with her brothers. Jessy felt she could do more than her parents were allowing her.

She had felt competent at the end of rehabilitation, but was having her competence, assertiveness and independence challenged by her parents.

TREATMENT

Jessy had clarified her long-term goals but was still unsure of the immediate future. Therapy time was spent doing values clarification and prioritizing short-term goals. Jessy would make a list of what she wanted to achieve by her next scheduled therapy when she would report her accomplishments or problems to the therapist. She developed lists incorporating her values and goals and became realistic concerning her current capabilities. Treatment also concentrated on increasing the function of her right UE through meaningful activities.

Two months after discharge, Jessy was admitted to a vocational training center for 6 months and participated in a computer training program. She continued to practice her habits and skills and worked towards her goal of financial and personal independence. During this time, in occupational therapy, she learned to drive again as she had not had a seizure for 1 year since the accident.

Outcome

After a period of a year and a half since her head injury, Jessy recognized her strengths and weaknesses and had partially achieved her goal of independence. She was no longer in the dependent role of an invalid and she felt competent in her occupational functioning.

Jessy's upper extremities' active range of motion was within normal limits except that the right hand remained limited in metacarpophalangial flexion and proximal interphalangial extension. Her sensation, coordination, and strength in both UEs was normal for her age and sex (although in the lowest range and with the left better than the right). Although Jessy's gait was affected she was ambulating with a cane.

Jessy was independent in self-care and basic homemaking and has developed good personal and work habits. She continued to demonstrate mild-to-moderate deficits in cognitive functions of problem solving, judgment and memory and she required minimal supervision. Jessy lived in a group home where she had her own room and shared household chores. She took the bus to her part-time job as a computer operator.

Jessy continued to make friends easily, had a new boyfriend and balanced her work and leisure time. She talked with her family on a bimonthly basis and has demonstrated her ability to be semi-independent. Though Jessy recognized she was unable to be the chemist she thought she would be, she continued to pursue her interest by volunteering in a junior high chemistry class. Jessy was content with her life for the present, but had the future goal of living totally by herself and owning a car.

CANCER

Cancer is composed of a large number of diseases characterized by an abnormal and uncontrollable growth of cells. Cancer strikes individuals of any age and it is estimated that one in four Americans will have cancer at some point in their lives (2). Cancer can include such pathology as sarcoma, melanoma and leukemia. It can affect a variety of body systems such as the brain, uterus, stomach and lungs. A cancer may be detected and cured at its primary site or it may metastasize to other body parts via the lymph or blood system (3).

Rehabilitation of the cancer patient is increasingly necessary as more effective treatments and earlier diagnosis result in survival (33). It is expected that 46% of cancer patients will be alive 5 years after diagnosis (3).

When an individual is diagnosed with and treated for cancer, there may be a wide range of impacts on occupational behavior. Consequently, occupational therapy may include such diverse efforts as maintaining function during treatment for cancer, enabling a cancer survivor to adapt to an amputation, or supporting optimal functioning of the terminal individual.

PERFORMANCE: SKILLS

Depending on the site of the cancer and the preferred treatment, the effect on an individual's skills can vary tremendously. Surgery remains, in most instances, the primary treatment for cancer; it can be curative or palliative (33). The disruption of skills associated with cancer may include permanent functional loss, intermittent loss of skills, the need to acquire new skills, or a continuous decline in skills.

Permanent functional loss occurs when there is damage to some somatic structure impairing the ability to function. Examples are amputations secondary to bone or soft tissue tumors and hemiplegia, paraplegia, and quadriplegia associated with a primary brain tumor or spinal cord tumor.

The side effects of chemotherapy or radiation treatment may impose an intermittent loss of skills. Possible effects of radiation include fatigue, skin irritation and alopecia (79). Side effects commonly associated with chemotherapy are a decrease in blood counts, fatigue, alopecia, nausea, vomiting, and parasthesias. These side effects vary depending on areas and doses of radiation and the specific drugs used for chemotherapy. A decrease in energy is usually temporary and will generally subside once the treatment is completed.

Some surgical procedures performed for cancers require that the individual learn new skills (4). These procedures include ostomies and laryngectomies. The patient with a colostomy will need to learn to care for the stoma and change colostomy bags. Patients who have undergone laryngectomies need to learn a complete new method of communicating either with an electrolarynx and/or esophageal speech (29).

Patients with advancing cancer and the patients entering the terminal stage of the disease will likely have a steady, continuous decline in skills. They may not be able to predict what they will be able to do from day to day (113). As the disease progresses and significant changes in function occur, frequent re-evaluations will be necessary (5).

HABITUATION

The effect of cancer and its treatment on habits and roles is also dependent on prognosis, degree and type of treatment, side effects of treatment, need for convalescence, and residual disability secondary to treatment.

Habits

A change in one's habits may occur secondary to a functional loss associated with treatment for cancer. For example, a man who was diagnosed with cancer of the larynx had been swimming a mile a day for exercise. Following a laryngectomy, he was no longer able to swim and experienced a disruption in his leisure habit pattern.

Patients who spend long periods of time in the hospital receiving treatment may experience an atrophy of habits. Hospitals tend to have regimented schedules and to disallow access to many activities which may have been components of an individual's habit pattern. As a result of a long hospitalization, it may be necessary for the patient to re-establish habit patterns after discharge.

For example, a 19-year-old man was admitted to the hospital with a relapse of his leukemia. Because of low blood counts, it was necessary for him to be placed in strict isolation. It took 6 weeks for him to respond to treatment and be discharged from the hospital. Prior to the hospitalization, he was up early in the morning and attended college. Following discharge, he felt unable, and was reluctant, to resume his prehospitalization habits.

The individual receiving long courses of treatment with debilitating side effects may experience intermittent disruption of habits. This could be compounded by frequent returns to an outpatient clinic for treatment with occasional admissions to the hospital. With the uncertainty of hospitalization and frequency of clinic visits, it may be difficult to establish and/or maintain habits. the individual with advancing disease may find it necessary to alter habits by changing the daily routine to include rest periods and less strenuous activities as strength and stamina wane.

Roles

An individual treated surgically for cure (e.g. a mastectomy for breast cancer) may find it necessary to delegate the roles of homemaker, worker and/or caregiver to another on a temporary basis. Without complications, the individual should be able to resume all former roles once the convalescent period is over (19).

Some treatments may cause or lead to a permanent role loss. For example, a young woman who worked as a dancer, lost that role secondary to a hemipelvectomy for a bone tumor. In many such cases, treatment may cure the cancer, but a permanent role loss ensues.

A decline in energy and function secondary to treatment, may lead to an intermittent role loss. For example, a mother of four diagnosed with breast cancer required chemotherapy once every 4 weeks for a year. Following the chemotherapy, she experienced nausea and vomiting and felt fatigued for a week after each treatment. During this week neighbors and relatives assisted her with homemaking tasks; hers was, thus, an intermittent disruption of roles.

During the terminal phase for the cancer patient, it may be necessary for the patient to relinquish some of the more active roles (i.e. worker and homemaker roles). At this time, it is also important to encourage the patient to maintain some roles. Even in a bedbound state,

it is possible for one to maintain the roles of parent and spouse (20).

In the event of relinquishing roles to others, the patient may be able to instruct others in their roles. One young mother diagnosed with terminal cancer found meaning in instructing her sister in the rearing of her daughter (40).

VOLITION

The effect a diagnosis of cancer will have on an individual's volition is dependent on a variety of factors. Prognosis, treatment and its effects and the impact on the body system affected by the cancer influence the degree of interruption of volition status.

Interests

A patient may exhibit a decline in interests secondary to the fear associated with a diagnosis of cancer. The diagnosis of cancer and the fear of death may immobilize an individual. Fatigue associated with treatment or advancing disease may lead a patient to abandon some interests despite their importance for morale and quality of life. A gentleman with a liver cancer, while in the hospital receiving chemotherapy, was angry and irritable. Described by his wife as an avid fisherman, he was encouraged to engage in fly tying while in the hospital and his irritability markedly decreased (19). Also a disability secondary to the cancer can affect the potency of one's interests. For example, an avid backpacker diagnosed with an osteosarcoma was unable to pursue this interest following an amputation.

Values

When diagnosed with cancer, the individual may feel a need to reassess valued goals (20). Even when treated for cure, the word, cancer, often signifies death to the individual (31). For the patient dealing with the possibility of death, it is probable that aspects of life formerly taken for granted will be magnified in importance. At this time personal relationships may become significantly more important than financial or business matters (20). The dying patient may be faced with resetting priorities which may cause a significant change in values. In order to ensure quality of life, the individual needs to have the opportunity to define what is important to him or her (113).

Personal Causation

Personal causation in many instances is the first subsystem impacted by cancer. The individual who learns that he or she has cancer is faced with a diagnosis of questionable outcome. Although many cancers are curable or can be controlled for long periods of time, cancer continues for many persons to denote fatality and finality. In fact, an individual with cancer is often considered terminal from the time of diagnosis (20). Knowledge of the diagnosis can make a person feel out of control and precipitate concerns regarding survival. The individual may also feel the threat of dependency and of being useless (31). On the other hand, many people with a strong sense of internal control may immediately take charge and play instrumental roles in planning and managing their treatment.

Another group of cancer patients must adapt during the process of dying. Maintaining a sense of control during the terminal stages can significantly affect their quality of life. This may be deciding to forego any further palliative treatments except those that would make the dying process more comfortable (19). It may also include taking control of where and how they will live for their remaining time and planning for the significant others who will be left after their death.

The belief one has in one's skills and a strong sense of control will have a direct influence on the quality of life one will experience during the terminal stages of the disease. For the patient with advancing disease with a resulting decrease in function, belief in skills may begin to deteriorate. Such factors as no longer being able to bathe oneself or control bowel habits may lead to an increased sense of dependency on others and loss of control (19).

ENVIRONMENT

A diagnosis of cancer may bring about a change in an individual's social environment. Cancer is viewed by many as a death sentence and few diseases bring with them the degree of anxiety that cancer does. The belief by many people that cancer is contagious will often cause significant others to abandon the cancer patient (31).

In addition, cancer is very often an illness of chronicity, often marked by remissions and exacerbations. With the need for long periods of time in the hospital, the patient becomes even more isolated (31).

Family members, friends and co-workers may anticipate and exacerbate a role change in the cancer patient. Once diagnosed, the cancer patient is often automatically placed in a sick role by significant others (20). Patients treated for cure for a localized cancer may experience difficulty leaving the sick role (20). They may be perceived as "sick" long after treatment is complete. Unfortunately the stigma associated with a diagnosis of cancer can persevere for many years.

Assessment and Treatment

Assessment and treatment of the cancer patient are dependent on a number of variables. Both will differ depending on the diagnosis, the treatment and the disease state. For example, the patient undergoing surgery for an upper extremity amputation will require a more detailed assessment of upper extremity function than the patient with generalized weakness.

While the assessment of performance will necessarily vary according to the particular physical problems, a more uniform evaluation of other subsystems is possible. In evaluation the therapist is seeking to determine temporary or permanent disruption of habits, roles, interests, values, and personal causation. Table 14.19 outlines possible status of occupational behavior, recommended evaluations and treatment considerations.

Treatment of the cancer patient falls into three major categories. The first category is rehabilitation for patients with functional losses secondary to treatment. Included in this category are upper extremity amputations, mastectomies and radical neck dissections. Treatment of patients with quadriplegia, paraplegia and hemiplegia will parallel that discussed in the spinal cord injury and brain damage sections of this chapter.

The second major category is treatment of the patient with periods of remissions and exacerbations. This category encompasses a large number of disabilities. Treatment may involve teaching one-handed daily living tasks to the individual with a pathological fracture of the humerus or instruction of work simplification principles to the woman receiving radiation therapy to bone metastases secondary to breast cancer. Often with the treatment for cancer, energy levels may fluctuate and the goal of treatment will be to enable the patient to maintain an optimal level of activity (43).

Table 14.19.
Persons with cancer: occupational status, recommended assessments and treatment considerations

Occupational status	Recommended assessments	Treatment-considerations
VOLITION		
Values		
Since diagnosis often implies death to many, valued goals may be abandoned. With the terminal patient, goals may be reassessed. Uncertain disease course may disrupt time orientation and future goals	Occupational Therapy Functional Screening Tool (OTFST) Occupational History (OH) Occupational Questionnaire (OQ) Activity Questionnaire (AQ)	Support and opportunities for pursuit of values Education concerning disease process
Personal Causation		
Knowledge of the disease may lead to feelings of loss of control	OTFST, OH, OQ, AQ	Allow individual to maintain control in goal setting and choosing treatment
Questionable outcome of the disease also leads to a sense of a loss of control. With questionable course of disease and decrease in skills, a loss of belief in skills may result		Enhance actual control through enabling successful engagement in meaningful tasks compatible with functional losses
Interests		
Changes dependent on prognosis, treatment of choice and the body system affected. Fear associated with the diagnosis may result in a decline in interests. Disability associated with treatment may bring about a change in interests	OTFST, OH, OQ, AQ Interest Checklist (modified)	Modifications to allow participation in interests. Exploration of new interests
HABITUATION		
Roles		
Both disease and treatment may affect roles. Role loss may be permanent secondary to treatment, temporary during convalescence or intermittent with exacerbations and remissions. Others may place the individual in a "sick" role	OTFST, OH, AQ Role Checklist	Adapting physical and social environment to allow for continuation of roles in whatever capacity possible
Habits		
Changes in habits may result from permanent functional losses secondary to treatment, atrophy of habits as a result of long hospitalizations or treatment regimes. Intermittent habit changes may occur secondary to exacerbations and remissions	OTFST, OH, OQ, AQ	Time management and development of schedules to enhance maximal function within limitations. Provide opportunities to practice new habits and to maintain old adaptive ones as much as possible within constraints of disease and treatment regime

Table 14.19.—Continued

Occupational status	Recommended assessments	Treatment-considerations
PERFORMANCE		
Skills		
Motor skills are affected variously depending on disease state and treatment of choice. Some may experience permanent functional losses secondary to advancing disease or treatment. Some persons are required to acquire new skills for self-care following treatments	OH, OTFST Depends on type of performance problems	Depends on type of performance problems, but generally includes activities to increase motor skills, adaptations and instruction in alternative methods in self-care, and adaptive equipment to increase performance
ENVIRONMENT		
The physical environment may become difficult to handle. Other's perceptions of the individual may be negative and effect his/her pursuit of interests and roles	OH Informal home evaluation	Adaptations to immediate environment. Instruct family and others in disease process and in handling of appropriate attitudes toward the person with cancer

The last category deals with the treatment of the terminal patient. The therapist at this point is concerned with continuing to allow or help the patient attain and/or maintain independence in self-care, play and work. This is done within the limitations of the patient's physical condition (113). This goal may be achieved through the use of adaptive equipment and alternative ways of performing daily living tasks.

It is important to include all cancer patients in treatment goal setting. By allowing the patient as much choice as possible, loss of control and feelings of worthlessness are diminished. When the patient is involved in goal setting an increase in motivation is often seen which directly influences outcomes (31).

CANCER CASE: MRS. HUGHES

Mrs. Hughes is a 63-year-old right-handed lady who was diagnosed with multiple myeloma approximately 12 years prior to this hospital admission. She had done well without problems until just prior to this admission when she developed pain in the right shoulder and episodes of confusion. She was admitted to the hospital and was found to have a pathological fracture of the right humerus. The confusion was attributed to hypercalcemia. While hospitalized, she was treated with radiation to the right humerus and received chemotherapy.

Assessment

Evaluation of Mrs. Hughes included an upper extremity evaluation, a self-care evaluation, the Interest Checklist, the Role Checklist, and a home assessment. Table 14.20 summarizes the findings from this assessment battery.

PERFORMANCE

Mrs. Hughes' left upper extremity range of motion and muscle strength were within functional limits. Her right upper extremity range of motion and muscle strength were not tested because of the fracture and the resulting pain. She had a significant decrease in endurance; she ambulated independently only for short distances with the assistance of a cane. Mrs. Hughes was oriented at the time of the evaluation but experienced some difficulty with memory and concentration.

Mrs. Hughes was independent in feeding with her left hand, but required assistance to cut her food. She performed her morning care and sponge bathed with minimal assistance. She required minimal to moderate assistance with dressing and experienced some difficulty transferring on and off the commode. Mrs. Hughes was independent in bed mobility and required minimal assistance to rise from sitting on low surfaces.

She was unable to write with her right hand

secondary to the pain and could only sign her name with her left hand. She was independent in communication with the telephone.

OCCUPATIONAL HISTORY

Mrs. Hughes was a college graduate and had been employed as an art teacher in an elementary school. She retired 3 years ago. She has two grown daughters both of whom are living outside the city and are employed. Mrs. Hughes was widowed when she was 40 years old.

ROLES

Mrs. Hughes lived independently in an apartment. She has two grown daughters. She identified her roles as being a mother, hobbyist, friend, family member, and home maintainer. She seemed most concerned with whether she would be able to carry on as hobbyist and home maintainer. She was pleased with the roles she had occupied and did not identify any others she would like to pursue.

INTERESTS

Mrs. Hughes' strong interests included weaving, knitting, pottery, cooking, and going to museums. Up until the onset of the shoulder pain and confusion, she had been actively engaging in all these interests. However, she was no longer doing so.

HOME ASSESSMENT

Mrs. Hughes lived in a second-story apartment by herself. The apartment consisted of a large family/dining room, two bedrooms, kitchen and a bathroom. The apartment was accessible to a bus line and Mrs. Hughes owned a car.

One of Mrs. Hughes' daughters was living with her temporarily. The daughter was supportive of Mrs. Hughes and facilitated her independence by allowing her to attempt tasks. The home was obstacle free and Mrs. Hughes was able to ambulate about it with her cane. She independently maneuvered the steps to the apartment using her cane and the hand rail.

Treatment

Mrs. Hughes was seen in occupational therapy during her inpatient stay and also through home care once she was discharged. Table 14.20 illustrates specific treatment strategies.

Initial occupational therapy treatment included immobilization of the right shoulder to enable healing of the fracture. She was fitted with an immobilization sling and was begun on a series of exercises for elbow, wrist and fingers. Instruction was also started on one-handed daily living tasks. Adaptations were made to enable her to attempt to write with her right hand. These included raising of the writing surface and supporting the right forearm.

Mrs. Hughes was provided with a raised toilet seat and tub seat to facilitate easier and safer transfers while she was unsteady. She was also provided with a long scrub sponge, rocker knife and nonslip surface materials to increase one-handed self-care.

During the course of the hospital stay, as her calcium level decreased, an improvement was noted in her mental status. The daughters, on the suggestion of the therapist, decorated her room with familiar objects and brought in scrap books with family pictures. This appeared to aid the patient and family in reality orientation.

Mrs. Hughes was discharged home following the radiation treatments to her shoulder. At that point, she was continuing to ambulate short distances with the cane, and was independent in all self-care with the exception of meal preparation, home maintenance and shopping. One of her daughters planned to stay with her until she regained her independence.

Following discharge from the hospital, Mrs. Hughes was followed by a home health agency which included occupational therapy. Treatment of Mrs. Hughes at home included increasing independence in self-care and encouragement in pursuit of roles and interests. She no longer needed the raised toilet seat and was able to transfer independently. She continued to use the tub seat independently.

Mrs. Hughes continued to wear the immobilization sling and kept up the exercise program established in the hospital. She had become increasingly more comfortable writing with her right hand. She was instructed in work simplification techniques to use at home and, with the therapist's encouragement, began to engage in more activities around the house; e.g. assisting with meal preparation and light housework.

After reviewing the bus schedule, Mrs. Hughes began to use public transportation. She started with short trips and increased the distances. Friends were available to take her to the store and to the museum, but Mrs. Hughes was not comfortable with relying on friends and was able to arrange for a college

Table 14.20.
Mrs. Hughes' occupational status, treatment goals and interventions

Occupational status	Treatment goals and interventions
VOLITION	
Personal causation	
In control within physical limitations	Build on her sense of control and allow her to establish goals
Values	
Has identified values, but not incorporating them into daily routine	Encourage pursuit of values
Interests	
Lack of participation in interests	Reactivate interests with necessary modifications
HABITUATION	
Roles	
Temporary loss of roles	Instruction in alternative methods of performing roles
	Encouragement of pursuit of roles
Habits	
Temporary disruption of habit patterns	Develop routine and grade activities as improvement in condition is noted
	Instruct in work simplification techniques
PERFORMANCE	
Skills	
Decreased right upper extremity range of motion secondary to fracture	Fit with sling to decrease pain associated with movement
	Exercises to maintain elbow and hand range of motion
Low endurance	Graded activities to increase time in activities
Decreased self-care status	Instruct in one-handed daily living tasks and provide equipment
Altered mental status	Reality orientation with family involvement
ENVIRONMENT	
Supportive family and accessible environment	Provide support to family and encourage involvement with the patient
Physical distance of resources she wished to use required transporation	Explore available resources to include bus and hiring of someone to drive her car

student to take her shopping several times a week. Again with encouragement of the therapist and her daughter, she also started knitting and crocheting again.

One month postdischarge from the hospital, Mrs. Hughes was independent in her activities of daily living. She was getting out of the apartment at frequent intervals and was taking daily walks of 1 mile without her cane.

She no longer needed the tub seat for bathing and was preparing her own meals. She was again engaging in her roles and interests.

ACUTE, GENERAL MEDICINE AND SURGERY PATIENTS

This section will consider the model of human occupation as it applies to persons in an acute care hospital (often referred to as general medicine and surgery patients). These persons have physical problems which impair ability to return immediately to their former roles. These impairments generally do not cause major changes in roles, abilities or life-styles over an extended period of time. Physical problems seen in this category include: hip fractures, total hip replacement, multiple trauma, debilitating illness such as pneumonia or hepatitis, various abdominal or thoracic surgeries or injuries, and some types of burns. The results of occupational therapy for these patients are measured by reduction of stress on the patient and the family system, rate of recovery, length of hospital stay, and intensity of posthospital care needed.

Impact on the Human System

Since there is substantial variability in this population, only a general analysis of the dynamics affecting the model components can be proposed. (See Table 14.21 for a summary of this analysis, which follows.)

PERFORMANCE

The major area affected is the performance subsystem. Problems affecting musculoskeletal, and occasionally neurological, function interrupt performance. Examples include the inability to walk following a hip fracture, to bring hand to mouth for feeding with upper extremity trauma injuries, to bend down to put on one's shoes following hip replacement, or to sit up long enough to bathe following severe pneumonia. Interpersonal/communication and process skills are generally not affected. Nonetheless, the person's level of capabilities in these skills affects their capacity to compensate for perceptual motor problems. For example, when there is a sensory loss due to a fracture or nerve injury, the patient must be able to understand implications of loss, to adhere to safety precautions and to problem solve how to do routine tasks such as cooking and adjusting water temperature.

HABITUATION

Problems in the performance subsystem have a constraining effect on the roles and habits of the habituation subsystem. Habit patterns are interrupted, and normal activities such as eating and self-care become more time consuming and difficult. Role changes in the habituation subsystem can occur. Family or hospital staff may

have to assume roles or role tasks formerly held by the patient, such as financial management and child care. Though such changes are likely to be temporary, the patient may be at risk to develop occupational dysfunction. Modified perceptual motor function, weakness from illness, surgery or prolonged immobility, the requirements for prevention of further injury, and pain may negatively influence a patient's return to adaptive habits and roles upon discharge.

VOLITION

The volition subsystem may not be affected as much as other subsystems, but it cannot be assumed that no volition problems are occurring.

The area of personal causation is most vulnerable. Pain, fear and uncertainty associated with the illness or injury, combined with the frustrations from inability to perform routine activities or roles impacts on a patient's feelings of control. Illness or injury raises concerns over one's ability to perform efficaciously and may elicit fear of failure upon returning to former life roles. The concerns may be augmented when the patient sees family members or others taking over the patient's own functions and roles. While values and interests are generally least affected by a short-term medical/surgical problem, each individual is unique in how an injury or illness may affect his or her own life-style. This is readily seen in the situation of a total hip replacement in which a patient must follow precautions in hip movement for at least 3 months after surgery (76, 97). To a retired machinist, no problem may exist when he must install a commode extender and commode safety frames in his bathroom, following surgery (96). But to an interior decorator, a serious problem could exist at all levels due to a different set of interests and values. The result may be dependence on others for maintaining self-care habits and possible further injury due to unsafe environmental conditions and improper use of body mechanics.

The importance of volition in the ultimate adaptation of patients can also be seen in the following example. The patient was a 53-year-old woman who suffered multiple fractures of her lower extremity in a car accident. After several complicated but unsuccessful surgeries, the leg had to be amputated below the hip. The patient was convinced she would be unable to function normally if the leg were lost. In her own value system, as a robust wife of a farmer, to have such a loss was irremediable. She never successfully used a prosthesis and spent the remaining 17 years of her life in a wheelchair, unnecessarily restricted in mobility.

On the other hand, volition characteristics of the patient may be important resources to identify and mobilize in the interest of enhancing recovery. A patient's values and long-standing sense of personal causation may be a source of strength of maintaining courage in the face of uncertainty, pain and risk. Interests may motivate the patient to keep active during hospitalization, maintaining a mental attitude and physical condition which facilitates recovery.

ENVIRONMENT

The environment of the acute care hospital plays a very important part in a patient's recovery process. Loss of security, privacy, self-identity, and self-esteem are factors which may be disruptive to self-care and role skills (44, 45). Within the ambience of acute care, the patients' understanding of their condition and the implication of their condition for function can easily be overlooked. This can contribute to feelings of loss of control and disallow opportunity for a patient to explore adapted techniques for independence. The hospital environment may intensify disability by decreasing opportunities for adaptation during convalescence.

Assessment

In acute care the therapist typically faces the challenge of making an adequate assessment of the patient in a relatively brief time. See Table 14.21 for a summary of recommended assessments. Assessment begins with informal screening. Chart review and contact with nursing or other personnel involved with the patient provides information about physical history, special problems and precautions as well as rehabilitation status.

Next, through an informal initial interview, the therapist should seek to determine strengths and problems related to: (a) fears over losing control and loss of function, (b) interests and values that are threatened or that can be used as assets in therapy, (c) personal goals for future performance beyond hospitalization, (d) past and anticipated future roles and possible impediments to return to role function, (e) aspects of the daily routine that may be disrupted, and (f) impact of the present condition on functional

ability in self-care, work and recreation tasks which the individual has performed in the past and expects to perform in the future.

The format and focus of each interview will vary with the patient's age, diagnosis, emotional state, expected length of stay in the hospital, and discharge plans. The goal of the information gained from this screening interview is to provide a general orientation to the patient's occupational status, to identify strengths and problem areas, and to note areas for further specific evaluation. Further evaluations of performance will depend on the patient's diagnosis and life roles. Basic biomedical, neurodevelopmental and rehabilitative evaluations (52, 84, 114) are selected as necessary to determine functional limitations. The brief length of stay may sometimes prevent detailed assessment of volitional and habituation traits, however, the Role Checklist, Interest Checklist, and a brief activity configuration can often be filled out by patients on their own and may serve not only as further data, but also as tools for mutual problem solving with the patient. Where functional limitations exist beyond hospitalization, a home and family evaluation may be necessary.

Assessment of the acute patient can be made more efficient when interviews are conducted in concert with certain treatment. For example, a therapist may interview a patient about concerns over loss of control while making a splint, or in the course of teaching the use of adaptive equipment. This also alerts the patient to the therapist's concern about the patient's practical everyday functioning, paving the way for patients to raise issues or seek help for these things. Otherwise patients may tend to see these things as outside the concerns of medical personnel.

Treatment

Treatment of the acute patient tends to focus on recovery from the immediate cause of hospitalization (Table 14.21). The therapist provides interesting and meaningful activities aimed at restoring or maintaining physical function and maintaining a positive mental attitude. The therapist also assists the patient in identifying and overcoming concerns about future problems, provides adaptive equipment and teaches adaptive strategies for overcoming limitations, and mutually plans and problem solves with patients for resuming old interests, roles and habits. In short, occupational therapy helps the patient

Table 14.21.
Occupational status, recommended assessments and treatment considerations for acute care patients

VOLITION

Personal causation

Personal causation may be affected by fears over recovery, pain and future risks	Informal interview and skilled clinical observation	Provide information about medical status, prognosis factors and timing of recovery. Identify areas of concern for control and skill and provide appropriate training, adapted equipment and practice to maximize control and success
If there is any residual limitation, personal causation may be negatively impacted		

Values

Generally unaffected. Fears over ability to maintain standards or attain goals may arise	Informal interview to determine standards and goals as well as meaningful activities	Identify possible conflicts of values with rehabilitation goals and provide opportunities to set priorities

Interests

Generally unaffected. May have temporary inability to pursue interests	Interest Checklist Informal interview	Support engagement in interests during hospitalization. Incorporate interests into occupations used to remediate performance deficits

HABITUATION

Roles

Temporary loss of roles; possible requirements for extended role adjustment after discharge	Role Checklist Informal interview	Identify role expectations and any problems of difficulty in performance. Plan for and practice role behaviors

Habits

Interruption of habit pattern by hospitalization. May be temporary or permanent limitations imposed on habits	Interview Simple activity configuration	Examine predisability habits to determine feasibility of return to prior life-style Plan time use upon discharge Identify and practice needed habits for managing disability/recovery

PERFORMANCE

Skills

Since a variety of diagnoses may be represented, impact on skills may be variable. Generally the focus is on loss of strength, range of motion, coordination, and stamina and the impact of these on performance of daily living tasks, play and work	Skill assessment will depend on the diagnosis; may be quite variable	Generally the focus is on restoration of temporarily impaired skills. Adaptive equipment may be given to compensate for temporary or indefinite limitations Emphasis in treatment is on functional activities oriented primarily to short-term goals for recovery

make a smooth transition back to a valid life-style and make needed adjustments because of limitations imposed by the disease or trauma.

AN ACUTE CARE CASE: MRS. HARRIS

Mrs. Harris is a 62-year-old housewife admitted to an orthopedic unit for a total hip replacement. The history of her illness began when she experienced incapacitating pain 10 years earlier and was diagnosed as having osteoarthritis of the right hip joint. A right cup arthroplasty was done at that time. After a slow recovery, she returned to full function. Six months later, she began to have pain with weight bearing, and 16 months following her first surgery, she was readmitted for a right total hip replacement. Mrs. Harris experienced no further problems for 7 years, until recently she began again to suffer severe pain on weight bearing. She was admitted to the hospital with a diagnosis of loosening of the femoral component of the hip joint replacement and was given a new replacement.

Typically, persons undergoing this surgery do so following a period of increasing impairment of ambulation, self-care and role performance. Many have had to adapt techniques and temporarily adjust roles within their family. The surgery typically involves a 2- to 3-week hospital stay. Many persons resume former activities, with minor limitations to hip movement, within 3 or more months; this is variable though, depending on the amount of joint damage, condition of the surrounding tissue and the type of activity to which the person wishes to return.

Assessment

Mrs. Harris was referred to occupational therapy 7 days after surgery. Initial screening included chart review and discussion with physical therapy and nursing staff. When seen for an initial interview, Mrs. Harris was sitting in bed doing needlework. She appeared relaxed and comfortable, and responded openly to questions.

She had lived with her husband in a very large house and was responsible for only light cooking since she had assistance with housekeeping. She had some social involvement within her community, but no responsibilities outside the home. Her major leisure interest was needlework, which she pursued throughout this hospitalization. She expected to resume spouse and homemaker roles following discharge and would be alone most of the day.

When Mrs. Harris was first seen, she was unable to move her right leg alone and needed assistance with rolling and getting in and out of bed. She was doing a partial bath and upper extremity dressing with minimal assistance. Her return to mobility and ambulation was considerably slower than normal. She had poor endurance and her participation in rehabilitation was poor. Both physical therapy and nursing staff noted that she was very apprehensive, and nursing staff questioned whether or not she wanted to be able to ambulate and become independent. Because the initial screening indicated that there may have been a problem in the areas of her goals for independence and personal causation, these were explored in more depth.

A discussion with Mrs. Harris concerning her goals for returning home revealed that she did in fact wish to be independent. She reported that she and her husband had been recently married and it was very important to her that she not make any demands on him and that she did not appear "disabled" to him. On the other hand, Mrs. Harris was experiencing fear over possible failure in returning home. She felt that she did not have and may not regain functional skills. Finally, she was overaroused by the demands of participating in the rehabilitation program. Mrs. Harris was experiencing reduced belief in skill, uncertainty about the future, and feared she could not attain her goals of independence and satisfy what she perceived to be her husband's expectations of a new spouse. In sum, Mrs. Harris demonstrated traits at the inefficiency level of occupational dysfunction as summarized in Table 14.22.

Intervention

In keeping with Mrs. Harris' goals for independence and to deal with her loss of personal causation, treatment was designed to help her attain functional skills at the exploratory level in a safe environment without too much challenge. Anticipating and planning what habits she would need upon discharge in order to attain her goals and fulfill role expectations was also a major focus of therapy. Specific treatment goals and interventions are noted in Table 14.22.

Treatment began with training the patient to protect the hip joint while engaging in normal activity. She was to avoid hip flexion beyond 90°, hip adduction past the body midline, internal rotation of the hip, and full weight bearing. Mrs. Harris was given written instruction and a demonstration of positions to avoid, followed by practice moving without using prohibited positions.

Table 14.22.
Mrs. Harris' occupational status treatment goals and intervention

Occupational status	Treatment goals and intervention
VOLITION	
Interests and goals	
Well defined and centered around homemaker and spouse role	Affirmation of goals and interests
Personal causation	
Disrupted by fears of inefficacy and future failure	Supportive, exploratory treatment approach in which skills are developed and identified
HABITUATION	
Roles	
Clearly defined and expectations are realistic	Mutual identification of roles and their validity
Habits	
Disrupted by the disability and hospital routine; they will continue to be altered until full function returns	Activities to begin restoration of self-care habits and mutual planning of habits after discharge
PERFORMANCE	
Surgical replacement of a musculoskeletal component along with contraindicated movements limit motor performance and, thus, performance of daily occupations	Progressive activity to restore strength, endurance and protect the artificial joint. Adaptive equipment to compensate for musculoskeletal limitations

Treatment also included training in skills she needed for daily living tasks. Because of immediate problems with self-care due to the acute impact of surgery, immobility and hospital routine, Mrs. Harris was given opportunities to problem solve how to increase her level of self-care in her immediate situation with the goals of increasing her belief in skill and feelings of internal control. Mrs. Harris was given a leg lifter and encouraged to experiment lifting her leg and abducting it. She did this independently several times a day and soon felt comfortable with moving her leg. Next she practiced getting to the side of the bed. This was accomplished in stages, with the bed rolled partly up at first and during four 10-minute treatment sessions each day to allow optimum conditions for success despite Mrs. Harris' limited endurance. Within 2 days, she was getting out of bed, with only stand-by help. She also exhibited an increased belief that she would succeed in walking and decreased signs of anxiety and depression were documented in the nurses' notes.

When her motility increased and she was able to sit up easily, adapted techniques using a long-handled sponge, reacher, extended shoe horn, and stocking aide were presented (and practiced). Emphasis was placed on using these to increase independence, to increase her activity level for muscle strengthening, and to assure protection to her hip joint. Finally, she was encouraged and assisted to begin planning her future use of time and needed supports in the home environment after discharge from the hospital.

Outcome

Sixteen days after surgery, Mrs. Harris was discharged, walking with a walker independently. She was able to go up stairs with only stand-by assistance. She was independent in self-care and had worked out a schedule for housework, meals and resting periods which would allow maximum independence and require assistance from her husband only at times he would ordinarily be present. Importantly, while she was not highly dysfunctional, her lowered personal causation and subsequent inability to participate effectively in the rehabilitation program, coupled with her fear and avoidance of the future may well have led to a increasingly maladaptive pattern upon return home. Her treatment is thus not only restorative, but, just as importantly, preventative.

SUMMARY

This chapter presented applications of the model of human occupation to physical disabilities practice in general and, specifically, to a number of areas representing the patients, clients and settings with which the occupational therapist might interface. The chapter is neither intended as an exhaustive treatment of therapeutic approaches for the occupational therapist in physical disabilities practice nor as an indication of all possible physical disabilities applications of the model of human occupation. The purpose of this chapter was to introduce the model as a framework for organizing knowledge about persons with various kinds of physical disabilities and as a practical framework for choosing assessments and generating rational and holistic treatment plans.

The discussions in this chapter represent first-level applications of this theoretical model which will require additional refinement and empirical verification. For example, each of the discussions concerning the status of various subsystems in relationship to particular disabilities were based, as much as possible, on the literature. However, many gaps in knowledge were encountered and clinical experience, logic and extrapolation from related literature was used to fill in the gaps as much as possible. Still, much of the discussion of this chapter remains theoretical and will need to be put to empirical test in descriptive research which examines the system status and other variables discussed herein. Further, the various recommended treatment strategies will require examination in research both to validate their utility and to refine methodologies for treatment. The chapter is thus, in our opinion, a much needed, but preliminary step in the development of a coherent, systematic and demonstrably efficacious occupational therapy service for physically disabled persons.

References

1. Adsett CA, Bruhn JG: Short-term psychotherapy for postmyocardial infarction patients and their wives. *Can Med Assoc J* 99:577–589, 1968.
2. American Cancer Society: *1982 Cancer Facts and Figures*. New York, American Cancer Society, 1981.
3. American Cancer Society: *1983 Cancer Facts and Figures*. New York, American Cancer Society, 1982.
4. American Occupational Therapy Association: *Cancer*. Rockville, American Occupational Therapy Association, Inc., 1983.
5. American Occupational Therapy Association: *Hospice*. Rockville, American Occupational Therapy Association, Inc., 1980.
6. Baum B, Hall KM: Relationship between constructional apraxia and dressing in the head-injured adult. *Am J Occup Ther* 35:438–442, 1981.
7. Baum B, Meeder DL: Head injury in adults. In Pedretti LW (ed): *Occupational Therapy: Practice Skills for Physical Dysfunction*. St. Louis, Mosby, 1981.
8. Beeson PB, McDermott W, Wyngaarden JB: (eds): *Cecil Textbook of Medicine*, ed 15. Philadelphia, Saunders, 1979, vol 1.
9. Bender M, Valletutti PJ, Bender R: *Teaching the Moderately and Severely Handicapped: Curriculum Objectives, Strategies, and Activities-Communication, Socialization, Safety and Leisure Time Skills*. Baltimore, University Park Press, 1976, vol 2.
10. Ben-Yishay Y, Diller L, Gerstman LJ, Goodkin R, Gordon W, Weinberg J: Working approaches to remediation of cognitive deficits in brain-damaged patients. New York, New York University Medical Center, Rehabilitation Monographs No. 59, 60, 61 and 62, 1978–1981.
11. Blaskey J, Wahlstrom P: Physical assessment and goal setting. In *Rehabilitation of the Head-Injured Adult: Comprehensive Management*. Downey, Calif, Professional Staff Association of Rancho Los Amigos Hospital, Inc., 1980.
12. Bobath B: *Adult hemiplegia: Evaluation and Treatment*, ed 2. London, William Heineman Medical Books, 1978.
13. Booth BJ, Doyle M, Woodward J: Application of casts for control of spasticity. In *Rehabiliation of the Head-Injured Adult: Comprehensive Management*. Downey, Calif, Professional Staff Association of Rancho Los Amigos Hospital, Inc., 1980.
14. Brooks NA, Matson RR: Social-psychological adjustment to multiple sclerosis. *NY State J Med* 3:312–326, 1982.
15. Bruhn JG: Psychological predictors of sudden death in myocardial infarction. *J Psychosom Res* 18:187, 1974.
16. Bruhn JG, McCrady KE, du Plessis A: Evidence of "emotional drain" preceding death from myocardial infarction. *Psychiatr Dig* 29:34-39, 1968.
17. Brunnstrom S: *Movement Therapy in Hemiplegia*. New York, Harper Row, 1970.
18. Burish TG, Bradley LA: Coping with chronic disease: definitions and issues. In Burish TG, Bradley LA (eds): *Coping with Chronic Disease*. New York, Academic Press, 1983.
19. Burkhalter PK, Donley DL: *Dynamics of Oncology Nursing*. New York, McGraw-Hill, 1978.
20. Burns N: *Nursing and Cancer*. Philadelphia, Saunders, 1982.
21. Carter, LT, Caruso, JL, Languirand, MA, Berard, MA: Cognitive skill remediation in stroke and nonstroke elderly. *Clin Neuropathol*, 2: 109–113, 1980.
22. Carter LT, Caruso JL, Languirand MA, Berard MA: *The thinking skills workbook: a cognitive skills remediation manual for adults*. Springfield, Ill, Charles C Thomas, 1980.

23. Carter LT, Howard BE, O'Neil WA: Effectiveness in cognitive skill remediation in acute stroke patients. *Am J Occup Ther* 37:320–326, 1982.

24. Caywood T: A quadriplegic young man looks at treatment. *J of Rehabil* 40:22–25, 1974.

25. Cherry D, Weigand G: Plaster drop-out casts as a dynamic means to reduce muscle contracture. *Phys Ther* 61:1601–1603, 1981.

26. Cogswell B: Self-socialization: Readjustment of paraplegics in the community. *J Rehabil* 34:11–13, 1968.

27. Cordery J: Joint protection—a responsibility of the occupational therapist. *Am J Occup Ther* 19:285–294, 1965.

28. Dembo T, Leviton GL, Wright BA: Adjustment to misfortune: a problem of social psychological rehabilitation. *Rehabil Psychol* 22:1–100, 1975.

29. DeVita VT, Hellman S, Rosenbberg SA: *Cancer Principles and Practice of Oncology*. Philadelphia, Lippincott, 1982.

30. Dimsdale JE, Hackett TP, Block PC, Hutter AM: Emotional correlatives of type A behavior pattern. *Psychosom Med* 40:580–583, 1978.

31. Donovan MI, Pierce SG: *Cancer Care Nursing*. New York, Appleton-Century-Croft, 1976.

32. Dossey L: Medicine enters the 4th dimension. *Sci Dig* October:80–82, 1982.

33. Downie PA: *Cancer Rehabilitation: An Introduction for Physio-Therapists and the Allied Professions*. London, Faber & Faber, 1978.

34. Eson ME, Yen JK, Bourke RS: Assessment of recovery from serious head injury. *J Neurol* 41:1036–1042, 1978.

35. Farber S: *Sensorimotor Evaluation and Treatment Procedures for Allied Health Personnel*. Indiana University Foundation, 1974.

36. Fogel ML, Rosillo RH: Correlation of psychologic variables and progress in physical rehabilitation: IV. The relation of body image to success in physical rehabilitation. *Arch Phys Med Rehabil* 52:182–186, 1971.

37. Friedman E, Katcher AH, Lynch JJ, Thomas SA: Animal companions and 1-year survival of patients after discharge from a coronary care unit. *Public Health Rep* 95:307–312, 1980.

38. Friedman M, Rosenman RH: *Type A Behavior and Your Heart*. New York, Fawcett Crest Books, 1974.

39. Furst GP: *Rehabilitation Through Learning: Energy Conservation and Joint Protection: A Workbook for Persons with Rheumatoid Arthritis*. Bethesda, Md, National Institutes of Health, U.S. Department of Health and Human Services, 1982.

40. Gammage SL, McMahon PS, Shanahan PM: The occupational therapist and terminal illness: learning to cope with death. *Am J Occup Ther* 30:294–299, 1976.

41. Gatz AJ: *Manter's Essentials of Clinical Neuroanatomy and Neuro-Physiology*, ed 4. Philadelphia, FA Davis, 1970.

42. Glass DC: Stress, behavior patterns and coronary disease. *Am Sci* 65:177–187, 1977.

43. Glasser DB, Franco PC, Mellette SJ, Griffith ER: *Learning to Live with a Dynamic Disability*. (Unpublished paper, Medical College of Virginia, 1979.)

44. Gray M: *Depersonalization and Loss of Occupational Skills During Hospitalization*. (Unpublished master's thesis, University of Southern California, 1969.)

45. Gray M: The effects of hospitalization of work-play behavior. *Am J Occup Ther* 26:180–185, 1972.

46. Gray RM, Reinhard AM, Ward JR: Psychosocial factors involved in the rehabilitation of persons with cardiovascular diseases. *Rehabil Lit* 30:354–359, 1969.

47. Gullege DA: Psychological aftermaths of myocardial infarction. In Doyle WD, Williams RB (eds): *Psychological Aspects of Myocardial Infarction and Coronary Care*. St. Louis, Mosby, 1979.

48. Hagen C, Malkmus D, Durham P: Levels of cognitive functioning. In *Rehabilitation of the Head-Injured Adult: Comprehensive Physical Management*. Downey, Calif, Professional Staff Association of Rancho Los Amigos Hospital, Inc., 1979.

49. Harris ED: Rheumatoid arthritis: the clinical spectrum. In Kelly WN, Harris ED, Ruddy S, Sledge C (eds): *Textbook of Rheumatology*. Philadelphia, Saunders, 1981.

50. Heilman KM, Valenstein E: *Clinical Neuropsychology*. New York, Oxford University Press, 1979.

51. Holme I, Helgeland A, Hjermann I, Loren P, Lund-Larsen PG: Physical activity at work and at leisure in relation to coronary risk factors and social class. A 4-year mortality follow-up. *Acta Med Scand* 209:277–283, 1981.

52. Hopkins H, Smith H: (eds): *Willard and Spackman's Occupational Therapy*, ed 5. Philadelphia, Lippincott, 1983.

53. Ibrahim M, Feldman J, Sultz H, Staiman M, Young L, Dean D: Management after myocardial infarction: a controlled trial for effect of group psychotherapy. *Int J Psychiatry Med* 5:253–268, 1974.

54. Jenkins CD: The coronary prone personality. In Gentry WD, Williams RB (eds): *Psychological Aspects of Myocardial Infarction and Coronary Care*. St. Louis, Mosby, 1979.

55. Jenkins CD: Psychologic and social precursors of coronary disease. *N Engl J Med* 284:307–317, 1971.

56. Jenkins CD, Zyzanski SJ, Ryan TJ, Flessas A, Tannenbaum SI: Social insecurity and coronary-prone type A responses as identifiers of severe atherosclerosis. *J Consult Clin Psychol* 45:1060–1067, 1977.

57. Jennett B, Bond M: Assessment of outcome after severe brain injury. *Lancet* 1:480–484, 1975.

58. Jennett B, Teasdale G: Aspects of coma after severe head injury. *Lancet* 2:878–884, 1977.

59. Jennett B, Teasdale G: *Management of Head Injuries*. Philadelphia, FA Davis, 1981.

60. Jones R, Giddens H, Croft D: Assessment and training of brain-damaged drivers. *Am J Occup Ther* 37:754–760, 1983.

61. Kaplan J, Hier DB: Visuospatial deficits after right hemisphere stroke. *Am J Occup Ther* 36:314–321, 1981.

62. Kern N: Staff expectations for disabled persons: helpful or harmful. In Stubbins J (ed): *Social and Psychological Aspects of Disability.* Baltimore, University Park Press, 1977.

63. King TI: Plaster splinting as a means of reducing elbow flexor spasticity: a case study. *Am J Occup Ther* 36:671–673, 1982.

64. Koppa RJ, McDermott M, Leavitt LA, Zuniga EN: Handicapped driver controls operability: advice for clinical evaluation of patients. *Arch Phys Med Rehabil* 59:227–231, 1978.

65. Levin HS, Grossman RG: Behavioral sequelae of closed head injury. *Arch Neurol* 35:720–727, 1978.

66. Litman TJ: Physical rehabilitation: a social-psychological approach. In Jaco EG (ed): *Patients, Physicians and Illness: A Sourcebook in Behavioral Science and Health* ed 2. New York, The Free Press, 1972.

67. Lundberg V, Theorell T, Lind E: Life changes and myocardial infarction, individual differences in life change scaling. *J Psychom Res* 19:27–32, 1975.

68. Luria AR: *Restoration of Function after Brain Injury.* New York, Macmillan, 1983.

69. Lynch WJ, Mauss NK: Brain injury rehabilitation: standard problem lists. *Arch Phys Med Rehabil* 62:223–227, 1981.

70. MacDonald J: An investigation of body scheme in adults with CVA. *Am J Occup Ther* 14:75–79, 1960.

71. Malkmus D, Booth BJ, Kodimer C: *Rehabilitation of the Head Injured Adult: Comprehensive Cognitive Management.* Downey, Calif, Professional Staff Association of Rancho Los Amigos Hospital, Inc., 1980.

72. Mayou R, Williamson B, Foster A: Outcome 2 months after myocardial infarction. *J Psychom Res* 22:439–445, 1978.

73. McAlpine D: Course and prognosis. In McAlpine D, Lunsden CE, Acheson ED (eds): *Multiple Sclerosis: A Reappraisal.* Baltimore, Williams & Wilkins, 1972.

74. McCarty DJ: *Arthritis and Allied Conditions: A Textbook of Rheumatology,* ed 9. Philadelphia, Lea & Febiger, 1979.

75. Meenan RF, Yelin EH, Nevitt M, Epstein WV: The impact of chronic disease: a sociomedical profile of rheumatoid arthritis. *Arthritis Rheum* 24:544–549, 1981.

76. Melvin J: *Rheumatic Disease: Occupational Therapy and Rehabilitation.* Philadelphia, FA Davis, 1977.

77. Miller JD: Early evaluation and management. In Rosenthal M, Griffith ER, Bond MR, Miller JD (eds): *Rehabilitation of the Head Injured Adult.* Philadelphia, FA Davis, 1983.

78. Monteiro LA: *Cardiac Patients Rehabilitation: Social Aspects of Recovery.* New York, Springer, 1979.

79. National Cancer Institute. *Radiation Therapy and You.* (NIH Publication No. 80-2227, U.S. Department of Health and Human Services.) Washington, DC, National Cancer Institute, August 1980.

80. Nelson LM, Thompson DS, Heaton RH, Burks JS, Walker SH: Cognitive deficits in multiple sclerosis. *Society for Neuroscience Abstracts,* 1982.

81. Oddy M, Humphrey M: Social recovery during the year following severe head injury. *J Neurol Neurosurg Psychiatry* 43:798–802, 1980.

82. Paap WR: The social reconstruction of reality: the rehabilitation of quadriplegics and paraplegics. (Doctoral dissertation, University of Missouri, 1971). *Dissertation Abstracts International,* 1972, vol 33, 415-A. (University Microfilms No. 72-19, 234).

83. Panikoff LG: Recovery trends of functional skills in the head injured adult. *Am J Occup Ther* 37:735–743, 1983.

84. Pedretti LW: *Occupational Therapy: Practice Skills for Physical Dysfunction.* St. Louis, Mosby, 1981.

85. Rabinowitz HS, Mitsos SB: Rehabilitation as planned social change: a conceptual framework. *J Health Soc Behav* 5:2–13, 1964.

86. Rogers JC, Figone JJ: The avocational pursuits of rehabilitants with traumatic quadriplegia. *Am J Occup Ther* 32:571–576, 1978.

87. Rogers JC, Figone JJ: Psychosocial parameters in treating the person with quadriplegia. *Am J Occup Ther* 33:432–439, 1979.

88. Romano M: Family response to traumatic head injury. *Scand J Rehab Med* 6:1–4, 1975.

89. Romano MD: Social skills training with the newly handicapped. *Arch Phys Med Rehabil* 57:302–303, 1976.

90. Rosenman RH, Brand RJ, Jenkins CD, Friedman M, Straus R, Wurm C: Coronary heart disease in the western collaborative group study: Five-year follow-up experiment of eight and a half years. *JAMA* 223:872–877, 1975.

91. Rosenman RH, Friedman M, Straus R, Wurm C, Jenkins CD, Messinger HB: Coronary heart disease in the western collaborative group study: a follow-up experiment of 2 years. *JAMA* 19:776–782, 1967.

92. Rosenthal MR, Griffith ER, Bond MR, Miller JD: *Rehabiliation of the Head Injured Adult.* Philadelphia, FA Davis, 1983.

93. Russek HI: Role of emotional stress in the etiology of clinical coronary heart disease. *Dis Chest* 52:1, 1967.

94. Sarbin TR: Role theory. In Lindzey G, Aronson E (eds): *The Hand-Book of Social Psychology* Reading, Mass, Addison-Wesley, 1954, vol 1.

95. Schiffer RB, Rudick RA, Herndon RM: Psychologic aspects of multiple sclerosis. *NY State J Med* 3:312–316, 1983.

96. Seeger M, Fisher L: Adaptive equipment used in the rehabilitation of hip arthroplasty patients. *Am J Occup Ther* 36:503–514, 1982.

97. Shillam LL, Beeman C, Loshin P: Effect of occupational therapy intervention on bathing independence of disabled persons. *Am J Occup Ther* 37:744–748, 1983.

98. Siegrist J, Dittman K, Rittner K, Weber I: Psychosocial risk constellation and first myocardial infarction. In Siegrist J, Halhuber MJ (eds): *Myocardial Infarctions and Psychosocial Risks.* Berlin, Springer-Verlag, 1981.

99. Siev E, Freishtat B: *Perceptual Dysfunction in the Adult Stroke Patient.* Thorofare, NJ, Charles

B. Slack, 1976.

100. Siller J: Psychological situation of the disabled with spinal cord injuries. *Rehabil Lit* 30:290–296, 1969.

101. Silverman EH, Elfant-Asher IL: Dysphagia: An evaluation and treatment program for the adult. *Am J Occup Ther* 6:382–392, 1979.

102. Simmons O: *Work and Mental Illness*. New York, Wiley, 1965.

103. Skelton M, Dominion J: Psychological stress in wives of patients with myocardial infarction. *Br Med J* 2:101–103, 1973.

104. Smith CA: Body image changes after myocardial infarction. *Nurs Clin North Am* 7:663–668, 1972.

105. Smith RO, Okamoto GA: Checklist for the prescription of slings for the hemiplegic patient. *Am J Occup Ther* 35:91–95, 1981.

106. Spencer EA: Functional restoration/specific diagnosis. In Hopkins H, Smith H (eds): *Willard and Spackman's Occupational Therapy*, ed 6. Philadelphia, Lippincott, 1983.

107. Stern MJ, Pascale L, Ackerman A: Life adjustment post-myocardial infarction: determining predictive variables. *Arch Int Med* 137:1680–1685, 1977.

108. Strauss A, Glaser BG: *Chronic Illness and the Quality of Life*. St. Louis, Mosby, 1975.

109. Suinn RM: Type A behavior pattern. In Williams, Jr, RB, Gentry WD (eds): *Behavioral Approaches to Medical Treatment*. Cambridge, Ballinger, 1977.

110. Suinn RM, Brock L, Cecil AE: Behavior therapy for type A patients. *Am J Cardiol* 36:269, 1975.

111. Thiel HG, Parker D, Bruel TA: Stress factors and the risk of myocardial infarction. *J Psychom Res* 17:43–57, 1973.

112. Thomas EJ: Problems of disability from the perspective of role theory. *J Health Hum Behav* 7:2–14, 1966.

113. Tigges KN, Sherman LM: The treatment of the hospice patient: from occupational history to occupational role. *Am J Occup Ther* 37:235–238, 1983.

114. Trombly CA (ed): *Occupational Therapy for Physical Dysfunction*, ed 2. Baltimore, Williams & Wilkins, 1983.

115. Turk DC, Sobel HJ, Follick MJ, Youkilis HD: A sequential criterion analysis for assessing coping with chronic illness. *J Hum Stress* 6:35–40, 1980.

116. Tyzenhouse PS: Myocardial infarction: its effect on family. *Am J Nurs* 73:1012–1013, 1973.

117. Versluys HP: Psychosocial adjustment to physical disability. In Trombly CA (ed): *Occupational Therapy for Physical Dysfunction* ed 2. Baltimore, Williams & Wilkins, 1983.

118. Versluys HP: The remediation of role disorders through focused group work. *Am J Occup Ther* 34:609–614, 1980.

119. Waldren I: The coronary-prone behavior pattern, blood pressure, employment, and socioeconomic status in women. *J Psychosom Res* 22:79–87, 1978.

120. Warren M: Relationship of constructional apraxia and body scheme disorders to dressing performance in adult CVA. *Am J Occup Ther* 35:431–437, 1981.

121. Weiner CL: The burden of rheumatoid arthritis: tolerating the uncertainty. *Soc Sci Med* 9:97–104, 1975.

122. Weissman R, Kutner B: Role disorders in extended hospitalization. *Hosp Admin* 12:52–55, 1967.

123. Werner-Beland JA: (ed): *Grief Responses to Long-Term Illness and Disability*. Reston, Virginia: Reston, 1980.

124. Williams RB: Physiological mechanisms underlying the association between psychosocial factors and coronary disease. In Gentry WD, Williams RB (eds): *Psychological Aspects of Myocardial Infarction and Coronary Care*. St. Louis, Mosby, 1979.

125. Wilson DJ, McKenzie MW, Barber LM: *Spinal cord injury: a treatment guide for occupational therapists*. Thorofare, NJ, Charles B. Slack, 1974.

126. Winstein C: Evaluation and managment of swallowing dysfunction. In *Rehabilitation of the Head-Injured Adult: Comprehensive Physical Management*. Downey, Calif, Professional Staff Association of Rancho Los Amigos Hospital, Inc., 1979.

127. Wright BA: *Physical Disability: A Psychological Approach*. New York, Harper & Row, 1960.

128. Zane MD, Lowenthal M: Motivation in rehabilitation of the physically handicapped. *Arch Phys Med Rehabil* 41:400–407, 1960.

CHAPTER 15

Psychosocial Dysfunction*

Roann Barris, Gary Kielhofner, Anne M. Neville, Frances Maag Oakley, Cheryl Salz, and Janet Hawkins Watts

Although occupational therapists have traditionally worked with patients with psychosocial disorders, their role and focus of treatment has undergone considerable change. This change has largely been in response to the changing conceptualizations of the etiology and prognosis of mental illnesses and to the changing treatment of people with psychosocial problems by other professionals in the health care system (9, 74, 138). Occupational therapists have similarly had to revise their view of the role of activities in treatment in order to accommodate different views of mental illness.

However, by conceptualizing psychosocial disorder in terms of occupational dysfunction as articulated in Chapter 5, it is possible to arrive at a consistent, logical and unique role for the occupational therapist. This role complements and supplements the roles of other professionals, but it is predicated on a way of thinking that begins by looking at the *occupational* nature of persons. In this chapter, the model of human occupation is used to explore the dynamics of occupational dysfunction and implications for assessment and intervention in several categories of clients typically seen by therapists working in psychosocial settings: the borderline

---

* The first two authors had responsibility for the content and organization of the entire chapter. Ann Neville made primary contributions to the section on depression, Frances Oakley to the schizophrenia section and Cheryl Salz to the borderline section. Cheryl Salz' contribution was based in part on an article that was originally published in *Occupational Therapy in Mental Health*, vol. 3, No. 3, 1983 (198) and is reprinted here with permission of the publisher. The authors also wish to acknowledge Jeff Lederer, Emily Perkins, and Lynn Smyntek, whose analysis and synthesis of the literature on juvenile delinquency, anorexia nervosa, and adolescent psychosocial disorder for their master's degree research projects provided a useful beginning to the work in various sections of this chapter. Finally, the authors want to thank Jan Bracalente and Terry Waters for providing the cases for the anorexia nervosa and juvenile delinquency sections, respectively.

person, the depressed person, the adolescent exhibiting anorexia or juvenile delinquency, and the person with chronic schizophrenia.

These categories have been chosen because of their prevalence in settings where occupational therapists are likely to work, or because they pose unusual or challenging problems for the therapist. This chapter does not aim to present a comprehensive picture of psychosocial practice, but by demonstrating the applicability of the model to several different types of patients and clients it should enable readers to begin conceptualizing and addressing other forms of psychosocial disorder in a similar fashion.

In this first general discussion we overview systems and environmental conditions which are typical for the person with psychosocial dysfunction. In reading this and later discussions, it should be kept in mind that psychosocial dysfunction is generally a very complex entity of which the occupational dysfunction is a component. Patients and clients may have problems in other areas of their life—e.g. in psychosexual identity, in family conflicts, and so on. These problems may contribute to problems in occupational performance or they may result from occupational dysfunction. The focus of this chapter, however, is on achieving an understanding of the occupational dysfunction that inheres in psychosocial dysfunction since this is the domain of occupational therapy.

GENERAL CHARACTERISTICS OF PSYCHOSOCIAL OCCUPATIONAL DYSFUNCTION

Persons with various types of psychosocial dysfunction are characterized by a unique pattern of system disturbances. However, these individuals share the general characteristics of maladaptive output—either a cessation of occupational behavior, or engagement in activities that hold no meaning for them, or an extreme increase and consequent imbalance in occupational activities.

Volition

Volitional problems are a critical component in most categories of psychosocial dysfunction. Decreased personal causation, unrealistic goals or an inability to identify goals, and an inability to find meaning or interest in leisure and work are typical areas of dysfunction.

PERSONAL CAUSATION

One of the most fundamental characteristics of persons with mental illness is their self-perception of inadequacy or helplessness (229). This belief in personal dependency and inability underlies other problems such as difficulty identifying goals or organizing behavior to accomplish goals.

A number of psychosocial disorders first become manifest during adolescence, and feelings of inefficacy may be pivotal in hindering adolescents' ability to cope with the demands for new roles and relationships that they face. Thus, belief in self-competence for handling problems has been found to distinguish normal adolescents from emotionally disturbed adolescents (69, 91, 148, 196, 242).

Moderately and severely psychologically disturbed adolescents have been found to be more externally oriented in their locus of control than their nonhospitalized peers (221). Hospitalized college students have similarly been found to be more external and to demonstrate a greater expectancy of failure in future tasks than nonhospitalized college students (37). Emotionally disturbed adolescents also indicate feelings of incompetence regarding the tasks in which they do engage (214). Because of this decreased sense of personal causation, adolescents with psychosocial disorders often prefer solitary tasks whose results are less easily judged by others (4).

In adults, researchers have consistently found that the greater the belief in external control, the greater the degree of psychological disturbance (34, 42, 49, 90, 213). Individuals who do not believe they are in control of their lives are: (a) less well adjusted; (b) less socially competent; (c) less likely to perceive themselves as active, independent, effective; (d) less content with life; (e) more apt to hold irrational values; (f) prone to mood disturbances; (g) likely to display behavior indicative of social maladjustment; and (h) less likely to pay attention to feedback. While the other dimensions of personal causation have not been as systematically investigated, writers have also referred to the expectancy of failure and a belief in personal ineffectiveness as concomitants of mental disturbance (90, 139, 223, 245).

Regardless of age, the patient role itself may contribute to a decreased sense of personal causation (78). However, because feelings of inefficacy are also prevalent in nonhospitalized persons at risk for mental illness (222), it seems probable that the decreased personal causation found in hospitalized persons both precedes and is enhanced by hospitalization.

VALUES

Identifying values and setting goals requires the ability to conceptualize and evaluate one's past experiences, assess one's skills and anticipate their relevance to the future. Individuals with psychopathology, however, generally have a maladaptive orientation to time, viewing the past in a disorganized and confused manner (161) or experiencing it as distant and removed, and regarding the future as hopeless and menacing (82). Emotionally disturbed adolescents, in particular, appear to have little sense of themselves in the future, and to be unable to anticipate or set goals (23, 24, 39, 177). This inability to set goals and lack of future orientation, combined with an absence of belief in self-efficacy, may lead to a crisis of belief in the worth of life, or extreme alienation (167, 202).

In general, people who do not experience a sense of connectedness to their past, present or future will not find hope and meaning in their lives. Both hope and meaning are necessary for successful adaptation—the lack of hope about one's life leads to feelings of impending despair and, in extreme cases, the inability to survive what appear to be insurmountable odds (119, 165). Similarly, the inability to find meaning in events can lead to a sense of purposelessness in one's life (67). This emptiness of meaning can contribute to the etiology of mental illness (67, 233).

Occupational values also include standards of performance. Both institutionalized and deinstitutionalized psychiatric patients often show minimal conformity to socially acceptable standards of behavior. However, this may actually represent an internalization of expectations in the social surroundings. For example, the patient in a back ward, or a resident in a community facility, may encounter and internalize expectations for passivity, isolation, and so on (44, 78).

INTERESTS

The ability to discriminate interests and to use these as a guide to engaging in occupations may show more variation in psychosocial clients than do the other components of volition. Problems may range from a current short-term inability to find interest in activities to a history of never having been able to identify and enact interests (4).

Research suggests that adolescents who have been hospitalized for psychiatric problems express few interests and engage in few activities of interest (85), and may make inappropriate use of leisure time choosing socially unacceptable interests (123, 238). Other research has found that alcoholics enact fewer of their interests than normals (201); and that chronic psychiatric patients have a paucity of interests (216).

Habituation

Problems with role performance and routines are frequently the fundamental area of disturbance in a variety of psychiatric dysfunctions, e.g. substance abuse and alcoholism. Most persons with mental illness manifest disorganization in the habituation subsystem; this disorganization, which leads to inability to enact roles, is the major impetus for their entry into the mental health care system (19, 157).

ROLES

Role dysfunction may be either or both a consequence and an etiological factor in psychosocial dysfunction. A disruption of role performance may occur when a person has failed to internalize roles; when internalized roles are incompatible with the person's values, interests and personal causation; when there is a conflict or imbalance in the demands of internalized roles; or when the internalized role is a deviant role (9, 40, 73, 81, 84, 113, 180, 250). *Role strain* (81) may occur when a person cannot meet the multiple obligations of several roles or when a person feels compelled to achieve highly in all roles. For instance, women who try to be "supermom," "superwife," and "superprofessional" may be at risk for role strain and failure in some or all of their role demands (17). However, involvement in too few roles is often more likely to be detrimental to psychosocial health than involvement in too many (150, 206, 217).

The loss of the worker role and chronic work role problems are especially implicated in psychosocial dysfunction. Many consequences of unemployment have been suggested: suicide; emotional problems (especially depression); stress-related health problems (ulcers, heart disease, renal problems); interpersonal problems; wife and child abuse; increased crime; maternal and infant mortality; and increased substance abuse (21, 25). A frequently cited concomitant of unemployment is the disorganization of daily routine. Unemployment means the loss of not only money and status, but also one's major form of daily activity. Work structures time, in both the present and future—one gets up to go to work, plans weekends and vacations around work, and develops long-term career timetables. Without work, many people find themselves unable to sleep or eat, and feeling aimless and restless (21). The problems of employment are complicated by the fact that once someone is labeled as mentally ill, it is often exceedingly difficult to find unbiased employers (58).

Adolescents with psychosocial disorders are frequently less involved in academic, leisure and work roles than are their peers (94, 152, 177). It is unclear whether this lack of involvement precedes or follows the inability to successfully make an occupational choice; however, the lack of meaningful work certainly contributes to the problem of having few internalized roles and contributes as well to decreased personal causation and increased isolation. Adolescent girls, in particular, seem more apt to stay home in unproductive roles, if they are unemployed and no longer in school (48).

HABITS

Habit disorganization can clearly result from role disruption; however, habits themselves can be dysfunctional and then constrain role performance. Habit disorganization may manifest itself in terms of habit patterns that are too rigid, and hence do not allow for changes in routine; in habits that lack any consistency whatsoever; and in habits that do not meet the demands of either the environment or the individual (112). For example, substance abuse is a habit that does not meet social requirements (in mainstream society). Consistently arriving late for work is a habit that does not meet either social requirements or the needs of a person who wants to maintain a job.

The habits of individuals with psychosocial dysfunction may include difficulty organizing oneself for work, dressing to meet the demands of different social situations, and maintaining a balance of work, play, rest, and self-care in daily routines. In some cases, the breakdown of habits may be interwoven with affective disturbances, whereas in other cases dysfunctional habits may precede psychosocial disorder. For example, the adolescent with habits of truancy coupled with poor study habits is at risk for failure, loss of self-esteem and entering a maladaptive cycle. Extreme habit dysfunction may be manifest in totally aimless behavior or in near complete withdrawal from activity.

Individuals with dysfunctional habits and roles may not only find that these routines are preventing the satisfaction of personal or societal values, but may also rely on these disordered habits to keep from feeling badly about not living up to their own or others' goals.

Performance

Deficits of skills and their constituents have been widely noted in psychosocially dysfunctional adults and adolescents. In adolescence the lack of skills for competent daily living may precipitate psychopathology (94), while in adulthood the lack of skills may contribute to a high recidivism rate (229).

Learning disabilities (deficits in symbolic and neurologic skills) occur with high frequency in psychosocially disordered adolescents. Learning-disabled adolescents may be at risk for psychopathology and a cycle of failure because their inability to succeed in school can undermine their confidence in both academic and extracurricular activities, leading to a decreased sense of efficacy and unsatisfying use of leisure time (39).

Although particular skill deficits vary with diagnostic groups, problems that have been observed in both adults and adolescents include deficits in coping skills (229), neurological and sensory-integrative problems (94, 116), and difficulties in forming and maintaining interpersonal relationships (4, 89, 100, 229). Communication is often disorganized in certain forms of mental illness, as is the ability to keep ideas organized and coherent (89, 94). Mentally ill persons are also often unable to discriminate between environmental cues (190).

A major problem area for most psychiatric clients is an inability to modulate levels of stress or arousal (89, 229). This inability leads to a high vulnerability to stressful situations.

Although skill deficits may contribute to the etiology of mental illness, it is critical to realize that they may also be sequelae to the illness or its treatment. For example, certain medications may render the person unable to concentrate or attend to tasks. Similarly, the person who once held a technically demanding job may be unable to make plans or complete small tasks following unemployment and the onset of an affective disorder.

The Environment and Psychosocial Dysfunction

Persons with psychosocial problems may be treated in hospitals and institutions and in the community. Current forms of alternative treatment settings include foster care, in which one or two patients are placed in a family setting; halfway houses, or proprietary homes for adults that may provide few or no services; satellite housing or supervised apartment programs associated with hospitals; partial hospitalization programs, in which patients spend either the day or the night in the hospital; and vocationally oriented programs, often based on the Fountain House model (32, 229). In addition, some individuals may never have more than outpatient contact with mental health professionals. This array of treatment options has developed for several reasons. First, the emphasis on deinstitutionalization, concomitant with the community mental health movement, created a large pool of long-term patients who suddenly found themselves discharged but with no place to go and no community support structures (101, 203, 226). Second, the increasing costs of health care have created incentives for finding ways to contain costs or to shift them from the federal and local governments to other parties (203, 229). Finally, there is evidence that hospitalization may be no more effective—and may actually be less effective—than other forms of treating mental illness (229).

Acknowledging the existence of these alternatives, however, says little about their qualities. Indeed, many of the environments associated with treatment of psychosocial dysfunction may contribute to the very problems they seek to alleviate, in part because they represent a discontinuity with "normal" environments, and in part because of physical and psychosocial properties inherent in these settings (56, 111, 203, 229).

OBJECTS

The context of hospitals and board-and-care settings is frequently devoid of interesting objects. Walls are often barren; patients' clothes are ill-fitting and unstylish; personal possessions may be considered dangerous or unsafe and thus taken from the patient for safekeeping. The deprivation created by such contexts can contribute to apathy and indifference to one's surroundings, to feelings of helplessness and dependency (84, 143), and to the continued maladaptive use of those objects that are present. In addition, the scarcity of objects that are readily accessible in other settings may give them a status that they ordinarily do not have, again contributing to a deviant symbol system. The absence of everyday objects in a setting can also foster apparently bizarre types of behaviors. For example, adults who scrounge for cigarette butts in ashtrays and garbage cans may do so because they lack money and a supply of their own (44).

The arrangement of objects can also constrain or influence task performance. For example, arranging groups of tables and chairs in a room encourages patients to engage in more social activities in their free time than other room arrangements (93). Or, serving food family style, rather than in trays, has been shown to lead to improved eating and social habits during meals (162).

TASKS

The task orientation of hospital wards is a modifiable factor that may play an important role in recidivism rates. Programs that have been shown to have good success in preparing patients to return to community living generally have a high practical orientation and emphasize order, organization and patient participation in tasks (169). Programs that have had poor success in keeping patients in the community tend to have a low emphasis on involving patients in social activities and also have poor planning of patients' activities (157, 169).

Because maladaptive behavior can be a response to either insufficient or too much challenge, the demands of tasks must be commensurate with patients' or clients' abilities (8). This may be particularly important when patients are discharged to community settings that often do not require the level of competence they may have developed in such areas as food preparation, clothing care and other areas of daily living tasks. However, a number of studies have shown that these patients can improve or maintain their level of performance if they are provided support on an ongoing basis (229). Further, there is some support for the idea that persons'

skills increase as the level of expectations increases (32).

Competitive tasks are often too arousing for seriously mentally ill persons. Some persons may perform competently in sheltered workshops but not in competitive employment because they are unable to control their level of arousal in the latter situation (229).

The meanings of tasks may also differ importantly for current and former patients. These differences may be a response to the role of certain tasks in their setting. For example, "passive waiting," an act which appears useless to most observers, may be sensible and meaningful to individuals whose days are structured around receiving medications and going to meals, and are otherwise filled with large blocks of empty time (115). To be therapeutic, the treatment environment must create the same temporal expectations and demands for quality of performance in work, play and self-care that most people experience routinely (9, 193).

SOCIAL GROUPS AND ORGANIZATIONS

Once persons are hospitalized, they lose access to the social groups to which they belonged prior to hospitalization. Their primary social environment becomes the hospital. Although some hospitalized patients may be fortunate enough to retain their occupational position, their corresponding role relationships terminate. With extended absence from work and home, others are forced to assume the patient's role responsibilities. Extended hospitalization alters community ties and social relationships by increasing physical distance between patients and their family and friends. Whereas interaction with significant others prior to hospitalization may have been frequent, spontaneous and emotional, during hospitalization it is confined to visiting hours. Display of emotion may be restrained due to lack of privacy and the possible negative effects an emotional change may have on patients. The result is that patients must rely on the hospital for social existence in the areas of friendship, intimacy and social approval (235).

Hospitalization may also place patients in a larger social group than they have previously experienced. This can have detrimental effects on their development of competent behavior if they do not have adequate opportunities to assume leadership roles. For example, a study of the environment of a psychiatric ward observed that there were too few activities or groups for the number of patients, and that those activities that were available were considered unimportant or inconsequential. Hence, patients were actually being "encouraged" to continue in passive, marginal roles, rather than to take on positions of responsibility (219).

The stigma of psychiatric hospitalization may also make it difficult for former patients to attain membership in community organizations. However, without resumption of meaningful roles, these persons are at risk for rehospitalization.

The social environment of community settings tends to be relatively homogeneous, in that patients are often grouped by diagnosis and have minimal contact with nonpatients (32). Yet, there is some evidence that when nonpatients are included in the living setting, patients perform at a higher level than otherwise (32).

Regardless of placement in a hospital or the community, many mentally ill persons experience (or have experienced) impoverished social environments (89). These persons frequently have fewer nonkindred relationships. In addition, the network of relationships among these other persons is often weak. The result is that the mentally ill person may be living in an understimulating environment, which then reinforces or encourages a tendency toward social withdrawal (89).

CULTURE

The cultural environment has a pervasive impact on what is recognized as healthy and appropriate or bizarre and unhealthy behavior (157, 204). Differing value orientations render behaviors that are acceptable in one culture unacceptable in another. Further, they influence the tolerance of society for deviant or unusual behaviors and, consequently, where and how persons manifesting these behaviors will be treated.

Once someone is identified as being mentally ill, he or she becomes a member of a new subcultural group, one with values that often conflict with those of the mainstream culture. For example, work and leisure typically do not have the same meanings within the hospital that they do outside, and generally only certain forms of these occupations are sanctioned by the hospital environment. At the same time, there is often a strong patient subculture, or underlife, in institutions, and the norms of this subculture may

lead to behaviors that are bizarre outside the hospital (78). Community settings, as well, are often not truly integrated into the social mainstream. These settings may therefore be equally promulgating values about work and play that differ from those of society. For example, in board-and-care facilities it is not uncommon for residents to spend most of the day idle and out of sight of staff. However, as long as these persons do not create "trouble" in the setting, such behavior is not deemed unproductive or inappropriate (56).

SUMMARY AND CHAPTER OVERVIEW

It is apparent from this discussion that occupational dysfunction can readily be identified in psychosocially disabled persons. Also apparent is the repercussive nature of the disorganization underlying occupational dysfunction; i.e. problems in any of the subsystems reflect and influence the status of the other subsystems. Consequently, it is not sufficient for the therapist to identify isolated deficits such as cognitive or neurological problems without considering the impact these will have on feelings of effectiveness, interests, goals, roles, and habits. Similarly, it is not enough to know a person's interests and values—one must also know whether these are supported by habits and skills, the environment, and so on.

The particular pattern of system disorganization that underlies occupational dysfunction may vary with different diagnostic groups. Thus, the therapist can develop a more specific set of expectations for likely occupational dysfunction related to various diagnoses. In the following sections of this chapter, discussions of specific diagnostic groups and the occupational dysfunction they exhibit are presented along with implications for assessment and intervention and with case illustrations.

BORDERLINE PERSONALITY DISORDER

Jill is a 30-yr-old single woman who has nearly completed a degree in philosophy with a straight A average but has been hospitalized with severe suicidal ideation during each of several attempts to complete her last semester. She cooks and makes jewelry on an expert level but derives almost no pleasure from these activities, valuing them only as mechanical exercises for reducing anxiety. She has at various times cut or starved herself and has episodically abused drugs. While many people like and admire her for her skills, her attractive appearance, her intelligence and her sense of humor, they are usually quickly put off by her lack of social initiative, her highly critical nature, and her episodic furious outbursts. She herself reports feeling empty, hopeless, confused, or angry almost all the time.

Jill is typical of patients who have been diagnosed as having a borderline personality disorder. Such patients have perplexed occupational therapists with their intact cognitive functioning, high skill levels and history of achievement coupled with erratic, angry, impulsive behavior; subjective feelings of emptiness or rage; and inconsistent work, leisure and social patterns.

While there is still disagreement over the critical diagnostic features of the borderline personality, and many efforts are currently being made to delineate subtypes (108, 158, 159), it is generally agreed that borderline pathology has its genesis in a failure of the separation/individuation process which normally takes place between the child and the primary caretaker at the age of 16–24 months (31, 144). This failure is due in part to the caretaker's need to maintain a dependent attachment to the child by rewarding dependent and clinging behavior and rejecting efforts at autonomy (195) or by withdrawing, leaving the child genuinely alone and vulnerable (145). It may also be influenced by constitutional features of the child, such as a high activity level, or difficulty in processing arousal (220). In short, the failure is in the open system of interaction between the child and the caretaker. Current research into the family histories of borderline patients shows that the most common parental configuration is a mother with an affective disorder and a passive or absent father, thus amounting to only one inconsistent caretaker (65).

The etiology of occupational dysfunction in individuals with borderline personality disorders appears to involve an interactional failure between caretaker and the child. The caretaker does not provide a safe arena in which the child can enact the urge to explore and master. Without a caretaker who can identify, support and value the child's attempts at exploration and autonomy, the child does not find a socially acceptable arena for enacting his or her own need for action. Further, because caretaker approval is not freely available and unconditional, the child comes to see performance solely as a means of seeking and obtaining approval from the caretaker. Thus, intrinsic enjoyment of ac-

tivity gives way to mechanical performance devoid of inner worth and pleasure and oriented to satisfying external expectations.

Diagnostic criteria point to major disturbances in the volition subsystem as distinguishing characteristics of the borderline person (4). Fluctuations between dependency and self-assertion, a chronic and pervasive sense of meaninglessness, emptiness and boredom are volitional traits that characterize borderline individuals. Yet, because the borderline individual often develops high levels of skill, these persons manifest a pattern of occupational functioning that alternates between achievement and helplessness.

Volition

PERSONAL CAUSATION

The person with a borderline disorder typically feels helpless and pessimistic (4, 159). This helplessness particularly extends to a persistent anticipation of defeat when attempting to achieve goals.

The borderline patient's impaired sense of personal causation is complicated by vacillating feelings of total dependence on others and total control over them (108). Because of these contradictory feelings, most everyday relationships remain very superficial, while attempts at close relationships involve dependency, self-devaluation and passive manipulation (86). This profound dependency leads to the situation in which the borderline person feels no internal desire for accomplishment, only the approval which accomplishment brings (60). Thus, personal belief in skill and belief in the efficacy of skill become secondary to the intensity of the need to win the approval and admiration of others. The consequence is that the sense of identity as a doer is incompletely developed and concomitant skill acquisition and improvement (even when they are substantial) are not perceived as leading to future success (60).

VALUES

Values are a primary area of dysfunction for borderline persons. Their central problem is an incapacity for meaningful and positive investment in occupations. The literature emphasizes that despite their achievements, these individuals feel a pervasive sense of emptiness, boredom and meaninglessness (4, 31, 184).

To understand this deficit it must be recalled that value images are internalized through interaction with the social environment from earliest childhood on. Originally it is the caretaker's appreciation of, and attunement to, the baby's playful explorations which give the child a sense of self as authentically and boundlessly creative (241). With continued nurturance the child can gradually move from the expansive, open-ended arena of exploratory play toward realistic goal-directed activity in constructive and other play forms. To do this, the child must give up the sense of unlimited potential and begin to focus on developing skills necessary to achieve realistic successful outcomes.

The interactive failure between mother and child which has been noted as a crucial determinant of borderline personality disorder mitigates against such growth. The child's efforts to please an erratic parent lead to disengaged, extrinsically motivated patterns of rote skill performance. The exploratory and mastery impulse is not enculturated. That is, it does not find its expression in attaining values mutually recognized by the person and the social environment. Instead the borderline person clings to unrealistic, grandiose values. For example, the borderline person may develop an idealized fantasy image of him or herself as suddenly becoming a great creative artist or a renowned performer. Because this ideal image exceeds what is possible or represents a level of attainment possible only after many years, the borderline person always falls short of his or her ideal. At the same time, the borderline person is unable to recognize the value of less dramatic accomplishments or of progress in attainment.

This pattern of devaluing task performance and overvaluing creativity combined with lack of belief in the efficacy of skills has several consequences. The borderline person is oriented toward the future, but the future is colored by pessimism and persistent fears that highly cherished fantasies will never be realized. Occupational goals shift unrealistically from unachievable grandiosity—"I think if I put my energy into it I could rival Picasso"—to total helplessness—"I know I'm going to end up a bag lady anyhow." In a similar manner personal standards also vacillate from the unachievably perfectionistic to careless and superficial.

INTERESTS

As noted above, creative, rather than goal-directed, activity is of major importance to the borderline individual, due to its closer relationship to the boundless pleasure of infancy. Yet, even in the artistic sphere, borderline persons are often uninterested in the reality-based skills and chores which support artistic work (60). Pleasure is derived, not from creative performance, but rather from fantasized performance. Actual outputs of talent or skill, while often quite impressive to others, are perceived as boring and unimpressive by the borderline person. In addition, their interest patterns are often narrow and unbalanced with a corresponding low potency of interest revealed in a lack of enthusiasm for present or past everyday activities.

Habituation

Unfueled by the deficit volition subsystem, the habituation subsystem does not develop adequate means of guiding effective behavior. Both roles and habits of the borderline person are impaired.

ROLES

The borderline patient never develops a sense of identity as a doer because autonomous doing is subsumed in the struggle to be nurtured by, yet separate from a caretaker. Adults come to be seen only as caretakers and not as occupational role models. This ongoing struggle does not allow for the development of internalized expectations consistent with adult occupational roles, e.g. the need to earn a living or the need to do one's fair share of a group task. This impairment in meaningful identification with role models is a key feature of borderline personality disorder (159).

Identity diffusion (57) characterizes the role configuration of the borderline patient. Identity diffusion occurs at a time when developmental experiences require commitment to physical intimacy, occupational choice, energetic competition, and psychosocial self-definition. Because the borderline person has no clear sense of values, interests, and personal causation, making decisions and succeeding in any direction are perceived as potentially constricting further tentative choices. Thus the borderline person may have a sense of being pushed into a role which does not feel "real," or which is too demanding. However, the borderline person's attempts to avoid choice lead to a sense of outer isolation and inner vacuum. Although painful, this avoidance of roles allows the borderline person to maintain indefinitely a condition of continuing possibility, dependence and freedom from the demands of reality. In so doing, the borderline person never satisfactorily assumes the roles of worker, student, friend, and so on.

HABITS

Because the borderline patient has not fully assumed roles, they do not serve as an organizing framework for the development of habits. The state of identity diffusion is expressed behaviorally in patterns of procrastination and postponement of role obligations. Study and work habits are poor, marked by an inability to consistently apply effort. Response patterns become limited and rigid or, conversely, unmodulated and impulsive (198). Impulsive habit disorders such as substance abuse, eating disorders, kleptomania and self-mutilation have been widely noted in borderline persons (4, 86, 184).

Performance

SKILLS

The performance deficits of borderline patients are fairly subtle, leading to the impression that borderline patients could perform but rebelliously refuse to do so. This is only partly true. Cognition and perceptual motor functioning remain intact, intelligence and talent are often obvious, and a superficial social adaptiveness is maintained (86). However, process skills are impaired (198). For example, the borderline patient can often "talk a good show," acting out the outer manifestations of a role sustained by an inner fantasy (60). However, this masks a deficit in the ability to establish an orderly and meaningful sequence of steps toward goal attainment. When such problem solving is required, the person may become rigid or impulsive, or unable to concentrate on required tasks (57).

Environment

For most children, there is an obvious advantage to growing up, because getting older means being able to participate in a wider range of occupations and environmental settings. The borderline person, however, is not prepared to cope with changing occupational and environmental demands. However, as long as the caretaker and the environment remain consistent, the child's functioning appears fairly normal and well adapted. The child takes cues from adults such as the mother or teacher and is able to adequately fulfill task demands. Warning signals such as overinvolvement in fantasy, outbursts of rage and general unhappiness are often overlooked because the child is "functioning" or "doing well in school."

It is only during adolescence, when the environmental press for role internalization increases dramatically, that the disorder becomes glaringly apparent. The achievement of adult roles requires a level of autonomy the borderline person has not attained. As the adolescent moves from the structure of home and school and can no longer rely on strong environmental cues, the deficits of habituation and skill and the central lack of volitional identity become obvious. With few exploratory strategies, the borderline person becomes extremely impulsive and erratic. Meaningless skills can no longer be incorporated into meaningful roles and the sense of emptiness and futility becomes unbearable. Unable to assume an autonomous role, the borderline person continually fails to respond to the press of social groups and organizations.

The task environment becomes a further source of overarousal when demands for complex skills and flexibility of performance increase. Because the borderline individual may approach all tasks with the need to achieve, rather than viewing them as opportunities for playful exploration, the consequences of failure are perceived as extreme and highly arousing.

Assessment

Establishing mutual collaboration is the key to successful evaluation of the borderline patient. Because the borderline person has the dual impulse to please and to frustrate a perceived authority, there is a likelihood that in the absence of a trusting relationship, the therapist will be unable to obtain accurate data. The borderline person may color or falsify self-description to impress or mislead the therapist.

Because the borderline person must attain insight into his or her patterns of internal organization, assessment should allow the patient, with the therapist, to explore characteristics of his or her interests, values, personal causation, and so on. Both the therapist's knowledge of the patient and the patient's self-knowledge are important for the therapeutic process. When an exploratory environment is maintained the patient can more comfortably examine these painful issues and begin to set nonthreatening goals related to change.

Once a safe context of exploration has been established, a variety of evaluation tools (Table 15.1) which provide an opportunity for the client to organize historical information independ-

Table 15.1.
Occupational status, recommended assessments and treatment considerations for the borderline patient

Occupational status	Recommended assessments	Treatment considerations
VOLITION		
Personal causation		
May not develop belief in skill or in the efficacy of skill	Internal/External Scale Initial Vocational Screening Form (IVSF) Occupational History (OH)	Establish a safe play environment as a context for exploring and developing new skills
Because achievement is aimed at obtaining approval, may feel helpless and be externally oriented	Occupational Questionnaire (OQ)	Develop parameters for goal setting which enable awareness of gains in skills and efficacy of skills
Values		
May perceive work/task behaviors as meaningless and overvalue creative pursuits	IVSF, OH, OQ	Stress a dual focus on engagement in activity and observation of one's reactions to activity
Personal standards vacillate from perfectionistic to inappropriately low Tendency to form unrealistic occupational goals		Therapist should not allow meaningless activity to go on too long without assisting client in establishing a meaningful context Values clarification and occupational choice activities may help development of realistic occupational goals
Interests		
Interests are often fantasized rather than real, leading to low potency Range of interests narrows Creative interests may predominate	OH, IVSF Self-Directed Search Interest Checklist	Encourage open-ended exploration of various occupations in different graded settings including workshop, home, volunteer job and classroom, with emphasis first on discovering what is intrinsically pleasurable, then increased competence
HABITUATION		
Roles		
Adults are not utilized as occupational role models	OH, IVSF Role Checklist Role Performance Scale (RPS)	The occupational therapist should function as mentor and role model for joyful, productive activity
Sustained identity diffusion results in avoidance of commitment to any adult roles		The therapeutic milieu should provide many opportunities to practice roles and obtain feedback regarding role performance
Habits		
Habits are consistent with the avoidance of role obligations and tend to include procrastination, impulsivity, rigidity, and inability to sustain effort	OQ, RPS	Treatment program should emphasize enactment of routine behaviors related to acceptable work peformance

Table 15.1.—*Continued*

Occupational status	Recommended assessments	Treatment considerations
Study and work habits especially suffer		Relationship between maladaptive habit patterns and inability to successfully internalize a worker role should be explored
		Client should develop awareness of effects of destructive habit patterns and explore and practice replacements for these habits

PERFORMANCE

Skills

Cognitive, perceptual and motor skills intact	IVSF, OH, RPS	Problem-solving skills should be taught and practiced in individual and group settings; application of these skills to real life situations should be emphasized
Verbal expressive abilities are generally excellent and may mask deficient problem-solving skills, causing client to appear more functional than he or she actually is	Clinical observation	
Interpersonal skills may be deficient as relationships tend to be superficial		Skills for new and unfamiliar roles should be taught

ENVIRONMENT

Childhood often did not take place in safe and playful arena	OH, IVSF, RPS	Treatment program must communicate that it is safe to try new behaviors and take risks
When environmental press remains consistent and unchanging, child often performed well		Level of press for skilled performance should be consistent with level attained by client
During adolescence, involvement in wider range of settings with increasing demands for flexible behavior leads to erratic and impulsive behavior		New roles and skills should be practiced in a variety of settings, to increase spontaneity and flexibility of behaviors
Demands for skilled performance are often overarousing		

ently and then to share conclusions with the therapist can be effectively used. The *St. Lukes A. M. Day Center Initial Vocational Screening Form* was developed expressly for this purpose. Vocational interest assessments, which the client can grade and interpret independently are also helpful as a basis for treatment planning.

Principles of Treatment

The primary occupational dysfunction of the borderline patient occurs at the level of exploratory play and becomes evident in the inability to perform autonomous adult roles. The purpose of occupational therapy treatment is the modification of the system's maladaptive cycle by allowing for the development of a solid exploratory base; graded and diversified experiential occupations must be provided which allow for movement from exploration to competence to achievement. Specific treatment strategies are noted in Table 15.1.

When a data base is identified, initial treatment goals and a time frame can be set. This also involves collaboration. For example, a patient who has failed three times at school and whose only explanation is, "I get bored, I lose my motivation," may wish intensely to return immediately to school. The therapist acknowledges and supports the importance the patient places on school, but points out that the cause of repeated failure is not clearly understood and failure could recur. The agreed upon plan might be that the patient will spend 3 months in the student group doing assignments and noticing his or her own reactions to the process carefully to discover what gets in the way of school achievement. Further decisions about school may be made at that point.

Because exploration is so central to the therapeutic process, principles of treatment concern the creation of a safe, interesting and playful context. To allow for the development of adaptive cycles of occupational behavior, a setting which makes clear, consistent functional demands within a specific time frame is necessary. This provides both the safe environment necessary for the emergence of spontaneous work and play, and a predictable setting to practice adult roles.

Within such a setting, the therapist acts as a mentor to genuine playful exploration, appreciating patients' play efforts and their struggle with meeting and failing to meet expectations. In the case of the borderline patient, this means the occupational therapist must constantly unhook him/herself from being the object of the patient's need and rage to help the patient notice and focus on the doing experience. This may involve honest confrontation of maladaptive behaviors. For example, in a therapeutic group designed as a classroom learning experience, a patient, Ann, hears the assignment and responds, "I want to throw spit balls at you! I forgot my pencil. What if we all refuse to do it?" The occupational therapist asks Ann if she has always tended to respond rebelliously when faced with a new school demand. Ann becomes thoughtful and answers, "I guess so, I always

find it very threatening." The occupational therapist suggests that Ann try to notice what happens to that rebellious feeling as she struggles with the new work and Ann is able to begin the project.

The level of activity must be neither over- nor underarousing, since these persons have difficulty regulating arousal for themselves. In either case, poor performance would result. To further curiosity, goals can be process oriented, rather than concerned with achievement of functional results. In other words, the purpose is exploration, to find out what activities are interesting and meaningful to the person, to be able to choose realistic, pleasurable occupations.

The logic of this treatment approach follows from the hierarchical nature of the exploration to achievement continuum. In the normal person achievement level occupational behavior builds upon prior successful exploratory experiences. Because the borderline person has had an early unsuccessful and dissatisfying experience with exploration, proceeding to the achievement level is constrained by incomplete and distorted conditions in the system resulting from the poor exploration experience. By returning to an exploratory level and allowing success within it, the patient is enabled to enter the achievement level for intrinsic reasons and thus to derive satisfaction from achievement.

BORDERLINE PERSONALITY DISORDER CASE: ANNA

Anna, who is 28 years old, was referred to day treatment after inpatient treatment for severe and debilitating bulimarexia of 3 years duration. She has a primary *Diagnostic and Statistic Manual* (*DSM*)-III diagnosis of anorexia nervosa and a secondary diagnosis of borderline personality disorder.

History

Anna is the only child of older parents who were both involved in the theater. She remembers her father as being very passive and distant. Her alcoholic mother appears to have been simultaneously devouring and devaluing. Anna recalls her mother telling her repeatedly, "You're me and I'm you. I'm the only one who will ever love you," and, "Aside from your music you're worthless." She also reports periods of sexual abuse from her mother. Anna's parents are still alive, but she left home at an early age and maintains only superficial contact with them.

Anna was a child musical prodigy with several early performing successes. While she initially found composing fun and natural, she came to resent the tremendous pressure to produce placed on her by parents and teachers. Practicing took the place of play in her childhood. She gradually developed an image of herself as ugly and lonely with her music her only means of attracting attention. As a young adult she successfully composed for a rock musician and made several recordings. She did not develop any enduring close relationships and began the escalating cycle of binge eating and vomiting which resulted in her hospitalization.

Assessments

At the beginning of day treatment Anna had returned to binge eating and vomiting. The use of a semistructured interview format and the St. Luke's A. M. Day Center Initial Vocational Screening Form yielded the following information.

While Anna strongly believed in her musical ability, she had for several years felt totally blocked in using her talent. She did not feel she had anything else to offer. Her external locus of control was revealed in a persistent tendency to feel helpless and victimized, and in her attempts to embellish or distort accounts of her actions in order to gain praise.

Anna complained of feeling empty and worthless. She overvalued musical achievement and devalued any other use of time. She was also far more concerned with "finding love," than with any values related to activity. A newly emerging value since her hospitalization was the wish to "find out who I am."

Anna's range of interests was extremely narrow. As with values, she was primarily interested in music and establishing a loving relationship. Currently, she did not actually engage in any interests.

For the past 3 years all role-related behavior had disappeared due to the strength of her habit disorder. Recently, in the hospital, she had assumed the patient role and become concerned about the severity of her illness and the extent to which it limited and even threatened her life.

Anna's bulimarexic symptoms dominated her life. Here is her own account of a day alone: "wake up, prepare food, binge and vomit, wash dishes, pass out, wake up, call up whomever I've made plans with and cancel, prepare food . . . ." She rarely followed through on plans to socialize or engage in leisure activities. She often lied to cover up the extent of her eating disorder and the inordinate sums of money spent on food.

Anna had above average intelligence and reported good musical and typing skills. Process and problem-solving skills were rigid and ineffective. For example, when a friend put pressure on her to repay a loan, her only response was, "I don't have the money so I might as well kill myself."

Anna had been a performer since her childhood. Her musical talent and her incessant lying were both used to please or impress the audience and obtain the desired loving response. Having never developed an authentic sense of self or means of self-expression, she felt enormously empty inside; her excessive binge eating and vomiting seemed to be a frantic effort to fill the emptiness. Anna's occupational status is summarized in Table 15.2.

Treatment

Day treatment in a specialized program for borderline patients gave Anna an opportunity for safe exploratory activity. Slowly, she was able to develop a sense of her own identity and effectiveness. This proceeded in several stages. Table 15.2 summarizes treatment.

PHASE 1

The first issue for Anna was attendance. Her preference was to stay home and binge and vomit. However, staff and member encouragement, pleasurable socialization with other members, and positive feedback from her beginning explorations in groups led to regular attendance within several weeks.

Anna and her therapist agreed that she would choose the groups she felt were important for herself and would set her own time frame for goal achievement and discharge. She was required, however, to pick specific times and stick to them. She agreed to try a broad array of activities to discover what she enjoyed. There was no staff pressure to return to music.

Over a year and a half Anna was involved in several activity and vocational groups led by the occupational therapist and other activity staff.

In collaboration with the occupational therapist, Anna began working on fingerpainting. She and the therapist painted together and for the first time she enjoyed an expansive, messy, exploratory activity in the presence of an accepting, participating adult. After this she experimented with writing. She began

Table 15.2.
Anna's occupational status, treatment goals and intervention

Occupational status	Treatment goals and interventions
VOLITION	
Personal causation	
Externally oriented; felt controlled by others and did things more for the praise from others than for intrinsic pleasure	Increase feelings of internal control by emphasizing exploratory, playful nature of activities rather than relationship aspects
Values	
Overvalued music, although new value of self-discovery was emerging	Explore role of music in her life and ways of drawing on talents without making music a major life commitment
Interests	
Major interest was music; currently did not enact any interests	Participate in variety of new leisure activities to develop interests
HABITUATION	
Roles	
Except for patient role, no roles organized present life	In prevocational group, identify and practice skills necessary to work role; assimilate work role through part-time job and continued support from day center
	Explore additional roles, such as volunteer, and ways in which musical abilities can be used in such roles
Habits	
Habits dominated by cycles of eating, binges and purging	Identify ways in which these habits interfere with performance of new roles
PEFORMANCE	
Skills	
Above average cognitive skills; musical talent; good typing skills	Increase planning skills by giving responsibility for setting time frames for goal achievement
Poor problem-solving skills manifested in inability to plan sequence of steps, to identify alternative solutions, and to follow through with plans	Provide opportunities for decision making related to assumption of new roles

with "bad" poems, then writing "bad" songs, and finally, moved to writing good songs, all at her own pace and with a minimum of anxiety. The occupational therapist soon learned to engage with Anna but to provide a minimum of feedback regarding her productions, as this quickly caused a regression to Anna's previous mode of focusing on the relationship to the exclusion of the activity.

In a prevocational group, Anna initially felt unable to work at all. After several months of treatment she was in serious financial diffi-

culty which was contributing to suicidal feelings. With staff help in identifying all possible solutions to the problem, she finally chose to take a part-time typing job, fearing she would despise it. In the prevocational group she was invited to explore her feelings and reactions to the job as fully as possible. Within several months she began to take pride in her extremely fast typing and in her learning capacity. Soon she was calling her job the one neutral relaxing area of her life. In this group, her use of the occupational therapist as a "worker" role model was a key factor in her vocational development.

Anna spent many months grappling with her feelings about music, finally concluding that she did not have to be a musician to have a worthwhile life. Toward the end of her treatment she was able to use her musical talents to prepare and run a series of sing-alongs as a volunteer at the day center and other hospital programs. This was both successful and rewarding to her. She was particularly proud of her much improved ability to make a commitment and follow through a logical sequence of steps to meet a realistic goal. Near the time of discharge she was offered and accepted a commission to write the music for a university show.

Outcomes

At the time of discharge Anna had significantly improved. Her increased self-regard was expressed through a more stylish and mature mode of dress, better grooming, greater participation in large community meetings, and a dramatic decrease in lying. She was more aware of her skills and able to use them in productive ways (the part-time job and the sing-alongs). She was better able to make decisions and to work toward goals. She had a more realistic sense of the role music could play in her life. Her range of interests had widened to include reading, clothes shopping and intellectual conversations. In addition to her role as day center member she had resumed the roles of worker, volunteer and friend.

Problems remained however. Anna was not able to stop binge eating and vomiting for longer than a 1½-month period. At discharge she binged and vomited about once a day. Her social network remained limited and she still tended to isolate herself when upset. The separation from the day center and her close relationships with staff and members was a big adjustment. Continued individual outpatient therapy will be necessary to help Anna maintain the gains she has made. A piece of writing shortly before discharge shows Anna's recognition of her progress and of her continuing difficulties:

"Getting better" shows itself in the most surprising ways. For the first time I saw a task through, on my own time, without overwhelming myself or becoming angry and feeling "put-upon." Even the collating and photocopying, which to me was always so odious I wouldn't do it, was simply a task that needed to be done.... This way I was not paralyzed, as I would have been if I went about it the other way.

This is only a song sheet for a 20-min sing along—no big deal—but to me it is a symbol of the definite change in the way I go about doing things. The world isn't so black and white any more ... although sometimes it is. But when I see it that way I know something's wrong!

DEPRESSIVE DISORDER

In the United States, more people seek mental health services for depression than for any other problem (62). Not only is depression widespread as a primary diagnosis, but it often underlies other significant disorders (117, 170). Suicide, alcoholism and drug abuse all show a significant link to depression.

While there is extensive literature and research on adult depression, only recently have authors studied and identified depression in children and adolescents as a clinical phenomenon which is similar to adult depression but manifested differently (171, 191, 236). Clinicians and researchers now recognize that truancy, running away from home, aggressive behavior, stealing, and sexual promiscuity may be associated with childhood and adolescent depression (4). Thus, not only is depression manifested differently at different life stages but the tumultuous life changes related to adolescence may make the individual particularly vulnerable to a depressive disorder (117).

There are numerous ways to classify depression. One view places depression on a continuum, ranging from a normal mood state of feeling blue or sad to severe depression characterized by psychotic features and a total breakdown in occupational functioning. Another conceptualizes depression as a disease, distinct from normal grief or sadness (5, 107).

Theories of biochemical and genetic etiology endorse the view of depression as a disease (174, 248). Psychoanalytic (2, 16, 164), behavioral (12, 20, 130, 207), sociological (52, 182), and existential models (11, 43, 66, 243) support the view of depression as a continuum.

Ultimately, a multidimensional theory positing an interaction between social, motivational and biochemical factors may be the most useful to understanding depression (2). For example, stressful experiences or an inability to explore one's environment and experience success may precipitate biochemical changes in the nervous system, leading to depressed affect. Similarly, a biochemical predisposition toward depression may impair a person's ability to find pleasure in life events (2). Use of the model of human occupation to view the depressed individual addresses that part of the total complex of factors in depression that is most relevant to occupational therapy.

Because the severity of depression may vary widely, in one individual and across individuals, occupational dysfunction in depressed persons may range from helplessness to achievement. Depression may express itself in the workplace with decreased productivity and motivation, in school with failing grades, in daily living activities by a disregard for grooming and hygiene, and in leisure activities by a lack of participation and/or a lack of enjoyment. While some individuals may experience a disruption in all areas of occupational behavior, others may be able to maintain high levels of achievement. However, these individuals are engaged in a constant struggle between their attainments and their fear of failure and feelings of incompetence (67). High achievers may also be at risk for depression because of their stressful and unbalanced lifestyles.

Volition

PERSONAL CAUSATION

Depressive behavior is associated with the belief that one lacks control to successfully master the environment (126). The depressed individual typically sees him/herself as a victim of external events, and the effects of personal actions are seen instead as being the result of luck or chance. The depressive person who lacks belief in personal control is unable to choose a course of action.

Studies of locus of control in depressed individuals (1, 14, 127) found severe depression and an external orientation to the environment to be significantly related. Similarly depressed children often perceive their failures as being caused by external uncontrollable events and, lacking self-confidence, they become unable to solve problems that they have previously completed successfully (50, 51).

External orientation may be reinforced by hosptalization, the medical interventions of antidepressant medication and electroconvulsive therapy, and loss of responsibility for daily occupations. That is, depressed persons may come to see themselves as incapable of managing their lives and influencing their mood if external interventions are emphasized by medical personnel. For example, a severely depressed woman who felt very helpless was advised by her psychiatrist to stay in bed and rest until the medication worked. Such a recommendation only serves to reinforce feelings of external control.

The issue of locus of control is not clear-cut, however. Individuals who have a need to control activities and choices completely and who score at the extreme end of internal control also can experience depressive disorder (188). In these persons, the extreme internal orientation seems to lead to rigid and inflexible behavior patterns in work, daily living and leisure. This imbalance in system output (i.e. all work and no play) may be a factor in depression for some persons. Further, these persons may have an unrealistic expectation for internal control which leads to negative self-assessment and a self-critical attitude.

INTERESTS

Depressed persons frequently indicate few current interests, even though past enjoyment and participation in interests may have been substantial (4). Researchers have found a significant relation between depressed mood and decreased enjoyment in activities (87, 128, 129, 142, 231). In addition, they have found that when subjects increased their activities in certain spheres their mood improved as well (231).

There are varied expressions of discrimination, pattern and potency of interest in depressive disorder. For example, a person may discriminate or pursue interests exclusively in the area of work. This imbalanced patterning of interests may contribute to depression because, if work becomes difficult or nonpleasurable, the person has no other area of interests from which to derive satisfaction. Similarly, the person who has focused all his or her interests on work has no source of replacement if retirement or other events necessitate giving up work.

Often, the loss of interest in activities may be precipitated by other events in the person's life. For example, one patient who recently lost his wife stopped participating in all activities that had been joint interests of both him and his wife. The child and adolescent may show decreased interest in school and play activities (6, 147). Although young depressed children can often be easily engaged in playful and interesting activities, when left to their own resources they become withdrawn and show little activity.

VALUES

Along with decreased interest and lack of control over events, the depressed individual may either question, completely give up, or rigidly adhere to previously held values regarding occupation. Because many depressed persons see the future as hopeless, occupations that were previously valued often come to be regarded as meaningless (243). When this occurs, previous standards of performance also become unimportant. Many adolescents express this value loss or lack of meaning and purpose by taking drugs or joining various religious sects or a delinquent peer group which may provide the adolescent with an identity otherwise lacking (3). One study of college students who had attempted suicide showed that despite many social contacts, good academic performance and positive family relationships, these students found life to be meaningless (67).

Overall, depressed individuals tend to experience time as moving slowly or being monotonous and lacking meaning (160). Orientation to the future is particularly deficient in depressive disorder; depressed individuals show extreme limitation in the years projected into the future (46, 246). In addition, their goals or plans for the future become limited (23, 46). Other depressed persons may set unrealistic goals which are unattainable using an "all or nothing" standard (156).

Habituation

ROLES

Usually, the inability of depressed individuals to meet the demands of current roles leads to hospitalization. While severe depression may involve total disruption of role behavior, less severe depression may be associated with role imbalance, a failure to match internal and external expectations for role performance (e.g. the individual occupying a new role as a student who finds expectations for time use, study habits, etc., were not as anticipated), or role loss.

In depressed children and adolescents, change in a family role due to the loss of a parent or significant other is particularly critical. A study of adolescent suicide attempts found that parents of these adolescents had died, left the home or remarried in 3 times as many cases as compared to a control group (227). In addition, adolescent suicide attempters appear to have a high incidence of separation from their mothers early in their life (228).

Women are particularly vulnerable to depression through role loss, especially in middle age (68). As children grow up and leave home, and parents die, both the mother and daughter role become suspended. Because many older women currently do not work, they lack other roles to substitute for this loss. The interaction of cultural values complicates the meaning of this loss, since Western society traditionally values the roles of wife and mother for women and the worker role for men. Thus, even for women who work, the loss of family roles may lead to the development of depression. Similarly, when men lose the worker role, they are at risk for depression. Although these cultural standards are changing, the implication is that it is critical to occupy more than one meaningful role, so that if one role is lost, there are other roles from which to derive satisfaction (68).

An illustrative case is that of Olivia (68), a middle-aged, divorced woman living alone in a new city. Her three children had been her primary interests and source of satisfaction while other social interactions consisted of infrequent contacts with individuals in a religious organization. Because she did not value her job as a caretaker for children of a neighboring family, she had little opportunity to experience competence and pleasure in her life and subsequently became depressed.

HABITS

Because time seems to be passing slowly to the depressed person (160), normal routines may be experienced as being inordinately long. Further, typically automatic routines may instead require constant effort to complete and maintain as the depressed person feels lethargic and unmotivated (4). Eventually, the depressed person may disregard routines rather than expend the energy; this may affect habits related to a number of roles. For example, if one neglects grooming and then goes to work or school, problems may quickly develop around the inappropriate grooming for work and social interactions. Peers and co-workers may ridicule or shun the individual leading to further isolation and withdrawal by the depressed person. Or, if the sleeping habits of the depressed individual are disrupted, he or she may be unable to rise on time for work. Because the depressed person may be working more slowly than usual, he or she may not be able to complete a day's work in the time required.

Performance

Depressed adults and adolescents typically have a prior history of adequate performance skills relevant to major life roles. However, these skills can be temporarily disrupted in depression, and it may even appear that the depressed individual is deficient in certain skills. For example, decreased concentration often accompanies depression and can lead to poor performance on work or school tasks (120). Poor performance, in turn, can frustrate and exacerbate the depressed mood.

In children and adolescents, depression may interfere with the development of performance skills that need to be mastered at a particular age. Conversely, hyperactive or learning-disabled children who are unable to acquire successful academic skills may be particularly vulnerable to depression (120). Therefore, in children, adolescents and adults, depression can both lead to the disruption or interruption of skills, as well as reflect existing skill deficits.

Depressed children and adults may experience psychomotor retardation or a slowing of purposeful movement (4, 77). Movement may be so slow as to impair all areas of occupational performance. Conversely, adolescents often show an increase in motor activity, evidenced in aggressive and self-destructive behavior (3).

Social and interactional skills are also often a problem in depressive disorder (41, 88, 134). Conversation styles tend to be self-centered, negative and pessimistic (156), and depressed individuals tend to be unassertive in their interactions (156). Individuals who attempted suicide are often characterized by decreased social involvement (135). Depressed children and adolescents also demonstrate deficient social skills (186). This failure to establish interpersonal relationships with peers and significant others leads to a vicious cycle of increased withdrawal and isolation (3).

Environment

Interestingly, depression may initially appear to be unrelated to the surroundings of the person. For instance, depressed persons often reside in comfortable, well furnished homes, their families may be supportive, and opportunities for involvement in stimulating tasks may be prevalent. Nevertheless, the depressed person may not be interacting with this environment. Further, as the person becomes increasingly depressed, he or she may begin to find the press communicated by these surroundings to be inconsistent with his or her own expectations for behavior. For example, someone who is convinced that she is too old to do anything may find the sociocultural stimulation of a large city to be threatening. In some cases, the person's response may be to physically shut out the external environment, e.g. retreating to bed.

In other cases depression may clearly be related to a mismatch between the person's abilities and environmental press. For example, a woman with residual physical deficits from a stroke attempted to maintain a volunteer role in an organization that apparently highly valued physical competence. Her inability to fit into this setting contributed to her feelings of inadequacy and depression. However, after being trained for a clerical task in another organization, she was able to carry out and enjoy her volunteer role.

With children and adolescents, the environmental level of social groups and organizations may be particularly critical in the development of depression (187). For example, parental restrictions on play and exploration or unrealistic expectations for school achievement may dampen the desire to explore and experiment with new behaviors and skills.

Assessment

Because of the extreme sense of hopelessness and doom experienced by the depressed person, engaging the individual in the assessment process can be quite difficult. Frequently patients will refuse an occupational therapy assessment stating they have no interests, no future, and want to be left alone. A strategy to deal with this extreme hopelessness is to first acknowledge the patient's depression and accompanying lack of occupational behavior, indicating a desire to know about those occupations that were enjoyable prior to the depression. In addition, the atmosphere for the assessment should be one in which the patient's feelings of responsibility and control are maximized.

Due to the short-term nature of most treatment of depressed persons, assessment and intervention occur simultaneously. It is important to begin as soon as possible to support the depressed individual's innate urge to explore and master.

While volition appears to be the primary subsystem affected directly in depression, the status of both habituation and performance also needs to be addressed during assessment. Table 15.3 illustrates recommended assessment procedures.

An occupational history is in many cases the best first choice of assessment. This can even be done at bedside and it can be part of the initial rapport-building process. Through this interview the therapist gains an overview of the patient's occupational participation and general status of all three subsystems. While the patient may be describing him or herself as totally incompetent, this type of assessment usually uncovers areas in which the person has been functioning quite competently and successfully in the past.

Treatment

Assuming that the person has adequately developed skills, adaptive occupational behavior in the depressed individual will be enhanced as volition becomes more organized. In general, then, treatment should emphasize the renewal or stimulation of interest in activities and the establishment of commitments to realistic life goals.

As soon as possible, interests and activities compatible with the individual's previous occupational roles should be engaged in by the patient since volitional change can only occur through feedback on behavior. These activities should be graded to increasingly represent the social and task demands inherent in daily life. Along with the revitalization of interest, habits need to be renewed. A goal for hospitalization is to reestablish occupational routines. For example, providing the patient with a schedule of hospital therapies, library times, and gift shop times, and expecting proper attire to therapy helps reactivate habits. In addition, some settings enable patients to transport themselves to and from therapy. This is important in giving the patient control and responsibility in a hospital environment that typically denies patients control of their lives. Specific treatment strategies are described in Table 15.3.

DEPRESSION CASE: MARY

Mary is a 45-year-old mother of six children aged 5–25 years. She, her husband, and their four youngest children live comfortably on the husband's income in a house which they own. The two oldest children are married and live nearby. Mary has a major affective disorder, major depression, and a history of substance abuse. On this occasion, Mary was hospitalized for persisting insomnia, loss of energy, indecisiveness, impulsive behavior, and psychomotor agitation.

The medical record revealed a history of suicidal attempts involving overdoses on prescribed medication. She has also abused street drugs and alcohol. In addition to a review of her past medical record, Mary's assessment included the Occupational History, the Internal/External Scale, the Time Reference Inventory—Shortened Form, the Expectancy Questionnaire, the Interest Checklist, the Role Checklist, and a simplified Occupational Questionnaire.

Prior Psychiatric Treatment

Mary has had seven short-term hospitalizations over the past 6 years, four of which occurred within the last 2 years. Although Mary has intermittently been involved in therapy with several different therapists for the last 10 years, she has engaged in therapy on a regular basis with the same psychiatrist for the past 1½ years.

Within the structure of occupational therapy, Mary had performed at a very competent level. However, when the structure was removed, Mary's performance deteriorated. She was unable to independently set goals. If she established goals with staff assistance, she was unable to follow through or sequence her behavior to attain goals.

Assessment Results

OCCUPATIONAL HISTORY

Mary grew up with her parents (who both had an eighth grade education), her two older brothers and two younger sisters. As a child, Mary never thought about what she wanted to be—this was discouraged by her family. She felt that her parents did not value education and described them as "perfectionists who were overly neat and clean." She had little responsibility at home because her parents felt that she could not do anything right or fast enough. She recalled often feeling sad and spent the bulk of her time sleeping. She

Table 15.3.
Occupational status, recommended assessments and treatment considerations for persons with depressive disorder

Occupational status	Recommended assessments	Treatment considerations
	VOLITION	

Personal causation

Occupational status	Recommended assessments	Treatment considerations
Extreme external orientation (which may be reinforced by hospitalization and medical interventions) leads to a loss of responsibility for daily living	Internal/External Scale	Provide opportunities for personal control and responsibility in hospital; share results of assessments with patient; discuss goals for hospitalization giving patient some control and input concerning selection of goals
Extreme internal orientation may lead to rigid and inflexible behavior patterns in work, daily living and leisure	Occupational Questionnaire (OQ)	
	Occupational History (OH)	
	Automatic Thoughts Questionnaire	
Expectations of defeat, disappointment and failure lead to a tendency to give up and avoid further performance	Hopelessness Scale	Maintain an atmosphere of expectation for performance that also conveys confidence in patient's ability to perform
Negative self-evaluation; positive feedback regarding performance may be turned into negative evaluations	Occupational Case Analysis Interview and Rating Scale (OCAIRS)	Engage the patient in occupations in which he or she can expect to succeed and that show some tangible evidence of successful performance; as self-evaluations become more positive, complexity of tasks should be increased
Feelings of incompetence, belief that skills are no longer adequate to perform in various roles, and that these skills are depleted and can never be regained		Provide positive feedback for small successes; check patient's perception of feedback
		Identify activities in prehospitalization daily schedule that patient experienced as successful and satisfying

Values

Occupational status	Recommended assessments	Treatment considerations
Patient identifies few or limited goals	OCAIRS, OH, OQ	Values clarification exercises to identify and modify unrealistic goals
Discrepancies exist between goals and achievements; goals may be unrealistically high and grandiose, rigid or perfectionistic	Time Reference Inventory	
	Role Checklist (RC)	Encourage setting of behavior goals that can be worked on actively in hospital
Because time is perceived as moving slowly, self is likewise perceived as moving slowly and inefficiently		Encourage identification of long-range goals and intermediate steps necessary to attainment
Extreme limitation in future orientation		Explore reasons for choices of activities and meanings attached to their performance
Activities no longer meaningful		

Table 15.3.—*Continued*

Occupational status	Recommended assessments	Treatment considerations
Interests		
May have few current strong interests with limited participation in them, or, may express little enjoyment in an average number of activities in which participated Interest pattern may be narrow, e.g. emphasizing only work-related interests; if these interests then become unavailable, person has no other interesting activities from which pleasure can be derived	OH, OQ, OCAIRS Interest Checklist Pleasant Events Schedule III Unpleasant Events Schedule	Support and provide opportunities for participation in prior interests that are related to a valued role Monitor pleasure or enjoyment experienced in different events from Pleasant Events Schedule III and decrease participation in activities that are unpleasant; increase participation in activities found pleasurable Explore new interests and opportunities for participation in community Analyze current uses of time to identify ways of increasing time available for leisure occupations

HABITUATION

Occupational status	Recommended assessments	Treatment considerations
Roles		
May be total disruption of roles Lack of role balance, when one role, such as worker or family member, is overemphasized Loss of a valued role, through such events as retirement, divorce or other transitions; this can be especially problematic when first role is highly valued by one's cultural group	RC, OH, OQ, OCAIRS Role Performance Scale (RPS)	Encourage participation in occupations that support valued roles Use time management techniques to improve balance among roles Establish participation in new roles that can offer feelings of efficacy associated with previous roles
Habits		
Normal routines are no longer automatic as daily living tasks require constant effort Habits for grooming, housekeeping or work may be disregarded	OQ, OH, OCAIRS, RPS	Reestablish routines of daily living in the hospital Have balanced schedule of activities for hospital which supports valued roles Provide positive feedback and support for habits

PERFORMANCE

Occupational status	Recommended assessments	Treatment considerations
Skills		
Motor activity may be slowed Decreased concentration, inability to think clearly	OH, OCAIRS, RPS Clinical observation	Engage in sports, movement games, or exercise routines Set up specific time schedules for performing routine tasks

Table 15.3.—Continued

Occupational status	Recommended assessments	Treatment considerations
Inability to problem solve to accomplish goals		Assist patient in problem solving related to goal accomplishments, e.g. setting priorities and devising sequential action plans to accomplish goals
Interaction styles are self-centered, negative and pessimistic		
		Assertiveness training related to occupational roles
		Participation in groups relevant to interests to increase social interactions
	ENVIRONMENT	
Lack of interaction with environment; incongruency between environmental press, person's skills or self-perception of skills	OH, OCAIRS, RPS Family and Work Climate Scales Behavior setting observations	Expectations that others have may need to be modified Exploration of new settings that optimize persons' skills; use of graded activities so that press and skills are congruent

had no friends, spent little time with her siblings and, in general, felt uncomfortable around others.

Mary dropped out of school in the tenth grade because it became "boring." She worked as a receptionist in a physician's office for 2 years, a job she found satisfying and at which she felt competent, until she was married. After her marriage she moved with her husband who accepted a promotion out of state. She entered the homemaker role and eventually gave birth to six children. She attempted to be a "supermom" and a "super wife" but found caring for the children and maintaining the home overwhelmed her.

Mary enjoys homemaking responsibilities such as cleaning and laundry, and believes she is competent in these tasks but her performance has been sporadic. When depressed, which is frequent, she loses all desire to do anything and spends the bulk of her day in bed. Her family is appreciative when she performs homemaking tasks, but assumes the responsibility when she is depressed. She reported that she does not visit with neighbors and has no friends.

She stated she would like to pursue something else, in addition to being a homemaker, if her depression and anxiety did not interfere. She would like to return to school and become a nurse's assistant.

She reports past interests including ceram-

ics which she purused on and off for several years, but stopped 2 years ago because she felt she no longer "did it well." In addition, she was a member of a bowling league for 7 years which she stopped 5 years ago due to a knee injury. When her knee healed, she did not resume bowling. She also likes to read and collect figurines. At present she is unable to relate to the word "fun." For Mary, fun is "getting away" from whatever bothers her via sleep. For the past several years, she has done very little with her husband and children in terms of leisure. The family does not take vacations.

INTERNAL/EXTERNAL SCALE

Mary's score of 15 on this scale indicates a moderately external locus of control.

TIME REFERENCE INVENTORY— SHORTENED FORM

Responses to the Time Reference Inventory are presented in Table 15.4. Basically, Mary is more past than future oriented.

EXPECTANCY QUESTIONNAIRE

When asked what she planned to be doing a year from now, Mary responded "Have my house in order the way I always wanted it to be," and "Going to school either part time or full time." Five years hence she planned to be "working as a nurse" and in ten years to be "working and traveling." In 15 years she expected to be "working." Her responses indicate a strong desire to enter a worker role or at least to move beyond her present homemaker role by returning to school and getting preparation for work. Since her overall temporal orientation is to the past, these goals may represent wishful thinking more than clearly planned out objectives for the future.

MODIFIED INTEREST CHECKLIST

Mary was able to discriminate among interests. In the past year, she expressed strong interest in clothes, hairstyling and fishing, but did not pursue them on a regular basis. When Mary stopped bowling (one of her past strong interests), she lost both an avocational activity and a social support system.

Table 15.4.
Mary's responses to the Time Reference Inventory—Shortened Form

	Past	Present	Future
Negative items	4	1	0
Positive items	4	1	0
Neutral items	1	1	0
Years projected into the future	0		
Years projected into the past	21		
Average age focus	24		

Mary does not indicate strong interest in the past year in any of the activities associated with her primary role of homemaker (i.e. home decorating, home repairs, child care, cooking, shopping, mending, house cleaning). The lack of homemaker-related interests is congruent with her report on the Occupational Questionnaire that she does not like to prepare meals.

ROLE CHECKLIST

Mary's responses to the Role Checklist are presented in Table 15.5. Mary's primary occupational role is homemaker—a role she has conflicting feelings about. Mary reported no continuous roles and she lacks a balance of other roles in her life.

Mary indicated future participation in all roles except participant in organizations which she identified as not valuable. Mary's anticipation of future incumbency in almost every role indicates a possibility of future role conflict, and reflects her difficulty in setting goals and priorities for herself.

OCCUPATIONAL QUESTIONNAIRE

When data from this instrument and the Interest Checklist were compared, they revealed that prior to hospitalization Mary spent 60% of the time sleeping, 10% of the time watching television, 10% of the time getting her children ready for school and 10% visiting with her husband; she indicated some interest in these activities. The remaining 10% of the time she spent preparing meals, an activity in which she had no interest. She enacted no activities which were highly interesting and felt that she performed all activities average or well.

Table 15.5.
Mary's responses on the Role Checklist

Role	Past	Present	Future	Value of the role		
				Not at all	Some-what	Very
Student	X		X			X
Worker	X		X			X
Volunteer			X			X
Caregiver	X		X			X
Home maintainer	X		X			X
Friend			X		X	
Family member	X		X			X
Religious participant	X		X			X
Hobbyist/amateur	X		X		X	
Participant in organizations	X			X		

Occupational Status

Mary's occupational status is summarized in Table 15.6. Her performance in the homemaker role—her major role—is mood dependent as she often surrenders homemaking responsibilities to family members because she is "too depressed." When she did attend to homemaking tasks, she felt her performance was adequate, but her routine very unsatisfying. The homemaker role does not provide her with a sense of worth or meaning and she lacks a healthy integration of roles which could provide her meaning. Mary abandoned her previous leisure roles of ceramics and bowling and it has been difficult for her to resume participation because of her tendency to be overly critical of her performance coupled with her anticipation of unsuccessful outcomes.

Occupational Therapy Interventions

Since it was unrealistic to Mary to abandon the homemaker role, the long-term goal of occupational therapy was to assist her in selecting, pursuing and performing other gratifying occupational roles and to maintain a balance among roles.

Another goal was for Mary to perform roles and habits despite her mood. Treatment was addressed in three phases. Mary gave input, agreed upon the sequence and the treatment team (psychiatrist, nurses and social worker) supported the plan.

PHASE 1

Mary began participating in the regular occupational therapy program on the unit. During this phase, she learned problem solving, planning, and time-management skills. The discrepancies among her valued roles and role performance were explored and clarified. She established realistic long- and short-term goals, prioritized future roles and identified the behaviors necessary to attain goals. Mary decided to pursue her roles related to homemaking (i.e. family member, caregiver, home maintainer) as well as roles of hobbyist and volunteer.

She explored and generated new interests in woodworking, cross-stitching, and caning, and resumed her past interest in ceramics in an atmosphere that allowed her to be successful but not critical of her performance.

She explored ways of attending to homemaking tasks and performing roles despite her mood. For example, she identified that instead of cooking a gourmet meal when depressed, she could prepare simpler meals with a minimum of effort and yet not forego her responsibilities.

PHASE 2

The objective of the second phase was to allow Mary the opportunity to independently implement what she had learned in the first phase by enacting roles she planned to perform upon discharge. Mary thus eased out of the structured occupational therapy program and was responsible for scheduling time for her homemaker and hobbyist roles (first in the hospital, then at home), and for carrying out such tasks as laundry, leisure interests and planning and preparing nutritious meals. During this phase, Mary kept a schedule that outlined her daily plans. At the end of each day she filled out a second schedule detailing what she had actually done. Both schedules were reviewed with her by the occupational therapist.

PHASE 3

In the third phase Mary performed the additional role of volunteer, working 3 times a week as a nurse's aide. She pursued leisure interests, maintained a balance among roles and went home on leaves of absence to attend to homemaking and caregiving responsibilities.

Outcomes

Mary rapidly progressed from phase 1 to phase 2. In the beginning of phase 2, she opted to plan and prepare lavish lunches on a daily basis in addition to following her busy occupational therapy and ward schedules. This proved to be overarousing and she experienced increased symptomatology. Rather than cutting back her schedule which she may have viewed as a failure, simpler lunches and time-management skills were reviewed and alternatives explored. For example, Mary decided to prepare a basic lunch that could be served several ways. This enabled Mary to continue to prepare lunches 7 days a week, which thus became a successful experience for her. Her symptomatology concurrently subsided.

Three months postdischarge, Mary was successfully functioning in the roles of caregiver, family member, part-time volunteer, and hobbyist despite bouts of depression.

ANOREXIA NERVOSA

Anorexia nervosa is an eating disorder that is characterized by an intense and unrealistic fear of becoming fat, distorted body perception and

Table 15.6.
Occupational status, treatment goals and intervention for Mary, a depressed woman

Occupational status	Treatment goals and intervention

VOLITION

Personal causation

Historically and currently does not believe in efficacy of her skills; anticipates failure

Expresses a feeling of loss of control due to her mental illness; is externally oriented

Explore new activities in a setting where outcomes are inconsequential; reality-test appropriateness of short-term goals and plans to ensure success

Provide opportunities for decision-making in activities and in planning treatment

Values

Holds excessively high personal standards

Discrepancy between role performance and valued roles

Although she is oriented to past, she can identify future goals; however, may not be able to sequence behavior to attain goals

Provide feedback regarding high standards; help monitor appropriateness of expectations for performance

Through values clarification explore discrepancies between values and actual performance

Treatment program should be relevant to future goals, e.g. begin volunteer role as nurse's aide to gain experience related to future work goals

Interests

Able to discriminate interests

Decreased potency; does not enact many prior interests and many current activities are considered strong interests

Incorporate past interests in treatment program; identify ways to pursue these, as well as new interests, following discharge

HABITUATION

Roles

Primary occupational role of homemaker causes conflicting feelings; lacks a balance or healthy integration of other roles in daily life

Internalized expectations for homemaker role are to be a "supermom" and "superwife"

Role performance is mood dependent

Possible future role conflict

Develop additional occupational roles while still in hospital (hobbyist, volunteer) and plan ways to continue their enactment following discharge

Provide opportunity to learn that role obligations can be met flexibly; plan alternative behaviors that will allow her to meet role responsibilities when depressed

Through values clarification, help prioritize future roles

Habits

Does not carry out routine tasks when depressed

Imbalance between work, play, leisure, and rest—was sleeping more than half the day

Encourage responsibility for scheduling daily plans while in hospital; compare with actual accomplishments

Maintain realistic balance among activities while in hospital

PERFORMANCE

Skills

Impaired process skills; interpersonal and perceptual-motor skills intact

Maintain existing skills while in hospital through group and individual activities

Develop process skills through such activities as daily scheduling, problem solving, and so on

Table 15.6.—*Continued*

Occupational status	Treatment goals and intervention
ENVIRONMENT	
Family is supportive, but currently is the only social group to which Mary belongs	Develop roles that will involve Mary in other social groups, e.g. bowling league
New or complex tasks initially appear over-arousing, leading to poor performance and other symptomatic behaviors	Through task simplification, help her to recognize her ability to modulate task demands

a weight loss of approximately 25% of the original body weight (4). While no physical disease precipitates the disorder, the severe weight loss often leads to metabolic and other physical changes. These changes are usually responsible for bringing the individual to medical attention, since, as a rule, the person denies that anything is wrong and is resistive to treatment (4).

Anorexia nervosa generally afflicts female adolescents,† many of whom come from middle- and upper-class families (72, 100). Anorexia has also been observed in women in young adulthood and is frequently a secondary diagnosis with another psychiatric disorder, e.g. depression or borderline personality disorder. In addition, anorexic behaviors are very prevalent among women who may not come to the attention of the health care system (218), suggesting that a spectrum of disordered eating behaviors may be clinically more useful than merely diagnosing the presence or absence of anorexia nervosa.

While the aspect most focused on in anorexia is the eating disorder and its biological consequences, the anorexic person typically exhibits an occupational dysfunction which makes occupational therapy intervention relevant. In as much as this occupational dysfunction is interwoven with the overall personality traits that precipitate the disorder, the occupational therapist may make a contribution to remediation of the anorexic condition. Because of its multidimensional nature, anorexia is certainly a problem requiring interdisciplinary effort.

Writers have typically focused on the family system as playing an important etiological role in anorexia, hypothesizing that these persons are overly dependent on their families and have difficulty developing autonomy while striving to

___

† Because anorexia nervosa afflicts a much higher percentage of females than males, this section will use the female pronoun throughout.

meet parental expectations (28, 168, 179). More recent formulations propose that an interaction of several factors contributes to the development of anorexia. These include a biological predisposition toward losing weight during periods of stress (more often a characteristic of females than males), a culture that values both thinness and achievement, and a lack of meaningful peer relationships (100). Both early and current perspectives recognize the struggle for identity and autonomy as key issues for the anorexic person.

Anorexics are frequently highly competent and achieving persons, who, in effect, appear to have an almost exaggerated need for occupation. They are often involved in a tremendous amount of physical activity (27), are very competitive, and excel in scholastic work (72, 137, 141). However, apart from the physical exercise which is seen as a route to weight control, their conceptualization of the relationship between means and ends may be faulty (224). In other words, the anorexic person may believe that by controlling her body weight, she will attain a sense of being an independent, competent person in all aspects of her life. Ironically, the effects of starvation may prevent her from successfully interacting with the environment. Thus, inefficacy and achievement are interwoven for those individuals.

Volition

PERSONAL CAUSATION

Traditionally, the anorexic female has been described as being involved in a struggle to attain internal control. Presumably, persons develop overly rigid eating patterns in response to feelings of helplessness (27, 35). By reducing their food intake to the point of starvation, they strive to achieve a sense of control and feelings of worthiness from having done something "extraordinary" (30).

Current research, however, is offering conflicting evidence to the assumption that anorexic persons are highly external. In fact, younger anorexic patients may score more internally than norms given for their age peers (95). However, those anorexic patients who do score highly on external locus of control seem to be more apt to score highly on other measures of psychological disturbance (95, 224). Whatever their internal/external orientation, these persons lack belief in the efficacy of their skills. This lack of belief in efficacy is found across a whole spectrum of persons with eating disorders. For example, college women who admitted that they engaged in anorexic behaviors but were not actually diagnosed as having the illness all reported feelings of being inadequate to maintaining their own high standards or expectations (218).

VALUES

The values of anorexic persons appear to be strongly shaped by the mass media and by their parents. By starving themselves, they carry the media image of the slender woman to its extremity (194). The anorexic teen-ager is also typically locked into her family system (28, 168), and finds it difficult to resist the family's high valuation of achievement. Unfortunately, the goal of perfection which she sets for herself becomes entwined with her attempt to establish control over her body (29).

Aimee Liu (138), a young woman who was anorexic from about the age of 12 until her college years, illustrates this interaction. When Aimee initially began dieting, it was in response to being slightly overweight for her age. After losing 15 pounds she felt that, for the first time, she had been in control of her life. Although Aimee was a top student, she felt that she was never as perfect as her parents and others expected her to be; losing more weight became her solution to the problem of perfection. As she became thinner, her dieting allowed her to achieve further independence in the form of job offers from modeling agencies. Of course, the modeling jobs only reinforced the notion that being thin was desirable.

The tendency to conform to social goals may also be manifested by conforming to subcultural group goals. Many of the anorexic-like women on college campuses are sorority members and influenced by these groups' strong emphasis on physical attractiveness (218). Anorexic and anorexic-type women are also overrepresented among dance and modeling students (72), two other subcultural groups that highly value thinness.

Although anorexic females are often perfectionists who set high standards of performance for themselves, their occupational goals are frequently unclear (22, 218). For many of these young women there may also be a conflict between traditional feminine occupational values and changing cultural notions of feminine success (22, 100). Thus, not knowing what their goals are or whether they can even attain them, they seize on the solution of changing their physique.

Finally, the anorexic person appears unable to find meaning in occupations when food- and weight-related concerns begin to dominate her daily life (27). Normal concerns with leisure, work and daily living tasks are overshadowed by a pathological concern for mastering body weight.

INTERESTS

Anorexic adolescents frequently have a wide range of interests, although athletic pursuits tend to be predominant (75, 138, 141, 183). These adolescents are also often quite creative, but such interests may eventually become subordinate to preoccupations with dieting and exercise (75, 151). Despite her own avoidance of eating, food-related activities, such as reading recipes and preparing gourmet meals for friends and family, also may become dominant (75, 124, 138). The anorexic adolescent may also engage in far fewer social leisure activities than other adolescents (100, 124, 183).

Although the anorexic woman typically can discriminate interests, their potency seems to wane as she becomes excessively preoccupied with aimless physical activity in order to "burn off calories" (Ref 75, p 112).

HABITUATION

ROLES

The family unit of anorexic adolescents tends to be highly self-contained. Family members are often strongly invested in one another and struggle to keep conflict and differences beneath the surface. Because of this self-containment and over-investment, these families are somewhat isolated from the larger social structure (100).

Since the role of family member prevails in the life of the anorexic female, other roles may be less important or not as well internalized. The role of friend, for example, is often a marginal one for these adolescents (100, 124). In addition, although they have completely fulfilled the obligations of the student role, they often have difficulty making the transition into an adult worker role (100). For some anorexic adolescents, starvation may become a means of resolving the conflict between wanting to remain enmeshed in the family while realizing the need to prepare for a worker role (100).

Certain occupational roles, however, may place the female at risk for developing anorexia. Occupations in which physique is pivotal, such as dancing, may have a larger than expected prevalence of anorexic members (72).

Adrian, a young woman who had been anorexic for many years, exemplifies the overinternalization of the family role at the expense of other roles. Although Adrian was married and working, her primary adult work role was as a freelance artist. Interestingly, this work was carried out in collaboration with her father, despite the fact that working with him was stressful for her. Socially, she mentioned having several friends, but in actuality her primary social companion appeared to be her husband, whereas her other relationships remained superficial.

HABITS

In many areas of her life, the anorexic person recognizes and conforms to socially expected habits. Academic habits, for example, are often highly effective. However, in the area of body weight, her habits are likely to be characterized by ritual and rigidity (27, 98). Food rituals include not eating during family meals, playing with food on her plate so as to simulate eating, studying caloric values of food, preparing elaborate or gourmet dishes for others to consume, and secret eating binges. Weight-related rituals may consist of self-induced vomiting or the use of laxatives following the ingestion of food, and repeated weight checks to make sure she has not gained. The anorexic person often becomes excessively rigid in her food-related habits because of her fear of losing all control should she relax her vigil against weight gain (27). This rigidity appears to be more characteristic of externally oriented anorexic persons than those who are more internal (224).

The emergence of pathological habits related to the anorexic syndrome also signals the breakdown of normal everyday occupational habits.

There appears to be a synergy between growing obsession with weight loss-oriented habits and the loss of everyday habits of work, play and daily living tasks, coupled with a loss of the security, reality orientation and satisfaction that routine performance affords. Thus, loss of a reality producing and satisfying routine may well augment the growing distortion of habits in the anorexic person.

Performance

SKILLS

Because the anorexic individual is bright, creative and active, she superficially appears to have no skill deficits. In reality, however, she may have deficits in perceptual and interactional skills. First, the anorexic individual may misinterpret or incorrectly perceive bodily sensations, so that she denies feeling hunger or fatigue (27), and after eating small amounts may feel unrealistically bloated. Perceptually, she does not recognize that she is emaciated and has an extremely distorted body image (22, 27, 95). Finally, anorexic persons often have poor social skills. Unlike "normal" individuals, they have few ties with peers, and the friendships that they do have tend to be short-lived (100).

Environment

Anorexia nervosa seems to emerge in response to particular properties of the social and cultural environments. At the level of social groups, the family environment is pivotal for the anorexic adolescent. Because these families tend to have impermeable boundaries, risk taking and change are not encouraged, and the growing child does not playfully explore her surroundings or interact with peers. Hence, the environment is one which does not promote competence or a sense of mastery in the adolescent (100).

Further, the values of the family may conflict with cultural views. While her family tacitly does not encourage or expect independence, cultural norms do expect increasing independence during adolescence. The gap between family and societal values can be more easily resolved when the adolescent has a strong peer network (100). The anorexic adolescent, however, is socially isolated, and finds it difficult to resolve the conflict productively (100).

The cultural environment is also implicated in anorexia through the values it transmits about standards of feminine beauty (100) and which tend to recognize the worth of women for this physical attractiveness as opposed to their accomplishments (22). The impact of skewed cultural values creating the plight of the modern women cannot be discounted as an important factor in the etiology of anorexia. That is, the young woman desiring recognition of her worth is torn between desiring recognition for achievement (the typically male avenue to external recognition) and finding that recognition is more readily available for physical beauty. Because her accomplishments may go unrecognized and unrewarded in a society that does not yet fully recognize and value accomplishment, the anorexic woman may view control of her body through starvation as a means of subverting this cultural norm (22).

Assessment

A key issue for the anorexic person may be her feelings of being manipulated or controlled by others in the treatment setting (27, 141). Therefore, the occupational therapist should view the assessment process as an attempt to collaborate with the anorexic person to identify situations in which she has typically felt out of control or incompetent, and situations which contradict these feelings of inefficacy. The use of a semistructured interview to explore her history of involvement in leisure and work should enable creation of an atmosphere of discovery. Within this context, such themes as the extent to which past activities pursued were solitary or social, reasons for engaging in activities, playfulness experienced during activities, skills developed or dropped, and other patterns can be identified. In addition, the history should also assist in determining where the person is in the occupational choice process since difficulty in choosing and entering an occupation is frequently a problem.

Because anorexia nervosa has strong sociocultural associations (72, 100), another focus for assessment should be the person's perceptions of the major environments in which she interacts. This should help to identify sources of conflict emanating from the values communicated by these settings. Finally, assessment should consider her present use of time to reveal the extent to which eating habits may be interfering with the enactment of her interests and values and with occupational habits.

Treatment

Although skills and habits may be disordered the inability to find pleasure and meaning in occupations may be a more significant component of dysfunction from the perspective of occupational therapy. The anorexic person needs to increase her feeling of comfort in situations requiring risk taking and flexibility without the necessity of achieving; play is an essential medium for accomplishing this. In addition, she must begin to visualize herself as moving into an independent adult worker role. To this end, the pleasurable experience of both work and leisure occupations is necessary, so that she can perceive herself as efficacious and capable of entering the occupational choice process.

The development of more extensive peer networks is another area for occupational therapy intervention. Situations in which the anorexic person can enact the friendship role should be identified and incorporated into the therapeutic process.

Table 15.7 presents a summary of the status of subsystem components along with more specific examples of assessments and treatment strategies for the anorexic person.

ELISE: AN ANOREXIC ADOLESCENT

Elise is a small and attractive 17-year-old who has been hospitalized six times in the past 5 years. Her current hospitalization, for anorexia nervosa, was precipitated by a weight loss of 30 pounds, from 103 to 73.

Elise's early development was normal; however, her parents separated when she was 5. She lived with her mother (who remarried when she was 10), and her sister, until the age of 14. At this time, Elise decided to live with her father. Her father had remarried for the second time when Elise was 13.

Admitting notes described Elise as being a good student, sociable although she had never dated, and interested in sports and arts and crafts. During this current hospitalization she has had several mood swings, with her most recent depression following a vacation taken by her psychotherapist. Nevertheless, she has regained most of her weight.

Elise was very eager to participate in occupational therapy and willingly completed a battery that consisted of the Interest and Role Checklists, Leisure Satisfaction Scale, Automatic Thoughts Questionnaire, Occupational Questionnaire, the student role portion of the

Table 15.7.
Occupational status, recommended assessments and treatment considerations for a female patient with anorexia nervosa

Occupational status	Recommended assessments	Treatment considerations
VOLITION		
Personal causation		
May feel extremely controlled, although this is not always true	Internal/External Scale	Use collaborative approach to treatment planning, so that client does not feel manipulated
Typically lacks belief in efficacy of her skills and does not think she can maintain her own high standards	Automatic Thoughts Questionnaire	
	Female Adolescent Role Development Questionnaire (FARDQ)	Explore examples of situations in past occupational and leisure activities that contradict feelings of inefficacy and external control
	Occupational Questionnaire (OQ)	
	Self-Esteem Scale	
	Occupational History (OH)	
Values		
Has internalized an exaggerated version of sociocultural valuation of slimness, as well as sociocultural tendency to devalue women for their accomplishments and overvalue them for their physical attractiveness	FARDQ, OQ, OH	Use values clarification activities to identify work and leisure-related values
	Leisure History Interview (LHI)	
Sets perfectionistic standards for self and is very achievement oriented		Explore current projects, their importance and their relevance to long-term goals; identify new projects in which to become involved
Occupational goals are frequently unclear		
The meaning of occupations becomes secondary to desire to lose weight		Through analysis of projects explore reasons for engaging in occupations and satisfactions derived from their pursuit
Interests		
Has a wide range of interests, although athletic and creative pursuits may prevail; has few social interests	LHI, OH, OQ	Experiment with new leisure interests in a playful setting; emphasis should be on performance for pleasure, not for achievement, and mistakes should not have serious consequences
	Interest Checklist	
Although interests are discriminated, potency may be weak since they soon become subordinate to food-related preoccupations	Leisure Satisfaction Questionnaire	
HABITUATION		
Roles		
Family role is pivotal in lifestyle; anorexic adolescent may avoid transition to worker role in effort to maintain centrality of family role	OH	Examine connections between long-standing interests and occupational roles
	Role Checklist	
Certain occupational roles, such as dancer or model, may create a greater vulnerability to anorexia	Role Performance Scale (RPS)	Opportunity to "apprentice" new roles should be made available, e.g. volunteering in areas related to interests
Friendship role is often marginal in overall life-style		Explore possibilities for enacting interests in social groups

Table 15.7.—*Continued*

Occupational status	Recommended assessments	Treatment considerations
Habits		
Although many habits are effective and socially acceptable, food-related habits are characterized by ritual and rigidity, and do not conform to social conventions	OQ, OH, RPS	Encourage experimentation with more flexible behaviors; identify realistic consequences of changing habits
Concern with weight and food-related habits diverts attention away from other occupational habits		
PERFORMANCE		
Skills		
Although task skills are often competent, deficits are apparent in interpersonal skills	OQ, LHI, FARDQ, OH, RPS	Assertiveness training may counteract feelings of being manipulated and discomfort in social situations
Usually misinterprets perceptions of feedback and has a distorted body image		
ENVIRONMENT		
Family environment is highly impermeable and does not encourage risk taking, exploration or mastery of surroundings	OH, RPS Family and School Climate Scales	Examine perceptions of values communicated by family and school and identify discrepancies with her own; values clarification may help solidify confidence in her own values
Family valuation of dependence generally conflicts with cultural valuation of independence		
Cultural ideal of feminine role emphasizes physical appearance over occupational accomplishments and contributes to value conflict		

Occupational History, and a Leisure History Interview. This battery was completed several months after her admission to the hospital.

Assessment Results

AUTOMATIC THOUGHTS QUESTIONNAIRE

This instrument measures a component of personal causation—belief in personal effectiveness. Although norms are not available, Elise's score of 133 is well above the mean for a group of depressed patients and reflects extremely negative beliefs about herself and her ability to accomplish things in her life.

INTEREST CHECKLIST

Elise showed a large decrease in the number of her interests from the past 10 years to the past year. Whereas in the past 10 years there were 20 activities in which she had no interest at all, in the past 1 year and in the present there were 40 such interests. However, her future interests reflect a return to the previous level, in that once again, only 20 interests are rejected. Notable for an adolescent girl who expresses interest in clothes, hairstyling and other social activities is her lack of interest in dating.

LEISURE SATISFACTION INDEX

Elise appears to gain a great deal of satisfaction from her leisure. In particular she derives feelings of competence and emotional well-being from her leisure, and identifies leisure as an opportunity to be with other people and to be physically active. However, Elise's responses to this questionnaire may more accurately reflect her current leisure (in the hospital) than her feelings about leisure before hospitalization. This possibility is supported by her responses to the Occupational Questionnaire and by the strong distinction which she made between "leisure" and "free time." Elise described her "free" time as frustrating and lonely.

ROLE CHECKLIST

Most of Elise's roles have been interrupted by hospitalization; student, friend and hobbyist are the only continuous roles she identified. Although religious participant is not a past role, it is identified as a future role, while organization participant is terminated. Elise added a role to the checklist—that of exerciser. Elise did not value the role of organization participant, and only somewhat valued the role of caregiver, home maintainer and friend. All other roles were very valuable, including the role of "maintaining physical health" which she added to the list.

OCCUPATIONAL QUESTIONNAIRE

Elise held a job in a fast-foods restaurant and worked after school and on weekends. On a typical Saturday she spent some time in the early afternoon engaged in exercise and shopping with her friends; then she worked for about 8 hours. While recreation activities were sources of competence and pleasure, work on the weekend was something Elise disliked and did not feel competent doing. Meals and sleep were similarly rated negatively.

On a schoolday, Elise was involved in vocational training to be a data processor. She was in this program because sitting still in class made her highly anxious. This took up most of her morning and was an evident source of satisfaction; however, her afternoon academic classes were rated considerably less positively. Elise worked in the evenings, but did not feel quite as negative about working on schooldays as she did on the weekend. Nevertheless, she still felt she did her job poorly.

OCCUPATIONAL HISTORY— STUDENT ROLE

Elise changed schools several times between kindergarten and ninth grade. Her reactions to school are similar to those of most adolescents—she likes the opportunity to be with friends, finds some classes interesting and dislikes others. Her grades are As and Bs and her major area of interest is science. Elise wants to attend college and to major in either physical therapy, animal science or premedicine. Elise's future plans include living with friends in an apartment, possibly marrying, having a job, taking better care of herself, and doing volunteer work with handicapped children. Elise identified current strengths as being art projects and personal hygiene.

LEISURE HISTORY INTERVIEW

Elise reported participation in a wide range of leisure activities from early childhood through the present. These included playing with toys and dolls, going to the zoo and amusement parks, playing outdoor games such as hopscotch and jump rope, doing things with her mother and grandmother (shopping or going to eat), being a Girl Scout and, more recently, dancing, taking exercise classes, belonging to a church youth group, and cooking for other people. Most of her favorite leisure activities were chosen either because her friends did them or her family and, consequently, tended to be group-oriented activities. Even babysitting, although not done with peers, is an activity which she appeared to enjoy because of the involvement with children. Except for babysitting, Elise generally equated doing well in something with being praised by others. She also felt that her parents had high expectations for her performance in many activities, and that her mother was very concerned with Elise's image as an attractive young girl.

Summary of Occupational Status

Elise has many assets. She has a wide range of interests, can identify future occupational goals, has enacted the worker and student role successfully in the past, and derives feelings of competence from her vocational program at school and many of her leisure activities. However, these assets are interwoven with her problem areas. For example, despite her good performance in school and work, she feels ineffective in most areas of her life. Many of her feelings of competence seem to come from external ratings of her behavior. Although she

Table 15.8.
Occupational status, treatment goals and interventions for Elise, an anorexic adolescent

Occupational status	Treatment goals and intervention
VOLITION	

Personal causation

Feels competent in prevocational activities at school and in some leisure; yet considers herself ineffective in many aspects of life	Identify in daily life experiences contradictions to feelings of inefficacy
Competency feelings seem to come from external feedback rather than intrinsic satisfaction with performance	Participate in enjoyable activities where outcomes are not important—emphasize self as source of feedback

Values

Values most roles although caregiver, home maintainer and friend are not strongly valued	In feminine identity group, develop friendship role in a variety of activities
May overvalue approval from others as few occupations are pursued for clearly intrinsically motivating reasons; believes others have high expectations for her	In values clarification group, explore reasons for choice of activities; peer approval may not be as critical as she believes
Identifies future goals related to work	Develop plans for attaining future occupational goals (e.g. part-time work and college)

Interests

Wide range of interests enacted in past; has had many past leisure interests	Begin to discriminate which interests are especially satisfying from those done because others do them; focus on ways to pursue the former while in hospital, on weekends and after discharge
Currently, decreased interests; did not enact many interests prior to hospitalization	

HABITUATION	

Roles

Has participated in most roles in past; has held several jobs and belonged to youth groups; roles currently disrupted by hospitalization	Explore plans to resume roles following discharge, especially worker role—identify possibilities for part-time job more relevant to areas of interest
Previous worker role not overly satisfying; did not think she performed well	Test reality of occupational plans by starting to take some college courses while still in hospital

Habits

Considers her personal hygiene a strength	Maintain grooming habits
Balance of leisure and work on weekend did not reflect her interests	While in hospital, begin spending weekends in a variety of personally chosen activities with other members of feminine identity group
Does not feel comfortable with unstructured time	In values clarification group, examine meaning of free time and the difference between time alone that is productive and that which is unproductive; identify satisfying uses of solitary time—separate need to feel in control from need to be busy

PERFORMANCE	

Skills

Does well in school; performs well in most activities	Support level of skills through continued involvement in activities, but emphasize playfulness rather than need to do well

Table 15.8.— *Continued*

Occupational status	Treatment goals and intervention
ENVIRONMENT	
Family environment appears unstable; school history reflects frequent changes in environment	Develop independent living skills so that she can realistically begin to plan to live away from home; develop peer network while in hospital so that alternative social groups are available

has many interests, she seems to rely on group activities, to feel threatened by unstructured or solitary time, and to choose activities so that she can be busy, rather than for their intrinsic meaning. Notably, a typical weekend day for her prior to hospitalization did not include a variety of pleasurable activities or provide her with feelings of effectiveness. Her previous job was not enjoyable to her and probably did not give her a chance to use the occupational skills and interests which she is developing. Thus, Elise's feelings of inefficacy seem to arise from engagement in activities that are not highly valued by her at the expense of participating in valued activities, and by her reliance on external feedback for feelings of competence. Elise's occupational status is elaborated in Table 15.8.

Treatment Goals and Intervention

Occupational therapy addressed problems related to Elise's occupational behavior. Treatment goals for Elise focused on increasing her reliance on self-evaluation for feelings of competence, helping her clarify values, further developing her creative skills, exploring the meaning that leisure has for her, and developing a peer network. Table 15.8 summarizes goals and methods of intervention.

Elise was initially referred to a creative skills group where she was able to try out various crafts and art activities in an unthreatening atmosphere. This group emphasized the pleasurable experience of activities rather than the nature of the end product. This was important for Elise in order to provide her with opportunities to play without having to meet others' expectations or having to judge her work in any way.

Elise was also referred to a feminine identity group, made up of all the girls on her unit. This group gave her a chance to focus on issues related to body image, self-esteem, and to develop relationships with peers that were not based solely on a need for acceptance. In this group, Elise revealed that she really had not been especially close to her school friends

and was uncomfortable in the role of friend. Because she lacked peer support and did not confide in her mother, she approached the idea of dating with much trepidation. She was also uncomfortable with plans to just "hang out" with friends, thinking that she would either be boring or bored, and that she would gain weight. Thus, within this group she began to focus on making joint plans for weekends with one or two group members. Members were encouraged to choose projects that ranged in amount and type of activity called for—e.g. sewing, going on a bird-watching walk, roller skating, or photography.

As Elise began to make progress in her groups, the emphasis changed from exploration to clarification of values and goals. In a values-clarification group, she began to examine her reasons and motivations for engaging in various activities. A critical issue for her in this group concerned her reasons for feeling "panic" when faced with unstructured time. She explored her feelings about not meeting others' expectations and how this led her to avoid certain occupations (such as academics). As part of this group, she began keeping a diary, recording her reactions to the activities in which she participated.

Outcome

Elise has been in the hospital for 8 months but has begun to make progress in many of the problem areas that were identified. For example, through the process of values clarification, she is beginning to recognize differences between time alone that is productive and time alone that is not. As she identifies meaningful ways of using her solitary time, she is learning that she can feel in control of her life without always being "busy," and that she can derive feelings of satisfaction and competence without having feedback from others.

Elise is aware that her environment has not been a source of stability for her and is now making plans to live alone or with friends when she leaves the hospital. To prepare for this step, she is now in an independent living skills group.

Elise wants to work and has a clear idea of the kind of work she would like to do. Currently she is exploring the possibility of taking some classes at a local college in order to get a taste of college life and to test her vocational plans. This is something she will be able to pursue while still in the hospital, if necessary. She is also investigating potential part-time jobs for discharge, in the hope of finding something more relevant to her future plans.

Of course, not all of Elise's problems are occupational in nature. Elise's depression and feelings of low self-esteem are tied to her family life, and not eating may be a means of generating the attention and caring she wants from others. These issues are being addressed in individual and family therapy. In addition, she has begun attending a community group for women with eating disorders. This group focuses on the sociocultural background of eating disorders and women's perceptions of themselves. In occupational therapy, however, Elise has been able to focus on how she can feel in control of, and intrinsically satisfied with, her leisure and work.

JUVENILE DELINQUENCY

The term juvenile delinquency may be viewed from several perspectives. First, as a legal classification it refers to the commission of crimes for which one would receive jail time as an adult (felonies and petty offenses) and, in some states, it may include such offenses as curfew violations and running away (200). Second, as a psychiatric diagnosis, juvenile delinquency usually refers to individuals diagnosed as having a conduct disorder. Typical maladaptive behaviors warranting this diagnosis are: the violation of others' rights or societal norms (e.g. thefts, attacks, chronic rule breaking), difficulties at home and in the community, sexual precocity, the tendency to blame others and reject responsibility, low self-esteem, poor academic achievement, and substance abuse (4).

Juvenile delinquency is a serious problem. In the United States, at least 12% of all youths‡ are likely to actually acquire a juvenile court record during adolescence (38); however, probably 90% of all adolescents have committed at least one act for which they *could* have been

---

‡ Research has tended to focus on the male juvenile delinquent; this section will therefore use the male pronoun.

arrested (232). While the term juvenile delinquency is generally limited to those who have actually been through the legal system, the much higher rate of probable delinquent behavior attests to the pervasiveness of the problem.

Juvenile delinquency is also a complex problem and a wide range of etiological theories have been proposed to explain its prevalence. Classic causation theories suggest that family problems (131), an inability to cope with emotional problems (221), faulty socialization experiences (36, 208), neurological deficits including perceptual-motor and cognitive skill deficits (15, 131, 132, 247), and/or a deviant value system (199) underlie juvenile delinquency. Common to these theories is the emphasis on the person as the source of etiology. More recent theories point to the social system instead, suggesting that certain social processes, such as the labeling of particular individuals as deviant (249), or a mismatch betwen environmental properties and the needs of persons (33, 121), result in delinquent behavior patterns. This latter perspective suggests that the occupational dysfunction of juvenile delinquents may arise from an inability to lead an efficacious life-style in terms of normative criteria for success. Unable to master the environment in more acceptable ways, they then engage in deviant behaviors that yield the feelings of success and mastery.

Volition

PERSONAL CAUSATION

Although a minority viewpoint suggests that delinquent adolescents develop a strong sense of internal control in early childhood and later make a deliberate decision to become delinquent (244), the predominant evidence indicates that juvenile delinquents do not develop a strong sense of internal control.

Several locus-of-control studies have identified a tendency for juvenile delinquents to score more externally than nondelinquents (122, 149). This external orientation is reflected in both general life situations as well as situations related to achievement (such as school) (122). The belief that they have only limited control over their environment may lead juvenile delinquents to view life as an "endless series of problems without solutions in sight" (Ref. 177, p 210), and it may also make them quick to deny responsibility for failure (55, 208, 209). The latter tendency has been especially noted in the game-playing of delinquent youths (209). For example, when caught cheating, delinquent adolescents were significantly more likely than nondelinquent adolescents to deny their cheating. In addition, they were more likely to deny having made mistakes and to avoid accepting responsibility for losing. At the same time, they were less accepting of the mistakes of others and quick to attack their peers about cheating.

In addition to an external orientation, juvenile delinquents may not possess feelings of self-efficacy. A large study of junior high school students found that several dimensions of self-esteem related to later acts of school vandalism and deviance (103). Students who perceived themselves as failures at home or at school, and students who tended to avoid responsibility for self-devaluing situations, were likely to perform a variety of deviant acts during the following year. Importantly, these students had not engaged in these acts during a specified time period prior to the study.

INTERESTS

The limited literature describing the interests of juvenile delinquents suggests that they are similar to those of nondelinquents. However, while both delinquents and nondelinquents may enjoy games and sports, differences exist in the types of games preferred by each. Juvenile delinquents may prefer games of chance as opposed to games of strategy, games with few rules, and games which provide an opportunity to express aggression (208, 209). Additionally, delinquency may itself reflect a search for excitement and adventure in risky situations not otherwise satisfied through more socially acceptable interests (123, 238).

Juvenile delinquents may be less able to discriminate their interests than are nondelinquents. Observations of juvenile delinquents in a vocational training program revealed that a common characteristic of this group was a lack of knowledge of their own work-related interests (181).

VALUES

Value formation is believed to be of particular importance in the choice of a delinquent lifestyle (54, 99). Certain theorists see delinquency as resulting from society's failure to properly socialize some individuals to mainstream values (36, 96, 208). Others have postulated that juvenile delinquents may hold middle class "subterranean" values which, unlike most individuals in the middle class, they then act out. These values include a premium on excitement and adventure, a disdain for work goals and idealization of the notion of machismo (155). Delinquent youths may also value the student role less than other adolescents, and choose values for hedonistic, rather than altruistic reasons (125). However, other research contradicts the notion of decreased altruism, finding instead no differences in delinquent and nondelinquent adolescents' values of idealism, altruism or concern for others (176).

There is some evidence that future time perspective differs for delinquent and nondelinquent persons. These differences, however, relate primarily to vocational goals (45, 176) and may actually reflect a realistic, although pessimistic, appraisal of the future.

Standards of performance, particularly relating to moral development, have received considerable attention in studies of juvenile delinquents. Findings, however, tend to be contradictory. For example, although junior high school students who later committed deviant acts were found to hold contranormative attitudes when compared with their peers (103), juvenile delinquents are not tolerant of rule-breaking in others (209). Part of the conflict may reflect differences in attitudes toward prosocial and antisocial norms of behavior. Thus, another study found that although juvenile delinquents endorsed socially prescribed behaviors, they were also more tolerant than their peers of socially unacceptable behaviors (e.g. drug use, shoplifting, and so on) (102). Studies of moral development are equally ambiguous in their results (102). Such studies suggest that juvenile delinquents vary in their level of moral development, and that situational, psychological and parental upbringing styles may account for some of these differences (53, 102). In sum, while no particular value pattern appears to characterize delinquents as a group, values do appear to be a factor in delinquent behavior.

Habituation

ROLES

Organized role behavior helps to establish a person's social worth; however, juvenile delinquents have trouble fulfilling certain socially acceptable roles and may instead choose a delinquent role in which to achieve a sense of belonging, identity, status, or self-esteem. Juvenile delinquents, especially, have difficulty in filling family, peer and student roles (80), and may experience considerable role conflict between peer and family roles. If their peers are members of the delinquent subculture, then juvenile delinquents will be forced to choose between the irresponsible behavior valued by peers and the more conventional expectations usually held by the family. Additionally, just being labeled "delinquent" may perpetuate delinquent behavior as the individual internalizes society's expectations for deviant behavior (105).

In addition to the conflict between peer and family roles, the delinquent may be involved in fewer roles than other adolescents. In particular, the delinquent appears less likely to internalize the role of hobbyist/amateur (125). One reason for involvement in fewer roles may be that the juvenile delinquent does not recognize or perceive that he has access to certain roles (249).

While juvenile delinquents may have greater difficulty imagining themselves in some more conforming roles, once they do leave ineffective roles, such as being a problem student, to enter legitimate roles such as husband or worker, delinquent behavior often decreases (76, 200).

HABITS

Although the habits of juvenile delinquent adolescents have not been extensively studied, it appears that disorganization and unproductivity exist. Juvenile delinquent adolescents spend much of their leisure time "hanging out" or engaging in socially unacceptable behaviors such as smoking, drinking or gambling (176, 239). In addition, some of the deviant acts engaged in by predelinquent junior high school students (103)—cheating, failing, and truancy—suggest that juvenile delinquents may have poor academic habits. Finally, juvenile delinquents have been observed to have deficits in daily living habits such as grooming and budgeting (181).

Performance

Skills

Learning disabilities have been widely noted in juvenile delinquents. Reading problems, poor verbal skills and overall poor performance on standardized intelligence tests are some of the documented problems (15, 83, 131). Because a much higher percentage of learning disabilities exists among juvenile delinquents than in the general population (140, 247), it is possible that delinquent behavior may be a response to the frustration over school and academic demands.

Some juvenile delinquents also appear to have deficits in their ability to process sensory stimuli (47, 197). For example, these adolescents may have difficulty screening out extraneous environmental stimuli, and may be less likely to attend to social cues than to other forms of information (197). This may lead them to ignore or misperceive facial cues, a factor that may relate to their observed deficits in social skills. Some writers have also suggested that juvenile delinquents may have reduced perceptions of sensory stimulation (47). Because they perceive less stimulation, juvenile delinquents may be more likely to engage in behavior that others would perceive as being overarousing or overstimulating.

Social skill deficits are common in juvenile delinquents. Both delinquent boys and girls have been found to perform less competently than nondelinquent adolescents in solving problems that require the use of social skills (70, 71).

Environment

Although the stereotyped image of juvenile delinquents portrays them as the products of a low socioeconomic, minority background (54), this stereotype may in fact reflect a tendency of society to label lower-class youths more often than middle- and upper-class youths as delinquent (249). Accordingly, it may not be possible or realistic to characterize the juvenile delinquent's environmental background. However, several theorists and researchers do suggest that delinquency is context-dependent, in that it reflects an interaction between characteristics of the person and characteristics of the environment (33, 121).

For example, within most social settings there are a limited number of roles that require active, responsible behaviors, and a larger number of passive behavior roles. People who fill these passive roles are both less likely to learn normative behaviors for that setting and more likely to be considered only marginally relevant to the setting (7, 33). However, by disrupting the setting (through some deviant act), one may actually achieve a position of social influence or, at the very least, attract attention to oneself (33).

Another perspective on the relationship of person-environment fit to delinquent behavior proposes that when a person subjectively or objectively lacks the ability to respond to environmental demands, or that when the environment does not contain the resources necessary to satisfying an individual's goals, some form of maladaptive behavior may result (121). An empirical examination of the relationship between school crime and student-school fit found some modest support for these hypotheses (121). For example, students' perceptions that school was not relevant to their future occupational needs correlated with school avoidance and classroom misbehavior, while discrepancies between students' abilities to respond to student role expectations showed a relationship with school crime, as well as avoidance and misbehavior.

Assessment

The delinquent adolescent, faced with possible punishment for behavior, incarceration and having had to conceal deviant acts or otherwise avoid being "caught," may pose a particularly difficult problem for obtaining reliable and valid data. Even performance on standardized tests may be affected by the adolescent's feelings of inadequacy from failure in the student role. As a result, assessment should proceed in an atmosphere of trust where the adolescent is shown opportunities for positive experiences and where a nonjudgemental, open, exploratory attitude is maintained.

Interviews such as the Occupational History may be particularly useful in establishing rapport with the adolescent and for demonstrating the therapist's genuine concern for his or her desires, dilemmas and so on. Specific recommended assessments are noted in Table 15.9. The assessment procedure may be best implemented as a gradual and ongoing process in which self-discovery along with therapist feedback is emphasized.

Treatment

Treatment of the delinquent adolescent must begin with an appreciation of the delinquent's current values, interests and personal causation. The delinquent adolescent who does not see the possibility of satisfying work, who feels incompetent in the student role and who is chronically bored may experience a sense of competence, excitement and group belonging when engaging in a delinquent behavior—in the context of gang membership, for instance. Changing the adolescent involves an honest, but respectful confrontation of the maladaptive nature of the overall pattern. Respect for the delinquent's values, interests and personal causation means recognition of the adolescent's perspective and the fact that he or she is gaining a sense of competence, enjoyment and so on in a way that works for him or her. Changing delinquent behavior thus entails providing opportunities that challenge the delinquent's view of the best way he or she can be competent and that provide an alternative perspective. Once the adolescent discovers that he or she can *both* derive personal satisfaction and satisfy societal expectations, the delinquent behavior pattern is more likely to change.

The area of role acquisition is also of particular importance. Socially acceptable role involvement is important for therapy, and roles should be commensurate with the adolescent's skills. The treatment setting should provide and require participation in a variety of roles similar to legitimate roles outside the facility. Valued and effective role models should be available in the treatment setting and others outside the facility should be identified by the client.

While intervention at the volition and habituation levels is important, skill areas also need to be assessed and may require treatment for several reasons. First, remediation may be needed for specific learning disabilities and perceptual-motor problems that may respond to treatment. Second, skills of primary importance for survival (e.g. consumer skills, dealing with emergencies, etc.) or skills that are not easily compensated for (e.g. certain social skills) may be targeted as treatment priorities. The therapist should also help clients recognize skill strengths and weaknesses, match these with demands for performance, and help them compensate in less developed skill areas. In particular, the individual's competencies should be matched with role demands during treatment and with role demands anticipated upon release. Finally, a general problem-solving approach should be used, and its application to a variety of life situations be made clear. This can be accomplished through the occupational choice counseling process as well as through everyday collaborative decision-making in therapy. Specific treatment strategies are noted in Table 15.9.

Table 15.9.
Occupational status, recommended assessments and treatment considerations for the juvenile delinquent adolescent

Occupational status	Recommended assessments	Treatment considerations
VOLITION		
Personal causation		
Generally lack a sense of internal control and expect failure because problems are perceived as insurmountable	Occupational Questionnaire (OQ) Occupational History (OH)	Provide graded opportunities to take responsibility for decision making
Have a tendency to emphasize luck over skill and effort and to avoid personal responsibility	Internal/External Scale Adolescent Role Assessment (ARA)	Emphasize collaborative and problem-solving nature of treatment program
Have difficulty identifying personal skills that would be acceptable to society at large	Self-Attitude Questionnaire (SAQ)	Emphasize importance of personal responsibility; provide opportunities for self-satisfaction to accrue from responsible behavior
		Provide positive feedback on any current skills as well as opportunities to learn socially appropriate skills; acknowledge deviant skills while pointing to their inefficacy in developing social competence
Values		
May hold values which emphasize machismo and excitement, and disdain for school and work	OH, ARA, SAQ, OQ	Collaboratively examine values related to everyday occupations and identify negative consequences of deviant values
Evidence is mixed but may hold immature or antisocial values which are reinforced by a deviant peer group		Engage in leisure activities combined with discussion of importance of rule following
		Review occupational choice process and provide opportunities to explore the worker role with emphasis on satisfaction in genuine efforts
Interests		
May prefer games of chance to those of strategy to avoid responsibility	OH, ARA, OQ Interest Checklist	Provide opportunities to develop interests in occupations requiring skill and effort
May hold deviant interests and/or lack of work-relevant interests		Provide participation in a variety of socially acceptable activities appropriate for developmental level
HABITUATION		
Roles		
May have trouble fulfilling socially-acceptable roles and may choose a delinquent role to achieve a sense of	OH, ARA Role Checklist	Identify strategies for success in socially acceptable roles such as student and organization participant

Table 15.9.—Continued

Occupational status	Recommended assessments	Treatment considerations
belonging, identity, status, or self-esteem		Provide opportunities to participate in roles during treatment program which correspond to legitimate roles that exist outside facility
Tend to experience considerable role conflict between peer and family roles when forced to choose between delinquent peer behavior and more conventional family expectations		
May internalize fewer roles, in particular may not internalize hobbyist/amateur role or worker role		
Labeling as "delinquent" may also perpetuate delinquent behavior		
Habits		
Disorganization and unproductivity may exist	ARA, OQ	Provide support and planning for participation in routine occupational behavior
Leisure time use may be maladaptive		Explore alternatives for leisure
Habits of truancy and cheating, and poor academic habits, may exacerbate problems in the student and other roles		Examination and planning of time use; emphasis should be on the positive feelings that can accrue from good time use
PERFORMANCE		
Skills		
Learning disabilities may be present	Bruininks-Oseretsky Test of Motor Performance	A general problem-solving approach should be used and its application to life situations should be demonstrated
Underlying problems of processing sensory stimulation and perceiving stimulation may be present	The Assets Program	
	Let's Talk Inventory for Adolescents	Develop work and leisure skills
May have social skill deficits, particularly in problem-solving situations	Group Interaction Skills Survey	Provide social skills training through group treatment
ENVIRONMENT		
Social groups may not make central roles of importance and responsibility available to many members	School Climate Scales	Identify environmental groups and situations that lead to or support delinquent behavior and explore ways of avoiding or modifying these settings as appropriate
May be incongruency between opportunities offered in social settings and adolescent's perceptions of needs	Family Climate Scales	
May be incongruency between press of social settings and adolescent's skills		Explore alternative settings that support adaptive occupational behavior

JUVENILE DELINQUENCY CASE: KEN

Ken, a 16-year-old, was referred by his probation officer for treatment at a private psychiatric hospital. While on probation for stealing a truck "to go joy riding" and forging checks, he broke house arrest and was placed in detention.

On hospital admission, the following behaviors were noted: sleep and appetite disturbance, crying spells, acting out behaviors, heavy substance abuse, poor school performance, withdrawal from family and peers, nervousness and anxiety, and difficulty relating to authority figures.

Ken is the youngest sibling, living with his mother, two sisters, and two brothers. His parents were divorced when he was 5 years old, and Ken lived with his father until a year ago. Difficulty functioning in daily living (i.e. substance abuse, delinquent acts, school difficulties) became evident 1 year ago. At this time, his grandfather, with whom he was especially close, died, leaving Ken emotionally devastated. Subsequent disagreements with his father led to Ken's decision to live with his mother.

During occupational therapy, Ken completed a battery of assessments that included some self-report questionnaires (the Occupational Questionnaire, the Role Checklist, the Locus of Control Scale for Adolescents) and the Occupational History.

Evaluation Findings

Ken is an attractive, healthy adolescent. He has good gross and fine motor coordination. Interactions with peers vary depending on the cohort group, while interactions with authority figures fluctuate from mistrustful and guarded to resistive and manipulative. His intellectual functioning is estimated to be above average.

OCCUPATIONAL QUESTIONNAIRE

Ken's typical weekday is structured by school attendance. His typical time use for a 24-hour day is: 40% sleeping, 25% at school, 15% cruising, partying or playing, and 12% eating, showering, sitting, listening to music or watching television, and smoking. After school, he spends time "cruising around or playing" and partying before listening to music and going to sleep at 8:30. He feels that he does the following activities either "well" or "very well": sleeping, smoking a cigarette before school, eating lunch, leisure time at

school, briefly sitting around home, watching television, and partying. He rates his effectiveness in school as "poor." Effectiveness at other routine tasks was rated as "about average."

Ken is indifferent to many daily activities, rating them as "rather not do" or "total waste of time." The following he considers "extremely important": getting dressed and smoking a cigarette in the morning, lunch, leisure time, briefly sitting around home after school, and listening to music after school. The following are considered "important": sleeping, dinner and partying. He rated most of his activities, which include school, cruising around, or playing and watching television, as "take it or leave it."

Ken's degree of interest in daily activities ranges from indifferent to liking them very much, except for waking up and showering, which he strongly dislikes. He neither likes nor dislikes school and watching television. He "likes" cruising or playing after school and partying and "likes very much" sleeping, smoking a morning cigarette, lunch, leisure time, briefly sitting at home after school, dinner and listening to music.

Overall, one of Ken's major activities is school attendance, which he considers "work," perceives himself as doing poorly, and is indifferent to as a value or an interest. His other time is spent preparing himself for school, in leisurely breaks before, during or after school, and at evening parties—all of which he perceives himself as doing well, values highly and in which he has a high degree of interest.

LOCUS OF CONTROL SCALE FOR ADOLESCENTS

Ken's score was 8 out of 20 possible answers. Thus, his locus of control seems to be neither extremely external nor internal.

ROLE CHECKLIST

Ken expects to have continuous participation in the following roles: student, caregiver, home maintainer, friend, family member, and hobbyist/amateur. The worker role is currently disrupted. He noted the possibility of future role participation as a volunteer in an organization by entering a "?" in the future column; he has never participated in this before. Religious participation and organizational participation were checked "not at all valuable." Student, volunteer, and hobbyist/amateur were considered "somewhat valuable," and worker, caregiver, home maintainer, friend and family member were "very valuable."

OCCUPATIONAL HISTORY

Ken's major occupational role is that of a high school student majoring in English. His education has been disrupted by several moves from school to school. He likes the peer interaction, learning and playing basketball at school, but dislikes being dependent on teachers. He states that he does, however, like one teacher who just gives him his work and lets him do it on his own. His performance in school has been variable, failing when he takes drugs, and getting "As" and "Bs" when he does not.

Although Ken could not recall what occupational fantasies he had as a child, his current fantasy is to be an artist or an architect. He enjoys art, has chosen to pursue it independently, and finds that others admire his work. Nevertheless, Ken does not really relate his present activities to this future goal. For example, although he does well in art, math, English and science, he does not see these courses as preparing him for a future job. Similarly, when Ken was later asked about future plans, he listed joining the army, going to college, learning about refrigeration, and marriage "sometime, but not too soon." In addition, his plans for future education are ambivalent and he expresses a lack of confidence in his ability to succeed in college.

During the interview, Ken indicated that he admires such characteristics as kindness, being socially adept, achieving in school, honesty, and independence. Ken's interests and skills include model building, drawing, basketball (as participant and spectator), and sleeping. Although he did not mention these activities on the Occupational Questionnaire, he stated that he currently enjoys bowling, sports, playing pool, and dating.

Ken has no specific responsibilities at home; rather, he helps out when needed. In the past, Ken worked as a fast-foods cook, but quit because he did not like the manager.

Occupational Status

Ken's occupational status is summarized in Table 15.10. He is currently at risk for continued failure; however, Ken possesses many strengths and with guidance could be helped to pursue a more successful occupational career.

His major occupational role is that of high school student, although his performance in this role is inconsistent. He has several iden-

tified occupational goals, and he highly values the worker role. Yet, he has no clear plans to achieve these and no role models. He does not see school as preparing him for these and acknowledges a lack of motivation to pursue future plans. Although Ken seems to have the basic skills for goal pursuit, he lacks history of success, seems to feel quite ineffective (except his artwork), and does not have habits supportive of adequate role performance. Ken has strengths in his valuing of socially acceptable attributes, balance of interests and skill level. Thus, although Ken has the capacity to perform at a level of competence or achievement, his current performance is characterized by incompetence and inefficacy.

Occupational Therapy Interventions

Intervention in occupational therapy, along with other mental health disciplines, focused on alleviating Ken's depressive symptoms and helping him control his impulsive behaviors. The occupational therapist involved Ken in structured group activities (such as volley ball) in which he could interact with peers and take increased responsibility for his behavior. In this early treatment phase, Ken was resistive and angry about hospitalization, in addition to being severely depressed about his family situation and the death of his grandfather. As he received more support from the staff and became involved in activities, his depression decreased, and he became more cooperative.

In the next stage of treatment, Ken's positive attributes (the presence of skills, values, interests) were emphasized as the therapist provided opportunities for Ken to explore interests in the community, use and develop skill areas and articulate values. For example, in the area of art Ken experimented with different media that he had not previously used, deriving personal satisfaction and expanding his skills at the same time. He tried some new physical recreation activities (weight lifting and ping-pong) and continued to play volley ball and basketball. In these activities, Ken was able to develop his leadership skills to instill good sportsmanship in peers. Field trips relating to leisure resources in the community included bowling and a trip to a science museum.

Ken also participated in an independent living skills group in which members took responsibility for planning each week's activity. These activities ranged from meal planning to role-playing family interactions to completing job applications.

On the unit, Ken was elected president for

Table 15.10.
Ken's occupational status, treatment goals and intervention

Occupational status	Treatment goals and intervention

VOLITION

Personal causation

Feels most effective when performing activities that do not require meeting any standards, for example, smoking and meals; feels ineffective at school and, even in his artwork, expresses doubts about future efficacy

Maintain involvement in art-related activities to provide continuing experiences of success

Challenge Ken's feelings of inefficacy with concrete evidence of contradiction (e.g. he can make good grades in school)

Explore new activities and roles requiring more responsibility in a playful environment

Values

Admires socially acceptable traits in others

In daily life, most values smoking, partying, and meals

Although future plans are vague, does mention goal of being an artist or architect

Through role modeling and prompting, encourage expression of positive values

Help Ken identify relationships between present and future plans, and to begin taking steps (e.g. obtaining information, making contacts) toward future goals

Interests

Has several strong and enduring interests (basketball, drawing, music) but currently is enacting few of these

Re-establish involvement in these interests during occupational therapy (e.g. playing volley ball, drawing projects, and so on) and explore ways to continue after discharge

HABITUATION

Roles

Performance in major role of student fluctuates, depending on substance use

Has internalized balance of roles related to family, leisure and school, but has not begun worker role

Increase awareness of link between current student role and future worker role

Explore possibilities for beginning worker role on part-time basis

Habits

Current use of time does not support good performance as student; does not carry out regular chores at home; leisure time seems unstructured and contingent on drug use

Treatment program should require behaviors necessary to student role (e.g. punctuality, regular attendance at groups, time in day allotted for studying)

Develop satisfying uses of leisure time that are seen as alternatives to drug use

PERFORMANCE

Skills

Good motor and congitive skills; interpersonal skills vary with situation

Provide opportunities to develop leadership skills among peers (e.g. being team captain)

Support continued use of existing skills in art, science and sports

ENVIRONMENT

Physical and social environment have been in flux (moving from father's house to mother's, changing schools, etc.)

Expectations for task performance at school and home are inconsistent

With family and Ken, plan daily routine in which Ken has regular responsibilities for household tasks

Part-time work and increased involvement in school sports teams may counteract family instability several week-long terms. Here again, he improved his leadership skills and began to relate to adults in a more mature fashion.

Ken began to improve his performance in school in the hospital and talked about returning to school after discharge (which he eventually did). While Ken occasionally abused substances on weekend passes, he finally stopped this drug use. Overall, his behavior became notably more adaptive in the clinic.

In the final phase, preparations were made for Ken's discharge. Ken was discharged to day-patient status for 3 weeks to test his ability to function in a less structured environment. In the 1st week, he showed more regression in terms of limit testing and defiant behavior. Gradually, he adjusted and, by discharge time, he was functioning well. His depression had lifted, and substance abuse had ceased; he was involved in regular leisure activities with friends. He also had a better idea of his skills, values and interests and had developed a more adaptive habit pattern.

Although treatment helped Ken to restore balance in his daily functioning, he was discharged before additional treatment goals related to future plans were addressed. For example, one of Ken's strongest values is to become established in a career. He is struggling with several options and seems to have no method for examining these. With more time, counseling in the process of occupational choice could have helped Ken identify benefits of school (course content, role models, skill development, etc) useful to later job performance or career development. Ken could further begin to identify prerequisite steps, information sources, role models, contacts, skills, and so on, needed to accomplish future plans, and he could explore ways to begin partial involvement in the worker role while still in school. Strategies such as these would link his current major life role to a valued future goal and serve to make aspects of the current role more meaningful.

CHRONIC SCHIZOPHRENIA

Longstanding psychosocial dysfunction and numerous psychiatric hospitalizations are typical of the person with chronic schizophrenia. Individuals with chronic schizophrenia usually have made several unsuccessful attempts at community living. Hospitalized or not, these individuals are usually socially isolated, unmarried, divorced or separated, and have minimal family contact (59). At best, the chronically ill person has a sporadic work history, tends to be undereducated, and usually comes from an economically or socially deprived background (59, 216). Many of these persons who have had substantial periods of institutionalization face, upon deinstitutionalization, such obstacles as isolation from the rest of the community, lack of meaningful activity, decreased income and, often, an unsatisfactory living environment (185).

The diagnosis of a schizophrenic disorder is based on the presence of certain psychotic features such as persecutory or self-referential delusions, the belief that one's thoughts are externally controlled, delusions of grandeur, and illogical or incoherent thinking associated with blunted affect and/or auditory hallucinations (4). In addition, deterioration from a previous level of functioning in such areas as work, social relations and self-care, and continuous signs of the illness for at least 6 months are also considered in making the diagnosis of schizophrenia (4). Other symptoms frequently noted in persons with schizophrenia include a loss of their sense of self-identity, a cessation of goal-directed activity, and a decrease in spontaneous psychomotor behavior (4).

Predominant theories of chronic mental illness have focused on various etiological factors, e.g. a genetic biological predisposition (particularly an imbalance of neurotransmittors), and dysfunctional family transactions (10, 118). Because of the complexity of the disorder, in all likelihood a combination of etiological factors is involved.

The occupational status of these persons may vary from extreme disorganization to a level of organization sufficient for daily survival. However, more so than the other disorders included in this chapter, chronic schizophrenic persons are likely to exhibit helpless or incompetent levels of occupational functioning. The continuum of functioning generally corresponds to the living environments of these persons. Thus, the most severely disorganized patients are usually found in public institutions, while those persons capable of functioning somewhat independently may now reside in community settings.

Volition

In chronic mental illness, volition may be disrupted or disorganized, leading to poor decisions or the inability to decide to act. The consequent disruption or cessation of occupation contributes to further maladaptation (61, 109, 110, 113, 114).

PERSONAL CAUSATION

People with chronic schizophrenia score significantly higher in external locus of control than nonschizophrenics (34, 42, 49, 90). Consequently, they lack the motivation to change the manner in which they act within their environment. In addition to the tendency toward external locus of control, chronic schizophrenic persons may be especially vulnerable to decreased expectancies of success and a diminished sense of personal effectiveness. For example, a 43-year-old woman who had been hospitalized on several occasions for chronic schizophrenia had repeatedly experienced failure regardless of whatever combination of medication, therapy, work, and schooling she pursued. Each hospitalization further evoked a deep sense of shame about her life becoming out of control, leading her to a self-fulfilling prophecy in which she always expected a "lousy" outcome to life events.

VALUES

In general, people with chronic schizophrenia have a decreased sense of the future and tend to be more past oriented than a normal population (82). Because they often do not work, their temporal orientation tends to reflect their unstructured daily lives (173). Furthermore, conceptualization and organization of future events may be chaotic (161, 173, 234). Goal-setting requires more internal organization and higher level process skills than many people with chronic schizophrenia demonstrate (104).

Occasionally, a distorted appraisal of skills leads to unrealistic goal setting. For example, David, a 27-year-old chronic schizophrenic male with an eighth grade education who has never worked, planned in 1 year to be "working as a ticket taker for a major airline," in 5 years to be enrolled in medical school, and in 10 years to be an "associate professor of drama and psychiatry."

People with schizophrenia may display a sense of aimlessness, meaninglessness and hopelessness in their lives (118). They fail to find worth, satisfaction and value in how they spend their time and perceive themselves as unable to successfully shape their future (46, 173, 234). This relationship may exist because a lack, reduction, or disruption of occupation eliminates a source of meaning for the individual (61). Further, institutionalization itself may lead to a breakdown of morale and the sense of self-worth, identity and purpose (78).

INTERESTS

People with chronic schizophrenia may lack interests, resulting in their inability to organize time in a meaningful way or to maintain their attention or commitment to occupations (118). Often their attention is focused on themselves rather than directed outward. One study proposed that outpatients with chronic schizophrenia are, in general, dissatisfied with their leisure activities (146). Schizophrenic adolescents have also been described as showing little pleasure in activities (94). Other research has found that chronic mentally ill persons in the community tend to engage in a higher percentage of passive activities (such as watching television, listening to the radio, or sitting), small chores and sleep than other people (216). However, this passivity may reflect the medicated life-style, lack of opportunities to pursue interests, and the low expectations typically made of these persons.

Habituation

ROLES

People with chronic schizophrenia often lack access to normal life roles, especially the role of worker (58). High levels of unemployment can make the possibility of working unlikely for these persons. In addition, people with chronic illness appear to perform fewer life roles on a continuous basis (175). Thus, they commonly find themselves cast in deviant roles with the expectation by others that they are unfit for normal role performance (9, 175). Deviant roles not only are peripheral to the mainstream of society, but also may be openly devalued and thus cannot serve as a source of self-worth (79). The person with chronic mental illness lapses into a state of rolelessness which is accompanied by societal stereotypes and the stigma of being a social parasite. Rolelessness leads to feelings of ostracism, incompetence, helplessness, emptiness, low self-esteem, lack of identity and, most important, the loss of an adaptive vehicle for organizing behavior (175, 192). This process may further exacerbate problems of internalized roles for the chronic schizophrenic person.

HABITS

Recognition of habit deterioration in schizophrenic persons is longstanding (166, 212). People with chronic schizophrenia are unlikely to have adaptive habits and routines (112). Typically they are unable to report how they spend their time (173) and their daily existence consists of a series of chaotic, disjointed events as opposed to a satisfying routine. Similarly, young adults hospitalized with schizophrenia have a substantially higher incidence of poor work and academic habits, poor planning and poor use of leisure time than other young adults (94).

Marian typifies the habit disorganization of schizophrenia. She is a 42-year-old female who lives alone and has a long history of chronic schizophrenia. With prompting, Marian describes a typical day that consists of watching TV, smoking and eating meals. What is striking in her report are the large blocks of unaccounted time.

Performance

SKILLS

People with chronic schizophrenia evidence impairment in the areas of interpersonal/communication, process and perceptual-motor skills. It is a common observation that individuals with chronic schizophrenia display marked deficits in interpersonal/communication skills (92, 106). It has been proposed that a lack of interpersonal skills is accompanied by isolation and high levels of social anxiety (189) and that goal achievement is hampered by deficient interpersonal/communicational skills (133). Perhaps this deficit is due to the failure to learn the rules or nuances of conduct underlying appropriate social behaviors or responses. For example, a person with schizophrenia may respond to the social inquiry "Hi, how are you today?" with a long-winded tirade of somatic complaints.

Deficiencies in process skills regarding sequencing behavior, problem solving, and planning as well as in perceptual-motor skills are common in chronic schizophrenic persons (116, 118, 230, 237). In addition, they exhibit deficiencies in the neurological, musculoskeletal, and symbolic constituents of skills (64, 172, 178). For example, schizophrenic adolescents often demonstrate slower motor development and inferior coordination (94), and infants and children at risk for adulthood schizophrenia appear to have visual-motor and vestibular-processing deficits (64, 237).

Inadequacies in both the dimensions and constituents of skills underlie what are observed as impairments in basic living skills—e.g. grooming, personal hygiene, meal planning and preparation, financial management, shopping, domestic chores, work skills, use of public transportation, and use of leisure time (26, 136, 225).

Environment

Although chronic schizophrenic patients no longer reside only in institutions, community facilities often create an environment that does not differ considerably from that of the long-term hospital (56). These environments, rather than promoting adaptive behavior, often serve to undermine occupational performance. For example, in the hospital, meals are prepared by the dietary department; domestic chores are performed by housekeeping; and personal hygiene, dress, sleep, and leisure are regimented by staff. As a result, patients lack the opportunity to learn, develop and/or practice those habits and skills necessary to return to the mainstream of life. In fact, it has been argued that many chronic patients may have more skills than they are encouraged to exhibit during hospitalization (154); further, if preexisting habits and skills are not maintained they will atrophy from disuse (84, 193, 210).

In addition to undermining skills, these facilities may create some of the problems that have been commonly assumed to be part of the disease process. Hospital furniture, poorly fitting clothes, inadequate nutrition, and inactivity may contribute more to the poor postural patterns and diminished muscle tone of schizophrenic patients than neurological deficits (13). Other research has shown that much of the isolated, passive behavior exhibited by chronic psychiatric patients is a direct function of physical attributes of the environment (93, 97).

The culture of community facilities and public institutions often exacerbates the lack of meaning in the lives of chronic schizophrenic persons. Typically, there are few sources of tradition and meaning available for persons in these facilities; what rituals there are tend to reflect the values of the hospital or board-and-care home rather than those of the traditional culture. Further, these settings often contain few items of interest and thereby contribute to a loss of interest in activities (18, 63, 78, 163, 215, 240, 250).

For many schizophrenic persons the social environment may have been impoverished or dysfunctional since childhood (10, 89). Schizophrenic persons often come from families in which the parents themselves had few social connections or were only marginal role models for their children (89). Thus, the schizophrenic person may have been deprived of the opportunity to learn competent behaviors, both within and outside the family.

Assessment and Treatment

Occupational therapy assessment and treatment for those with chronic schizophrenia depend upon the level of occupational dysfunction. Assessment and treatment should typically be addressed in phases. For example, a hospitalized individual with occupational dysfunction at the helplessness level, who is regressed, withdrawn and isolated, would not be able to participate in a formal assessment battery as it would only serve to overwhelm the person, reinforce his or her feeling out of control and highlight his or her incompetence. Rather, assessment at this phase should focus upon collecting data from skilled observation, family, peers, and past occupational therapy intervention. Therapy should be aimed toward organizing a safe environment with a low level of arousal, in order to evoke interest in the environment and exploratory behavior. In a later phase, as the individual became more organized, an assessment battery would be indicated in order to determine strengths to be maintained as well as dysfunctional areas to be remediated or modified (Table 15.11 presents recommended instruments from which a battery can be constituted.)

The chronic schizophrenic person often has maladaptive habits and routines and typically lacks access to traditional roles to organize daily routines. Although assessment and treatment attends to all subsystem components, the habituation subsystem is a primary target area for occupational therapy intervention. The occupational therapist guides the individual in pursuing alternative productive roles that are not only congruent with interests, goals and values, but also compatible with skills.

Because the schizophrenic person is typically inactive and lacks spontaneity, games involving physical movement are an important part of treatment. In addition, compensatory interactional and daily living skills must be taught. However, if these skills are not incorporated into habit patterns, they will not be maintained (106, 153).

The development of adaptive habit patterns and successful role performance provides positive feelings of self-confidence and competence. Although this process may begin during hospitalization, it must continue beyond discharge and throughout community reintegration. People with chronic schizophrenia may need ongoing treatment which may last indefinitely (185, 205). If traditional roles are unavailable in the community, alternative roles under the auspices of psychosocial rehabilitation, day treatment, and so forth should be pursued. Occupational therapy intervention within these settings is long-term and aims at maintaining a balance of productive roles within the mainstream of society. See Table 15.11 for further elaboration of treatment strategies.

CHRONIC SCHIZOPHRENIA CASE STUDY: CARL

Carl is 32 years old, single and has a diagnosis of chronic schizophrenia. He has an eighth grade education and has always lived with his parents and older brother in a two-bedroom apartment in a low income neighborhood in a major city. None of the family members is employed—each received supplemental social security. Both parents have a history of mental illness. Carl has a long history of psychiatric hospitalizations dating back to when he was 16 years old.

Carl stopped taking his medications approximately 6 weeks prior to this acute care hospital admission and, according to his parents, his behavior has gradually deteriorated. At the time of his referral to occupational therapy, he demonstrated occupational dysfunction at the level of helplessness. He was disoriented and reported hearing voices. He often wandered into other patients' rooms taking their plants and flowers into his room. He was extremely withdrawn, was not responsive to verbal approaches, and required staff assistance for personal hygiene, grooming and eating. He was unable to articulate his interests or his goals and preferred to stay in his room in the dark.

Occupational Therapy Intervention

Assessment and treatment were addressed in phases. At admission, Carl's occupational behavior was too disorganized for him to participate in a formal assessment battery. Data were therefore gathered from observation and from talking with Carl's parents. They related

Table 15.11.
Occupational status, recommended assessments and treatment considerations for persons with chronic schizophrenia

Occupational status	Recommended assessments	Treatment considerations
	VOLITION	

Personal causation

Inability to assess skills and the environment leads to decreased belief in skill	Occupational History (OH)	Identification of intact skills which can serve as source of competence; successful participation in activities of increasing complexity
Lack of success and personal achievement experiences result in a belief in personal ineffectiveness accompanied by increased anxiety, decreased self-concept, and decreased competence	Internal/External Scale Occupational Questionnaire (OQ) Occupational Case Analysis Interview and Rating Scale (OCAIRS) Occupational Functioning Tool (OFT)	Opportunity to attempt interesting, realistic activities which have a high probability of success; activities should match the person's level of skill and be of an appropriate level of arousal; identification of past successes which can serve as a source of encouragement for future action
External locus of control		Increased opportunity for independent decision making such as choosing activities

Values

Inability to establish priorities among goals; inability to identify and execute behavior required for goal realization	OH, OCAIRS, OFT Role Checklist (RC)	Goal-setting group emphasizing identification of short-term concrete goals, whose attainment can be readily ascertained
Possible temporal dysfunction with deficient future orientation; difficulty conceptualizing and ordering future events		Break down long-term goals into sequences of shorter steps
A sense of hopelessness and meaninglessness		Goals of treatment groups and relationship to long-term plans should be made clear
Inability to internalize societal values and establish priorities among these		Occupations used in treatment should be personally relevant and meaningful to client
		Daily routine should include opportunity for developing and/or maintaining skills, habits, and roles necessary to goal attainment

Interests

Dissatisfaction with leisure or inability to discriminate interests	OH, OQ, OCAIRS, OFT Interest Checklist	Opportunities to explore and generate new interests should be provided; however, these interests should realistically reflect socioeconomic and environmental constraints
Paucity of interest or high occurrence of passive interests (TV, sitting, etc.) which may reflect opportunities in setting		

Table 15.11.—*Continued*

Occupational status	Recommended assessments	Treatment considerations
		Skills for leisure planning should be taught and practiced; patient should be assisted in identifying community resources for continuing pursuit of new interests
		In hospital, patients should be given responsibility for planning leisure and social activities at nights and on weekends

HABITUATION

Roles

May lack a major occupational role such as worker or family member	OH, RC, OCAIRS, OFT	Use graded, work-oriented groups to develop skills necessary for assumption of worker role
Access to traditional occupational roles is often blocked after person acquires a history of mental illness		In the community, programs based on Fountain House model can help entry into worker role
Social support system may be weakened, decreasing chances to enact friendship role		Explore opportunities for participating in other occupational roles, e.g. hobbyist, volunteer, participant in religious groups, and so on
May not have fully internalized expectations for role performance		Role play situations associated with new roles so that client can learn and internalize expectations for performance

Habits

Habits do not support performance of roles	OQ, OH	Opportunities to learn and practice habits and skills necessary to role performance should be provided
Time may be chaotic and disorganized, or large amounts of time may be spent idle		Hospital should communicate expectations for routine occupational habits such as wearing street clothes, being on time for groups, and so on
Attention to habits of grooming, punctuality and other social conventions may be lacking		Schedule should include a balance of work, play and daily living tasks

Table 15.11.—_Continued_

Occupational status	Recommended assessments	Treatment considerations
	PERFORMANCE	

Skills

Occupational status	Recommended assessments	Treatment considerations
All areas of skills may be deficient; deficits reflected in motor retardation, unconventional social behavior, inattention to environmental and social cues, and unusual communication	OCAIRS, OFT Bay Area Functional Performance Evaluation	Social skills training, incorporating videotape and role playing, in order to learn rules of conduct, appropriate behaviors and responses; clear feedback regarding performance should be given Training and practice in steps of problem solving with application to a variety of situations Use of sports, dancing and games to encourage awareness and use of body

Occupational status	Recommended assessments	Treatment considerations
	ENVIRONMENT	
Hospital and community programs may not communicate expectations for maintenance of occupational roles, thus contributing to loss of roles, habits and skills Treatment may reinforce external locus of control Decay and/or lack of cultural tradition in treatment setting undermines meaning in occupations Social stigma related to mental illness makes reentry into society difficult	OH, OCAIRS Climate Scales (for ward or community program) Environmental Questionnaire Inventory of Depersonalization and Role Loss	Treatment should be a normalizing experience affording choices with consequences such as increased responsibility, increased self-management and increased decision making; e.g. the person selects meals, collaborates in setting goals, monitors progress, and has control over personal space Environment should replicate societal values as well as sanctions for inappropriate behavior Cultural traditions, including festivities, should be maintained; traditions should relate to client's cultural background Links between hospital and community programs and community advocates may help transition and acceptance into society

that Carl had never worked nor had friends, and spent the majority of his time at home watching television. Occasionally, he would ride the bus to the local park where he would pick flowers and bring them home. When his illness was in remission, he was able to attend to his self-care and help around the house.

The short-term goal (phase 1) was to en-courage Carl to interact with the environment and to develop adaptive habits. Plants seemed to be the only thing that evoked Carl's interest. Since there were several plants in the occupational therapy room, Carl was invited to care for them during therapy. Gradually, he began to repot plants, plant seeds and water and prune plants—all of which he did very well. His behavior became more organized and he started performing personal hygiene and dressing without staff intervention. He preferred to work alone, remaining on the fringes of the group with little interaction with others. As Carl became increasingly organized, he was administered the Interest Checklist, the Role Checklist, and an activity configuration. This began the second phase of assessment and treatment.

INTEREST CHECKLIST

So as not to overwhelm Carl, the original, simpler version of the Interest Checklist was administered to Carl. He reported strong interest in gardening/yardwork, macrame (which he had never performed), and listening to the radio; some interest in woodworking, (performed during past hospitalizations), television, ceramics (which he had never performed), housecleaning, laundry, and home repairs. All other activities were of no interest. Thus, he not only had few interests, but the potency of his interests was low.

ROLE CHECKLIST

Carl's responses on the Role Checklist are presented in Table 15.12. He has no continuous roles, but indicates past and future role incumbency in the roles of home maintainer and hobbyist—both of which he checked as very valuable roles.

SIMPLIFIED OCCUPATIONAL QUESTIONNAIRE

Carl was asked to record, in 1-hour intervals, how he spent his time. His typical day was the same as described by his parents—at home watching television.

Further Treatment Interventions

The long-term goal of occupational therapy was to engage Carl in an occupational role which was meaningful to him, which matched his level of skill, and which would serve to organize his daily life. Carl was encouraged to pursue the role of hobbyist. It was a role he had performed in the past, anticipated performing in the future and one he rated as very valuable. The hobbyist role was built around his interest in plants and flowers. In occupational therapy, Carl participated in increasingly complex projects. He learned to make wooden hangers for his plants. He also learned to macrame plant hangers, and to make ceramic pots. He seemed very pleased with his accomplishments and received positive feedback from the patients and staff. Carl's occupational status and treatment interventions are summarized in Table 15.13.

Outcome

Toward the end of his hospitalization, Carl began to attend a psychiatric day treatment center 5 days a week. Prior to Carl's arrival at the center, the staff was alerted to his progress and interest in plants so that he could

Table 15.12.
Carl's Role Checklist responses

Role	Past	Present	Future	Not at all	Some-what	Very
				Value		
Student	X				X	
Worker					X	
Volunteer				X		
Caregiver					X	
Home maintainer	X		X			X
Friend			X		X	
Family member					X	
Religious participant					X	
Hobbyist/amateur	X		X			X
Participant in organizations				X		

Table 15.13.
Carl's occupational status, treatment goals and interventions

Occupational status	Treatment goals and interventions
VOLITION	

Personal causation

Lack of successful experiences	Opportunity to attempt interesting, realistic activities with a high probability of success. Activities should match his level of skill and be of an appropriate level of arousal. Identification of past successes which can serve as a source of future action

Values

Deficient future orientation	Assist in goal formation with identification of behaviors needed to attain goals. Use occupations which have meaning for him
Sense of meaninglessness	

Interests

Decreased potency of interests. Primary area of interest is plants and flowers. Does express interest in activities never performed—ceramics, macrame. Has done woodworking during past hospitalizations	Opportunity to explore and generate new interests and to maintain past interest in plants. Interests pursued should be congruent with his economic status and potential opportunities beyond hospitalization

HABITUATION

Roles

Lacks a major occupational role. Lacks access to traditional occupational roles	Encourage participation in alternative role of hobbyist centering around his interest in flowers and plants

Habits

Maladaptive habit pattern; skills not organized into habits	Opportunity to develop and maintain habits and skills which support occupational role performance and that are congruent with volition

PERFORMANCE

Skills

Perceptual motor skills intact	Opportunity to practice problem solving and planning skills
Process skills impaired	
Deficient interpersonal/communication skills	Include in groups, to assist in development of increased interpersonal skills

pursue this at the center. It was also suggested that Carl be assigned tasks to perform over the weekend (when the center was closed) related to his interest. Carl was discharged home after 30 days of hospitalization. At 1 month postdischarge, Carl was regularly attending the day treatment center Monday through Friday. Occasionally, on weekends, he went to the park with a friend from the center to collect plants and flowers to take to the center on Monday.

References

1. Abramowitz SI: Locus of control and self-reported depression among college students. *Psychol Rep* 25:149–150, 1969.
2. Akiskal HS, McKinney WT, Jr: Depressive disorders: toward a unified hypothesis. *Science*, 182:20–29, 1973.
3. Allchin R: Some observations on depression and suicide in adolescents. In Meyerson S (ed): *Adolescence and Breakdown*. London, George Allen and University Ltd., 1975.

4. American Psychiatric Association: *Diagnostic and Statistical Manual of Mental Disorders*, ed 3. Washington, DC, American Psychiatric Association, 1980.
5. Andreasen NC: Concepts, diagnosis, and classification. In Paykel ES (ed): *Handbook of Affective Disorders*. New York, Churchill Livingstone, 1982.
6. Annell AL: Depressive states in childhood and adolescence. In Annell AL (ed): *Depressive States in Childhood and Adolescence*. New York, Halsted Press, 1972.
7. Barker R, Gump P: *Big School, Small School*. Stanford, Calif, Stanford University Press, 1964.
8. Barris R: Environmental interactions: an extension of the model of human occupation. *Am J Occup Ther* 36:637–644, 1982.
9. Barris R, Kielhofner G, Watts J: *Psychosocial Occupational Therapy: Practice in A Pluralistic Arena*. Laurel, Md, Ramsco Publishing Company, 1983.
10. Bateson G, Jackson DD, Haley J, Weakland JH: Toward a theory of schizophrenia. In Bateson G (ed): *Step to An Ecology of Mind*. San Francisco, Chandler, 1972.
11. Battista J, Almond R: The development of meaning in life. *Psychiatry*, 36:409–427, 1973.
12. Beck AT: *Depression: Causes and Treatment*. Philadelphia, University of Pennsylvania, 1967.
13. Beck MA, Callahan DK: Impact of institutionalization on the posture of chronic schizophrenic patients. *Am J Occup Ther* 34:332–335, 1980.
14. Becker EW, Lesiak WJ: Feelings of hostility and personal control as related to depression. *J Clin Psychol* 33:654–657, 1977.
15. Berman A, Siegel AW: Adaptive and learning skills in juvenile delinquents: a neuropsychological analysis. *J Learn Dis* 9:583–590, 1976.
16. Bernstein AE, Warner GM: *An Introduction to Contemporary Psychoanalysis*. New York, Jason Aronson, 1981.
17. Beutell NJ, Greenhaus JH: Integration of home and nonhome roles: women's conflict and coping behavior. *J Appl Psychol* 68:43–48, 1983.
18. Bhaskaran K, Dhawan N: A comparison of the effects of hospitalization on long stay and recently admitted female schizophrenic patients. *Int J Soc Psychiatry* 20:72–77, 1974.
19. Black M: The occupational career. *Am J Occup Ther* 30:225–228, 1976.
20. Blaney PH: Contemporary theories of depression: critique and comparison. *J Abnorm Psychol* 66:203–223, 1977.
21. Borrero IM: Psychological and emotional impact of unemployment. *J Sociol Soc Welfare*, 7:916–934, 1980.
22. Boskind-Lodahl M: Cinderella's stepsisters: a feminist perspective on anorexia nervosa and bulimia. *J Women Cult Soc* 2:342–356, 1976.
23. Braley LS, Freed N: Modes of temporal orientation and psychopathology. *J Consul Clin Psychol* 36:33–39, 1971.
24. Brandt R, Johnson D: Time orientation in delinquents. *J Abnorm Soc Psychol*, 51:343–45, 1955.
25. Briar KH: Helping the unemployed client. *J Sociol Soc Welfare*, 7:895–906, 1980.
26. Brokema M, Danz K, Schloemer C: Occupational therapy in a community aftercare program. *Am J Occup Ther* 29:22–27, 1975.
27. Bruch H: Changing approaches to anorexia nervosa. *Int Psychiat Clin* 7:3–24, 1970.
28. Bruch H: *Eating Disorders*. New York, Basic Books, 1973.
29. Bruch H: Psychological antecedents of anorexia nervosa. In Vigersky RA (ed): *Anorexia Nervosa*. New York, Raven Press, 1977.
30. Bruch H: *The Golden Cage: The Enigma of Anorexia Nervosa*. Cambridge, Mass, Harvard, 1978.
31. Buie DH, Adler G: Definitive treatment of the borderline personality. *Int J Psychoanal Psychother* 9:51–87, 1982.
32. Carpenter MD: Residential placement for the chronic schizophrenic patient: a review and evaluation of the literature. *Schizophr Bull*, 4:384–398, 1978.
33. Carr TH, Strain PS, Cooke TP, McMillan D: An ecologically oriented approach to youth deviance. *J Community Psychol* 4:389–400, 1976.
34. Cash T, Stack J: Locus of control among schizophrenics and other hospitalized psychiatric patients. *Genet Psychol Monogr* 87:105–122, 1973.
35. Casper RC, Davis JM: On the course of anorexia nervosa. *Am J Psychiat* 131:974–978, 1977.
36. Cavan RS, Cavan JT: *Delinquency and Crime: Cultural Cross-Perspectives*. Philadelphia, Lippincott, 1968.
37. Coehlo G, Silber E, Hamburg D: Use of the student-TAT to assess coping behaviors in hospitalized, normal, and exceptionally competent college freshman. *J Pers Soc Psychol* 18:305–310, 1971.
38. Conger J: A world they never knew: the family and social change. In Kraemer H (ed): *Youth and Culture: A Human-Development Approach*. Monterey, Calif, Brooks/Cole, 1974.
39. Cook L: The adolescent with a learning disability: a developmental perspective. *Adolescence*, 14:697–707, 1979.
40. Coser L: *Greedy Institutions*. New York, Free Press, 1974.
41. Coyne JD: Depression and the response of others. *J Abnorm Psychol* 85:186–193, 1976.
42. Cromwell R, Rosenthal D, Shakow D, Zahn T: Reaction time, locus of control, choice behavior, and descriptions of parental behavior in schizophrenic and normal subjects. *J Pers* 29:363–380, 1961.
43. Crumbaugh JC, Maholick LT: An experimental study in existentialism; the psychometric approach to Frankl's concept of noogenic neurosis. *J Clin Psychol* 20:200–207, 1964.
44. Diamond T: Nursing homes as trouble. *Urban Life*, 12:269–289, 1983.
45. Dillig P: (Future perspective of young prisoners and peers as well as resulting resocialization goals and methods). (English abstract) *Z Klin Psychol Forschung und Praxis*, 11:16–32, 1982.
46. Dilling C, Rabin A: Temporal experience in depressive states and schizophenia. *J Consult Psychol* 31:604–608, 1967.
47. Donnelly P: Athletes and juvenile delinquents: a comparative analysis based on a review of literature. *Adolescence*, 16:415–432, 1981.
48. Donovan A, Oddy M: Psychological aspects of

unemployment: an investigation into the emotional and social adjustment of school leavers. *J Adolesc* 5:15–30, 1982.

49. Duke M, Mullens M: Preferred interpersonal distance as a function of locus of control orientation in chronic schizophrenics, nonschizophrenic patients, and normals. *J Consult Clin Psychol* 41:230–234, 1973.

50. Dweck CS: The role of expectations and attributions in the alleviation of learned helplessness. *J Pers Soc Psychol* 31:674–685, 1975.

51. Dweck CS, Reppucci ND: Learned helplessness and reinforcement responsibility in children. *J Pers Soc Psychol* 25:109–116, 1973.

52. Eaton WW: *The Sociology of Mental Disorders.* New York, Praeger, 1980.

53. Eisikovits Z, Sagi A: Moral development and discipline encounter in delinquent and nondelinquent adolescents. *J Youth Adolesc* 11:217–230, 1982.

54. Elliot DS, Ageton SS, Carter RJ: An integrated theoretical perspective on delinquent behavior. *J Res Crime Delinq* 10:3–27, 1979.

55. Elliot DS, Voss HL: *Delinquency and Dropout.* Lexington, Mass, Heath, 1974.

56. Emerson RM, Rochford EB, Shaw LL: The micropolitics of trouble in a psychiatric board and care facility. *Urban Life*, 12:349–366, 1983.

57. Erikson EH: The problem of ego identity. *J Am Psychoanal Assoc* 4:15–121, 1956.

58. Erikson KT: Notes on the sociology of deviance. In Becker HS (ed): *The Other Side: Perspectives on Deviance.* New York, Free Press, 1973.

59. Ethridge D: The management view of the future of occupational therapy in mental health. *Am J Occup Ther* 30:623–628, 1976.

60. Fast I: Aspects of work style and work difficulty in borderline personalities. *Int J Psychoanal* 56:397–403, 1975.

61. Fidler G, Fidler J: Doing and becoming: purposeful action and self-actualization. *Am J Occup Ther* 32:305–310, 1978.

62. Fieve RR: *Moodswing.* New York, Bantam Books, 1975.

63. Fink H: The relationship of time perspective to age, institutionalization, and activity. *J Gerontol* 12:414–417, 1957.

64. Fish B, Hagin R: Visual-motor disorders in infants at risk for schizophrenia. *Arch Gen Psychiatry* 28:900–904, 1973.

65. Frank H, Paris J: Recollections of family experiences in borderline patients. *Arch Gen Psychiatry* 38:1031–1036, 1981.

66. Frankl V: *Man's Search for Meaning.* Boston, Beacon Press, 1963.

67. Frankl VE: *The Unheard Cry for Meaning.* New York, Touchstone Books, 1978.

68. Freden L: *Psychosocial Aspects of Depression.* New York, Wiley, 1982.

69. Freedman B, Donahoe C, Rosenthal L, Schlundt D: A social-behavioral analysis of skill deficits in delinquent and nondelinquent adolescent boys. *J Consul Clin Psychol* 46:1448–1462, 1978.

70. Freedman BJ, Rosenthal L, Donahoe CP, Jr, Schlundt DG, McFall RM: A social-behavioral analysis of skill deficits in delinquent and nondelinquent adolescent boys. *J Consult Clin Psy-*

chol 46:1448–1462, 1978.

71. Gaffney LR, McFall RM: A comparison of social skills in delinquent and nondelinquent adolescent girls using a behavioral role-playing inventory. *J Consult Clin Psychol* 49:959–967, 1981.

72. Garner DM, Garfinkel PE: Socio-cultural factors in the development of anorexia nervosa. *Psychol Med* 10:647–656, 1980.

73. Gerson EM: On "quality of life." *Am Soc Rev* 41:793–806, 1976.

74. Gillette ND: Changing methods in the treatment of psychosocial dysfunction. *Am J Occup Ther* 21:230–233, 1967.

75. Gladston R: Mind over matter. Observations on 50 patients hospitalized with anorexia nervosa. *J Am Acad Child Psychiatry* 13:246–263, 1974.

76. Glaser D: Economic and sociocultural variables affecting rates of youth unemployment. *Youth Soc* 11:53–82, 1979.

77. Glazer HI, Clarkin JF, Hunt HF: Assessment of depression. In Clarkin JF, Glazer HI (eds): *Depression: Behavioral and Directive Intervention Strategies.* New York, Garland STPM Press, 1981.

78. Goffman E: *Asylums.* New York, Doubleday, 1961.

79. Goffman E: *Stigma: Notes on the Management of Spoiled Identity.* Englewood Cliffs, NJ, Prentice-Hall, 1963.

80. Gold M: Juvenile delinquency as a symptom of alienation. *J Soc Issues* 25, 121–135, 1969.

81. Goode WJ: A theory of role strain. *Am Sociol Rev* 25:483–496, 1960.

82. Gorman B, Wessman A: *The Personal Experience of Time.* New York, Plenum Press, 1977.

83. Goshen CE: *Society and the Youthful Offender.* Springfield, Ill, Charles C Thomas, 1974.

84. Gray M: Effects of hospitalization on work-play behavior. *Am J Occup Ther* 26:180–185, 1972.

85. Grob M, Singer J: *Adolescent Patients in Transition: Impact and Outcome of Psychiatric Hospitalization.* New York, Behavioral Publications, 1974.

86. Gunderson JG, Singer MT: Defining borderline patients: an overview. *Am J Psychiatry*, 132:1–10, 1975.

87. Hammen CC, Glas DR, Jr: Depression, activity, and evaluation of reinforcement. *J Abnorm Psychol* 84:718–721, 1975.

88. Hammen CL, Peters SD: Interpersonal consequences of depression: response to men and women enacting a depressed role. *J Abnorm Psychol* 87:322–332, 1978.

89. Hammer M, Makiesky-Barrow S, Gutwirth L: Social networks and schizophrenia. *Schizophr Bull* 4:522–545, 1978.

90. Harrow M, Ferrante A: Locus of control in psychiatric patients. *J Consult Clin Psychol* 33:582–589, 1969.

91. Hauser S: The content and structure of adolescent self-concepts. *AMA Arch Gen Psychiatry* 33:27–32, 1976.

92. Hersen M, Bellack A: Social skills training for chronic psychiatric patients: rationale, research findings and future directions. *Compr Psychiatry* 17:559–580, 1976.

93. Holahan CJ: Environmental psychology in psy-

chiatric hospital settings. In Canter D, Canter S (eds): *Designing for Therapeutic Environments: A Review of Research.* New York, Wiley, 1979.

94. Holzman P, Grinker R: Schizophrenia in adolescence. *J Youth Adolesc* 3:267–279, 1974.

95. Hood J, Moore TE, Garner DM: Locus of control as a measure of ineffectiveness in anorexia nervosa. *J Consult Clin Psychol* 50:3–13, 1982.

96. Hudak MA, Andre J, Allen RD: Delinquency and social values. *Youth Soc* 11:353–368, 1980.

97. Ittelson WH, Proshansky HM, Rivlin LG: The environmental psychology of the psychiatric ward. In Proshansky HM, Ittelson WH, Rivlin LG (eds): *Environmental Psychology: Man and His Physical Setting.* New York, Holt, Rinehart, & Winston, 1970.

98. Jeammet P: The anorectic stance. *J Adolesc* 4:113–129, 1981.

99. Johnson RE: *Juvenile Delinquency and Its Origins.* Cambridge, Mass, Cambridge University Press, 1979.

100. Jones D: Structural discontinuity and the development of anorexia nervosa. *Sociol Focus* 3:233–247, 1981.

101. Jones RE: Street people and psychiatry: an introduction. *Hosp Commun Psychiat* 34:807–811, 1983.

102. Jurkovic GJ: The juvenile delinquent as a moral philosopher: a structural-developmental perspective. *Psychol Bull* 88:709–727, 1980.

103. Kaplan HB: Antecedents of deviant responses: predicting from a general theory of deviant behavior. *J Youth Adolesc* 6:89–101, 1977.

104. Kaplan K: *The Directive Group.* (Unpublished paper, 1982.)

105. Kelly PH, Fink WT: School commitment. Youth rebellion and delinquency. *Criminology* 10:473–485, 1973.

106. Kelly J, Urey J, Patterson J: Improving heterosocial conversational skills of male and psychiatric patients through a small group training procedure. *Behav Ther* 11:179–188, 1980.

107. Kendall RE: The classification of depression: a review of contemporary confusion. *Br J Psychiat* 129:15–28, 1976.

108. Kernberg O: *Borderline Conditions and Pathological Narcissism.* New York, Jason Aronson, 1975.

109. Kielhofner G: A model of human occupation, part 2. Ontogenesis from the perspective of temporal adaptation. *Am J Occup Ther* 34:657–663, 1980.

110. Kielhofner G: A model of human occupation, part 3, benign and vicious cycles. *Am J Occup Ther* 34:731–737, 1980.

111. Kielhofher G: An ethnographic study of deinstitutionalized adults: their community settings and daily life experiences. *Occup Ther J Res* 1:125–142, 1981.

112. Kielhofner G, Barris R, Watts J: Habits and habit dysfunction: a clinical perspective for psychosocial occupational therapy. *Occup Ther Ment Health* 2:1–22, 1982.

113. Kielhofner G, Burke J: A model of human occupation, part 1. Conceptual framework and content. *Am J Occup Ther* 34:572–581, 1980.

114. Kielhofner G, Burke J, Igi C: A model of human occupation, part 4. Assessment and intervention. *Am J Occup Ther* 34:777–788, 1980.

115. Kielhofner G, Takata N: A study of mentally retarded persons: applied research in occupational therapy. *Am J Occup Ther* 34:252–258, 1980.

116. King L: A sensory-integrative approach to schizophrenia. *Am J Occup Ther.* 28:529–536, 1974.

117. Kline NS: *From Sad to Glad.* New York, Ballantine Books, 1974.

118. Kolb LC: *Modern Clinical Psychiatry,* ed 9. Philadelphia, Saunders, 1977.

119. Korner I: Hope as a method of coping. *J Consult Clin Psychol* 34:134–139, 1970.

120. Kovacs M, Beck AT: An empirical clinical approach toward a definition of childhood depression. In Schullerbrandt JC, Raskin A (eds): *Depression in Childhood: Diagnosis, Treatment and Conceptual Models.* New York, Raven Press, 1977.

121. Kulka RA, Klingel DM, Mann DW: School crime and disruption as a function of student-school fit: an empirical assessment. *J Youth Adolesc* 9:353–370, 1980.

122. Kumchy CI, Sayer LA: Locus of control in a delinquent adolescent population. *Psychol Rep* 46:1307–1310, 1980.

123. Lambert BG, Rothschild BF, Atland R, Green LB: *Adolescence: Transition from Childhood to Maturity,* ed 2. Monterey, Calif. Brooks/Cole, 1978.

124. Larson R, Johnson C: Anorexia nervosa in the context of daily experience. *J Youth Adolesc* 10:455–471, 1981.

125. Lederer J: *The Model of Human Occupation Applied to Delinquent and Nondelinquent Adolescents.* (Unpublished master's project, Virginia Commonwealth University, 1983).

126. Lefcourt HM: *Locus of Control: Current Trends in Theory and Research.* New Jersey, Erlbaum, 1976.

127. Leggett J, Archer RP: Locus of control and depression among psychiatric patients. *Psychol Rep* 45:835–838, 1979.

128. Lewinsohn PM: Engagement in pleasant activities and depression level. *J Abnorm Psychol* 84:729–731, 1975.

129. Lewinsohn PM, Graf M: Pleasant activities and depression. *J Consult Clin Psychol* 41:261–268, 1973.

130. Lewinsohn PM, Hoberman HM: Behavioral and cognitive approaches. In Paykel ES (ed): *Handbook of Affective Disorders.* New York, Churchill Livingstone, 1982.

131. Lewis DO: *Vulnerabilities to Delinquency.* New York, Spectrum Press, 1981.

132. Lewis DO, Balla DA: *Delinquency and Psychopathology.* New York, Grune & Stratton, 1976.

133. Liberman R: Assessment of social skills. *Schizophr Bull* 8:62–83, 1982.

134. Libet J, Lewinsohn PM: The concept of social skill with special references to the behavior of depressed persons. *J Consult Clin Psychol* 40:304–312, 1973.

135. Linehan MM: A social-behavioral analysis of suicide and parasuicide: Implications for clinical assessment and treatment. In Clarkin JF, Glaser HI (eds): *Depression: Behavioral and Directive*

Intervention Strategies. New York, Garland STPM Press, 1981.

136. Linnell K, Stechmann A, Watson C: Resocialization of schizophrenic patients. *Am J Occup Ther* 29:288–290, 1975.

137. Liu A: *Solitaire: A Narrative.* NY, Harper & Row, 1979.

138. Llorens, LA: Changing methods in treatment of psychosocial dysfunction. *Am J Occup Ther* 22:26–29, 1968.

139. Lovejoy M: Expectations and the recovery process. *Schizophr Bull* 8:605–609, 1982.

140. Lynn R: *Learning Disabilities: An Overview of Theories, Approaches and Politics.* New York, Free Press, 1979.

141. MacLeod S: *The Art of Starvation.* London, Virago, 1981.

142. MacPhilany DJ, Lewinsohn PM: Depression as a function of desired and obtained pleasure. *J Abnorm Psychol* 83:651–657, 1974.

143. Magill J, Vargo J: Helplessness, hope and the occupational therapist. *Can J Occup Ther* 44:65–69, 1977.

144. Mahler MS, Kaplan L: Developmental aspects in the assessment of narcissistic and so-called borderline personalities. In Hartocollis P (ed): *Borderline Personality Disorders: The Concept, the Syndrome, the Patient.* New York, International Universities Press, 1975.

145. Mahler MS, Pine F, Bergman A: *The Psychological Birth of the Human Infant.* New York, Basic Books, 1975.

146. Malm U, May P, Dencker S: Evaluation of the quality of life of the schizophrenic outpatient: a checklist. *Schizophr Bull* 7:477–487, 1981.

147. Malmquist CP: Depression in childhood. In Flach FF, Draghi SC (eds): *The Nature and Treatment of Depression.* New York, Wiley, 1975.

148. Manaster G: *Adolescent Development and the Life Tasks.* Boston, Allyn & Bacon, 1977.

149. Maqsud M: The relationship of sense of powerlessness to antisocial behavior and school achievement. *J Psychol* 105:147–150, 1980.

150. Marks SR: Multiple roles and role strain: some notes on human energy, time, and commitment. *Am Sociol Rev* 42:921–936, 1977.

151. Martin JE: Anorexia nervosa—A disorder of weight. In *Proceedings of the Seventh International Congress of the World Federation of Occupational Therapists.* Paper presented at the meeting of the World Federation of Occupational Therapists, Israel, March, 1978.

152. Masterson J, Washburne A: The psychiatric adolescent: psychiatric illness or adolescent turmoil? *Amer J Psychiatry* 122:1240–80, 1966.

153. Matson J, Stephens R: Increasing appropriate behavior of explosive chronic psychiatric patients with a social-skills training package. *Behav Modif* 2:60–76, 1978.

154. Matson J, Ziess A, Ziess R, Bowman W: A comparison of social skills training and contingent attention to improve behavioral deficits of chronic psychiatric patients. *Br J Soc Clin Psychol* 19:57–64, 1980.

155. Matza D, Sykes GM: Juvenile delinquency and subterranean values. In Cavan R (ed): *Readings in Juvenile Delinquency.* Philadelphia, Lippincott, 1969.

156. McLean P: Remediation of skills and performance deficits in depression. In Clarkin JF, Glazer HI (eds): *Depression: Behavioral and Directive Intervention Strategies.* New York, Garland STPM Press, 1981.

157. Mechanic D: *Mental Health and Social Policy,* ed 2. Englewood Cliffs, NJ, Prentice-Hall, 1980.

158. Meissner WW: Notes on the levels of differentiation within borderline conditions. *Psychoanal Rev* 70:179–209, 1983.

159. Meissner WW: Notes on the potential differentiation of borderline conditions. *Int J Psychoanal Psychother* 9:3–49, 1982.

160. Melges FT: *Time and the Inner Future: A Temporal Approach to Psychiatric Disorders.* New York, Wiley 1982.

161. Melges G, Fougerousse C: Time sense, emotions, and acute mental illness. *J Psychiat Res* 4:127–140, 1966.

162. Melin L, Gotestam G: The effects of rearranging ward routines on communication and eating behaviors of psychogeriatric patients. *J Appl Behav Anal* 14:47–51, 1981.

163. Mendel W: Effect of length of hospitalization on rate and quality of remission from acute psychotic episodes. *J Nerv Ment Dis* 143:226–233, 1966.

164. Mendelson M: Psychodynamics. In Paykel ES (ed): *Handbook of Affective Disorders.* New York, Churchill Livingstone, 1982.

165. Menninger K: Hope. In Doniger S (ed): *The Nature of Man in Theological and Psychological Perspective.* New York, Harper Brothers, 1962.

166. Meyer A. The philosophy of occupational therapy. *Arch Occup Ther* 1:1–10, 1922.

167. Mitchell JJ: *The Adolescent Predicament.* Toronto, Holt, Winston 1975.

168. Moore JH, Coulman RN: Anorexia nervosa: the patient, her family and key family therapy interventions. *J Psychol Nurs Ment Health Serv* 19:9–14, 1981.

169. Moos RH: *Evaluating Treatment Environments: A Social Ecological Approach.* New York, Wiley, 1974.

170. Motto JA: The recognition and management of the suicidal patient. In Flach FF, Draghi SC (eds): *The Nature and Treatment of Depression.* New York, Wiley, 1975.

171. Moyal BR: Locus of control, self-esteem, stimulus appraisal, and depressive symptoms in children. *J Consult Clin Psychol* 45:951–952, 1977.

172. Myers S, Caldwell D, Purcell G: Vestibular dysfunction in schizophrenia. *Biol Psychiatry* 7:255–261, 1973.

173. Neville A: Temporal adaptation: application with short-term psychiatric patients. *Am J Occup Ther* 34:328–331, 1980.

174. Nurnberger JI, Gershon ES: Genetics. In Paykel ES (ed): *Handbook of Affective Disorders.* New York, Churchill Livingstone, 1982.

175. Oakley F: *The Model of Human Occupation in Psychiatry.* (Unpublished master's project, Virginia Commonwealth University, Richmond, Va, 1982.)

176. Offer D, Marohn RC, Ostrov E: Delinquent and normal adolescents. *Comp Psychiatry,* 13:347–

353, 1972.

177. Offer D, Ostrov E, Howard K: *The Adolescent: A Psychological Self-Report.* New York, Basic Books, 1981.

178. Ornitz EM: Vestibular dysfunction in schizophrenia and childhood atutism. *Comp Psychiatry* 11:159–173, 1970.

179. Palazzoli MS: *Self-Starvation.* New York, Jason Aronson, 1978.

180. Parsons T: Illness and the role of the physician: a sociological perspective. In Kluckhohn C, Murray H, Schneider O (eds): *Personality in Nature, Society, and Culture,* ed 2. New York, Knopf, 1953.

181. Paulson CP: Juvenile delinquency and occupational choice. *Am J Occup Ther* 34:565–571, 1980.

182. Paykel ES: Life events and early environment. In Paykel ES (ed): *Handbook of Affective Disorders.* New York, Churchill Livingston, 1982.

183. Perkins E: *The Patterns, Meanings and Need-Satisfication of Leisure Activities for Eating Disordered and Noneating Disordered Female Adolescents.* (Unpublished master's project, Virginia Commonwealth University, Richmond, Va, 1983.)

184. Perry JC, Klerman G: Clinical features of the borderline personality disorder. *Am J Psychiatry,* 137:165–173, 1980.

185. Peterson R: What are the needs of chronic mental patients? *Schizophr Bull* 30:610–616, 1982.

186. Petti TA: Active treatment of childhood depression. In Clarkin JF, Glazer HI (eds): *Depression: Behavioral and Directive Intervention Strategies.* New York, Garland STPM Press, 1981.

187. Petti TA: Depression and withdrawal in children. In Ollendick TH, Hersen M (eds): *Handbook of Child Psychopathology.* New York, Plenum Press, 1983.

188. Phillips WM: Purpose in life, depression, and locus of control. *J Clin Psychol* 36:661–667, 1980.

189. Pilkonis P, Feldman H, Himmelhoch J, Cornes C: Social anxiety and psychiatric diagnosis. *J Nerv Ment Dis* 168:13–18, 1980.

190. Polsky RH, McGuire MT: Social ethology of acute psychiatric patients: the influence of sex, hospital environment, and spatial proximity. *J Nerv Ment Dis* 169:28–36, 1981.

191. Puig-Antich J, Gittleman R: Depression in childhood and adolescence. In Paykel ES (ed): *Handbook of Affective Disorders.* New York, Churchill Livingston, 1982.

192. Rabinowitz H: Motivation for recovery: four social-psychologic aspects. *J Health Soc Behav* 5:2–13, 1964.

193. Reilly MA: A psychiatric occupational therapy program as a teaching model. *Am J Occup Ther* 20:61–67, 1966.

194. Rickarby GA: Psychological dynamics in anorexia nervosa. *Med J Austr* 1:587–589, 1979.

195. Rinsley DB: An object-relations view of borderline personality. In Hartocollis P (ed): *Borderline Personality Disorders: The Concept, the Syndrome, the Patient.* New York, International Universities Press, 1977.

196. Rosenberg M. *Society and the Adolescent Self-Image.* Princeton, NJ, Princeton University Press, 1965.

197. Rosenthal RH, Lani F: Selective attention and self-control in delinquent adolescents. *J Youth Adolesc* 10:211–220, 1981.

198. Salz C: A theoretical approach to the treatment of work difficulties in borderline patients. *Occup Ther Ment Health,* 3:33–46, 1983.

199. Samenow SE: The criminal personality. *Clin Proc* 36:14–22, 1980.

200. Sanders WE: *Juvenile Delinquency: Causes, Patterns, and Reactions.* New York, Holt, Rinehart & Winston, 1981.

201. Scaffa M: *Temporal Adaptation and Alcoholism.* (Unpublished master's project, Virginia Commonwealth University, Richmond, Va, 1982.)

202. Schiamberg LB: *Adolescent Alienation.* Columbus, Ohio, Merrill, 1973.

203. Scull AT: *Decarceration: Community Treatment and the Deviant—A Radical View.* Englewood Cliffs, NJ, Prentice-Hall, 1977.

204. Sedgwick P: Illness, mental and otherwise. *Hastings Cen Studies* 1:19–40, 1973.

205. Seeman M: Outpatient groups for schizophrenia—ensuring attendance. *Can J Psychiatry,* 28:32–37, 1981.

206. Seiber SD: Toward a theory of role accumulation. *Am Sociol Rev* 39:567–578, 1974.

207. Seligman MEP: *Helplessness: On Depression, Development, and Death.* San Francisco, Freeman, 1974.

208. Serok S, Blum A: A treatment vehicle for delinquent youths. *Crime Delinquency,* 25:358–362, 1979.

209. Serok S, Blum A: Rule-violating behavior of delinquent and nondelinquent youth in games. *Adolescence,* 17:457–464, 1982.

210. Shannon P: Work-play theory and the occupational therapy process. *Am J Occup Ther* 26:169–172, 1972.

211. Shybut J: Time perspective, internal versus external control, and severity of psychological disturbance. *J Clin Psychol* 24:312–315, 1968.

212. Slagle EC: Training aides for mental patients. *Arch Occup Ther* 1:11–17, 1922.

213. Smith C, Pryer M, Distefano M: Internal-external control and severity of emotional impairment among psychiatric patients. *J Clin Psychol* 27:449–450, 1971.

214. Smyntek LE: *A Comparison of Occupationally Functional and Dysfunctional Adolescents.* (Unpublished master's project, Virginia Commonwealth University, Richmond, Va 1983.)

215. Sommer R, Whitney G: The chain of chronicity. *Am J Psychiatry* 118:111–117, 1961.

216. Spivak G, Siegel J, Sklaver D, Deuschle L, Garrett L: The long-term patient in the community: Life-style patterns and treatment implications. *Hosp Commun Psychiatry,* 33:291–295, 1982.

217. Spreitzer E, Snyder EE, Larson DL: Multiple roles and psychological well-being. *Sociol Focus,* 12:141–148, 1979.

218. Squire S: Is the binge-purge cycle catching? *Ms. Magazine,* October 1983, pp 41–42, 46.

219. Srivastava RK: Undermanning theory in the context of mental health care environments. In Carson DH (ed): *Man-Environment Interactions; Evaluations and Applications, Part II.* Stroudsberg, Pa, Dowden, Hutchinson, & Ross, 1974.

220. Stern D: The first relationship: infant and mother. In Bruner J, Cole M, Lloyd G (eds): *The Developing Child*. Cambridge, Mass, Harvard University Press, 1977.

221. Stott DH: *Delinquency and Human Nature*. Baltimore, University Park Press, 1980.

222. Strassberg D: Relationships among locus of control, anxiety, and valued-goal expectations. *J Consul Clin Psychol* 41:319, 1973.

223. Strickland B: Internal-external expectancies and health-related behaviors. *J Consult Clin Psychol* 46:1192-1211, 1978.

224. Strober M: Locus of control, psychopathology, and weight gain in juvenile anorexia nervosa. *J Abnorm Child Psychopathol* 10:97-106, 1982.

225. Sylphe J, Ross H, Kedward H: Social disability in chronic psychiatric patients. *Am J Psychiatry*, 134:1391-1394, 1977.

226. Taube CA, Thompson JW, Rosenstein MJ, Rosen BM, Goldman HH: The "chronic" mental hospital patient. *Hosp Commun Psychiatry*, 34:611-615, 1983.

227. Teicher JD: A solution to the chronic problem of living: Adolescent attempted suicide. In Schoolar JC (ed): *Current Issues in Adolescent Psychiatry*. New York, Brunner/Mazel, 1973.

228. Teicher JD: The enigma of depression in infancy, childhood and adolescence. In Enelow AJ (ed: *Depression in Medical Practice*. West Point, Pa, Merck, Sharp & Dohme, 1970.

229. Test MA, Stein LI: Community treatment of the chronic patient: a research overview. *Schizophr Bull* 4:350-364, 1978.

230. Tucker GJ, Campion EW, Silberfarb PM: Sensorimotor functions and cognitive disturbance in psychiatric patients. *Am J Psychiatry*, 132:17-21, 1975.

231. Turner RW, Ward MF, Turner DJ: Behavioral treatment for depression: an evaluation of therapeutic components. *J Clin Psychol* 35:166-175, 1979.

232. Uncovic CM, Brown WR, Mierswa CG: Counterattack on juvenile delinquency: a configurational approach. *Adolescence*, 13:401-410, 1978.

233. Von Bertalanffy L: General systems theory and psychiatry. In Arieti S (ed.), *American Handbook of Psychiatry*. New York, Basic Books, 1966.

234. Wallace M: Future time perspective in schizophrenia. *J Abnorm Soc Psychol* 52:240-245, 1956.

235. Weissman R, Kutner B: Role disorders in ex-tended hospitalization. *Hosp Admin* 12:52-59, 1967.

236. Welner Z. Childhood depression: an overview. *J Nerv Ment Dis* 166:588-593, 1978.

237. Werry JS: The childhood psychoses. In Quay HC, Werry JS (eds): *Psychopathological Disorders of Childhood*, ed 2. New York, Wiley, 1979.

238. Werthman C: The function of sociological definitions in the development of the gang boy's career. In Giallombardo R, (ed): *Juvenile Delinquency: A Book of Readings*, ed 3. New York, Wiley, 1976.

239. West DJ, Farrington DP: *The Delinquent Way of Life: Third Report of the Cambridge Study in Delinquent Development*. London, Heinemann, 1977.

240. Wing J: Institutionalism in mental hospitals. *Br J Soc Clin Psychol* 7:38-51, 1962.

241. Winnicott DW: Ego distortion in terms of the true and false self. In Winnicott DW (collected papers): *The Maturational Processes and the Facilitating Environment*. New York, International Universities Press, 1965.

242. Wylie R. *The Self-Concept: Theory and Research*, revised ed. Lincoln, Nebr, University of Nebraska Press, 1979, vol 2.

243. Yalom ID: *Existential Psychotherapy*. New York, Basic Books, 1980.

244. Yochelson S, Samenow SE: *The Criminal Personality*. New York, Aronson, 1976.

245. Youkilis H, Bootzin R: The relationship between adjustment and perceived locus of control in female psychiatric in-patients. *J Genet Psychol* 135:297-299, 1979.

246. Yufit RI, Benzies B, Fonte ME, Fawcett JA: Suicide potential and time perspective. *Arch Gen Psychiatry*, 23:158-163, 1970.

247. Zinkus PW, Gottlieb MI, Zinkus CB: The learning-disabled juvenile delinquent: a case for early intervention of perceptually-handicapped children. *Am J Occup Ther*, 33:180-184, 1979.

248. Zis AP, Goodwon FK: The amine hypothesis. In Paykel ES, (ed): *Handbook of Affective Disorders*. New York, Churchill Livingstone, 1982.

249. Zober E: The socialization of adolescents into juvenile delinquency. *Adolescence*, 16:321-330, 1981.

250. Zusman J: Some explanations of the changing appearance of psychotic patients. *Int J Psychiatry*, 3:216-247, 1967.

CHAPTER 16

Pediatric Dysfunction*

Zoe Mailloux, Sue Hirsch Knox, Janice Posatery Burke, and Florence Clark

PEDIATRIC PRACTICE IN OCCUPATIONAL THERAPY

The occupational therapist working in a pediatric setting has many unique and challenging clinical and professional puzzles to face on a regular basis. Like each particular age group, childhood brings its own important milestones to be reached and mastered. But in childhood these milestones may be of long-term importance when the human is viewed as an evolving open system. The young child is truly in the formative years in which the behavior performed today provides the supportive structures on which tomorrow's life experiences will be built.

In childhood, the subsystem components of the system are being constructed, ordered and organized. The results of this process will have a major impact upon the trajectory patterns of future daily life performance. Similarly, the immaturity and flexibility of the constituents (neurological, musculoskeletal and symbolic) of the child's skills offers the therapist an excellent opportunity to have an immediate and far reaching impact on the child's adaptation.

Occupational therapists working with children have the opportunity to significantly prevent or lessen the impact of disability on the human system. Children are maturing human beings who, by the very nature of the developmental process, will be receptive to incorporation of new behaviors into their developing repertoire of role performance. In addition, most pediatric practices provide an opportunity for considerable involvement of family members, caregivers, and other significant people in the child's daily life. The ability to influence a highly flexible, maturing human system, coupled with the opportunity to interact with those in the child's environment, allows the occupational therapist to influence a wide range of critical coping skills and strategies in the young child.

Pediatric practice also carries with it unique and special problems. For occupational therapists involved in the care of young children, there is continual confrontation with others' perception of the questionable application of occupation to childhood. Teachers and school principals, hospital administrators, physicians and other health professionals, parents, and family members often have difficulty comprehending the role of occupational therapy in the care of a child who is years away from getting a job, much less embarking upon a career.

The complicated task of articulating the role of occupational therapy (on the habilitation and rehabilitation team) to other professionals as well as to family members is additionally compounded by the arena in which therapists address acquisition of role performance. In medical settings, where primary attention is focused on pathology, physical intervention and basic survival, the concern for play and optimal role performance is seen to be of lesser importance than the other elements of intervention that appear more technical or are more readily identifiable with traditional medicine. That play is a reflection of the individual's developmental integrity and a key opportunity to significantly influence the child's future interactions with the world is easily overlooked in a setting that is oriented to a more mechanical, symptom reduction, disease-focused approach. Likewise, parents may think of play as a behavior that all children do, regardless of their disease or disability, and are far more concerned with traditional questions related to their children's outwardly recognizable abilities such as walking and talking.

In light of these clinical and professional dilemmas, the therapist is faced with considerable

* The preparation of this manuscript has been partially supported by the U.S. Department of Health and Human Services, Bureau of Health Care Delivery and Assistance, Division of Maternal and Child Health, Grant MCJ-009048-01-0. Fictional names are used for patients and their relatives in this chapter.

problems, questions and concerns. The purpose of this chapter is to demonstrate how occupational therapists can make use of the model of human occupation to organize information that addresses the wide range of problems of children with disabilities and chronic diseases.

In order to utilize the model, the therapist must first integrate clinical knowledge with concepts of the model. In the first section of this chapter, we address general effects of disability on each of the human subsystems in relation to childhood occupation. Following this general orientation, clinical application will be considered in the following four categories of occupational dysfunction: (a) disorders which place the child at risk, (b) acute or temporary disorders, (c) chronic disability, and (d) progressive and terminal illness. This typology of disability was chosen in an effort to move away from a discussion centered on specific diagnostic categories and as a way of emphasizing the effects of disruption on each level of the human system and the environment when different types of disorders are present. Evaluation and treatment guidelines for each category are presented and are illustrated through specific case studies.

The Child as an Open System

As open systems, children are influenced by changes in the environment and, in turn, influence the environment as they change. The specific range of effects that a disability or disease has on an individual will vary, based on the type and severity of the problem, the integrity of the system prior to the incident and the life circumstances of the particular child. The degree of dysfunction that will occur cannot be predicted based on the child's medical diagnosis, age or particular living environment, or other such variables.

However, the model of human occupation specifies areas of functioning that are especially important to evaluate when a child is confronted with a disease or a disability. Further, theory and research concerning the development of human competence, cognition and creativity point out the importance of timing to the development of skills and abilities. According to such literature, these skills and abilities naturally develop at predictable periods of time based on the child's readiness.

This idea that the organism is poised or ready to accept new information and act on it in ways that it has not done so before is of primary concern for the pediatric occupational therapist. Treatment of a child who has not acquired skills that foster adaptation should include opportunities for the developing of compensatory skills. These skills, in a sense, bypass areas of dysfunction while ensuring that the child will be capable of effective interaction with the environment. The timing of such intervention is critical and assessment and treatment strategies must be habilitative, rehabilitative and preventive.

Disability resulting from disorders of childhood might be conceptualized as primary or secondary disorders. Primary dysfunction occurs as a direct result of the pathology present. For example, a child with muscular dystrophy may be unable to play with certain toys due to upper extremity muscle weakness which occurs as part of the disease process. A child, however, may develop disabilities which occur in association with a disorder, but not as a direct result. Problems of this kind can be considered secondary. The same child with muscular dystrophy may not develop particular coordination, perceptual, emotional, or social skills consequent to a reduction in opportunities for engaging in a wide range of activities necessitated by reduced vital capacity. The developing child is dependent on active involvement with the environment in order to flourish; thus any disorder limiting this involvement also holds the potential for compounding dysfunction.

With some children who have chronic illnesses and disabilities, it is often difficult to separate physical and psychosocial origins of the child's occupational dysfunction. Just as neurological, musculoskeletal and symbolic constituents of skills are developing simultaneously, so may both psychosocial and physical attributes of the child be affected in the presence of disease and disability. But this certainly is not always the case. In fact, many children seem to cope well with adversity, disability, and at-risk situations (9).

At the same time, a child's abilities to walk, move and handle objects are affected not only by disease and disability but also by the inner abilities to perceive and develop a sense of self and to formulate positive feelings associated with a sense of personal causation. The awareness of this interaction between the physical and symbolic aspects of behavior in the presence of dysfunction requires the therapist to have a commitment to a broad systems orientation of the child. In the following section the performance, habituation and volitional subsystems will be discussed for the purpose of providing a framework for evaluation and treatment of children with special needs.

THE PERFORMANCE SUBSYSTEM

Illness or disability can impair any or all of the constituents of skills at any time during the developmental process. The resultant reductions or delays in skilled behavior generally vary from child to child, even among those with the same condition. When skills are lost or compromised, remediation may be aimed at promoting greater efficiency in the constituents which underly the skills. In other instances, the child may be taught compensatory skills. For example, children with severe burns on their hands are prevented from manipulating toys or holding tools. These children need to develop alternate means of fine motor prehension including use of their mouth, feet or of specially fabricated adaptive devices. When problems such as these occur early in life, the result may be the inability to learn a specific skill or the learning of the skill in an atypical manner. Children with cerebral palsy, for example, who have abnormal muscle tone and associated atypical movement patterns will often use dominating motor reflexes to enable them to move about a room. While the movement may be adaptive in the sense that the child can move around, the repeated use of the primitive reflexes may inhibit the development of more mature motor patterns.

Illness may restrict or decrease opportunities (physical or environmental) for a child to explore or experiment with objects in the environment, often leading to distorted perceptions and limited information about the world and how one can act on and in it. Young children with rheumatoid arthritis are typically restricted in their movements due to decreased range of motion and associated pain when they do move. In turn, these children are likely to develop a fear of moving and of being on moving equipment on which their balance is challenged. These fears emerge as a by-product of their limited experiences as well as past negative experiences they have had with movement and pain. In contrast, the child who appears gravitationally insecure due to poor modulation of sensory input may express a similar fear of movement activities. Here, however, the cause is primary in origin (neurological) rather than secondary (i.e. due to painful or limited experience).

Communication and interaction skills may also be significantly affected when a child has a chronic disability or disease. Participation with peers is likely to be minimal or absent and other important social experiences such as family and recreational events, which are important influences on developing social and interactional skills, are likely to be significantly limited. Relationships with family members, hospital staff members, and others often foster dependent strategies at times when the development of skills for independence and autonomy are crucial.

The presence of a chronic disability or illness may also affect process skills including problem solving and decision making. Disturbances in these skills are commonly associated with decreased opportunities for the successful completion of tasks due to fatigue, pain, medical complications, drug reactions, etc. However, in some cases such as profound mental retardation, these disturbances may be a direct outcome of brain pathology.

THE HABITUATION SUBSYSTEM

The habituation subsystem is the critical link between the child and the everyday environment. The development of this system is shaped in the family context, in which the child is familiarized with the rhythms of daily of life and the ongoing cycles of human occupation and develops perceptions of his or herself as occupying a place in the social network.

The addition of a new member to a family instigates shifts in the routines of the overall family system. "The newborn has become recognized as a valued member of society and an entity to be reckoned with in the scientific world" (43). Findings of research revealing the active role of the neonate in the environment include recognition of the significance of the infant in determining the mother-infant relationship (42), and the effect of the neonate in patterning of the mother's behavior (36).

This interplay between the child and the environment, which probably begins before birth, leads to major transformations for both the child and the family throughout the developmental period. When dysfunction occurs, the development of habits and roles becomes an even more complex process and may be subject to disruption.

Habits

When dysfunction occurs at birth or early in life, basic regulatory functions such as breathing, sucking or heart rate may be disordered, in even the most elementary rhythms of the organism. For the premature or otherwise critically ill infant, disturbance in the first precursors to habits is disruptive for the routines of both the infant and the family because of the actual disorder, as well as the inevitable need for medical intervention. Future opportunities for developing regularity in these behaviors and a sense of routine in sleeping, feeding and playing are also likely to be affected.

The constraints of an extended hospital stay are likely to interfere with the usual adjustment period which occurs following the arrival of any new baby. The distress related to having a child with a dysfunction and the additional uncertainty of what the parents can expect are likely to become preoccupations eroding the potential for establishment of an effective habit structure for management of the child's care and other daily routines.

As the child grows older, more complex routines related to play and school performance may fail to develop normally as a result of disability in childhood. Again, parental expectations and perspectives will also influence the way in which the child's routines are shaped. Reactions to having a disabled child such as overprotection, self-blame, anxiety, acceptance, or rejection will affect the kinds of behaviors the child engages in and the types of activities performed for him or her (15, 52).

Many factors, including the ages of the parents, the type of disability present and the cultural perspective in the family, will contribute to the way in which the family and the child react to the disability (44). Additionally, special therapy programs, recurrent hospital stays, and other externally imposed medical regimens may significantly affect the evolution of habits. Children who spend the greater amount of their time in these medically supervised routines are less likely to develop an internalized sense of self-regulated routine.

Roles

The salient roles of childhood relate to play, school, self-care, family membership, and peer interaction. Just as habits are influenced in both parents and child from the earliest interactions, so too can roles be dramatically altered when individuals take on parenthood and children take their place within the family, community and culture.

Whether disability is present at birth or occurs during the developmental period, the process of internalizing roles for both parent and child is likely to be affected. Research related to the stigma of having a handicap sheds light on the degree to which perceived incumbency is affected when a disability is present. "The real trouble lies not so much with the disability, but in the extraordinary stigma that is such an inherent part of our culture" (Ref 11, p. 22). The status, rights and obligations of disabled children and their families are automatically colored by the presence of disability. Unfortunately, cultural attitudes about, and behaviors toward, dysfunction often make disability the most critical element of the perceived role of the child and other family members.

Beyond the stigma, specific limitations consequent to disability may also alter role perception for both the child and family; for example, inability to perform certain tasks may become internalized so that the range of role perfomance opportunities is seen as limited. Thus, the child with a disability may never develop an image of holding certain roles or achieving specific role requirements. There is, however, an interplay between social stigma and individual ability with each factor influencing the ultimate potential of the person with a disability within the society. It should be noted that many individuals with a disability follow a developmental trajectory that leads to constructive adaptation and, with it, life satisfaction (59).

The potential exists for the child with a disability to adopt the sick role, most likely leading to a maladaptive cycle. This is especially true, for example, in children who have diseases such as juvenile rheumatoid arthritis or leukemia. In such situations, large amounts of time are spent in the hospital or in acute stages of illness. The medical demands make it difficult for the parents and child to attend to other roles. Certain milestones seem to take on critical importance to all parents, but perhaps even more so when a child is disabled. The ability to walk and talk often becomes the focus of concern. Important everyday role behaviors related to play, self-care, peer interaction, and organization of behavior may be overlooked by the family or seen as secondary although these behaviors are vital for eventual adaptation.

A major problem for the family of a child with a disability centers on the excessive structure and demands that are often imposed by therapy schedules, special school programs and medical intervention, which leave few free hours for participation in the player role and family interaction. Occupational therapists employing the model of human oocupation will have the primary responsibility of rendering the family assistance in attainment of the delicate balance between allotment of time to medical and other necessary regimens and productive, growth inducing nondisability-related activity.

THE VOLITION SUBSYSTEM

As with the habituation and performance subsystems, a disability occurring during the developmental period may have either primary or secondary effects on the volition subsystem. The urge for exploration and mastery is critical to all aspects of childhood development. The sense of personal causation, the development of values, and the self-knowledge evidenced by interests contribute to choice, action and organization of behavior from the earliest parent-infant interactions through to the final stages of independence in adolescence and young adulthood. The effect of disability on these processes is a continuum influenced not only by factors from all other levels of the human system but also by the environment and the feedback received about system performance.

Some disorders, such as autism, could partially be described as a malfunction of the structures which are known to contribute directly to volitional capabilities. Ayres states " ... the 'I want to do it' system is working poorly in the autistic child" (Ref 4, p. 128). Children with this type of dysfunction may therefore have a distorted or insufficient urge toward exploration and mastery. Other disorders such as traumatic injuries create abrupt alterations in the volitional attributes which have started to define the essence of a child. For example, changes in skills and routines which result from disability may alter the urge toward action by changing the child's view of self. Since the volition subsystem is vital in initiating the child's active participation in occupational therapy, both primary and secondary disruptions of the volition subsystem have important implications for treatment.

Personal Causation

Beliefs about one's effectiveness in the environment are based on personal experience, therefore, the early presence of disability (i.e. that which is present at birth or in early childhood) has the potential to negatively impact upon the way in which those beliefs develop. Due to real or perceived limitations, a child with a disability may be less likely to acquire a sense of having control over and choice in the course his or her life will take (30).

Opportunities for risk taking which allow the child to acknowledge effectiveness and mastery are likely to be reduced as a consequence of limitations in skill, inadequate experience or overprotection from the family. There is, therefore, the potential for the development of a maladaptive cycle based on the child's lack of belief in his or her abilities. Early opportunities for developing a sense of control over the environment and mastery of skills are largely dependent on the types of objects played with by the child and the other characteristics of the play milieu (54). If it is assumed that a child with a disability would not derive meaning or enjoyment from play experiences, the opportunities for mastery are likely to be greatly diminished. Limitations on interactions with the physical and social environment may exacerbate the maladaptive cycle by obstructing the child's acquisition of a sense of security with physical challenges and the development of social initiative and social competence.

The parent of a disabled child is faced with a particularly challenging dilemma related to helping foster a sense of personal causation in the presence of the disability. Any such parent must struggle to achieve a balance between keeping a child safe and allowing a child to gain autonomy. The parent's ability to allow autonomy is greatly influenced when disability creates ever present risks to a child's physical or emotional safety.

Families who are able to overcome the tendency to overprotect and shield the child who has a disability must still be able to help that child with the reality of the limitations which may be present. Thus, belief in skill and expectancies of success or failure must be viewed within the context of the child's capabilities.

Values

The development of values occurs in concert with individual capabilities and cultural expectations. Children develop the rudiments of values by learning what is good, right and/or important primarily through their actions. When action is limited by reduced capabilities or opportunities, the process of acquiring values may occur in a more passive manner. Additionally, the cultural expectations of a person with a disability present from early childhood are likely to influence available choices and experiences of belonging within subgroups.

While the child with a disability may be only marginally aware of those images which could be called values, the family may be forced to critically analyze its values in several realms. In relation to temporal orientation, the parents of a child with a disability face difficult issues. They must grapple with questions concerning how much time they devote to their "special" child in relation to the amount spent with normal siblings, how much time they attend to their own needs in light of demanding therapy and school schedules and, perhaps, most difficult is the question of how their child, if severely handicapped, will survive and cope with the world, given the likelihood that the child will outlive its parents.

The way in which the family deals with these questions will serve to structure the future occupational objectives that the parents envision for the child. If the child achieves the ability to acquire occupational goals, these too will be at least somewhat based on the parents' early perspectives toward future orientations. The particular combination of values that will guide the child's choices of occupations is a by-product of the interplay between the child's own values and those that characterize his or her family.

Interests

The process of seeking activities which are pleasurable can probably be traced to life in utero where fetuses have been shown to respond more favorably to certain sensations than others. While these early indications of preference are largely based on the needs of the nervous system, individual differences are present and transcend a purely survival explanation. Even in premature infants, rudiments of interest can be discerned. As with all other components of the human system, however, the presence of a disability in a young child and the family's strategies for coping with it will have synergistic effects on the potential for interest formation in the child.

The ability to develop discrimination of interests, which requires differentiating expectations of enjoyment from a range of activity options, is initially dependent on the child's ability to register input, gain meaning and interpret feedback during an activity. Disabilities which limit sensory, motor or cognitive discrimination, for example, may also constrict or change the potential for gaining pleasure from an activity. A child with cerebral palsy may be attracted to a novel toy presented visually but may be unable to register the input provided by the toy, gain meaning from the input or interpret the feedback provided from interaction with the toy. In addition, poor motor performance may limit the range and quality of those interactions so that feedback is not only sparse but also exceedingly difficult to interpret.

In all children, the patterns and potency of interests which emerge are dependent on early discrimination abilities and the steps taken to broaden the child's opportunities and experience. Since interests both contribute to, and result from, action, they play an important role in occupational behavior. An example of satisfying interest development was observed in a boy with muscle disease which caused congenital paralysis. Growing up in a family with three brothers he was exposed to a great number of sports activities but was obviously unable to participate in them directly. Family efforts to foster this boy's interests in sports by providing opportunities for spectator involvement (subscriptions to sports magazines, wheelchair seating at sports events, remote control television with subscription to sports channels, etc.) allowed him to develop an interest in sports to the same magnitude his brothers achieved in participation. In this case, interests were strong enough to lead to an occupational choice of sports broadcasting.

The volition subsystem describes capabilities which are uniquely human. Children with disabilities can learn to take charge of their lives by developing this subsystem optimally. Their ability to do so will be contingent upon their own attitudes, their family's, and other elements of the environment in which they live and function.

THE ENVIRONMENT

Children develop within a range of environments, including those of the family and society-at-large. The result of an illness or disability in the child profoundly affects the family. Since the family is ideally the child's greatest support system, when the family prospers, so does the child. However, when the child has difficulty coping, then most likely the family also suffers. Additionally, the family's views of the child's condition will profoundly affect the child.

The parents', especially the mother's, adjustment to the birth of a child is a gradual process, starting when the mother first discovers she is pregnant. Many factors, such as self-esteem, attitudes and previous experiences as a mother, enter into the adjustment process and it usually follows a predictable sequence leading to attachment with the infant. The birth of a premature baby or child with a disability may, but does not necessarily, interfere with this process. Parents may go through stages similar to the stages of loss associated with death, such as (a) crisis, with shock and anxiety; (b) adjustment, with denial, guilt, and anger; and (c) reintegration with gradual acceptance. Their behavior towards the child during these stages may affect the child's subsequent adaptation.

In addition, illness or disability early in life often imposes separation of children from their parents and, because of this, may disrupt the attachment process. As the mother-child relationship develops, it is strongly dependent upon reciprocal interaction. Infants differ in their responsiveness to the nurturing behaviors of their mothers, but an infant with certain severe disabilities may be unable, or only minimally able, to indicate any reactions whatsoever. Additionally, if the infant requires special care, he or she may be separated from his or her mother, and both will be deprived of full days in which they can become comfortable and relaxed with one another. In the worst situation, the mother may withdraw from the maternal role. On the other hand, some mothers of children with disabilities will find nutring a child with disability satisfying and fulfilling as they strive to overcome the obstacles associated with disability.

As the child grows and develops, new challenges emerge. If these are viewed as problems rather than opportunities to overcome obstacles, a negative cycle can be established. Lamerowski (40), and Kornblum and Anderson (39) have presented the parental coping process as one of "chronic sorrow." They feel that the course of parents' grief is ongoing since the ways the disability will affect the child as a whole person

are unknown. Kornblum and Anderson (39) describe the child as a "living reminder" of the abnormality. New crises can occur as developmental milestones are not reached at expected times if parents are not helped to develop a positive attitude.

The ways that a parent deals with expectations, discipline, protection, stimulation, and consistency between the child who has special needs and siblings, all will impact on the child's overall system and especially on the development of self-esteem and feelings of competency. The feedback component of the open system provides individuals with information regarding the effect of their behavior or performance. Expected results are compared with actual outcome and the system is modified accordingly. The child quickly learns to expect certain responses to certain behaviors. Discrepancies due to privilege or special status are easily perceived and incorporated into the system as useful information for future interactions. The additional stresses of increased financial burdens, medical care and increased time necessary for child care and for seeking appropriate community supports all will effect the parent and, in turn, all other people involved with the person.

The reactions of siblings also affect the child's role behavior. A brother or sister with a disability will affect sibling reactions and demands on the parents. Reactions such as aggression or depressive anxious feelings are not uncommon.

Societal views of children with special needs will also have an effect on the childrens' perceptions of themselves. Sensky (51) explored the concept of "stigma" in children with congenital physical handicaps and in their families. The tendency is for society at large to endorse a normative stance and view individuals with disabilities as "different" and somewhat negative or shameful. The "different" individual is consequently stigmatized.

Parents assume "stigmas" with the birth of a child with a problem or when illness or injury results in their child having a disability. However, the child's understanding of stigma and its personal relevance grow with the development of body image. The way a child views and reacts to his or her special needs is highly dependent on many factors including: (a) age; (b) whether or not the problem first occurred at birth or later on, after having developed self-concepts; and (c) the coping mechanisms which the individual has subsequently developed.

CLINICAL APPLICATION OF THE MODEL OF HUMAN OCCUPATION IN PEDIATRICS

Thus far, this chapter has presented a general discussion of the possble effects of disability on the occupations of childhood. A major theme has been that the child with a disability has a better chance of living a productive and meaningful life if the internal hierarchy of subsystems and the environment encourage skill development, effective habit formation, opportunities for internalization of role, successful interactions, and a diversity of activity. However, the impact of disability on children will differ, in part, in accord with the nature of the disorder and the child's and the parents' reaction to it. In the following sections, clinical application of the model will be discussed in terms of four categories: (*a*) disorders which place the child at risk, (*b*) acute or temporary disorders, (*c*) chronic disability, and (*d*) progressive or terminal illness. Each of these categories represent different organizing themes or emphases for evaluation and treatment. An individual child, however, may present with elements of more than one disorder, and treatment, therefore, may combine elements of more than one category. Examples of this might be the child with juvenile arthritis who manifests acute disruptive episodes within the chronic disease process. Another child may become cerebral palsied following acute head trauma. Consideration of the organizing themes for all four categories is important in developing treatment programs to optimize occupational performance.

Disorders Which Place the Child at Risk

Many disorders, particularly those in the neonatal or early childhood periods, present not only with acute medical problems, but place the child at risk for future developmental problems and deficit role performance. Examples of these types of disorders are prematurity, child abuse, or neglect, and other metabolic, physical or neurologic problems occurring in infancy.

Factors which place the child at risk can occur both within the system (such as the immature physiological and nervous system of a premature infant) and from the environment (such as in child abuse). Treatment of these children encompasses all aspects of intervention from direct remediation of problems through preventive aspects, the primary theme of this category being prevention.

THE ENVIRONMENT

With infants and children at risk, the environment, particularly the caregiver-child interaction, is probably the most important consideration, as the young child can develop competently only if the environment fosters development. Therefore, in this section, discussion of environmental effects will be presented first in order to place the therapist's intervention into perspective.

Klaus and Kennell's (36) description of the attachment process serves as a framework within which such risk factors can be analyzed. They state that the parent and the infant both bring fixed and alterable behaviors to the relationship. The mother's behavior is dependent on such factors as her upbringing, culture and previous experiences. The infant's behavior develops from innate neurologic and physical attributes, and factors resulting from birth. Alterable factors include such things as hospital procedures, separation and management of the infant's responses. Results of the developing relationships between caregiver and infant can range from effective caregiving and attachment, through mild disturbances such as behavior problems, to severe disturbances such as abuse and/or neglect. Early intervention towards restoring or developing positive caregiver-child attachment serves to facilitate the development of optimum occupational performance of the child.

This process is also a major consideration with abused or neglected children. Researchers speculate that, with inadequate attachment, when parents undergo inordinate stress (either from their environment or from the child), they demonstrate inadequate coping mechanisms which may result in abuse and/or neglect (6, 24, 33). These studies are supported by the fact that, among populations of abused and neglected children, there are high incidences of medical problems, prematurity, multiple births, and separation following birth (6, 24).

In addition to separation from the mother postnatally, the high risk newborn also must cope with the artificial environment of the neonatal intensive care unit (NICU). Imposition of this environment on an infant whose own physiological and neurological systems are immature may have profound effects, although there exists great controversy in the field of neonatology on this issue. The NICU may be providing a combination of overstimulation in some areas and deprivation in others. More important, however, may be the fact that the input which the infant receives is noncontingent, i.e. it has little relationship to natural body rhythm or drives. Under normal circumstances, an infant and his mother develop their own patterns and timing, and care and stimulation is related to cues from the infant (contingencies) (29). This is generally not true in the NICU. The therapist may be providing a valuable service to young infants by helping others provide care that approximates that of normal mother-child interaction.

As the infant develops, persons and objects within the environment provide the press for development within the subsystems. When the environment is inadequate, such as with a neglected child, the child develops alternate coping mechanisms which may or may not be adaptive. For example, an environment devoid of toys, may force a child to utilize himself, peers or household objects to provide him with necessary sensory input. This may be adaptive in that he may create ingenious toys from other objects; or it may be maladaptive if he retreats into self-stimulatory behavior.

The following discussion of the subsystems provides additional examples of how the environment affects occupational performance.

THE PERFORMANCE SUBSYSTEM

The attributes that an infant or child brings to the caregiver-child interaction help shape that interaction. The newborn has been described as follows: "a biologically social and active partner in a feedback system with the caregiver, eliciting and seeking that ... organization from the environment that he himself needs in order to progress on his own course of self-actualization." (1).

The newborn's primary adaptive tasks are described as stages in behavioral organization (1, 29). Consideration of these tasks forms one of the bases for assessment and treatment of the newborn. These stages are described as follows:

1. Physiological—stabilization and integration of physiological functions
2. Motor—beginning of organized behavioral responses to sensory inputs
3. State—differentiation and modulated control of attentional state

4. Interaction—differentiation and modulated control of social interaction (29).

Disruption of these "tasks" by prematurity or later by neglect most profoundly affects the performance subsystem but it may also affect the habituation and volition subsystems as well. The premature infant initially shows great variability in internal regulation of physiological function and often requires an external life-sustaining support system. The occupational therapist's role in this case might be in helping to alter environmental inputs to help the infant regulate body function (i.e. suggesting the use of water beds as a way to receive motion or designing ways to decrease the constant light level usually present in a NICU).

As the infant gains physiological stability and begins to develop motor control, care needs to be taken to assure that appropriate patterns of movement are developing and that abnormal patterns are becoming inhibited. For example, a neonate who has been on a respirator for a prolonged time often develops strong extension patterns in the neck and trunk, partially due to efforts to keep the airway open and partially due to the position encouraged by the external apparatus. The therapist's concern in this example might be positioning and stimulation to facilitate neck flexion patterns while at the same time making sure breathing is not compromised. Likewise, the development of skills needed for state control and environmental interaction guide therapeutic intervention to enable the infant to develop competent behavioral organization.

As with the infant, the skills of the older "at risk" child may be compromised. Children who are neglected often do not receive the adequate nutrition needed for growth and lack environmental impetus for development. If the child is also abused, skills may not develop as a result of the injury or secondarily as a result of fear or punishment.

Studies have been conducted that suggest that the developmental characteristics of abused or neglected children that are most vulnerable to delay are in the areas of gross motor skills, adaptive performance and language acquisition (6, 24). These areas are all highly dependent on stimulation from humans and objects in the environment for optimal development. When they are deficient, therapy must focus on altering the environment as well as on direct remediation in order to give the child a firm base that will eventually contribute to coping.

THE HABITUATION SUBSYSTEM

The many aspects of the habituation subsystem can also be profoundly affected by "at risk" factors. In neonates, physiological stability as well as control over sleep/wake cycles are the beginnings of habits and temporal adaptation. The disruption of these normal habits by the NICU and by medical procedures has already been discussed. In addition to helping adjust infants' schedules and making care more contingent, the therapist may also provide direct inhibition or stimulation techniques to assist the infant in controlling his own behavior.

When considering the child in a neglected or abused situation, habits are usually profoundly altered. Often the parents are deficient in their own occupational performance, especially regulation of their own lives. They may have little time for, or interest in, their child's development of habits or skills. Decreased expectations or no expectations may be placed on the child. A child who is passive and/or nondemanding is often considered "good" and this type of behavior is encouraged. On the other hand, the curious, explorative child may often be perceived as spoiled, a nuisance, or "bad," and his behavior discouraged or even punished. The pattern of overexpectations, when applied to daily habits such as dressing and toilet training, is also seen in many abusive families. Inadequate knowledge about normal developmental milestones and timetables on the part of the parents and/or the belief that a child who is independent in self-care is less work for the parent may lead to premature training and unjustifiable discipline for inadequate performance.

The "at risk" population shows special problems related to the development of roles. When an infant is premature or sick at birth, the parents almost invariably undergo an immediate and profound grieving process. This often results in the parents perceiving the infant as an invalid. This is especially true of infants who have had life-threatening episodes. The role perceived by the parent often is adopted by the child, and the child learns to think of himself as sickly. Likewise, a child who is inconsistently disciplined or abused may come to think of himself as inadequate or "bad" and behave accordingly.

Additional problems arise with children who, because of an endangered environment, are removed from the family and placed in foster homes or institutions. They may undergo long periods of separation from parents and siblings and may change settings often. The variety of demands and expectations placed on them by the different living situations may add to role confusion.

One of the major roles of this age group, that of "player," often is disrupted. The infant learns about how his own body works and how he can interact with the environment through play. Often the restrictions imposed by necessary medical procedures and equipment (e.g. intravenous feeding, respirators, monitors) do not permit the freedom of movement to sense and explore adequately.

Children who receive little or inappropriate environmental stimulation may develop compensatory patterns of play, such as self-stimulation. Also common is increased solitary and fantasy play. One child hospitalized for abuse and neglect spent almost all of her play time with a toy dollhouse which had a closet under the stairs. She would scold and hit the dolls and shut them into the closet. In her play, she may have been attempting to gain some control over her environment. On the other hand, she was also practicing a deviant adult behavior. Statistics suggest that most abusing adults were abused in their childhood. Careful therapeutic intervention needs to be planned to break these cycles of deviant role acquisition.

THE VOLITION SUBSYSTEM

Early in life, infants show preferences for certain kinds of sensory input which may excite for some and tend to calm for others. However, the premature infant may have difficulty developing these preferences (precursors of interests) due to his or her immature system, or to external constraints. Also, medical routines may obscure the infant's preferences, manifested by his approach and withdrawal behaviors, and even when present these may go unrecognized. Instruction of NICU staff in recognizing and utilizing the infant's "cues" in daily care will help the infant develop and utilize the precursors of interests to motivate exploratory behavior.

Interests are further reflected in the play behavior of the young child, and are developed when play is fostered. Many of the deviations in

Table 16.1
Occupational status, recommended assessments and treatment considerations for the infant or child at risk

Occupational status*	Recommended assessments	Treatment considerations
VOLITION		
Personal Causation		
Decreased ability to control state in response to sensory input	Infant Temperament Questionnaire	Provide care contingent on infant's cues
Decreased reciprocal interaction with caregiver	Play History (PH)	Provide environment where child can safely take risks
Inconsistent feedback on actions	Neonatal Behavior Assessment Scale (NBAS)	
	Assessment of Premature Infant Behavior (APIB)	
	Bayley Scales of Infant Development (BSID)	
	Interview, and observation	
Values		
Inconsistent expectations	BSID, PH	Promote consistency in caregiving
	Interview; observations	
Interests		
Reduced components of conscious choice and interests	NBAS, APIB, BSID, PH	Provide sensory stimulation to develop preferences and interests
	Preschool Play Scale (PPS)	
	Interview, observation	Provide a variety of play materials and experiences
HABITUATION		
Roles		
Viewed as "sick"	Interview; observation	Promote parent/child attachment
Overprotection		
Inappropriate role models		Educate parents regarding developmental expectations
Habits		
Decreased establishment of routine patterns of behavior	NBAS, APIB, BSID	Promote environment that encourages normal cycling and routines
Input not contingent on cues	Interview	
Disturbed or inconsistent expectations in ADLs	Vineland Social Maturity Scale (VSMS)	Provide techniques to help infant control his own states and behaviors
	Gesell Developmental Exam (GDE)	
	ADL assessment	Develop age appropriate ADL
PERFORMANCE		
Skills		
Decreased development of components of skills	NBAS, APIB, GDE, BSID, PPS, ADL, VSMS	Develop skill components as appropriate
Decreased differentiation and modulation of skills	Miller Assessment for Preschoolers (MAP)	Grade sensory input to promote integration
Delayed development of skills	Clinical Play Observation (CPO)	Prevent further disability
	Parten Play Scale (PS)	Remediate skills

Table 16.1.—Continued

Occupational status	Recommended assessments	Treatment considerations
ENVIRONMENT		
Nonconducive to optimal role performance	PH	Alter sensory input and care in NICU's
Separation from parents	Interview	Promote parent/child attachment
Medical restrictions	Home visit	
Decreased opportunities and materials for play	Observation of maternal care	Build environments which foster curiosity and exploration

[a] Risk factors listed under occupational status do not necessarily apply to every child nor do they reflect the numerous strengths and assets a child may demonstrate when faced with dysfunction.

the play behavior of the child "at risk" have already been discussed and need not be repeated.

Children's belief in their own efficacy develops through personal experiences and through expectations placed on them. If they are viewed as invalids and not expected to do things for themselves, they may not develop a good sense of personal causation. Also if expectations are not consistent, or if they are arbitrarily punished, their sense of efficacy becomes diminished (Table 16.1).

Evaluation

The occupational therapist working with the neonatal or pediatric population usually is part of a multidisciplinary team. The therapist's evaluation is a portion of a comprehensive assessment from many disciplines' points of view. Just as the occupational therapist contributes to the total picture, so may other disciplines contribute to areas of concern for the occupational therapist. This is especially true when evaluating family involvement and needs.

Another aspect to consider in evaluation of pediatric populations is that many assessment tools require or recommend specialized training on the part of the therapist. For accurate use of these assessments and for a thorough understanding of them, it is important for the therapist to seek the additional training necessary.

An additional limitation to assessment with the "at risk" population is the medical stability of the child. Premature infants usually are not referred to occupational therapy until they are considered stable by the criteria set forth by the physicians. On the other hand, an abused child may have immediate medical needs such as burns, fractures or head trauma, which may affect the timing of involvement by the therapist.

The purposes of evaluation of the "at risk" infant or child are many. Evaluation provides a baseline, or picture of current functioning in occupational performance. It can also be used to assess progress. With neonates, serial evaluations are necessary as rapid changes occur in their behavioral organization. The predictive value of single developmental assessments has been questioned by many, but most authors agree that repeated tests can be helpful.

Another important purpose of the evaluation is to enable treatment planning and intervention. Areas of strength and deficits can be identified. The model of human occupation provides the structure for describing these and for planning treatment as all subsystems are considered. A number of standardized tests and clinical observations have been developed specifically for the neonate and young child (Table 16.1). These evaluations primarily assess the precursors to skills, such as neurological integration, reflexes, range of motion, and strength, and skills and habits. Some evaluate the quality of skills, while others assess role behaviors, such as play, and how they reflect all subsystems.

Most of the above assessment tools appraise the child's performance. Also critical to treatment is evaluation of the family. Crucial aspects to consider are the family's understanding of the problems, knowledge of mothering skills and developmental progression, expectations for the child, and direct interaction with the child. A few formal assessment tools are available in these areas but most of the information is gathered from informal interview.

A fourth purpose of evaluation is for staff and parent education. The Neonatal Behavioral Assessment Scale (NBAS), for example, has been used often to demonstrate an infant's skills and behavioral responses. Observation of how the infant performs, as well as explanations of the infant's cues, how stimuli are handled, and the response to different types of handling has proved very useful. Many parents report that, following observation of the examination, they begin to see their baby as an individual or as a "real person"; observation and explanation of an evaluation to a parent or staff member may serve the important purpose of enhancing attachment and increasing knowledge of children and performance in order to foster optimum role behavior.

Treatment

Treatment of the neonate and young child must again focus on two areas: (*a*) remediation of the child's deficits and enhancement of strengths and (*b*) building an environment which fosters curiosity, exploration and the development of optimum occupational performance.

Treatment of the neonate is quite specialized and each program must be individualized, taking into account the infant's stages of behavioral organization and needs. Intervention must be carefully graded and should be contingent on the infant's cues and on information gained from the external monitoring systems used on the unit. Examples of utilizing contingencies in treatment would be feeding when the infant is awake and hungry as opposed to feeding on a rigid schedule; or, utilizing calming methods to assist an infant in regulating a hypersensitivity to sensory stimuli. Controlled and graded sensory input is important in order to develop the sensory integration necessary for skills, for establishing routines and habits, and for developing interactive mechanisms.

Specific procedures may be utilized for remediation of neurologic and/or orthopaedic problems to prevent further complications and to provide a base for the development of skills and habits. Splinting, special positioning and utilization of neurodevelopmental techniques are all examples of this type of treatment. Another important aspect of neonatal treatment is fostering the development of oral control and feeding. Finally, considering the precursors to play development is vital to treatment of the neonate.

Early involvement and training of parents is of utmost importance with this population. Parents need to be helped to recognize their infant as unique and to develop appropriate interactions based on their infant's behavior. Interpretation of infant cues and education about the special problems of premature infants is vital.

Therapists must provide positive experiences for the parents and model techniques to help them care effectively for the infant. Discussion regarding developmental trends and specific needs is also necessary if the parents are to be able to foster optimal performance.

Treatment of the young child who has been abused or neglected is often complicated. Traditional occupational therapy techniques are routinely used to develop skills and habits, and these are necessary. However, one aspect of treatment particularly important for these children is that of utilizing a play approach for remediation. As already stated, many of these children will not have had good play opportunities or experiences and, as a result, are not in the habit of using play as an arena for skill development. Utilizing play as treatment requires the therapist to shift roles from one of "directing" an activity (as seen with more traditional techniques) to one of "participating" in the activity. It requires that the therapist set up situations to encourage play as well as meet treatment goals, but it is the child and the play itself that guides the therapy. The therapist encourages exploration and experimentation rather than repetition of a specific task. This type of approach encourages curiosity, exploration and intrinsic motivation on the part of the child, which is particularly important to develop in these children. It also helps build internal feelings of efficacy and a sense of responsibility (Table 16.1).

The importance of working with the parents or other caregivers cannot be overstressed. A recent study showed that these children showed developmental advances during periods of intense family support and instruction, but that they declined when active intervention was reduced (38). Family training must begin early and should not only consist of education regarding developmental and role expectations but should include opportunities for the parents to learn and practice behaviors that foster the development of optimal occupational behavior.

PREMATURE INFANT CASE: EDDIE

Background Information

Eddie was a black male, born at 30 weeks of gestational age. He was delivered via cesarean section due to fetal distress. His Apgar scores (a measure of fetal maturity) were 3 at 1 minute and 7 at 5 minutes (well below optimal scores of 8–10) and his weight was

1600 grams. He had difficulty breathing initially and was diagnosed as having bronchiopulmonary dysplasia. He was intubated and placed on a respirator at 100% oxygen. Because of severe agitation he was placed on phenobarbital and pancuronium bromide (Pavulon), which results in a neuromuscular block. On the second day he developed a left pneumothorax and a chest tube was placed. At 5 days of age he had a cardiac arrest and was revived. At 12 days of age, ultrasound revealed that he had had an intraventricular hemorrhage. At 1 month, he was taken off Pavulon. At this time, he was referred to occupational therapy because of limitations in range of motion and increased extensor tone in neck, trunk and extremities. The neurologist diagnosed him as having a spastic quadriparesis.

Eddie's mother was 19 years old, single and had a 4-year-old daughter. She had lived independently in the past but was, at the time of Eddie's birth, living with her mother. She saw Eddie's father often but had no plans to marry. The mother had a history of occasional alcohol use, regular smoking and questionable marijuana use. The psychological evaluation done by the social worker revealed an anxious mother who expressed feelings of confusion and concern for her baby. Although she had another child, she stated that she depended greatly on her mother for support and assistance.

Eddie was seen initially by the occupational therapist for evaluation at 1 month of age (or 34 weeks when age was corrected for prematurity). He was still on the respirator, but could be removed from the isolette for evaluation. Assessment included the Neonatal Behavioral Assessment Scale (NBAS) and further evaluation of range of motion, muscle tone, and oral function. Eddie's mother was not available for interview at the time. The NBAS scores are profiled into four dimensions, representing stages of neonatal behavioral organization. The scores are categorized into three levels: excellent, average or worrisome. Analysis of these dimensions show that three of them (interactive processes, motoric processes and response to physiological stress) relate primarily to the performance subsystem. The fourth dimension (state control) relates more to the habituation subsystem. The results of the NBAS and related observations will be described in terms of the subsystems.

PERFORMANCE SUBSYSTEM

Eddie's performance on the NBAS dimension of interactive processes was worrisome (lowest level). Primarily due to his difficulty with state control, his orientation to animate and inanimate visual and auditory stimuli was difficult to assess. He showed brief, variable periods of alertness and attentiveness. Within these brief periods, he showed some quieting and eye shifting to voices, and quieting only to a rattle sound. He made no attempt to turn or search for the sounds. He briefly focused on the examiner's face and on a red ball and followed the examiner's face and voice combined for 30° arcs. When he became upset, he was unable to console himself and he needed to be wrapped tightly and rocked. Because of increased muscle tone and irritability, it took a great amount of nestling, rocking and inhibitory handling in order for him to relax enough to try to cuddle against the examiner.

Motoric processes were also worrisome. Many developmental reflexes were abnormal or absent due to his increased tone. For example, he showed an abnormally high neonatal positive support reflex. Walking responses were absent because he could not break through the extensor tone elicited by the positive support. Eddie showed a hyper-responsive Moro response which was elicited by small changes in position, noises, and light touch. Muscle tone was hypertonic in the extensors throughout the neck, trunk and extremities. Movements were jerky in quality with limited arcs of motion. Passive range of motion was also limited in the shoulders and hips. There were no purposeful hand-to-mouth or defensive responses with upper extremities. When he was upset, he exhibited constant movements which perpetuated his crying. Movements could only be controlled by wrapping or restraining him.

Eddie also showed worrisome responses to physiological stress, as demonstrated by his hyper-responsive startle, tremors in extremities in most states, and marked color changes when he was upset.

HABITUATION SUBSYSTEM

The fourth NBAS dimension, state control, relates to the development of habits and daily routines. Again, Eddie's performance was worrisome and he could be described as very labile. He was unable to modulate his states and reacted in a disorganized way to most testing maneuvers. He became upset initially with the rattle stimulus and showed irritability to most stimuli. He made brief attempts to calm himself but was unsuccessful and needed intervention. When finally calmed, he had exhausted himself and retreated into sleep states. His ability to modulate his state and establish patterns of sleep/wake/interaction was deficient. Oral skills, precursors to feeding, were also tested. At the time, he was tube fed. However, he did show slight rooting responses and made weak attempts to suck on the examiner's finger, although this was inhibited by the respirator.

THE VOLITION SUBSYSTEM

At this time, Eddie did not display the physiological or neuromuscular maturity to interact with the environment on a preference basis, other than that he showed a preference for rocking by calming in response to it. As mentioned before, he was unable to exercise much control over his environment and needed intervention to help calm him.

In summary, Eddie was an infant who, due to immature physiological systems and abnormal neuromotor systems, was functioning at the lowest stages of behavioral organization. He showed deficits in many of the precursors to skills, such as reflexes and muscle tone, which led to deficits in basic motor and interactive skills. His inability to control his reactions to sensory stimuli, in combination with the above, made it difficult for him to regulate his states and develop more adaptive responses to handling.

ENVIRONMENT

Initially Eddie was in an isolette with a respirator and feeding and intravenous tubes. The respirator contributed to his extended posture and it, along with the abnormal muscle tone and hard flat surface of the bed, made it difficult to position him comfortably. The constant lighting and noise of the NICU also inhibited the development of normal sleep/wake cycles.

The persons in his environment were many, their handling of him was varied, and he underwent many medical procedures daily, most of which were uncomfortable or painful. In addition, his mother was seldom present. Even when she did visit, she seldom touched or handled him due to his fragile status and her insecurities. Her visits became further apart although she would call daily for progress reports.

Treatment Goals and Plans

The following goals and plans were established on the basis of the evaluation and are in terms of subsystems.

THE PERFORMANCE SUBSYSTEM

1. Increase physiological and neuromuscular stability through controlled sensory input and calming methods, thus enabling him to begin to control his responses.
2. Increase range of motion through passive ranging, facilitation of active movement and positioning.
3. Decrease abnormal tone and posturing through positioning and neurodevelopmental handling techniques.
4. Develop smooth coordinated purposeful movement through controlled sensory input and neurodevelopmental handling.
5. Provide education to the nursing and other staff regarding appropriate handling, calming techniques and positioning.
6. Provide education to the mother and grandmother regarding specific handling, positioning, etc.

THE HABITUATION SUBSYSTEM

1. Develop normal cycling of sleep/wake and interaction/withdrawal behaviors by utilizing the infant's cues as contingencies for intervention.
2. Develop prefeeding, and eventually feeding skills through oral stimulation and feeding techniques when medically ready.
3. Provide education to the nursing and other staff regarding reading infant's cues, timing procedures and other interactions contingent on these cues.
4. Reinstall the mother as a caregiver by the following methods:
   a. Help her become acquainted with her infant by helping her read his cues and respond appropriately to them.
   b. Provide interpretations of his behavior. For example, suggest to her that his arching into extension does not mean he does not like her.
   c. Recommend simple routines, such as rocking him, which may soothe him and train her in caregiving.

THE VOLITION SUBSYSTEM

1. Develop self-control and interests by the use of contingent behaviors as described above
2. Develop visual and auditory attention by providing visual and auditory stimuli in the crib to which he could alert or orient according to his wake/sleep cycle.

Course of Treatment

Occupational therapy involvement on the NICU was an integral part of a multidisciplinary team through weekly team meetings and informal discussion of progress, problems and plans. Initially, Eddie was seen in his isolette, but as he became more medically stable he was taken out for treatment. At 4 months chronologically, the respirator was removed and oxygen was given by nasal canulas facilitating handling. He was also moved to a crib.

Occupational therapy consisted of graded sensory stimulation, range of motion, neurodevelopmental handling techniques, and play/interactive activities during his awake periods; the length was dependent on his cues. Calming techniques were used to help him relax when he was upset or following medical procedures. Oral stimulation was provided, especially during tube feedings. At 4 months, when the feeding tube was removed, oral feeding (nippling) was started. At 7 months, spoon feeding was initiated. With all feeding, he had difficulty coordinating suck/swallow and he showed excessive vertical jaw movement; therefore, special feeding techniques were used.

Various positioning devices, consisting of small wedges, a crib cuddle (a hammock device), rolls, infant seat, and infant swing were used to decrease the hyperextended posture. The rhythmic rocking of the swing particularly helped calm him. As he grew, toys and mirrors in the crib provided visual and auditory stimuli.

Inservices and individual instructions were given to nursing staff regarding handling, calming methods, interpretation of his cues, and play activities. His mother was encouraged to visit; when she did, she was also shown therapy techniques, cues and behaviors were interpreted for her, and she was encouraged to play with Eddie.

Treatment Outcomes

At the time of this study, Eddie was 7½ months chronologically and 4 months corrected age. He was still an inpatient, but was approaching discharge. He was on 35% oxygen. His mother was beginning to visit more regularly but was still reluctant to play with Eddie or participate in other caregiving activities. Eddie's occupational performance at this time was assessed by use of the Revised Gessell Developmental Schedules and was as follows.

THE PERFORMANCE SUBSYSTEM

Eddie continued to show limitations in passive range of motion secondary to increased muscle tone. Range had improved. He could easily be moved out of the hyperextended position and he could maintain midline positions for extended periods. Muscle tone had decreased somewhat, but still markedly affected skills. He continued to show primitive reflexes but was no longer bound by them. Intermittently, he could break through with spontaneous movement. Movements remained jerky with limited arcs. All developmental skills were below age expectancy and were affected by tone. However, in gross motor areas, he was more symmetrical and was gaining control of head movements in prone and in the supported sitting position. He was also beginning to show purposeful upper and lower extremity movement out of patterns; e.g. in sitting, he could get his right hand to his mouth and was beginning to grasp and feel toys and attempt to bring them to his mouth. In interactive skills, he showed direct definite regard of persons, his mirror image and toys, and was able to turn his head slowly to follow them visually. He also turned towards, and sought out, animate and inanimate sounds. He did not demonstrate any vocalizations, although his cry was audible and strong. He smiled in response to stimulation.

THE HABITUATION SUBSYSTEM

Eddie showed an improved ability to control his state; however, he continued to need intervention to help calm him when upset. He was able to sustain an alert state and interact with an adult and with toys for up to 45 minutes. He continued to show startle responses to light touch, noise and position changes, but his behavior no longer disintegrated and he could calm immediately. He was improving with feeding but continued to need special techniques including jaw control to inhibit the vertical jaw movement and facilitate mouth closure.

THE VOLITION SUBSYSTEM

Eddie showed definite preferences for certain types of sensory stimuli, particularly vestibular input. He needed and responded positively to rigorous rocking and bouncing. He also was beginning to show preferences for familiar caregivers and therapists with smiling and increased social interaction.

Recommendations

Although Eddie showed progress during his hospitalization, he will continue to need prolonged, active, therapy intervention for his neurologic and developmental problems following discharge. The deficient mother-child relationship also makes him at risk for abuse and/or neglect. Therefore, intensive work with his mother needs to be done to help her attach to him and provide competent care for him, and provide the stimulation necessary for him to achieve appropriate role behavior.

Acute or Temporary Pediatric Disorders

Acute illnesses occurring during childhood usually strike suddenly with little notice. This section will examine the effects of acute pediatric dysfunction from the perspective of the model of human occupation. Disorders included in this category are viral and bacterial infections (e.g. meningitis), fractures, burns, poisonings, and other accidental incidents such as near drownings and head injuries. The organizing theme of this section is one of disruption and reorganization for the child and and the family. The acute phases of diseases such as juvenile rheumatoid arthritis, hydrocephaly, seizure disorders, asthma, diabetes mellitus and oncological conditions are also included here because of the similar disruption which occurs in these cases.

The role of occupational therapy in this area of practice is often largely preventive. Consideration of the developmental sequence and the potential effect of the disruptive nature of illness in childhood is critical. The immediate and most obvious effects of the disorders are often seen in the performance subsystem. The way in which the entire system is affected depends upon the severity of the condition, the prognosis, and the coping strategies of the child and family.

THE PERFORMANCE SUBSYSTEM

The components of the performance subsystem affected by an acute disorder will be determined by the type and extent of the problem. As discussed in the first section of this chapter, the problems may be considered primary or secondary. Examples of primary disorders in the performance system include decreased muscle strength, disrupted sensory processing, lessened range of motion, incoordination, poor cognitive processing, and disturbed language skills. These are the problems which occur as a direct result of pathology (e.g. inflammation of the meninges of the brain or spinal cord in meningitis) or trauma (e.g. a crush fracture of the radius). Additional performance level problems may occur due to disuse, lack of opportunity for developing a skill, or overprotection of the injured or sick child. For example, a child hospitalized following an automobile accident may develop muscle weakness as a function of prolonged

immobilization, or the same child may be kept from playing group sports at a later time (thus decreasing socialization opportunities) if there is concern for reinjury.

Often a very specific problem becomes the focus of attention when a disorder occurs suddenly. For example, when a child sustains a burn injury, the first concern of the occupational therapist may be to prevent contractures which occur consequent to decreased elasticity of the skin. Although longer term considerations would involve many other aspects of function, the critical nature of an acute stage of illness may necessitate initial focus on a more specific problem than is usual for a chronic disability. However, because dysfunction in performance level skills is often the most obvious and the most critical in an acute disorder, there may be a tendency to overlook the effects these problems have on other levels of the system. The impact on habituation and volition level components can be, in fact, significant.

THE HABITUATION SUBSYSTEM

While interest and energy may become focused on changes in performance level skills during acute illness, habituation level components may also undergo major disruption. A large body of research on the effects of hospitalization in childhood, originated in the 1950s and 1960s continues to evolve. Consideration of the effects of hospitalization is relevant because the acute nature of most of the disorders discussed in this section usually necessitates some type of hospital stay. Several of the classic studies from this body of literature will be discussed here as many of the ideas expressed in the hospitalization research are applicable to the ways in which the habituation system is likely to become disturbed when an acute illness state is present.

Cooke (22) proposed a typology of changes in routine which occur during hospitalization. Separation is considered the first major component of change. For example, the child hospitalized with a severe asthma attack or arthritis flare becomes separated from activities (e.g. school, play), people (e.g. parents, siblings, peers) and things (e.g. home, bed, toys). Separation is compounded by the existing illness, the deprivation of normal sensory and social experiences, and the usual suddenness of acute illness and hospitalization. The second major component of change described by Cooke is the introduction of many new elements to the child's environment. For example, the child who has survived a near drowning accident experiences many new activities (e.g. different routines, procedures, meals), people (e.g. nurses, doctors, therapists) and things (e.g. monitors, intravenous bottles, hospital clothes). Numerous other studies have cited similar disorganizing factors in childhood hospitalization (14, 16, 45). Since habits and roles in childhood are largely organized by daily life routines, changes occurring due to separation from the family and the presence of a new situation have the effect of disrupting the functioning of the habituation subsystem.

An additional complicating factor relates to the logic skills present in childhood. Younger children may have difficulty with time concepts relative to their daily schedule and the length of their hospital stay. Thus a child may view the new schedule as permanent. In other children, loss of participation in activities such as sports or social events may create great feelings of disappointment and frustration (23). Cognitive deficits accompanying disorders such as head trauma or meningitis may create further difficulty in coping.

Habituation components for all family members change when acute illness occurs. Glen (28) describes the existence of family "rituals" in relation to illness. He states, "a crisis encountered in an acute illness usually requires the family to reorganize" and notes that the family must determine caretaking roles and effects on family routines (Ref 28, p 954). Coordinating hospital visits (including possible overnight stays by one of the parents), meetings with medical personnel and therapy schedules with ongoing activities of the family can become complicated and exhausting. Increased numbers of working mothers and single parent families, in addition to decreased proximity of extended family members may also create a loss of traditional support systems for families when acute illness is present.

THE VOLITION SUBSYSTEM

The emotional impact of sudden serious illness will undoubtedly affect volitional attributes of the child as well as those of the family. When illness necessitates restrictions on movement (as in fractures) or on input to the system (as in burns when the possibility of infection limits the items allowed into a child's room), the child may be afforded very few choices. The suddenness of an acute situation also contributes to the feeling of loss of control over one's environment. Thus personal causation or believing in one's effectiveness is challenged.

The family may experience a similar loss in feelings of personal causation. The sudden introduction of numerous authority figures providing directions or advice may lessen the family members' sense of control over their lives. If the child has been previously free of any dysfunction (as in an accident victim) the family may be unprepared for the loss of control they are likely to encounter within the medical care setting. Families of children with recurrent disorders may search for mechanisms to promote their sense of control when an exacerbation occurs. In this case, the family's behavior may be interpreted as manipulation, aggression, or withdrawal unless the health care team is sensitive to the trauma inherent in such a situation.

The effect of acute illness on interests and values may be temporary or permanent, depending upon the severity of the condition and the prognosis. Some of the conditions discussed in this section, such as near drowning incidents or burn injuries, are likely to create long-term care considerations which would be similar to the conditions discussed in the chronic disability section. However, even a temporary traumatic event, such as a nonfatal poisoning, can activate a new set of interests and values within a family.

THE ENVIRONMENT

As discussed in preceding chapters, the environment is critical to recovery from acute illness. Lack of, or inadequate amounts of, sensory input within the hospital environment can lead to listlessness, indifference, poor appetite, etc. in the child (19, 55). Restoration of normalcy of routine and of opportunities for play are vital elements in the environment for promoting the emotional well being necessary as a foundation for recovery. Because the critical nature of an acute illness might focus attention on medical needs related to immediate survival, the occupational therapist may play a key role in structuring the environment to promote well being and prevent future problems related to occupational role performance (Table 16.2).

Evaluation

An occupational therapy evaluation of the child in an acute stage of illness serves several purposes. First, the information from the as-

Table 16.2
Occupational status, recommended assessments, treatment considerations for the child with an acute or temporary disorder

Occupational status	Recommended assessments	Treatment considerations
VOLITION		
Personal causation		
Limited opportunities for choice	Stanford Preschool Internal-External Scale (SPIES)	Provide opportunities to plan activities and make choices regarding plans
Feelings challenged by illness, medical care, restrictive movement, and input	Play History (PH) Interview, and observation	
Values		
Feelings of decreased worth	PH	Provide opportunities to participate in goal setting
Decreased ability to set goals and problem solve	Piers Harris Children's Self-Concept Scale (PHSC) Preschool Play Scale (PPS) Observation and interview	
Interests		
May be altered temporarily or permanently	PH, PPS Interest Checklist (IC) Interview and Observation	Provide activities to foster interests Provide temporary adaptations to allow expression of interests
HABITUATION		
Roles		
Disruption of school and player roles by illness and hospitalization	PH Role Checklist (RC) Vineland Social Maturity Scale (VSMS) Interviews	Provide opportunities for socialization Continue school activities as appropriate Provide expectations in self-care and simple chores
Habits		
Disorganizing effects of hospitalization	ADL, PH, VSMS Gesell Developmental Evaluation (GDE)	Restore normal routines and opportunities for play Involve child and family in planning daily routines
Disruption of normal routines and habits	Bayley Scales of Infant Development (BSID) Interview	
Time concepts disrupted		
PERFORMANCE		
Skills		
Disruption and reduction in skills with subsequent recovery	GDE, BSID, PH, PPS Range of motion	Remediation of constituents of skills Develop age appropriate skills
Recovery may be uneven or incomplete	Muscle test Reflex integration	Prevent further disabilties, due to disease, lack of opportunity, or overprotection
Disruption of skill components	Muscle tone	

Table 16.2—*Continued*

Occupational status	Recommended assessments	Treatment considerations
	Oral motor assessment	Provide opportunities for play and exploration
	McCarthy Scales of Children's Abilities	
	Bruininks-Oseretsky Test	
	Southern California Sensory Integration Tests	
	Southern California Postrotary Nystagmus Test	
	Clinical Play Observation	
	Parten Play Scale	
	Interview and Observation	
	Decision Making Inventory (DMI)	
ENVIRONMENT		
Separation from family environment and persons	PH	Involve family in daily care
Deprivation of normal sensory and social experiences	Home visit	Provide toys and play experiences
	Interview	
Introduction of new elements into the environment		Give suggestions to promote gains such as involvement in community programs

sessment may help to clarify the nature of the problem when compared to findings of other treatment team members. For example, a dressing evaluation of a child with an active brain tumor may reveal difficulties in visual perception or motor planning ability not previously observed. Assessment tools also help chart the progression or course of the problems. Repeated evaluation of dressing skills of the child in this example may demonstrate deterioration or improvement of performance level skills such as coordination, strength, problem solving, etc. In addition, through the evaluative interaction, the therapist may detect habituation disruption such as discomfort with unfamiliar clothes and dressing schedules, or the beginning of volition level problems such as loss of interest in self-care or a sense of lack of control over the situation. Finally, evaluation helps to set treatment goals by revealing verified as well as potential areas of dysfunction. Constraints associated with assessment of the child in an acute stage of illness include medical complications, hospital stays of short duration, and lack of appro-

priate referral to occupational therapy. Additionally, since therapy is based on the results of the assessment, all aspects of the system must be addressed. Therefore, evaluation of the habituation and volition system is equally important to assessment of the more obviously dysfunctional performance system (Table 16.2).

Treatment

The treatment approach utilized for the acutely ill child from the perspective of the model is dependent upon both the present dysfunction of the various levels of the system and the potential for further disruption. The overall goal of any intervention is to promote reorganization and adaptation within the system. Often initial treatment focuses on critical performance level components. For example, splints are often applied within 24 hours following a burn injury to prevent deformity. This immediate action is necessary to prevent future problems which would be likely to affect all levels of the system. The therapist must also consider (often within a very short time span) how, for example, loss of mobility in the burn injured child will affect developmental tasks related to the child's sense of efficacy, self-esteem and exploration. Play provides the vehicle for addressing components of all levels of the system and is, therefore, as important in the acute setting as in other longer term situations. Finally, involvement of the family even in the very early stages of intervention can serve to promote reorganization within the home and ensure consistency and carryover of therapeutic objectives (Table 16.2).

Therapeutic interaction in pediatrics always requires ingenuity and imagination on the part of the therapist in order to structure activities that both address the problem areas and interest the child. The presence of acute illness can be an additional challenge. However, intervention in the acute stage is often vital to prevent the development of chronic disability such as those discussed in the following section.

MENINGITIS CASE: KEITH

Background Information

This case is based on a real case; however, some of the evaluation findings and treatment methods are hypothetical in order to present a more complete example of intervention when using the model of human occupation in acute pediatric illness.

Keith is an 8-year-old boy who contracted aseptic (viral) meningitis thought to be related to group B Coxsackie virus infection. The onset was sudden with Keith demonstrating fever, headache, malaise and neck stiffness. Kernig's sign was evident upon admission and the diagnosis of meningitis was made after laboratory analysis demonstrated the presence of the virus in the pharynx. Keith was admitted to the ICU and started on antibiotic therapy. He was seen once in occupational therapy while in the hospital and was then referred for outpatient occupational therapy following discharge. This illness occurred in February, necessitating absence from school for the rest of the semester.

Evaluation

While in the hospital, Keith was evaluated for upper extremity range of motion and strength, coordination, cognition, and self-care abilities, and observed for general affect and interests. Assessment during the first outpatient visits included evaluation of sensory integration processing, a play history, and administration of a self-esteem measure and a modified interest checklist. An interview with Keith's parents was also conducted to gain information about the family and home environment.

THE PERFORMANCE SUBSYSTEM

Keith, who was right handed, demonstrated range of motion and strength within normal limits for his age in his right upper extremity. Although passive range of motion in the left upper extremity was normal, Keith displayed weakness in this extremity. Manual muscle testing revealed good muscle grade throughout the shoulder girdle, fair to fair-plus grade in elbow flexion and extension and in supination and pronation, and poor muscle grade in the wrist and hand musculature. Keith showed no signs of weakness in the lower extremities. Coordination was evaluated by observing Keith involved in activities such as ball catching and throwing, bead stringing and wood working. Keith's incoordination appeared much worse than would be expected due to the left upper extremity weakness alone.

Cognition was assessed by question and answer and by problem-solving games. Keith appeared quite bright with no apparent cognitive dysfunction. His parents verified that they had not observed any interference of cognitive abilities following his illness. Observations of self-care activities such as dressing, bathing, and grooming also revealed excessive problems which were beyond those that would be caused by weakness alone. In both coordination and self-care activities, Keith appeared to have the greatest difficulty with tasks which involved the use of his hands out of his visual range (e.g. putting a T shirt on over his head or combing the back of his hair). The outpatient evaluation of sensory integration helped to shed light on Keith's coordination and self-care problems. His scores on the Southern California Sensory Integration Tests were generally within normal expectations except his score on the Kinesthesia test (−2.6 standard deviations from the mean for his age). This finding was further validated by observation of Keith in motor activities. Motor planning, evaluated by the Imitation of Posture Test and clinical observations, appeared slightly dysfunctional. Thus, the major performance level deficits demonstrated by the assessments were left upper extremity weakness and generalized poor kinesthesia. Slight dyspraxia was also present.

THE HABITUATION SUBSYSTEM

Interviews with Keith and with his mother were the main source of assessment of the habituation level. The play history was incorporated into both interviews and also provided information on habits and roles.

Keith was an only child. His mother was an extremely obese woman who admitted to being very self-conscious of her weight and therefore uncomfortable with leaving the house very much. Keith's father worked as an electrician and often worked overtime in the evenings. Keith's social life occurred mostly at school as his home situation made extracurricular involvement in activities such as Boy Scouts or Little League difficult. Keith, who was mildly overweight himself, was not particularly involved in sports before his illness. Information from the interviews and play history revealed that a typical day involved school during the day, homework or television after school and after dinner, and a family meal at dinnertime. Keith's family lived in an apartment where there were few children his age. Keith had recently become friends with a 6-year-old neighbor. According to Keith, most of their play time involved indoor play with army men. Keith reported that he had friends at school but that he did not see them outside of school. Keith's household responsibilities included making his bed, cleaning his room and taking out the trash. Keith's habituation system was markedly disrupted by the onset of his illness. Since school activities constituted the major portion of Keith's habits and routines, hospitalization and the subsequent rehabilitation program represented a major shift of daily activity. After discharge from the hospital, Keith attended occupational therapy 5 days a week for 1 hour a day. The rest of his day was spent mostly playing alone at home and watching television. Keith expressed unhappiness over missing school and his mother reported that he had told her he felt clumsy and awkward and did not feel like seeing his neighborhood friend. Loss of performance level skills and a major change of normal daily activity had created disruption of habituation level functioning.

THE VOLITION SUBSYSTEM

At evaluation, Keith displayed a generally depressed affect and did not appear motivated to engage in the assessment activities. Although not tested specifically, Keith appeared to feel little control over his situation. When given choices, he often looked to his mother or told the therapist to decide. His mother reported that he had a tendency to depend on her in difficult situations before his illness but that his behavior at this time was much more dependent than in the past. A frequent response to questions was, "It doesn't matter." On the Piers Harris Children's Self-Concept Scale, Keith scored below the 50th percentile in all six of the domains measured, with his scores on "behavior, intellect and school status" and on "popularity" being the lowest. When a modified interest checklist was administered, Keith stated that he was interested in television and school but expressed no interest in other activities listed. He specifically said that he did not want to play with friends because he thought they would make fun of him.

The interviews and observations revealed that school activities were valued most by Keith and at that point active involvement in school had constituted his main occupation. Peer play and family activities had been less important but were also valued as part of his daily life. Having had his normal routines disrupted, Keith could find little in his current situation that seemed important or interesting. The effect on his personal causation and self-esteem had been negative with Keith feeling as though he could not do much to his current status.

Treatment Strategies

During the first 3 weeks after hospital discharge, Keith was in an outpatient occupational therapy department of a hospital five times a week for 1-hour sessions. For the following 4 months, Keith was seen in a private practice occupational therapy clinic two times a week for 1-hour sessions. Strengthening activities for the left upper extremity were incorporated first into simple play activities such as ball throwing and catching, and board games with weighted playing pieces. As his therapy program progressed, Keith became involved in constructing several craft projects (a toy box, a leather key chain and a tile tray for his mother). These activities were designed to further strengthen his left upper extremity as he began to regain muscle use. Self-care activities were encouraged while Keith was seen in the outpatient department, mostly through play activities such as dressing in costumes and water games in the pool after which he would shower, dress and comb his hair.

A great deal of proprioceptive input was

provided to Keith both at the hospital and throughout his therapy program at the private clinic. Joint traction was provided in the course of swinging, jumping and running activities. A weighted vest was also used to help give Keith more sensory information in relation to his body position. The vest was called a "back pack" and it was used as part of "camping" and "hiking" games. All of the activities involved coordination and motor planning.

Throughout the therapy program, Keith was encouraged to plan activities in his daily routine. He and the therapist in the private practice period devised a daily log in which he tried to do "five new things" each week. Keith worked on his craft activities partially at home and sometimes tried a new part of the activity on his own. Other "new things" included helping with cooking dinner, collecting different kinds of rocks from the neighborhood and writing a letter to his classmates at school. The daily log, as well as the craft and play activities, were designed to promote balance in the components of the habituation level. Keith's therapeutic intervention would have been considered "child guided," i.e. initiated based on the child's interests and needs, with the therapist assisting to make the activities successful experiences. When possible, Keith was encouraged to interact with other children in the private practice setting in order to also promote social interaction. Keith was a child with limited social experiences prior to his illness and he was considered "at risk" for future social withdrawal due to his current self-image. As discharge from occupational therapy approached, a home program was developed in conjunction with Keith and his mother to ensure continuity of his gains. Since therapy ended during the summer, the therapist suggested that Keith's mother explore a summer playground program. It was felt that this type of program would provide more varied activities for Keith, lessen the trauma of returning to school in the fall after missing a full semester, and increase Keith's opportunities for social interaction with children his own age. This strategy was aimed at enhancing Keith's environment in a family situation which was adequate for providing care but not enriched in terms of helping Keith to achieve his best potential.

Outcomes of Treatment

Keith's left upper extremity muscle strength and overall kinesthetic perception increased gradually throughout the therapy program to within normal limits by the 4th month of outpatient therapy. It was not pos- sible to determine how much of this gain was due to spontaneous recovery following the meningitis versus the effects of the therapeutic program. By the time Keith completed his outpatient program at the hospital, he was independent in all self-care activities.

Although Keith's daily routines had normalized somewhat by the time he was discharged from therapy, it was not certain how well he would organize his day once he did not have the therapist's guidance. A readministration of the Piers Harris test revealed cluster scores above the 50th percentile in each category although "behavior, intellect and school status" and "popularity" were still his lowest scores.

Thus Keith was still considered at risk for after-effects of his illness on the habituation and volition subsystems even though his performance level skills had basically returned to normal. The home program and suggestions for involvement in the summer school activities were designed to help ameliorate the potential for future success. The mother was asked to report back to the clinic at the end of the summer but she did not and Keith's long-term response to this disruptive, acute illness experience is unknown.

Chronic Disorders or Diseases

Some children will grow up with a disability and have it with them through the course of their lives. The chronic disabilities of childhood include, but are not limited to, cerebral palsy, spina bifida, autism, mental retardation, juvenile rheumatoid arthritis, congenital malformations, and learning disabilities. United States statistics have recently revealed that the proportion of children with disability due to chronic illness has increased markedly. In the noninstitutionalized population, the percentage of children with activity limitation has risen from 2.1% in 1967 (57) to 3.9% in 1978 (58). The increase partially reflects the impact of medical advances that enable children with severe disabilities to survive, but is also attributed to the trend for children with severe disabilities to be cared for in the home instead of in institutions (18). For the occupational therapist, these statistics suggest that in the future a greater proportion of therapy will be provided for children with chronic disabilities and their families who are now carrying the day-to-day burden of managing the care and coordinating the customary round of daily activity of their child. It also implies that treatment will be based to a lesser extent in hospitals and institutions and to a greater extent in homes and community settings.

The model of human occupation provides a useful framework for therapists confronting these changing times and challenges. It compels the therapist to view the child as an open system and to focus away from specific pathology. Not only must the system be addressed, but also its environment. The key to maximizing the benefit of occupational therapy for the child with a chronic disability centers on the theme of adaptation. Parents and child will need to learn to make adjustments to a chronic condition, and to share in the creation of an environment that is most likely to foster a meaningful and satisfying life for the entire family constellation.

At the outset, the therapist employing the model of human occupation must examine his or her own perspective on chronic disability. While there are special problems encountered by persons with disabilities, a large proportion of these individuals strive positively, adapt and live satisfying lives (59). All clinicians are in danger of becoming preoccupied with pathology in their work. This attitude can be particularly damaging to the very person the clinician is hoping to help, the child, who is regularly exposed to the clinician who becomes part of the environment affecting the system. Through repeated exposure, the child is vulnerable to absorbing this pathology-centered attitude as his or her own (10).

Instead, the therapist must convey to the child a balanced perspective on disability. This perspective would include the recognition that the majority of children cope well with adverse and disabling conditions (9). A chronic disability may simply be different, rather than bad or tragic (10). In fact, Blom and his colleagues (10) cite a number of sources that suggest that disabled persons (insiders), in contrast to the able-bodied (outsiders), view their condition as a fact of life to be dealt with realistically. Therapists utilizing the model of human occupation must initially adopt the premise that "while life growing up with disability is different, it does not have to mean abnormality or pathology" (10).

A perspective on the contributors to successful adaptation and how they are fostered must govern clinical reasoning. Children with a variety of at-risk conditions (including chronic physical illness and disability) identified by their teachers and principals as doing remarkably well in mainstream situations have been found to share common characteristics. They tend to be friendly, accepted by their peers, talkative, sensitive, insightful, inner directed, self-reliant, resistant to negative labeling, and achieve in school (9). Three concepts are suggested by Blom and his colleagues (10) to explain adaptation of individuals with disability: coping, competence, and quality-of-life. The first, coping, is described as a process, while competence and quality-of-life are outcomes. Coping is defined as the active psychosocial process through which persistent efforts are made to overcome and solve the problems and dilemmas of the person or imposed by the environment (10). Competence is defined, consistent with its meaning in the occupational behavior perspective. Finally, quality-of-life is defined as positive feeling states captured by concepts like happiness, well-being, and hope. As the occupational therapist employs the model of human occupation to intervene with the child with a chronic disability, the focus will be on the creation of an environment that will foster a constructive approach to disability (coping) and promote competence and quality-of-life. The model of human occupation is used as a guide to suggest how children can be rendered invincible while living with a chronic disability.

THE PERFORMANCE SUBSYSTEM

Most chronic disabilities with onsets in childhood will have deleterious effects on certain kinds of skill acquisition, although each may compromise different constitutents or types of skill or the same types or constituents with different degrees of severity. For example, both autism and childhood aphasia result in communication/interaction skill deficits, but autism is usually the more debilitating, probably because its pathologic process not only severely affects language but also interferes markedly with the acqusition of other types of skill. Motor skills are compromised directly by pathology associated with juvenile rheumatoid arthritis or congenital limb deficiency, but consequent to the primary pathology of autism, cerebral palsy, mental retardation, and learning disability, several types of skills may be impeded.

Even when the pathologic process does not directly affect a particular constituent of skill, the child's customary round of activity may not be particularly conducive to skill acquisition. Chronic disabling conditions in childhood can militate against a smooth interplay of musculoskeletal, neurological and symbolic phenomena for the production of a skilled act. The child with juvenile arthritis whose primary problem is in the musculoskeletal system (i.e. joint pain), may eventually become deficient in rule formation because, in refraining from movement, the child inadvertently forfeits the experience that would encourage acquisition of knowledge about people and objects. On the other hand, the child with a limb deficiency may seek out a variety of experiences that would result in rule-building but, because of physical limitations (e.g. the absence of a hand), may be unable to manipulate objects well enough to fully investigate their details.

The development of communication/interaction skills may be especially important for the chronically disabled child, but compromised because of a primary or secondary effect of a disability. Blom and his colleagues (10) believe that a socially competent person is more apt than others to persistently view his or her own diminished functional ability in certain areas of living as a challenge or inconvenience (as opposed to a tragedy) and to seek ways of overcoming its potential negative effects. If the chronically disabled child develops adequate communication/interaction skills, he or she may be more apt to develop friendships, withstand the negative impact of labeling, and overcome the feelings of alienation that may be associated with being considered by others as different or handicapped.

As already mentioned, children who appear to be invulnerable to the potential, but not obligatory, negative effects of chronically disabling or other at-risk conditions have been found to be talkative, friendly and accepted by their peers (9). These characteristics are fostered in childhood play, yet many children with chronic disabilities will spend less time in play than their able-bodied counterparts. At least one authority has observed that children with chronic conditions have greater television exposure and fewer peer contacts than other children (10). While departure from the normative mode is not intrinsically undesirable, when a pattern of this kind deprives a child of experiences that may lead to better coping, it probably should not be encouraged.

THE HABITUATION SUBSYSTEM

The acquisition of time and energy-efficient, or in other ways health-promoting, habits by the child with a chronic disability makes possible participation in the roles that characterize childhood. If the child with rheumatoid arthritis learns to utilize the larger joints or both hands when lifting or carrying items or to avoid activities that stress affected joints, time spent in the hospital in the acute sick role may be mitigated, and more time for participation in productive roles will be available. Similarly, if the child who is hyperactive can learn to make an effort to wait before responding to stimuli, he or she may be able to refrain from erratic actions and become more productive (34).

Habits

Habits govern the style with which children or their parents approach tasks. Any member of a family in which there is a child with a severe disability may be susceptible to the frustrations that can come with having to devote enormous amounts of time to routine care. Daily activities such as hair combing or grooming, while socially required, may subject the child to pain or stress and the caregiver to frustration. Basic routines may be so taxing or unpleasant that they may be the major impediment to the child's investment in other occupations. The daily care of a child with a severe chronic disability may deplete the energy of the parents, restrict family activities and cause withdrawal from social activities (17, 18).

Habits that are eventually acquired by a child with a chronic disability may interfere with adequate role performance. As an example, a child with a sensory integrative dysfunction may have learned to approach daily activity with obliviousness to the environment. If the child had been trained to attend to the details of the surroundings and how they differentially affect the "state" of his or her nervous system, functioning may have improved, despite the disability. The child may have developed strategies like selecting optimal lighting, constructing or seeking a well-organized work space, color coding, or withdrawing to calming environments when necessary. Generally, the habit of appraising an environment to determine how well it will optimize function will be useful for most children with chronic disabilities. A child who is disabled in one environment may not be in another.

Unfortunately, the very nature of a child's disability may make it especially difficult to develop the habits that organize daily activities or promote better functioning. Ayres (5) believes that children who have difficulty programing their motor actions (those with certain types of apraxia) may also have difficulty programming and sequencing their daily activity. Although most accentuated in conditions such as autism or mental retardation in which cognitive capacity is quite limited, this deficiency may also be evidenced in children with less severe disabilities, like sensory integrative dysfunctions. A child with a sensory integrative dysfunction may plan to do a hobby, but never get to it, because in his or her daily routine a great deal of time must be sacrificed to undoing the negative effects of previous actions. The child may break dishes when using them, lose many of the items handled and then have to invest enormous amounts of time searching for them, or work on many activities simultaneously so that none is ever completed. For any child, the presence of efficient routines is important; in children with chronic disability, they are vital. Without such routines the child may be unable to find time to participate in the roles that will shape identity while the family becomes exasperated with daily routines.

Roles

The foundation for internalization of role is laid in childhood. Although in this period the player, student and family member roles predominate, chores and activities engaged in begin preparation for the other occupational roles. Later, in adolescence, the child normally devotes more time than in early childhood to the hobbyist/amateur, participant in an organization, and worker roles. The model of human occupation suggests that for the child with a chronic disability, effective role performance is supported through the acquisition of skill and appropriate and flexible habits.

As already pointed out, the child with a chronic disability runs the risk of exclusively adopting the "sick role," or adopting disability as a total identity. This situation is counterproductive to adequate occupational functioning. If the child's parents support this view by being overprotective, and conveying hopelessness and the belief that their child will never be a contributing member of society, the problem may be exacerbated. In this case, the child's negative perceptions will be reinforced by parental attitudes and opportunities to gain a new and constructive perspective curtailed. On the other end of the continuum, if parental expectations are not achievable by the child, a state of family tension may ensue and the child's tendency to seek refuge in the sick role may inadvertently be promoted.

In the young child with a chronic disability, performance of the player role may be impeded by the child's problems with motivation, lack of time, environmental barriers, parental constraint, or physical and mental limitations. Because play is one of the primary vehicles through which the child learns flexibility, communication/interaction skills, problem solving/processing skills, and perceptual motor skills, potential compensations for the disabling condition may not be acquired consequent to insufficient exposure to the player role. The child may not learn to cooperate with other children, to exercise the repertoire of behaviors associated with different types of play, or to learn to problem solve and creatively structure time. In early childhood play, rudiments of the friendship role are established. Without this experience, the child with a chronic disability may become socially incompetent and lack social initiative.

THE VOLITION SUBSYSTEM

While a small percentage of children with chronic disabilities (e.g. autistic children) will seem to have a blocked neurogenic urge to explore the environment, the vast majority, if they have problems in the volitional system, will have them in the areas of personal causation, values and interests.

Personal Causation

The belief that one is empowered to influence events or control one's destiny is critical for coping with chronic disability and experiencing quality-of-life (10, 31). As they accrue life experiences, children with chronic disabilities are at risk for developing the view that they are unable to create observable changes in the environment. The antidote to this condition may be ensuring that the child's daily activity is characterized by achievable and challenging activity. The conflicts and struggles that the disabled child encounters will require persistent efforts to overcome and solve problems. These efforts will be made only if the child believes in his or her power to influence events.

Temporal Adaptation and Values

Children with chronic disabilities also need to acquire the values that will reinforce occupational functioning. The process of acquiring values is posited in the model of human occupation to begin in early childhood when parents convey the perceived worth or appropriateness of behavior. It is essential therefore, that parents first of all communicate to the child that they are pleased when the child makes efforts to overcome and solve dilemmas or exercise control over the environment. The parents should be encouraged to praise the child whenever the child strives positively, seeks solutions or discovers activities that are satisfying (59). When parents demonstrate that they believe these behaviors are good, right and important they are probably fostering the skills that enable coping.

Instead of devaluing their child for being disabled, parents may be encouraged to view the child's disability as a challenge that can further growth and self-actualization. If the child is physically disabled, the parents could underplay the need for whole body intactness and help their child to view disability not as an identity, but as a characteristic. Steps that the child takes to develop skills should be encouraged. It may be that placing a high value on education will be particularly useful for the child with a chronic disability since it appears that academic success is associated with better coping (9). On the other hand, if the child has a chronic learning disability, other areas of skill should be valued.

The child with a chronic disability is likely to grow up with different time schedules for developmental events and have different sorts of socialization experiences (10, 26). Instead of placing high value on normative standards, parents of children with chronic disabilities can be encouraged to accept the differences that will characterize their children's daily activities. It may be, as in the case of the mentally retarded child, that the parents will need to develop enormous patience as their child makes developmental gains in small increments and at a slower pace than nondisabled children.

Children with chronic disabilities will need to find importance, security, worthiness, and purpose in occupations. Blom and his colleagues (10) report that of the nine severely chronically disabled adults they studied who had been described as doing remarkably well and living satisfactory lives, seven were employed and the remaining two were heavily involved in community activities. In order to choose satisfying occupations in which they can be successful, children with chronic disabilities will need to go through an occupational choice process. A rich variety of play and activity experiences will enable the child to focus on the occupations from which he or she derives the most meaning. Eventually, the child will establish objectives and standards for personal accomplishments.

Interests

Blom and his colleagues cite several studies, including their own, that suggest that disabled adults derive satisfaction from their interests (2, 8, 20, 37, 48). Some of the interests from which disabled adults seem to receive pleasure are active leisure, opportunities for travel, outside-of-home activities, helping other people, belonging to disabled groups, and community involvement. The process of interest discrimination begins in childhood. If the disabled child is to mature into a happy and satisfied adult, early childhood experience should enable the child to acquire a feel for the occupations from which he or she derives greater and lesser amounts of pleasure. Since interests (as well as personal causation and values) are at least in part a consequence of action, children with chronic disabilities, if they are deprived of a diversity of activity, may not sufficiently sort out and discover interests (Table 16.3).

ENVIRONMENT

In the model of human occupation, the child with a chronic disability is viewed as impelled to explore and master the environment. Barris (7) points out that the model implies that the individual is perpetually involved in choosing, entering and exploring environments. Experience in one environment presumably develops the skills that will subsequently be needed in new environments. Through successive interaction in progressively more complex settings, the individual ideally develops greater competence and initiative. The first environment in which the chronically disabled child will encounter challenges is usually the home setting.

Unfortunately, research employing path analysis has shown that the presence of a disabled child in the home often has a negative effect on the family repertoire of activities which, in turn, seems to erode a mother's sense of mastery. The final outcome of this deleterious chain of events is maternal distress. The impact is far greater for blacks than for whites (18). These data imply that children with chronic disabilities may be

Table 16.3
Occupational status, recommended assessments, treatment considerations for the child with a chronic disability

Occupational risks	Recommended assessments	Treatment considerations
VOLITION		
Personal causation		
Distorted or depressed urge towards mastery	Play history (PH)	Involve child in decision-making opportunities
Decreased opportunities for risk taking and affecting environment	Stanford Preschool Internal/External Scale (SPIES) Interview and observation	Develop coping strategies
Values		
Feelings of decreased worth	PH	Develop the view that a disability is a challenge rather than an abnormality
	Preschool Play Scale (PPS)	
	Piers Harris Children's Self-Concept Scale	
	Decision-Making Inventory (DMI)	
Interests		
Pursuit of interests affected by illness	PH, PPS	Provide activities to foster interests
	Interest Checklist	
	Interview	Make adaptations to allow expression of interests
HABITUATION		
Roles		
Failure to develop routines related to play and school	Role checklist	Provide opportunities to develop role-appropriate behaviors
Perception of self as "sick"	Vineland Social Maturity Scale (VSMS)	
	Home visit	Promote sense of "wellness"
	Interview	
Habits		
Decreased or inappropriate parental expectations	VSMS	Develop time-efficient, energy-conserving habits
Disturbed routines due to the demands of hospital, therapy and medical regimes	Preschool Rating Scale Time logs	Train in ADL
Decreased ability to care for self	Gesell Developmental Scale of Infant Development (GDE)	Involve child and family in establishing daily routines that are realistic
Decreased opportunities to learn daily routines	Bayley Scales of Infant Development (BSID) Interview	
PERFORMANCE		
Skills		
Disruption and reduction in skills and components	GDE, BSID, PH, PPS, DMI	Remediate constituents of skills
Delayed development of skills	Range of motion Muscle test	Develop age appropriate skills

Table 16.3.—Continued

Occupational status	Recommended assessments	Treatment considerations
Decreased process skills such as problem solving and decision making	Reflex integration	Develop alternatives or adaptations when skills are lost
	Muscle tone	Prevent further deterioration of skills
	Oral Motor Assessment	
	McCarthy Scales of Children's Abilities	Provide opportunities for play and exploration
	Bruininks-Oseretsky Test	
	Southern California Sensory Integration Tests	
	Southern California Postrotary Nystagmus Test	
	Clinical Play Observation	
	Parten Play Scale	
	Observation and Interview	
	Riley Motor Problems Inventory	
	Test for Auditory Comprehension of Language	
ENVIRONMENT		
Decreased opportunities to explore environment	PH	Encourage caregiver/child habits that support role performance
Overprotection	Interview	
	Home Visit	Home and school modifications and adaptations
Negative effect on family's repertoire of activities	School Visit	
Reduced sensory and social experiences		Create environment to foster meaningful and satisfying life experiences

more prone than others to grow up in families that have limited activity repertoires. If extradomestic activities are not experienced and home life is dull and monotonous, the child's chances for developing an array of interests, goals and skills are compromised. When the child enters school, the reduced exposure to environmental challenges in the home environment may have militated against the development of coping skills that would enable smooth adjustment in the infinitely more complex academic setting.

Evaluation

THE PERFORMANCE SUBSYSTEM

The occupational therapy evaluation for the child with a chronic disability begins with as-

sessment of the performance subsystem. If the child has cerebral palsy, an assessment of reflex integration, patterns of movement and tone will be utilized. An oral-motor assessment will also be given. In the case of juvenile rheumatoid arthritis, active joint range of motion and muscle strength will be evaluated. Autistic children may be assessed for their responsiveness to sensory simulation while learning-disabled and higher level autistic children are likely to be given a test of the integrity of their sensory integration.

Regardless of the diagnosis, the child is also likely to be given a general developmental assessment or screening of skill in the fine motor, gross motor, language, social, and cognitive areas. Assessments which more specifically evaluate daily living skills are also given (Table 16.3).

THE HABITUATION SUBSYSTEM

The habituation subsystem evaluation can begin with asking the child's caregiver to fill out a weekly or daily time log indicating what activities were done in respective time periods. An alternative means of obtaining this information is through an interview of daily habit patterns. Some therapists will choose to make a home visit to observe the customary round of activity engaged in by mother and child and the style with which they approach common day activities.

The primary role of the child is that of player and role performance is, therefore, measured by the variety of play scales, histories and inventories that have been developed as part of the occupational behavior perspective. The play environment, the child's social and constructive play, his or her interaction skills, and the attitudes of caregivers toward play and their skills in facilitating the play of their child may be assessed. The reader is referred to Florey (27) for a thorough review of these instruments.

THE VOLITION SUBSYSTEM

Personal causation, interests and valued goals are commonly assessed by drawing inferences from the child's play. Self-esteem may also be evaluated. Instruments such as the Interest Inventory, Role Checklist, Internal-External Scale and Decision Making Inventory may be used with adolescents (see Appendix).

ENVIRONMENT

Various elements of the environment may be evaluated including the degree of press, its encouragement of play, its tendency to promote the overcoming of functional limitations which might otherwise be imposed by the disabling condition, and so on (Table 16.3).

Treatment Goals and Strategies

Treatment of the child with a chronic disability addresses all the levels of the system as well as the environment. The ultimate aim of therapy is to foster an adaptive cycle. This will entail the development of coping skills, competence and quality-of-life. In the treatment program, so far as possible, the child should be given opportunities to adapt to environmental demands.

Familiar activities may be performed in new ways and achievable new challenges should be confronted in progressively more complex environments (Table 16.3).

THE PERFORMANCE SUBSYSTEM

Each constituent of skill is addressed when appropriate. Children with arthritis and other musculoskeletal disorders may be encouraged to engage in activities that will strengthen muscles and increase or maintain ranges of motion. Splints may be fabricated and provided when they will promote function. Children with neuromuscular disorders in which the pathology is to upper motor neurons may be treated with the neurophysiological procedures described by Bobath (12), Bobath and Bobath (13), Farber (25), Rood (47) or others. The aim of these procedures is to normalize tone, improve sensorimotor processing, and reduce pathologic patterns of movement so that the child can move more normally. Insofar as possible, the model of human occupation suggests these techniques should be used within the context of playful or purposeful activity, in part because the focus is away from pathology. The symbolic component of skill is also worked on within the context of play in which rule building is fostered (46). Play settings and experience are also employed to facilitate acquisition of communication/interaction, problem solving and decision making skills.

Perceptual-motor skills are also promoted in a pressureless and playful environment. For the child with the types of sensory integrative dysfunction that are responsive to sensory integrative procedures, the procedures described by Ayres (3, 4) are recommended. These procedures make use of a pressureless and especially equipped environment in which the child must organize his or her behavior to achieve a goal, while at the same time receiving optimal amounts and kinds of sensory stimulation. It is hypothesized that the procedures enhance the efficiency with which the nervous system interprets sensory input and can respond adaptively to it. While these procedures are mistakenly often thought of as directed solely toward improvement of perceptual functioning, they are likely to also produce positive effects on the habituation and volitional systems. Improved sensory integration is thought to be related to better organization of behavioral routine and a sense of mastery and control over the environment.

In the early developmental period, children are infatuated with the learning of simple daily living skills. For many children with chronic disabilities, the preschool and early childhood period will be an optimal time to develop competence in this area. Fueled by their fascination with putting shoes on and taking them off, buttoning and other dressing skills, the 2- to 3-year-old chooses to spend a large portion of time practicing and fully absorbed in these seemingly mundane activities (21). If the child with a chronic disability demonstrates this kind of interest in self-care skills, the therapist is in the optimum position for capitalizing on this drive and helping the child learn ways of accomplishment.

As the child moves into adolescence, other independent living skills will need to be developed, while self-care skills are concurrently refined. Homemaking, social-recreational, school, and vocational skills will need to be developed. As already suggested, the development of social initiative, social intelligence and communication/interaction skills will be especially important for the child with a chronic physical disability.

THE HABITUATION SUBSYSTEM

The child with a chronic disability should develop habits that will support the player and student and eventually the worker roles. Early, the child and his or her caregiver should develop habits of daily care that will be time efficient, energy conserving, as pleasant as possible, and lessen the frequency of the need for hospitalization. Through knowledge of the disease process and expertise in the area of activity analysis, the therapist should help parent and child with habit formation and modification. The ultimate aim is the acquisition of a repertoire of safe, nonaversive and expedient habits.

All children need a balance of sleep, rest and activity, but this will be especially important for the child with a chronic disability. Irritability and poor performance consequent to insufficient rest, a common occurrence in normal children, can be misinterpreted as part of the pathology associated with a disease or as a psychological problem in the disabled child. Adequate utilization of the model of human occupation requires the therapist to work with parent and child to ensure that the child receives a proper balance of rest and activity, so that the child is able to muster his or her full array of resources for accomplishment of productive occupations.

As an adult, the individual with a chronic disability will need to organize his or her own time if independent living is his or her goal. Early childhood and adolescent experiences in developing daily and weekly plans of activity will provide a preparation for activity and time management in the future.

Habits

The habits of the caregiver and the child need to be shaped so that they will support role performance. If the child is in school, his or her performance will, in part, depend upon the methods he or she employs to function in this environment. The therapist may need to help the child develop the habit of using certain adaptive devices that may initially feel awkward. These devices may enable writing, carrying of books, or performance of other tasks required in the school setting. In addition, the therapist may assist the child who is hyperactive in learning more reflective approaches to daily tasks or may restructure the environment so that work space is organized and lighting, textures and decor are calming. Optimally, the child will eventually need to develop habits through which he or she can independently create, construct or discover environments that will promote optimal functioning. It may be that for some children the habit of secluding themselves for a few moments to become reconstituted will promote better performance.

Role

In early childhood, the player and student roles predominate and therapy is directed toward enabling the child to participate effectively in these statuses. Structured and unstructured play sessions with siblings and normal and disabled peers will usually be recommended. Initially, the sessions may need to occur in the presence of a therapist who can monitor interaction but eventually the child may be sufficiently competent to effectively interact in free play sessions with neighbors or in structured nontherapy-linked situations like Boy Scouts.

In play, the child is encouraged to risk take, problem solve and develop fine-motor, gross-motor, communication, and social skills. There may be particular skills required in school with which the child is having difficulty that could be practiced in the safe and secure, presumably fun-filled, playful therapy environment. Rehearsal of school-related skills in the therapy situation capitalizes upon the player role to support the student role.

The therapist using the model of human occupation will attempt to help the child with performance of the student role through other means as well. Observations of the child's adjustment to the school setting may lead to specific recommendations regarding the structuring of peer interactions, organization of work space, choice of activities, management of daily routine, use of adaptive equipment, and so on.

THE VOLITIONAL SUBSYSTEM

The volitional system is also addressed through encouragement of play experiences in which the child can experience a sense of control over the environment. A variety of types of enjoyable puzzles can be presented to the child that will encourage striving positively and solution seeking. The child may also be asked to develop the schedule of activities within the therapy session, thereby exercising temporal organization. The experience of encountering challenges, problem-solving, taking risks, and being successful will potentially result in the child's belief that he or she is empowered to influence the environment.

Interests will also be developed as part of the therapy plan. As the caregiver and child develop time-conserving habits, portions of the day will be freed for extradomestic interests. The child may be encouraged to go on outings, participate in activity groups in other settings, or develop interests through structured home study. In the preschooler or young child, fantasy may be encouraged as part of interest formation. In the adolescent, a move toward realistic appraisal of skills and interests will contribute to potentiation of an optimal occupational choice process.

ENVIRONMENT

The ways in which the environment is modified to be of therapeutic value have already been implicitly addressed. The environment may be restructured physically to support the player and student roles. If it is too boring the therapist may make recommendations for how it could be rendered more interesting, or if it is disorganized and confusing, strategies for rendering it calm-

ing might be proposed. Artifacts, lighting and color may be modified or added. Finally, the unspoken demands of the environment (press) will be analyzed to determine whether it provides a goodness-of-fit between the child's capabilities and the expectations others in the environment have for the child. Recommendations for alterations in the environment will be made so that the child is only required to do tasks in which success is likely.

CHRONIC DISABILITY (DEVELOPMENTAL DELAY AND APHASIA) CASE: MARIA
Background Information

This case study is based on a real case treated as part of a research study. However, some of the evaluations, treatment methods and outcomes have been fabricated for instructional purposes in order to comprehensively illustrate application of the model of human occupation.

Maria was 4 years, 8 months when she was referred by her Head Start teacher to the occupational therapist. The presenting problem was that she appeared to be behind the other preschoolers in her class in fine motor, gross motor and, especially, language skills. Four months prior to the date of referral, Maria had been evaluated at a large county hospital. The results indicated that she was delayed 15 months in language and was minimally delayed in the gross motor and personal-social areas. In the present referral, the Head Start teacher indicated that Maria had difficulty partaking in most classroom activities.

History

The medical chart revealed a history of birth trauma. Mrs. Gonzalez, Maria's mother, began labor in Mexico in the 7th month of her pregnancy. Maria was unable to suck at birth and was hospitalized for 1 month. She sat at 7 months, stood alone at 12 months, and walked at 18 months. Her mother reported that she first cried at 3 months when she also began sucking. Initially, it would take her mother 2 hours to feed her a 4-oz bottle of formula. In 1977, Maria was certified by a Head Start psychologist and speech pathologist as developmentally impaired and aphasic.

Evaluation

The following tests were used to assess the performance subsystem: Riley Motor Problems Inventory, Southern California Motor Accuracy Test, Southern California Postrotary Nystagmus Test, and the Test for the Auditory Comprehension of Language. The habituation subsystem was assessed through two home observations and the mother's recording of 3 days of daily activities. In addition, performance of the student role was assessed by Maria's teacher's ratings of her behaviors on the Preschool Rating Scale. Play performance was assessed using a modified version of the Standardized Clinical Play Observation (Kalverboer) and the Social Play Scale (Parten), as well as an observation in a domestic play setting. Finally, the volitional subsystem was assessed by noting the extent to which Maria demonstrated an urge to explore the environment, risk taking, and temporal organization in a free unstructured play period when other children were present.

During testing, Maris was fearful, shy and withdrawn. She refused to speak throughout the evaluation and needed encouragement from her mother to perform. It was felt that test scores probably reflected Maria's optimal performance and were indicative of her overall level of functioning.

Results

THE PERFORMANCE SUBSYSTEM

Perceptual-Motor Status

The tests that measured motor performance, postural responses, and eye-hand usage indicated that Maria was not functioning within age expectations. She scored in the second percentile on the Riley Motor Problems Inventory. Both right and left hand performance on the Southern California Motor Accuracy Test was below age-expectations with the left hand performing worse. When using a pencil, Maria used little pressure and an immature grasp. Duration of postrotary nystagmus was 10 seconds on the left and 11 seconds on the right. She was unable to draw a human figure. Overall, her perceptual-motor functioning was extremely delayed and it was noted that Maria seemed fearful of movement.

Communication/Interaction Skills

Maria scored in the 4th percentile on the Carrow Test for Auditory Comprehension of Language. On the Preschool Rating Scale, she was rated poorly in most areas with language and social relations the most deficient.

Problem Solving/Planning Skills

On the Preschool Rating Scale, Maria was rated as only moderately deficient in planning, organization and problem solving.

THE HABITUATION SUBSYSTEM

Two visits to Maria's home in which the therapist observed daily habits and routines indicated that there were many problems in this system. Mealtimes took excessively long as Maria appeared to lack sufficient oral-motor skill to chew food efficiently. Bath time was characterized by stress and tension as Maria cried when her body (and especially her face) was washed. Although Maria had two sisters, one 7 years old and the other 3, her mother seemed to have little time to devote to them. Often they would assume a caregiver role toward Maria. Maria was able to go to the toilet independently, feed herself and wash her hands unaided. Although Maria attempted to dress herself, she was observed to require considerable help from her mother. In the course of the day, Maria and her sisters would fight and Maria would frequently cry and seek comfort from her mother. Tantrums also occurred daily. The sisters seemed impatient with and intolerant of their sister's problems.

At home, Maria's only playmates were her sisters. Formal assessment of her performance in the player role revealed that she was well below age expectations in this area, functioning at about the 3-year-old level. When her free constructive play was observed, she spent most of the session (8 of 10 minutes) staring and fingering her dress on the floor. Only 75 seconds were used in block manipulation in which she simply stacked and made piles of a few. Play interaction with peers consisted of unoccupied behavior. Only in a few instances did she demonstrate on-looker, solitary or parallel play. In a free play situation in a play house, she demonstrated simple domestic mimicry (e.g. pushed a baby stroller) but neither incorporated objects imaginatively in her play nor used verbal communication to interact with her peers.

THE VOLITION SUBSYSTEM

Maria demonstrated a maladaptive cycle, characterized by being locked into safe but nonproductive activity, a lack of social initiative, and stagnation. She withdrew from essentially any new challenging activity, sometimes seeking refuge in a developmentally less demanding task. More often, she would refrain completely from purposeful activity. This pattern suggested that she did not feel in control of the environment. Withdrawal from purposeful and diverse activity lessened the probability that she would develop sufficient interests and goals to guide future occupational choice.

ENVIRONMENT

Maria lived in a small house with her two parents and siblings. Her mother appeared to have fallen asunder to a common pattern of mothers of children with disability: withdrawal from extra-domestic activity, devotion of an enormous amount of time to the disabled child and distress. Although Maria's father was employed, the family had limited financial resources.

The home situation did not encourage play. Few toys were available and although Mrs. Gonzalez did not encourage television exposure, neither did she foster the play of the children. She reported that her biggest problem was managing the tension among the children. When her sisters would ask Maria to do something, Maria would try, get frustrated, and cry to her mother, saying, "I can't." The siblings, in turn, would become angry that Maria was once again consuming their mother's attention.

Interpretation

Maria appeared to have a chronic physical disability that had disrupted all levels of the system. Gross, fine and oral motor skills were impaired. The most severe deficiencies were in communication/interaction skills. Problems in this system generated multiple disruptions in the habituation system which was characterized by ineffective habitual patterns and a consequent reduction in time for engagement in the player role. Repeated failures and tensions within a disrupted home environment had militated against the development of a sense of mastery over the environment, of interests and of goals. In a state of stagnation, it seemed unlikely that Maria would develop coping skills and competence and enjoy a qualitatively satisfying life.

Treatment Goals and Strategies

The following goals were established and treatment methods used.

THE PERFORMANCE SUBSYSTEM

Perceptual-Motor Skills

Goal 1: Decrease aversive reaction to touch

Strategy: Each therapy session began with exposure to tactile stimulation. Rather than imposing stimulation, Maria was asked to choose textures that felt good and apply the stimulation herself. Initially she used a soft carpet square on her arms and legs as she reacted aversively to all other textures. Eventually, Maria became receptive to a variety of carpet squares varying in their degree of roughness, to the vibrator and to light brushing. She was most defensive around the mouth and continued to be for the duration of therapy. She was taught to apply deep pressure to skin surfaces that were most defensive, and she obviously enjoyed doing this. Eventually, a box filled with styrofoam was presented in which she would locate hidden toys, registering delight in each new discovery.

Goal 2: Improve postural skills

Strategy: Maria was encouraged to interact on equipment that provided achievable challenges to her equilibrium and protective responses (e.g. foam cylinder). Eventually, when suspended equipment that moved was offered, she chose to interact with it. Bobath procedures were employed to encourage trunk rotation and rolling, but only within the context of playful and pleasureful rolling games.

Goal 3: Improve oral/motor skills

Strategy: One of Maria's most salient problems interfering with speech was dysarthria. Instead of applying traditional oral-motor stimulation and facilitation procedures, tongue lateralization and better coordination and control over the muscles of mastication and speech were encouraged through a variety of oral-motor games involving textured foods that Maria liked.

Goal 4: Improve fine-motor skills

Strategy: Constructive play activities (e.g. Play-Doh, simple weaving) were used to provide practice in hand use within the context of a pressureless environment. The symbolic component of these activities was fostered by encouraging Maria to make things (e.g. snake, pot) and to imitate the therapist in including a symbolic dimension to the objects created. Through interaction with objects with which she had not had any previous exposure, Maria was acquiring rules of objects. It should be noted that other elements of the program facilitated acquisition of rules of motion and people.

Processing/Planning Skills

Goal 1: Improve motor planning

Strategy: Observation of Maria in the evaluation suggested she had difficulty planning nonhabitual motor acts. In therapy, she was offered equipment that provided a range of potential challenges. Initially, she chose the barrel, but could not independently make it roll when she was inside it. After she had mastered this motor planning task, she chose to move on to an obstacle course and then to even more complex activities requiring sequencing, timing and planning.

Goal 2: Improve behavioral planning

Strategy: Maria was drawn toward domestic social play in which she could incorporate pretending. In therapy, this interest was capitalized upon as much time was spent in domestic play. Although initially she could enact only simple behaviors (e.g. pretend eating and drinking), with greater experience she eventually could chain a series of sequential elements of domestic roles and tasks.

Communication/Interaction Skills

Strategy: It was assumed that language skills would be fostered by elements of the treatment program that were aimed at improving oral-motor coordination and knowledge about objects and self (rule building). Incorporation of one, or no more than two, other children within the same play experiences fostered communication/interaction skills in an environment that would not be too threatening.

THE HABITUATION SUBSYSTEM

Habits

Goal 1: Develop skills that will foster better time management and energy conservation.

Strategy: The treatment strategies just described that were utilized to influence the performance subsystem had positive ramifications for the habituation system by enabling accomplishment of this goal. As postural reactions improved, Maria became more independent in managing the changes of position that are required in daily routines. She therefore consumed less of her mother's time and energy with requests for help. As another example, the reduction in her negative responses to tactile stimulation lessened, somewhat, the strain in the relationship between Mrs. Gonzalez and Maria as daily living skills were tackled.

Goal 2: Assist Mrs. Gonzalez in developing strategies for managing Maria that would lessen tension between them.

Strategy: Two sources of tension were excessively disturbing to Mrs. Gonzalez. The first was Maria's reactions to daily care. Mrs. Gonzalez had reported that Maria cried continuously during hair brushing, washing, bathing, and some elements of dressing and this was confirmed in the therapist's home observation. When it was time for these activities, Maria would act out and had developed a number of "avoidance" behaviors that just prolonged the enormous amount of time it took to care for Maria. Treatment involved educating Maria's mother about tactile defensiveness and making recommendations that would lessen the child's aversive reaction to being touched during daily routines (e.g. allowing the child to watch television or hear music during these activities to deflect attention, using the bath cloth on a wide area of the face with pressure, selecting a less aversive brush, etc.).

The second source of tension was an outcome of Mrs. Gonzalez's worry that her child would never improve, never talk well or never be like other children. The therapist demonstrated how modifications to the environment (e.g. work space and seating) had the immediate effect of enhancing Maria's competence and lessening the demands she made on her mother. The mother's own sense of stress and hopelessness lessened as she perceived her child's increased competence and had more time to devote to her other children and to other activities.

Goal 3: Develop a daily schedule in which Maria would acquire a healthful balance of rest and play and extradomestic activity.

Strategy: The therapist sat down with Mrs. Gonzalez and initially helped her develop balanced daily schedules for herself, Maria and the other siblings. In planning, it became evident that Maria was not getting sufficient rest daily and that this might, in part, account for her tantrums. The schedule developed for Maria ensured proper rest, as well as time for gross motor, fine motor and dramatic play with her siblings and other children. It also incorporated a daily time period when Mrs. Gonzalez would be able to devote full attention to her other children and to herself without interruption. Utilization of relatives and babysitters made implementation of the schedule possible on a regular basis and it was found that Maria responded well to the new individuals with whom she was regularly interacting in new settings.

Goal 4: Enrich home environment and daily activity to provide appropriate challenges.

Strategy: Mrs. Gonzalez was encouraged to take Maria and the other children to the park where Maria could explore the textures of dirt, sand and grass and engage in simple motor planning activities (e.g. like climbing up a hill) while the siblings located their own appropriate challenges. It was recommended that she invite a friend who had children to go on outings with her family so that her own social contact would be increased. At home, simple equipment that provided the appropriate demands on Maria's nervous system were suspended on a tree. Mrs. Gonzalez was taught to involve her children in the homemaking tasks (e.g. baking) she performed and how to interact playfully with Maria and the other children. While Maria was in preschool, Mrs. Gonzalez was encouraged to take walks and do social activities with her other children. Finally, an area of the house was partitioned to provide a comfort area supplied with textured remnants that appealed to Maria. The partition was made through rearrangement of furniture.

Goal 5: Create a home environment with the appropriate press

Strategy: Maria's older sister and parents were given a balanced perspective on what could reasonably be expected of Maria. They were taught strategies for lessening their own frustrations including focusing on Maria's accomplishments, engaging in activities they found satisfying and sharing the responsibility for helping Maria. They were also encouraged to find time for activities outside of the home.

Role

Goal 1: Improve Maria's performance in the role of preschooler

Strategy: It was expected that changes occurring in the other aspects of the habituation system and in the performance system would have positive consequences on Maria's performance in school.

Goal 2: Improve Maria's performance in the role of player

Strategy: As already implied, the treatment plan placed great emphasis on constructive play, social play and dramatic play both within therapy sessions and at home. It was reasoned that enhanced exposure to play would foster Maria's competence in the player role.

THE VOLITION SYSTEM

Goal 1: Promote a positive sense of personal causation and develop values and interests.

Strategy: In nearly every aspect of the treatment program, Maria was given the freedom to choose activities in which she would be successful. The therapist structured the environment to insure the successes that would lead to the view of being empowered to control the environment. One of the major obstacles to Maria's exploration appeared to be a primal fear of movement. In therapy, focus was on enabling her to become more secure with movement. Initially, Maria chose activities on stationary objects. However, she gradually became confident enough in her ability to control her own body and the environment to derive pleasure from swinging equipment, provided she could hold on tightly and move slowly. After having been in therapy for several months she freely interacted with a variety of suspended equipment with her body in a variety of positions. She seemed to have overcome her initial fear of falling and laughed when she did fall on a mat. As she engaged in a diversity of these activities and had the opportunity to playfully experience fantasy roles in sociodramatic play, it was assumed goals and interests were developing.

ENVIRONMENT

Goal 1: Create an environment that will foster Maria's occupational performance and lessen family distress

Strategy: The ways in which the environment was altered to foster occupational functioning in Maria and lessen maternal stress have been described in other sections of the treatment plan.

Outcomes

Maria had attended 21 out of 27 1-hour scheduled treatment sessions from January through May (5 months). She was reevaluated on the same instruments on which she was initially tested. It was felt that the scores on the final testing were an accurate reflection of Maria's ability in the areas tested. It is interesting to note, that despite Maria's presumably successful experiences in therapy, in the testing situation, she became frustrated and needed a great deal of encouragement to continue.

THE PERFORMANCE SUBSYSTEM

Maria improved in coordination as indicated by an improved standard score on the Southern California Motor Accuracy Test. Her accuracy scores which were below normal expectations were now within normative limits. Improvements were also noted on the other motor tests, however, performance on these tests had not yet reached age expectations. In communication/interaction skills, Maria showed some improvement. On the Carrow Test for Auditory Comprehension of Language she now scored in the 9th percentile (initially she was in the 4th). Scores on the Preschool Rating Scale indicated marked improvements in social skills.

THE HABITUATION SUBSYSTEM

Mrs. Gonzalez reported that daily activity was now going relatively smoothly. The methods to render daily activity less tactually aversive seemed to have contributed to a reduction in tantrums and tension, thereby getting each day off to a positive start. The other treatment strategies that addressed this system were enabling the whole family to engage in more satisfying activity and lessened familial distress.

Maria had clearly improved in her performance of the player role. Final testing revealed improvement in constructive and social play. She was now able to construct simple structures with symbolic content. Rather than being an onlooker, she would now initiate social play with other children, although infrequently.

Her teacher reported considerable improvement in her performance as student. She was described as now able to assist younger children (3-year-olds) with puzzles and to interact better with peers. She was also able to participate in relay races with other children and would jump from the jungle gym.

THE VOLITION SUBSYSTEM

The activities that Maria sought out suggested that she had become more courageous and had overcome her fear of movement. Although she still chose to spend a good deal of time alone, the amount of time had lessened. Beginning glimpses of social initiative and a sense of being in control of her own life and competent seemed to be appearing. As her parents witnessed these changes, their view of her potential was modified. It was expected that this renewed sense of hope would be absorbed by Maria and translated into a pattern of positive adaptation.

Progressive and Terminal Illness

In childhood, disabilities and diseases that are progressive and terminal present special challenges for the child, the family and the occupational therapist. The goal of all intervention is

maintenance of function and, as a result, often requires that the therapist be innovative in designing both equipment and environmental adaptations (50). Specific goals for each individual being treated will differ but, in general, the occupational therapist must also be concerned with providing the child with enriching quality-of-life experiences that will stimulate all levels of the human system. Further concerns are for providing strategies for coping with decreasing physical, emotional and psychological skills (53, 56).

Illnesses such as muscular dystrophy, renal disease, certain types of cancers, and cystic fibrosis represent diseases that fall into the category of progressive and degenerative. Children may be diagnosed with a particular disease as early as the first weeks of life or at any age throughout childhood. Characteristic of progressive diseases is a pattern of decreasing abilities and associated losses in skills. As motor abilities decline appropriate adjustments in the various roles and habits that the child enacts are necessary. Components of the volitional subsystem are also affected and the child is likely to benefit from intervention at this level.

Problems associated with muscular dystrophy will be discussed as representative of a progressive degenerative disease of childhood. Age of onset, age when muscles are first affected, rate of muscle deterioration and length of life will differ depending on the type of dystrophy and the individual child. Although the courses of the disease will be unique in each person, typically it is expected that the child will require long-term follow-up care as the disease progresses.

Muscular dystrophy is a muscle disease characterized by onset in early childhood with progressive degeneration of the muscles used for moving and maintaining posture (35). The most common type of dystrophy in young children is Duchenne's. This is an hereditary condition appearing between the ages of 2 and 6 years old. It begins in the muscles involved in standing and walking and progresses over time to involve all major and minor muscle groups involved in movement (49).

THE PERFORMANCE SUBSYSTEM
Skills

In muscular dystrophy (MD) motor skills are affected most profoundly by weakness and associated clumsiness and incoordination. Initially a child with MD will have some noticeable difficulties with walking, climbing and assumption of standing. As the muscles gradually weaken, the child will require assistive and adaptive equipment such as braces, crutches, a wheelchair, and dressing aides. Skilled performance in play, self-care and school-related behaviors are significantly affected as the disease progresses.

In some children, early onset of the disease may have resulted in limited opportunities to interact in a wide variety of contexts. These limitations may impact on the individual's ability to understand the surrounding world and may, in fact, mean that the child has a decreased repository of information or internal organization to guide action.

Process skills are not directly affected by the disease process. Children with MD tend to score lower on intellectual testing but whether this is due to actual diminished ability or a result of a restricted environment, experiences and emotional difficulties is unknown (56). For many children, process skills become a strength in light of increasingly impaired physical abilities. As the children become more limited in movement they must rely on their cognitive abilities to understand the world around them. In some cases a child may have had limited opportunities to acquire experiences in problem solving and is now faced with motor difficulties that prevent translating information into action or, vice versa, deriving information from action.

Communication and interaction skills are often limited in the child with MD due to reduced opportunities to interact in a variety of settings and with a variety of people. Additionally, parents may often feel guilt in relation to the hereditary aspect of the disease and may compensate for such feelings by overprotecting and over indulging their child. In turn, children may feel easily frustrated by their physical limitations appearing uncooperative aggressive or depressed (45, 56). Siblings and other close family members may feel jealous of the attention that the child with MD receives and may reduce or restrict their interactions with the child and parents. These complex environmental and interactive constraints to communication impact on the child's ability to be effective and competent in everyday activities that require interaction with others.

THE HABITUATION SUBSYSTEM

Habits

Habit patterns are significantly altered in the course of the muscular dystrophy disease process. Children who were once able to dress, play, feed themselves, and engage in other independent activities are confronted with dependence and gradually altered abilities as MD erodes their skills. Parental and environmental expectations that do not account for a child's decreasing abilities also present obstacles for the child with MD.

Old habit patterns must be carefully analyzed and adapted to ensure their utility in supporting currently practiced routines. It is also important to assist the child in acquiring new habit patterns for age-appropriate tasks and role behaviors. Opportunities for children to have a balance of productive, playful and restful activities in their daily life is a primary goal in habit formation and is best achieved when useful habit patterns and routines are in place.

Roles

The child with MD is particularly vulnerable in the area of role performance. The slowly progressive nature of the disease that presents ever increasing weakness, decreased mobility and decreased personal independence will mean relinquishing certain roles and adapting others.

By 10 to 12 years of age when we typically expect a young boy to be involved in roles of player, friend, group member, and student, the child with MD is facing increasing problems such as the need for a wheelchair, weakening arms that can no longer be raised over his head for dressing, weakening spinal muscles that result in taking abnormal postures to obtain support and the beginning of respiratory problems (56). These physical limitations along with psychological and emotional stress and decreased self-esteem that is associated with role stress and conflict (giving up roles, not meeting perceived expectations), severely impact on the child's role performance.

Parents, family members and friends provide important information to the child regarding role performance. Unrealistic expectations for role performance or for behavior associated with the sick role give the child a message about how he or she should behave as contrasted with how he or she may want to act.

THE VOLITION SYSTEM

Personal Causation

The rapid deterioration of skills and abilities that is associated with MD is particularly difficult for the young child who sees peers and siblings acquiring increasing proficiency in manual and motor performance. Increasing weakness that prevents carrying out preferred behaviors leaves the child feeling out of control and helpless. Interest in maintaining range of motion, preventing deformities and compensating for lost abilities may be met with feelings of hopelessness.

As the disease processess progressess, the child is faced with increasing losses as he is unable to perform favorite activities in familiar and successful ways. Participation in group activities with peers and playmates may become less frequent as the child is faced with unexpected failures as he becomes increasingly weaker.

Personal causation can be seriously disrupted in the presence of MD, as each of us bases our views of ourselves on belief in skills, the efficacy of skills and expectancy for success. Because of increasingly limited movement skills, the child is repeatedly faced with tasks that may have been successfully realized a year earlier but are no longer possible due to increased weakness, contractures or other musculoskeletal problems.

It is difficult for the individual to see himself or herself as a causal agent, and to believe in his or her own capacities to face what are becoming decreasingly successful interactions with the environment. When an activity is approached, these children are typically unwilling to participate, being unsure whether they may still possess the needed skills to ensure a positive interaction. Difficulties in anticipating outcomes and investing in activities and tasks that are challenging are common problems associated with MD.

Values

By middle childhood the individual has acquired familial, cultural and societal values that guide choices for action. In the child with MD, many values associated with good and right behaviors are difficult to act on. Typically young preadolescent boys are expected to value physical skills such as increasing strength, speed and endurance. Participation in peer-related activities such as team sports, secret clubs, bicycle riding, and similar activities are common pasttimes.

Physical abilities are greatly impaired by the time the young boy with MD reaches middle childhood. Interaction with peers may be reduced to one or two relatives or family friends who visit infrequently. By this age many children no longer attend school due to severe mobility and transfer problems, reducing further their opportunities to interact with peers. Opportunities to acquire skills in delaying gratification, becoming future oriented, and other standards of performance may be greatly limited.

Interests

Interests are guided by internal feelings of pleasure and satisfaction; for children, attention to certain kinds of play and hobbies is fueled by their individual preferences for such activity. Dysfunction or distortion in this area of interaction is more likely to occur when there are severe environmental restrictions or deprivations, or in the presence of severe emotional or cognitive deficits.

Participation in interests is impacted in the child with MD by decreasing mobility in the lower extremities, use of a wheelchair and, in later stages of the disease, decreased mobility in the upper extremities. Active engagement in areas of interest may be limited to spectator roles or may require combining skills with able-bodied friends and family members to assist in carrying out tasks. In later stages of the disease, adaptive equipment may be useful to encourage interest related activity.

ENVIRONMENT

For children with MD, the environment provides an important role in supporting and stimulating behavior at all levels of the human system. As physical abilities diminish there is a need to adapt the physical and social environments to insure active participation of the individual.

Adaptations to the home environment that will provide optimal opportunities for independence and for engaging in new activities will stimulate the child. Difficulties with small or narrow spaces that do not permit movement in or from the wheelchair will restrict the child in his exploration and interaction in the environment. Telephones, televisions and other frequently used items will need to be stored within easy reach to accommodate limited used of muscles of the shoulder girdle, upper arms and spine.

Daily living routines will require careful observation to minimize stress for family members involved in the care of the child. Increasing strength demands for transfers, daily living routines and play activities may cause family members to feel emotionally and physically exhausted. As mobility becomes more restricted the child will need adaptations to the physical environment. These adaptations are mainly designed to maintain function in self-care especially dressing and grooming activities.

Opportunities for excursions outside the home and immediate environment are important sources of stimulation for the child with MD. However, community and social access may be reduced as the child requires more and more assistance to maintain interactions. Adaptive equipment for car transfers and transportation mobility will assist the family in maintaining this interaction with the outside world.

In later stages of the disease, children are homebound due to maximum assistance needed in all areas of mobility. In such situations, social stimulation is limited to phone calls and visits from close friends and family relatives (Table 16.4).

Occupational Function and Dysfunction in A Chronic Progressive Disability

Children maintain interest and involvement within their environments as long as opportunities are available to arouse and engage them. Active involvement with objects and people help to offset dysfunctional behavior such as aggression and uncooperativeness. When opportunities for action are limited, the child and the family may feel trapped in a web of despair and frustration that is common in light of the increasing and severe physical difficulties that the patient is experiencing.

A maladaptive cycle of behavior is created when failure at an activity breeds feelings of ineffectance, lack of interest and helplessness. These feelings are appropriate associations for an individual to make in the presence of a disabling condition. In such a situation it is important to interrupt the cycle of failure by creating opportunities for the child to be successful. Activities that tap the child's abilities, allow for independence, creativity and choice provide sources for feelings of competence (Table 16.4).

Evaluation

The child with MD will require long-term care and continual reassessment for monitoring strength, range of motion, endurance and the effects of decreasing abilities on the performance, habituation and volitional subsystems.

At the level of the performance subsystem, assessment addresses skills in activities of daily living, perceptual motor skills, process, and communication/interactions skills. Assessment instruments used may include use of an activities of daily living checklist, Play History, Play Scale, Vineland Social Maturity Scale, muscle, and range of motion testing. The range of roles and habits that the child engages in and the degree of involvement may be assessed using the Vineland Social Maturity Scale, observation and interview with the child and family (Table 16.4).

Volitional components including personal causation, values and interests are assessed to determine the child's goals and appropriateness of strategies used to pursue them, the constellation of interests and opportunities for acting on them, and overall feelings of competence and effectance. Interview, the interest checklist, Stanford Preschool Internal/External Scale, Adolescent Role Assessment, Play Observation, Play History, and Play Scale are among the instruments that may be used for assessment of this subsystem.

Additional assessment focuses on external contraints and supports in the environment by addressing people and places that are part of the child's everyday life. By identifying areas of deficit, the therapist can offer support to family members, school personnel, and others who interact with the child. (Table 6-4).

Treatment

The occupational therapist working with children and their families facing progressive degenerative conditions is in the position of offering a wide range of treatment strategies. Most importantly, the therapist is able to offer families a systematic, practical and beneficial approach for coping with an individual's decreasing skills and abilities.

With long-term care, the therapist is able to build a strong and trusting relationship with the family. Clinic and home visits as well as telephone contacts are all part of providing comprehensive follow-up care. At the performance subsystem level, treatment is directed toward grading activities to accommodate for decreasing coordination and strength. Habituation level intervention focuses on adapting equipment and the home environment in order to assist the child in maintaining important habits to support acquired roles. Habits that support age-expected

Table 16.4.
Occupational Status, Recommended Assessments, Treatment Considerations for the Child with a Progressive or Terminal Illness

Occupational status	Recommended assessments	Treatment considerations
	VOLITION	
Personal Causation		
Frustration at inabilities may result in feeling "out of control"	Play history (PH)	Provide with strategies for coping with decreased skills
Decreased opportunities for risk taking	Stanford Preschool Internal/External Scale (SPIES);	
	Locus of Control	
	Interview and observation	
Values		
Previous acquired values challenged	PH, PPS	Provide outlets for expression of grief and sorrow
	Piers Harris Children's Self-Concept Scale	
	Decision Making Inventory Interview (DMI)	
Interests		
Decreased opportunities to pursue interests	PH	Provide opportunities to engage in activities that are exciting, interesting and challenging
Need to adapt interests	Preschool Play Scale (PPS)	
	Interest Checklist	
	Interview	Adaptations to allow pursuit of interests
	Time Logs	
	HABITUATION	
Roles		
Adjusted roles in light of decreased abilities	Role checklist	Provide opportunities to develop new or adjusted roles
Relinquishment of some roles and adaptation of others	Adolescent-role assessment	Promote continued contact with peers and others who are important to the child
	Vineland Social Maturity Scale (VSMS)	
Decreased school-related behavior	Home visit	
	Interview	
Habits		
Decreasing abilities in self-care	ADL, VSMS	Maintain important habits
Disturbed routines due to progressive nature of illness	Preschool Rating Scale Time Loop	Adapt routines and equipment
	Gesell Developmental Exam (GDE)	Analyze habit patterns
		Assist in acquiring age-appropriate new habits
	Bayley Scale of Infant Development (BSID)	
	Home visit	
	Interview	
	PERFORMANCE	
Skills		
Decreased abilities and associated losses in skills and components	GDE, BSID, PH, PPS, DMI	Monitor and grade the effects of illness on decreasing abilities
	Range of motion	
	Muscle test	Maintain skills
Process skills may be a strength	Muscle tone	Adapt tools, toys, and equip-

Table 16.4.—Continued

Occupational status	Recommended assessments	Treatment considerations
Limited opportunities to problem solve	Oral motor assessment	ment to allow skill development and maintenance
Delayed development of age appropriate skills	McCarthy Scales of Children's Abilities	Teach new age-appropriate skills
	Bruininks-Oseretsky Test	Provide opportunities for play and exploration
	Southern California Sensory Integration Tests	
	Southern California Postrotary Nystagmus Test	
	Clinical Play Observation	
	Parten Play Scale	
	Riley Motor Problems	
	Interview and observation	
	ENVIRONMENT	
Decreased opportunity to interact with peers	PH	Encourage involvement in peer, school, and community activities
Decreased ability to explore environment	Interview	
	Home visit	Problem solve issues of grief and sorrow with family
Overprotection	School visit	
Effects on other family members		Suggest home and school modifications

behaviors including assuming appropriate decision making and use of time responsibility are stressed (32).

Volitional level behaviors are addressed in treatment by providing opportunities for the child to engage in activities that are considered to be exciting, are interesting and challenging, give clear and positive feedback on the worth of the individual performing the activity, and are valued by the child.

For the family, school personnel and others who interact with the child, the therapist is able to provide continued resources that will support these important avenues of stimulation. Activity and equipment adaptation are starting points for consultation that may later include strategies for encouraging participation by a child who is depressed, and for solving personal issues of grief and sorrow that accompany long-term involvement with a child who is dying.

MUSCULAR DYSTROPHY CASE: ROBBIE

Background Information

Robbie is a 7-year-old boy with muscular dystrophy, Duchenne's type. This diagnosis was first made when he was 5 years old. At that time he had begun having difficulties keeping up with other children on the playground. He reportedly fell frequently during outdoor play and generally had trouble moving around. His parents were first suspicious that Robbie was having special problems when they noticed he seemed to be "getting worse" in his movement skills rather than better.

This child was initially referred to occupational therapy for an overall assessment, lower extremity dressing training and a home consultation in preparation for Robbie receiving a wheelchair.

Evaluation

THE PERFORMANCE SYSTEM

On initial evaluation, activities of daily living were found to be age appropriate with the exception of lower extremity dressing which required moderate assistance and bathing activities, in which Robbie required assistance for getting in and out of the tub. Areas of dependence appeared to be secondary to muscle weakness rather than a lack of awareness of task demands or poor problem-solving skills.

Findings on the Vineland Social Maturity Scale revealed the following. Robbie was able to fix simple snacks for himself. He used kitchen appliances independently including a juicer in which he made favorite drinks. He had a room of his own which, until recently, he had maintained independently requiring verbal reminders for daily ordering and cleaning activities. His mother reported that within the last 2 months, Robbie had been unable to reach for and retrieve objects that have fallen to the floor. He had also asked for assistance to complete bed-making activities.

Muscle testing revealed poor-to-fair muscle strength in hip, knee and ankle extensors. Active range of motion showed minimal limitations in all extension movements of lower extremities. Upper extremity strength was within normal limits with full range of motion in all planes of movement.

Robbie was able to walk short distances with minimal assistance for stability. His gait was slow and awkward and he had a tendency to walk on his toes. He tired easily and asked to rest frequently. Some lordosis was present as he ambulated and appeared to be associated with decreased knee and hip extension abilities.

Communication and interaction skills during assessment appeared age appropriate. Robbie answered all assessment questions, demonstrated skills when requested and volunteered additional information when needed. He was interested in finding out about other children attending the occupational therapy clinic and asked how he might meet them.

The Play History revealed limited gross motor "action" skills that would be appropriate for a child at the end of the dramatic and complex constructive and pregame epoch of play and transitioning into the game epoch. Robbie was unable to participate in hopping, skipping or similar play activities; he was also unable to use a bicycle or tricycle. Fine motor play skills were at age level as demonstrated by his ability to work with models and to participate in simple projects in his Boy Scout troop.

Robbie was found to be at risk in all areas of emerging play skills. He was unable to participate in gross motor sports and his decreasing muscle strength suggested that fine motor "actions" that emphasize skill and precision (especially use of tools) would eventually be limited.

THE HABITUATION SUBSYSTEM

Robbie participated in a variety of roles including age-expected family roles of son, grandson, brother, and cousin. At home Robbie had responsibility for regular chores which included setting the table for breakfast and dinner and watering several houseplants.

He attended a public school and appeared to fulfill most requirements of the student role with the exception of gross motor recreational/recess time behaviors. He had one close friend at school who was extremely shy and withdrawn, according to the mother, and who preferred to sit with Robbie during lunch and recess rather than be with the other children.

THE VOLITIONAL SUBSYSTEM

Among Robbie's favorite activities were model building, playing boardgames, and listening to stories about cowboys. He also reported an interest in "electronics" saying that he liked to take radios and clocks apart and that he hoped to repair televisions when he got to be older.

He appeared to have minimal interest in sports as evidenced by his lack of preference for any particular athletic game, position of play or major team. He was able to name sports that were played during different seasons but did not appear to be familiar with players or teams.

Robbie's log of daily activities included watching television, looking at pictures in books, and sitting at a favorite window. Play with peers occurred three to four times per week including Boy Scout troop meetings, a regularly scheduled church group meeting and arranged visits with family friends and relatives.

Robbie demonstrated many behaviors characteristic of a child who feels good about himself and in control of his actions. His preferences for board games appeared partially motivated by his skill in winning especially favorite games such as Chinese Checkers, Sorry, and Parchesi. His interest in model building also provided many opportunities for him to feel good about the outcome of his actions. Difficulties with motor skills did not appear to have impacted greatly on Robbie's concept of himself. Although he stated that he missed "running around with the other kids," he also indicated that it was "OK to sit and watch."

An interview with his mother and father included information on family patterns and values. Both parents were involved in work outside of the home, enjoyed family and church-oriented activities, and valued hard work and "sticking together to get things done." Robbie's parents were involved in hobbies and special interests which included woodworking for the father and quilting, doll-making, and gardening for the mother.

HOME ENVIRONMENT

Robbie lived with his parents and two younger siblings in a small house owned by the family. Robbie had his own room which was small and required significant modifications to accommodate a wheelchair. The house had limited wheelchair access due to doors between rooms and arrangement of furnishings. The bathroom was accessible but would require installation of grab rails for maintaining Robbie's present level in toileting and bathing. Entry to the front door was up three stairs; however, the back door was at ground level and would easily accommodate a wheelchair.

The family spends most of their free time in and around the home. Robbie's 4-year-old and 10-month-old sisters are active and noisy, providing many opportunities for Robbie to participate in their care (watching them) and their play (building castles, stringing beads, dangling simple music and sound toys).

Treatment Goals and Strategies

Treatment was initiated when Robbie was 7 years old. He demonstrated competence in fine motor action and material play with skills in gross motor and self-care skills beginning to show some atrophy due to increasing muscle weakness and range of motion limitations secondary to MD. The initial objective of treatment was to provide training and adaptive equipment to help Robbie maintain his functioning in self-care activities. Energy conservation techniques that would help Robbie continue to enact his chore roles were also given immediate attention.

Home consultation was given in an attempt to modify existing space to accommodate a wheelchair. Removal and rearrangement of furniture throughout the house and especially in Robbie's room was recommended. Bathroom modifications were also designed and a bathtub bench was purchased and training was given for transfer techniques.

Robbie was put on a 1-month follow-up program for occupational therapy and remained on that schedule for the next 6 months. At the end of that sequence Robbie showed increased deterioration of motor skills. He was dependent in lower extremity dressing and needed assistance for donning any clothing that required him to raise his arms over his head. Bathing activities required moderate assistance for transfers, maintaining balance and washing. Toileting activities required use of a portable urinal throughout the day and use of a bedpan. As Robbie's motor skills became worse, associated habituation and volitional behaviors followed suit. Spending most of his day in his wheelchair, Robbie was no longer able to carry out chore roles finding it impossible to leave

his chair for even brief periods. Because of the size of the rooms in his home, manipulation of the wheelchair around furniture and throughout the house was too difficult for Robbie to manage himself.

The impact of the continued degeneration of skills and capacities was especially startling at the volitional level. Robbie was much less cooperative during the occupational therapy consultation, often remaining silent when asked for information or simply answering "I don't know." His mother reported that he had recently become withdrawn and did not appear interested in any of his former hobbies or favorite activities and now preferred to watch others play, rarely becoming involved himself.

Occupational therapy intervention shifted to a one-time per week program. Robbie attended a preadolescent group three times a month and was seen at home on the 4th week.

Programming was designed to provide opportunities for Robbie to interact with other children who were having motor difficulties. Exercises and movement activities combined with crafts, games, and simple cooking activities provided a backdrop for exploring positive ways to engage in successful interactions with people and objects and exploring alternative ways to do the things that each child cared about.

Robbie became friends with another boy in the group who had a similar degree of impairment due to rheumatoid arthritis. Together they worked on airplane and car models with both boys compensating for decreased skill and reducing their frustrations by taking turns at completing one project. Their friendship and working partnership continued outside of the group with weekend and after school visits scheduled regularly.

Through this friendship, Robbie learned about CB and amateur (ham) radios. His parents recognized this interest and purchased a CB for their son. They reported that he spent "hours and hours" listening and tuning his radio in to conversations and enthusiastically sharing what he heard at mealtimes or when friends came to visit.

In the next year Robbie continued his interest in the CB radio. He listened to it frequently and was always eager to share what he had heard or to tell a story about a conversation he had with a "CB-er." Two years after initial evaluation Robbie was dependent in all self-care. Transfers to and from his wheelchair now required maximal assistance.

His "friendly" personality, ongoing participation in the occupational therapy group, establishment of a friendship, and avid interest in his radio hobby provided him with opportunities to feel good about himself in spite of his rapidly deteriorating physical condition. Robbie's parents reported that they continued to find their son "off to himself, just sitting and watching other kids" but that the majority of his time he was involved in activities of interest.

Robbie's role of big brother to his two sisters required "adjustments" to become valid. With support and training from the therapist Robbie shifted from a co-player and learned about "babysitting" responsibilities. He was able to manage verbal supervision and some simple play activities that allowed him to feel like he was "in charge of the girls" for short periods of time.

Three years after initial evaluation in occupational therapy. Robbie continued to be involved in treatment. Due to severe transfer difficulties, Robbie no longer attended group sessions but was seen in his home one time per month. Treatment focused on providing simple motor "assembly" projects, general stimulation and problem solving, and support to the family for Robbie's increasing dependency needs. Robbie had stopped attending school and was now being seen by an "in home" teacher. Consultation was provided to the teacher on use of space and placement of teaching materials so that Robbie would have opportunities for maximum successful interactions.

Over the course of treatment the human occupation perspective allowed the therapist to shift treatment goals and strategies in order to address the continuously changing needs of the child with a progressive degenerative disease.

CONCLUSION

Utilization of the model of human occupation in pediatrics can have positive effects on the spirit of the therapist, the child, his or her caregivers, and society-at-large. Therapists who endorse the model may feel liberated from the sense of hopelessness they experience when they are preoccupied with unalterable and sometimes unrelenting disease processes. Diseases and their outcomes cannot always be eliminated or even appreciably changed but fortunately, in the face of adversity, the young child is remarkably resilient. The model of human occupation provides guidelines on how the spirits of children and their parents can be lifted, how alleged incapacities can become metamorphosized into capacities through the ingenuity that creates compensation and environmental change, and how the dreams of children can become realized

through positive striving and initiative. When a child with a pediatric disorder benefits, their families benefit. When these children's potential to be productive is realized, society benefits. The model of human occupation requires the therapist to take on a multidimensional, multifaceted perspective that uniquely tailors the treatment plan for each child. Ultimately, the goal is that the child, his or her parents and the therapist create a partnership in which each member will experience competence, hope and positive striving.

References

1. Als H, Lester BM, Trovick E, Brazelton TB: Towards a research instrument for the assessment of preterm infants' behavior. In Fitzgerald HE, Lester BM, Yogman MW (eds): *Theory of Research in Behavioral Pediatrics*, New York, Plenum, 1980, vol 1, p 6.
2. Andersen SE, Holstein BE: Integration of blind children: the fulfillment of the needs for having, loving and being. *Proceedings of the Third European Regional Conference of Rehabilitation International.* Vienna, Austria, Austrian Workers' Compensation Board, 1981.
3. Ayres AJ: *Sensory Intergration and Learning Disorders.* Los Angeles, Western Psychological Services, 1972.
4. Ayres AJ: *Sensory Integration and the Child.* Los Angeles, Western Psychological Services, 1979.
5. Ayres AJ: *Aspects of the Somatomotor Adaptive Response and Praxis.* Audiotape available from the Center for the Study of Sensory Integrative Dysfunction, Pasadena, Calif, 1981.
6. Barbers J, Shaheen E: Environmental failure to thrive: a clinical view. *J Pediatr* 71:639–644, 1967.
7. Barris R: Environmental interactions: an extension of the model of occupation. *Am J Occup Ther* 36:637–644, 1982.
8. Bernstein NR: Medical tragedies in facial burn disfigurement. *Psych Annuals* 6:31–49, 1976.
9. Blom GE: Child nurturing in 1985. In Boger RP, Blom GE, Lezzotte LE (eds): *Child Nurturance.* New York, Plenum, 1984.
10. Blom GE, Ek K, Irwin S, Kulkarni M, Miller K, Frey W: *Coping with Handicaps: Implications for Adults with Physical Disabilities.* Paper presented at the National Rehabilitation Association Annual Meeting, Anaheim, Calif, September 20, 1982.
11. Bloom H: An aspect of social services for the handicapped child in the community. *Talk,* Spring, 79:22–25, 1976.
12. Bobath K: *A Neurophysiological Basis for the Treatment of Cerebral Palsy.* London, William Heinemann Medical Books, 1980.
13. Bobath K, Bobath B: The facilitation of normal postural reactions and movements in the treatment of cerebral palsy. *Physiotherapy* (England), 50:246–262, 1964.
14. Bowlby J: Childhood mourning and its implications for psychiatry. *Am J Psychiatry* 118:481–498, 1961.

15. Bowley A: A follow-up study of 64 children with cerebral palsy. *Dev Med Child Neurol* 9:172–182, 1967.
16. Branstetter E: The young child's response to hospitalization: separation anxiety or lack of mothering care. *Am J Public Health* 59:92–97, 1969.
17. Breslau N: Siblings of disabled children: birth order and age-spacing effects. *J Abnorm Child Psychol* 10:85–96, 1982.
18. Breslau N: Family care: Effect on siblings and mothers. In Thompson GH, Rubin IL, Bilenker RM (eds): *Comprehensive Management of Cerebral Palsy.* New York, Grune & Stratton, 1983.
19. Brooks M: Why play in hospitals. *Nurs Clin North Am* 5:431–441, 1970.
20. Campling J: (ed): *Images of Ourselves: Women with Disabilities Talking.* Boston, Routledge & Kegan Paul, 1981.
21. Coley IL: *Pediatric Assessment of Self-Care Activities.* St. Louis, Mosby, 1978.
22. Cooke R: The hospitalized child and his family. In Haller JA (ed): *The Hospitalized Child and His Family.* Baltimore, Johns Hopkins Press, 1967.
23. Crocker, E: Reactions of children to health care encounters: programs that can make a difference. In Robinson G, Clarke H (eds): *The Hospital Care of Children: A Review of Contemporary Issues.* New York, Oxford University Press, 1980.
24. Elmer E, Gregg G: Developmental characteristics of abused children. *Pediatrics* 40:596–602, 1967.
25. Farber SD: A multisensory approach to neurorehabilitation. In Farber SD (ed): *Neurorehabilitation: A Multisensory Approach.* Philadephia, Saunders, 1982.
26. Fliedman J, Roth W: *The Unexpected Minority: Handicapped Children in America.* New York, Harcourt, Brace, Jovanovich, 1980.
27. Florey LL: Studies of play: implications for growth, development, and for clinical practice. *Am J Occup Ther* 35:519–524, 1981.
28. Glen M: Family illness rituals. *J Fam Prac* 14:950–954, 1982.
29. Gorski P, Dawson M, Brazelton TP: Stages of behavioral organization in the high-risk neonate: theoretical and clinical considerations. *Sem Perinatol* 13:61–72, 1979.
30. Gruen GE, Korte JR, Baum JF: Group measure of locus of control. *Dev Psychol* 10:683–686, 1974.
31. Haan N: *Coping and Defending: Processes of Self-Environment Organization.* New York, Academic Press, 1977.
32. Hamant C: Pediatrics. In Hopkins HL, Smith HD (ed): *Willard and Spackman's Occupational Therapy,* ed 5, Philadelphia, Lippincott, 1978.
33. Kent M: A longitudinal study of physically abused children. (Unpublished grant reports, 1974–1977, Childrens Hospital of Los Angeles.)
34. Keogh BK, Margolis J: Learn to labor and to wait: Attentional problems of children with learning disorders. *J Learn Disabil* 9:276–286, 1976.
35. Kiernan SS, Conner FP, von Hippel CS, Jones SH: *Children with Orthopaedic Handicaps.* Washington, DC, U.S. Department of Human Development Services, 1978.
36. Klaus, Kennell J: *Maternal-Infant Bonding.* St Louis, Mosby, 1976.
37. Kleinfield S: *The Hidden Minority: A Profile of Handicapped Americans.* Boston: Little Brown, 1979.
38. Knox S: *Battered and Failure to Thrive Children: Developmental Analyses.* Lecture presented at AOTA Annual Conference, 1980.
39. Kornblum H, Anderson B: Acceptance: reassessed—a point of view. *Child Psychiatry Hum Dev* 12:171–178, 1982.
40. Lamerowski S: Helping families cope with handicapped children. *Top Clin Nurs* July, 41–56, 1982.
41. Lindquist I, Lind J, Harvey D: Play in hospital. In Tizard B, Harvey D (eds): *Biology of Play.* Philadelphia, Lippincott, 1977.
42. Osofsky J, Danzger B: Relationships between neonatal characteristics and mother-infant characteristics and mother-infant interaction. *Dev Psychol* 1:124–130, 1974.
43. Parker S, Brazelton TB: Newborn behavioral assessment. *Child Today* 3:2–5, 1981.
44. Philip M, Duckworth D: *Children with Disabilities and Their Families.* Windsor, England, NFER-Nelson, 1982.
45. Robertson J (ed): *Hospitals and Children.* London, Victor Gollancz, 1962.
46. Robinson A: Play: the arena for acquisition of rules for competent behavior. *Am J Occup Ther* 31:248–253, 1977.
47. Rood MS: Neurophysiologic reactions as a basis for physical therapy. *Phys Ther Rev* 34:444–449, 1954.
48. Roth W: *The Handicapped Speak.* Jefferson, NC, McFarland 1981.
49. Rusk HA: *Rehabilitation Medicine.* St. Louis, Mosby, 1971.
50. Scott A: Degenerative diseases. In Trombly CA (ed): *Occupational Therapy for Physical Dysfunction.* Baltimore, Williams & Wilkins, 1983.
51. Sensky T. Family stigma in congenital physical handicap. *Br Med J* 285:1033–1035, 1982.
52. Sheridan M: *The Handicapped Child and His Home.* London, National Children's Home, 1965.
53. Spencer EA: Functional restoration. In Hopkins HL, Smith HD (ed): *Willard and Spackman's Occupational Therapy,* (ed 5) Philadelphia, Lippincott, 1978.
54. Takata N: The play milieu. A preliminary appraisal. *Am J Occup Ther* 25:281–284, 1971.
55. Tisza B, Angoff K: A play program for hospitalized children: the role of the playroom teacher. *Pediatrics* 28:841–845, 1961.
56. Turner A: *The praction of occupational therapy.* Edinburgh, Churchill Livingston, 1981.
57. U.S. National Center for Health Statistics: *Current Estimates From the Health Interview Survey: United States 1967.* DHEW Pub No. 1000, Series 10, No. 52. Washington, DC, U.S. Government Printing Office, 1969.
58. U.S. National Center for Health Statistics: *Current Estimates from the Health Inteview Survey: United States, 1978.* DHEW Pub. No. (PHS) 80-1551. Washington, DC, U.S. Government Printing Office, 1979.
59. Wright BA: Developing constructive views of life with a disability. *Rehab Lit* 41:274–279, 1980.

CHAPTER 17

Dysfunctional Older Adults

Teena L. Snow and Joan C. Rogers

THE MULTIPLICITY OF PROBLEMS OF DYSFUNCTIONAL OLDER ADULTS

This chapter presents several case studies that illustrate the unique aspects of therapeutic interventions with older adults using the model of human occupation. Many of the treatment strategies used with the different disability groups discussed in this book are also appropriate for the elderly. However, treatment decisions are often complicated by the multiplicity of problems that confront older adults in their routines. The problems caused by specific diseases in older adults are compounded by the preexisting conditions that can occur in any or all subsystems. Older adults commonly have one or more chronic diseases. They frequently accept societal expectations of "slowing down" with age or have some sensory or musculoskeletal changes that necessitate such "slowing" and hence experience disuse atrophy. They may become victims of catastrophic illnesses. Table 17.1 briefly summarizes the typical occupational status of dysfunctional older adults.

The complex presentations of older adults' abilities and disabilities must be recognized and evaluated by the therapist to provide optimal treatment. The diminished ability of many older adults to meet the variable demands of their environments can impact on them in a highly specific and unexpected fashion. Incidents, which on the surface appear trivial, may serve to create dangerous imbalances in existing ecosystems of older adults. Minimal changes in a social support network that has made it possible for a severely impaired person to continue functioning in a complex environment may result in severe deficits and dysfunction in all subsystems. Changes in environmental demands due to relocation or alterations in established habit patterns may mean that the older adult can no longer adequately adjust. Critical incidents may involve the vacation time of a regular caregiver, an increase in rental costs for adequate housing,

or the worsening of an existing chronic health condition after a cold or flu.

Although the delicate balance by which many older adults adapt can be upset, the cases presented here demonstrate that this balance can also be reestablished. This requires a mixture of support and autonomy to promote a sense of control necessary to direct one's life and simultaneously meet requirements for safety and social expectations.

General problem areas seen in the older adults treated by therapists fall into four categories. Some problems are due to normal changes that occur with the aging process. Other difficulties are due to the presence of chronic diseases while others are caused by disuse or misuse atrophy. Finally, problems arise due to traumatic insults to one or more subsystems. Older adults who experience only the changes that occur normally with aging are most likely to have problems in the performance and habituation subsystems. Difficulties in the performance subsystem center around the subtle and gradual changes that affect sensory perception, mobility and endurance. These changes can eventually cause significant losses in performance abilities in many facets of daily life if a maladaptive cycle is begun. Visual losses often result in problems with the use of necessary appliances and information sources such as telephones, newspapers, telephone books, clocks, prescription labels, maps, street signs, and stoves. Hearing losses result in fewer social contacts, increases in problems with the comprehension of verbal information and the labeling of many older people as mentally impaired, forgetful or confused. The slowing of motor performance and the gradual reduction of endurance can necessitate revisions of daily schedules and activities. These alterations provide the older adult with concrete evidence of changes in performance skills, and impact strongly on the self-evaluation of ability to continue in previously enjoyed activities and roles. These changes also provide evidence of diminishing competence to family members, friends

Table 17.1.
Occupational status, recommended assessments, and treatment considerations for dysfunctional older adults

Occupational status	Assessments	Treatment considerations
VOLITION		
Personal causation		
Due to changes in roles and performance skills, feels lack of efficacy and external control	Occupational History (OH) Occupational Therapy Functional Screening Tool (OTFST) Occupational Questionnaire (OQ) Rotter Internal/External Locus of Control Scale	Provide opportunities to control the treatment program and environment. Promote decision-making opportunities and reinforce any appropriate involvement in internalizing locus of control
Values		
Changing abilities often result in inability to meet previous standards and difficulty planning for future tasks	OH, OTFST, OQ Values portion of Role Checklist Life Satisfaction Scale	Values clarification and counseling to reconcile current abilities with previously held standards. Involve person and social supports in goal setting and program implementation
Interests		
Disease processes and normal performance skills deficits may make participation in past interests no longer viable. Performance skills impairments may reduce potency or limit acceptable interests	OH, OTFST, OQ Interest Checklist	Use previous interests to develop new interests based on current skills Use past work roles to develop potential interest areas
HABITUATION		
Roles		
Changing environmental supports may cause repeated role losses and the adoption of negatively perceived roles	OH, OTFST Role Checklist	Resumption of previously valued roles is often possible with a restructuring of the environment. Positive aspects of currently available roles need to be explored. Counseling may be needed to help the person and the social support system to value the older adult and provide appropriate roles
Habits		
Strong lifelong habit patterns may encourage misuse or disuse atrophy. This then limits skills and abilities	OH, OTFST, OQ Daily schedules	The need to change habits should be weighed against the problem of altering lifelong patterns. Changes should be made carefully and deliberately. Restructuring of daily routine should be coupled with constant support

Table 17.1.—Continued

Occupational status	Assessments	Treatment considerations
PERFORMANCE		
Skills		
Perceptual-motor skills are negatively affected. Process and communication skills are affected by sensory changes resulting in impairment in these areas	Performance Activities of Daily Living Evaluation FROMAJE Mental Status Evaluation Set Test Parachek Geriatric Rating Scale Instrumental Activities of Daily Living Other appropriate assessments of strength, range, etc.	Identify baseline skills and determine the potential for improvement. Work with the person to determine the usefulness of improvement. Carefully assess the impairment of process and communication skills to determine appropriate intervention strategies. Improvement in these areas can cause changes in all other areas
Environment		
Objects may become difficult to use. Modified equipment or habits may be needed to perform familiar tasks. Social supports may become more critical for continued maintenance of the individual	OH Appropriate home evaluations and interviews with significant others	Assessment of objects, appliances, furniture, and equipment in the environment to determine need for modifications to promote safety, independence and/or ease of function

and health professionals, and raise questions regarding safety and independence. These losses tend to raise issues of rights and responsibilities for the continuation of self-determining behavior as opposed to societal or medical decision making for older adults with some deficits.

Changes that older adults experience in the habituation subsystem often result from the difficulty in balancing new routines and roles with previous habits, problems with selecting and successfully integrating new roles, and difficulty in changing behaviors that have been learned over a lifetime. Role losses and habit changes are often viewed by the older adult as originating from external sources and biased against their continued independence and personal preferences. Evaluation of the older adult's perception of new roles, changes in behaviors and ability and desire to fill allocated roles and modify habit structures is essential in determining successful adaptation to normal aging changes.

Older adults who experience problems due to chronic conditions can experience difficulties in all subsystems. The periodic exacerbations of persistent and incurable diseases cause many problems similar to those experienced by younger counterparts. Additional difficulties are encountered when more than one chronic disease is present or when the normal changes in various body systems amplify the problems. Occupational performance in the presence of a diabetic condition with resultant peripheral neuropathy is made more difficult when visual and auditory impairments exist and protective reactions are slowed due to musculoskeletal changes. For older adults with chronic conditions there is a continual need to provide periodic reevaluation of each subsystem. Changes may be identified secondary to disease processes, the normal changes that accompany aging and traumatic injuries.

Disuse or misuse atrophy are phenomena that impact principally on the performance or volition subsystems due to maladaptation within the habituation subsystem. Typical daily routines and individual decisions regarding role internalization create environmental constraints that promote or prevent activities that can maintain previous levels of motoric, cognitive and social performance. These changes resonate through all components of the open system and predispose older adults to more difficult and time consuming rehabilitation after traumatic insults or during flare-ups of chronic conditions.

When disuse or misuse atrophy exists it is often possible to enhance abilities with therapeutic intervention.

An older adult who is unable, initially, to make independent decisions regarding living arrangements, participation in therapeutic programming, or goal identification can improve substantially. Through practice and skill building, the person can regain feelings of efficacy and take control of planning and executing activities. Enhancement of physical skills, mental prowess, or social skills can dramatically affect the person's ability to be involved in self-determining behaviors.

Traumatic insults due to physical injuries such as strokes or hip fractures, role losses such as the death of a spouse or friend, or environmental changes such as relocation or institutionalization impact on all subsystems. The maladaptations that occur are much like those identified for younger populations with physical disabilities or mental illnesses. These difficulties are compounded by the problems that arise from maladaptations due to normal aging changes, the presence of chronic diseases or disuse atrophy. Societal and family expectations of rehabilitation potential, baseline performance skills and limited health and rehabilitation resources restrict and sometimes eliminate options for many older people regardless of personal needs and abilities.

Many of the assessment and treatment procedures found in this chapter are the same as those located elsewhere in this text, however, the decisions that lead to those interventive strategies are based on the accumulation of information on the older adult's abilities and problem areas. Goals for therapy include maintenance programs to retain existing skills, preventive programs to prevent deterioration or regression, restorative programs to regain or improve function and abilities, and progressive programs to enhance skills and improve premorbid conditions beyond baseline measures.

Occupational therapists frequently serve as holistic assessors of the functional status of older adults. They assume responsibility for investigating the complex interrelationships of medical diagnoses, physical abilities, mental processing, performance capabilities, and personal goals and needs when determining the possibilities and probabilities for meeting the complex needs of their patients. Table 17.1 illustrates recommended assessments and treatment interventions. Each geriatric case analysis is designed to illustrate the complex nature of assessing and treating older adults in their environments.

A RETURN TO INDEPENDENT LIVING: MRS. LEE

Mrs. Ester Lee was an 86-year-old woman who was referred to occupational therapy specifically to evaluate her potential to return to independent living after an extended stay in a long-term care facility. She had been admitted to the facility from an acute care hospital following a fall in her home. When admitted to the hospital, she was reported to be experiencing mental confusion and disorientation. Neither condition cleared during her hospital stay. She had been in the nursing home for 6 months and had been moved from a skilled nursing wing to an intermediate care wing after the first 4 weeks of rehabilitation efforts. During her stay in the facility she had consistantly raised the issue of going home. The feasibility of discharging her to her apartment was pursued at this time. This was due to a pending change in her financial eligibility from private pay to Medicaid. The use of Medicaid monies for institutional care would necessitate the loss of her government-subsidized apartment.

Medical diagnoses at the time of assessment were: chronic congestive heart failure, severe and chronic osteoporosis, multiple vertebral compression fractures in the lumbar portion of the spine, dependent edema in the lower extremities, chronic gastritis, and a history of transient ischemic attacks.

Mrs. Lee was first assessed in the long-term care facility and subsequently evaluated during a 24-hour visit to her apartment.

Performance Evaluation

PERCEPTUAL-MOTOR SKILLS

Mrs. Lee was evaluated for upper and lower extremity range of motion, endurance, strength, and general speed and accuracy of hand-eye coordination tasks. Range of motion in her shoulders was limited by pain. She was unable to raise her arms above shoulder height which resulted in her being unable to reach back-opening zippers on dresses. Bilateral hand function was adequate with fair-to-good strength and coordination in her hands, arms and shoulders. Mrs. Lee was able to manipulate small objects without difficulty, but could not use visual discrimination to perform any accuracy tasks. She stated that she "just can't see well enough, even with these new glasses, to do much."

Range of motion was significantly restricted in her lower back, hips and knees due to spinal compression fractures and osteoarthritis. She was unable to bend forward to reach the floor from a seated position due to back pain and trunk immobility. She was, therefore, unable to put on her stockings or shoes without help. Since she was unable to fully extend her hips, she ambulated with her hips flexed at approximately 30–40° and her knees flexed at about 20°. Stair climbing was precluded due to instability and fear of falling. She had great difficulty stepping over the 3-inch ridge in the shower stall at her apartment.

Mrs. Lee's endurance was poor. She became short of breath and required frequent rest periods after 15 feet of ambulation or 10 minutes of upper or lower extremity exercises. The nursing home staff was unable to identify specific reasons for her inability or unwillingness to ambulate, but assumed it had to do with her preadmission fall.

Mrs Lee demonstrated no losses in peripheral sensation in regard to light touch, two-point discrimination, hot-cold sensation, and sharp-dull discrimination despite a history of transient ischemic attacks.

A performance task consisting of locating a telephone number for a local grocery in the telephone book and dialing the correct number, demonstrated that Mrs. Lee had a loss of visual acuity and that her major visual complaint was of a central visual field loss bilaterally. She was also unable to read medication labels, meal preparation instructions, small calendars, or other instruction sheets or clock dials. Using a large magnifier, she was able to read the telephone book and dial the telephone with a moderate amount of difficulty. Mrs. Lee was able to read instructions if they were written on nonglare paper in 2-inch-high letters. As a result of this evaluation an ophthalmology consultation was requested and revealed that Mrs. Lee was suffering from progressive macular degeneration bilaterally.

Mrs. Lee did not have any difficulty with auditory perception, showing herself capable of following multiple verbal instructions which were spoken in a normal voice in the presence of assorted background noises.

PROCESS SKILLS

In the areas of problem solving and general mental abilities, Mrs. Lee demonstrated some impairment. She scored a 12 on the FRO-MAJE Mental Status Evaluation. The results indicated that she: (a) needed some supervi-

sion of activities of daily living performance for reasons of safety; (b) was able to demonstrate adequate reasoning skills in abstract problem solving tasks; (c) was oriented to person, place and time; (d) had difficulties with immediate and recent memory, but no difficulties with remote memory; (e) had intact mathematical skills, although these were very slow in view of the fact that she had been an accountant for a law firm until her retirement at age 60; (f) had some impairment of judgment in that she tended to overestimate her abilities and place herself in precarious situations unless supervised by others; and (g) had appropriately variable emotional affect. Mrs. Lee was slow in most of her responses involving emergency situations. These results indicate that some minimal-to-moderate impairment of mental capabilities was present, due possibly to depression or dementia.

Mrs. Lee had no difficulty with the Set Test. Her results, a score of 36 out of a possible 40, indicated that her performance on the FRO-MAJE was probably more closely related to depression than dementia.

COMMUNICATION/INTERACTION SKILLS

The social worker at the long-term care facility indicated that Mrs. Lee had rarely attended activities and actively chose to remain apart from other residents except for some hallway conversations that she initiated during her wheelchair trips to the dining area. Mrs. Lee stated that she "had little in common with the other people at the home," since she "originally came from a small town and had not gotten involved in any groups after she moved to the city 20 years ago."

Mrs. Lee had attended physical therapy sessions for 3 weeks after her admission to the facility, but discontinued the sessions after she experienced several episodes of urinary incontinence during ambulation training.

Prior to her institutionalization, Mrs. Lee indicated that she rarely left the floor of her apartment building to participate in the senior activities held on a daily basis in the building. She identified her reluctance as stemming from not knowing anyone well enough to want to eat or socialize with them. She noted that prior to the death of one of her close friends a year ago she had gone with that friend and others to many social functions and noon nutritional programs in the building and "enjoyed them a great deal." Mrs. Lee had continued to have lunch with a friend, Mrs. Quinton, once a week at a nearby restaurant until her fall and subsequent admission. Mrs. Quinton continued to visit once weekly at the facility and the two women ate together at that time.

Mrs. Lee showed no evidence of having problems communicating her needs or preferences to any of the staff or caregivers. She is skilled in using both verbal and nonverbal communication patterns.

Habituation Evaluation

HABITS

Mrs. Lee had developed several new habits in the institutional setting that impaired her ability to function at home. She had greatly reduced her general activity level and had become functionally nonambulatory and wheelchair dependent. She was treated as dependent in activities of daily living despite having ambulatory abilities and received help for all self-care activities except eating. She remained in her nightgown throughout the day. She called for assistance nightly to change the bedding, due to urinary incontinence. She was generally not responsible for maintaining any routine daily performance of self-care tasks, administration of medications or engagement in physical activities.

ROLES

Mrs. Lee identified the roles of daughter, friend and independent woman as her major life roles. She stated that two of these roles had been "taken away" from her, those of daughter and independent woman, and that her role as a friend was now lacking in substance.

After retiring, Mrs. Lee had returned to her small town home to care for her parents through several prolonged illnesses until their deaths about 20 years ago. She then sold the family home and left the town where she had grown up. She moved into an apartment in the urban area where she had worked as an accountant in a law firm for 38 years. Mrs. Lee renewed friendships with a small group of women, including Mrs. Quinton, after her return to the city. Along with several members of this group, she moved into a new government-subsidized apartment building. This move was precipitated by repeated, substantial rent increases over a 10-year-period.

Mrs. Lee has been living in her current apartment for over 8 years, but noted that most of her friends were no longer living in the building due to death or institutionalization. She noted that she had not made many efforts at developing new friendships with her new neighbors "because it took too much energy and you never knew how long they were going to be around."

Mrs. Lee volunteered that she had been married briefly in her twenties but was left by her husband after 2 years of marriage. She had obtained a divorce shortly thereafter and had never again been involved in any intimate relationship with a man, "since they just didn't respect a person's right to do things their own way without interfering."

Mrs. Lee indicated that her ability to be a friend to anyone had been greatly impaired by her illness and institutionalization. She felt that until her illness, she had been someone who could be counted on to help out and provide whatever kind of help was needed. She identified her current roles as: "dependent, sick, helpless, taker, worthless, and patient."

Volition Evaluation

VALUES

Mrs. Lee stated that one of the most important things for her was "to live as independently as possible and to not continue to live if she couldn't be independent." She noted that she disliked the nursing home intensely and resented having to stay there. She indicated that she would prefer to "take her chances at home rather than dying slowly in that place."

After the home visit and discussions with the therapist, she had been able to identify priorities and compromises in the area of total independence in activities of daily living and home maintenance tasks that would need to occur so that she would be able to return to her apartment. She was willing to accept help on a daily basis for supervision of activities of daily living and assistance with all of the housekeeping tasks that needed to be done routinely. She was willing to accept some modifications to make her bedroom and bathroom safer for her use, but was not willing to rearrange the furniture in her living room to allow a wider pathway for her walker. She was willing to raise the height of furniture and to replace one large stuffed rocking recliner with a high, firm, stable chair with armrests to accommodate her decreased ability to get up if her knees were flexed at more than 90°.

Personal Standards

Mrs. Lee demonstrated a major discrepancy between professed standards of personal appearance and personal performance of self-care and home care tasks. She stated that she wanted to be totally independent and wanted to look well dressed and neat. Her behavior indicated that she did not actively pursue any of these preferred outcomes.

Temporal Orientation

Mrs. Lee demonstrated little awareness of time and futurist thinking when evaluated. She noted that in the nursing home nothing changed and no one went anywhere.

INTERESTS

Mrs. Lee had great difficulty identifying any leisure interests. She indicated that she had never done much in this area, preferring instead to spend her time helping her friends or keeping her house clean and neat. She was clear that at this time her focus was on taking control of removing herself from an undesirable environment and returning to her familiar apartment. The interests that she could identify centered around being able to maintain herself in her home environment and developing the type and degrees of support that would allow her to remain at home.

PERSONAL CAUSATION

During the initial evaluation, Mrs. Lee seemed to feel that she had little control over anything. For example, she commented that "there is nothing I could do to change where I am, what people do for me and what I am allowed to do for myself." She could best be described as being externally controlled.

Output: Occupational Performance

Mrs. Lee's self-care capabilities were unknown to the nursing staff at the initial evaluation, consequently the aides had been assisting her in all activities except feeding. Mrs. Lee was assessed using the Instrumental Activities of Daily Living Scale. Mrs. Lee's score on the evaluation indicated minimal to no impairment in physically performing the tasks, however, some supervision was needed to assure that she did not overestimate her abilities. This was especially true in the areas of mobility and stability while ambulating, judging fatigue and scheduling adequate rest periods during daily activities. Based on this information, it was judged that further evaluation was needed to determine what she was capable of doing in the home.

Mrs. Lee's ability to perform in her home was then assessed by taking her to her apartment and asking her to perform self-care tasks for a 24-hour time period according to her normal routine prior to institutionalization. The therapist observed her performance of specific tasks. The reports of a close friend, who remained with Mrs. Lee during the entire 24-hour period, were also considered. The home evaluation indicated that she was independent in most personal care activities such as toiletting, bathing, dressing, eating, and grooming. Standby assistance and supervision was required for safety in the areas of transfers, ambulation, meal preparation, and medication intake. Mrs. Lee demonstrated some impairment in sequencing tasks and problems with immediate and recent memory. These impairments affected greatly her safety in self-administering medictions, preparing cooked meals, getting up from seated positions (especially since she also suffered from some postural hypotension), and bathing in her glass-partitioned shower stall. She was found to be unable to perform housework, shopping or laundry tasks due to poor endurance, lower back pain, instability in ambulation, difficulty in sequencing and completing tasks, general fatigue, and problems arranging and managing transportation.

Mrs. Lee had three episodes of urinary incontinence during her stay at home. Two of these occurred after she had been sitting for some time and began to ambulate. The third occurred during the night. Mrs. Lee indicated that the major reason she had remained in the wheelchair at the facility was because of her incontinence. She expressed extreme embarrassment and reluctance to ambulate due to her inability to control her urine. She began to use adult incontinence pads during the home trial, which caused her to be willing to ambulate more frequently.

Environmental Supports

SOCIAL ENVIRONMENT

Mrs. Lee had no living relatives. She had one very close, elderly female friend. Mrs. Quinton, who was 72 years old and had assumed power of attorney for Mrs. Lee upon her admission to the long-term care facility. Mrs. Quinton wanted Mrs. Lee to make her own decision about returning home or remaining in the nursing home, but felt that Mrs. Lee would be safer in the nursing home. Mrs. Quinton was willing to assume responsibility for financial management for Mrs. Lee and was willing to visit one time weekly on the weekend to ensure that everything was going well, if Mrs. Lee decided to go home. Mrs. Quinton was unable to assist Mrs. Lee in performing any homemaking tasks due to her own poor health, but felt that Mrs. Lee would need that type of assistance.

Mrs. Lee also had some neighbors on the floor of her apartment building who indicated that they were willing to check in on Mrs. Lee on a daily basis "to make sure she was up and about."

HOME ENVIRONMENT

Mrs. Lee's apartment was in a high-rise building with adequate elevator access. Her entire apartment was walker and wheelchair accessible except for the bathroom. The living and bedroom areas were carpeted and some practice ambulating and maneuvering her wheelchair on this surface was identified as necessary. The toilet was of standard height and lacked safety rails. There was no tub and the shower stall had a glass partition and lacked adequate handrails.

Table 17.2 summarizes Mrs. Lee's occupational status at the time of assessment and proposed goals and interventions.

Goals and Treatment

GOALS

The home visit helped Mrs. Lee recognize that she need not be helpless. Subsequently, she accepted responsibility for removing herself from the institution and returning to her apartment by planning for her discharge and concretely preparing herself for that event. The primary goal was identified by Mrs. Lee and the therapist as the return of Mrs. Lee to her apartment with as many safety measures in place as possible.

The goals for the management of Mrs. Lee's case were to provide adequate environmental supports to promote safety in the home environment, to determine the appropriate treatment strategy for her urinary incontinence, to provide necessary referrals to other health professionals, and to assist Mrs. Quinton in providing support for Mrs. Lee.

The goals for occupational therapy intervention regarding Mrs. Lee's situation were to adapt the apartment to improve safety, to improve Mrs. Lee's endurance and physical performance skills, to optimize Mrs. Lee's ability to be independent in self-care and home care tasks, and to train the caregiver in providing appropriate assistance to Mrs. Lee.

Mrs. Lee returned to her apartment with the following plans being activated. Daily chore and personal care assistance was arranged and provided to supervise Mrs. Lee's performance of all activities of daily living and to perform all housekeeping and home maintenance tasks, such as shopping, cooking, cleaning, laundry, and emptying the bedside commode. This help was available 4 hours a day, 6 days a week. The helper prepared food for Sunday and Mrs. Quinton visited on that day to check on Mrs. Lee's situation.

Adapted equipment was added to the bathroom and bedroom to improve safety in these areas. Items included a bedside commode for nighttime continence problems; a night-light to facilitate safety in movement at night; a raised toilet seat and a grab rail marked with fluorescent tape for toiletting in the bathroom; a shower curtain to replace the glass partition; a shower bench with rails for the shower stall; a bed with partial side rails to provide handholds when coming to a standing position; a raised height bed to facilitate ease in standing from a seated position; and a fracture pan for urgency incontinence in the evening or early morning hours.

LifeLife, an emergency call system, was installed to improve Mrs. Lee's ability to summon help if she should fall and be unable to reach the phone.

Mrs. Quinton agreed to work with Mrs. Lee on managing finances, arranging for discharge from the facility, making funeral arrangements and planning social outings or visits on a weekly basis. She worked with Mrs. Quinton to arrange and finance her funeral arrangements prior to her discharge from the facility, since Mrs. Lee identified a proper burial as necessary for peace of mind before returning home.

Biweekly nursing visits were ordered by the physician to check on Mrs. Lee's compliance with her medication regimes and that her physical and medical conditions remained stable. The nursing visits were paid for by Medicare Home Health coverage for a short period of time. The funding source was changed to Medicaid for nursing visits twice a month.

Occupational therapy treatment was initiated on a weekly basis to improve endurance, increase performance skills in the areas of self-care and home maintenance tasks, and involve Mrs. Lee in leisure activities as her physical endurance improved. This service was to be paid for by Medicare Home Health coverage. Follow-up to reinforce new habits and scheduling was to be done by the chore and personal care supervisor.

Urology consultation was arranged to evaluate and treat Mrs. Lee's incontinence as aggressively as possible, since her emotional reaction to this problem interfered with her

Table 17.2.
Mrs. Lee: Occupational status, goals and interventions

Current occupational status	Goals and interventions

VOLITION

Personal causation

Lacks feelings of control in all spheres	Promote sense of personal control in daily routine, medication administration, etc.
No responsibility for personal care and physical well-being	Promote resumption of personal responsibility for self on a daily basis
Unaware of physical health problems and methods to minimize effects	Educate regarding medications and daily programming to control conditions

Values

Incongruency between stated values and current living situation	Provide opportunity to develop a living situation consistent with values
Conflict for implementing goal of returning home and being totally independent	Clarify primary goal and methods to achieve the primary goal
Lack of preparation for burial arrangements	Develop burial arrangements in accordance with stated values

Interests

Exclusive interest in resuming independent lifestyle	Facilitate safe return to apartment living
No leisure interests identified	Identify leisure interests after resolving current situation

HABITUATION

Roles

Views self as dependent, helpless and worthless	Promote reentry into valued roles

Habits

Normal habit structure modified by institutional routines	Develop appropriate habit structure for resumption of apartment living
Dependency on caregivers to schedule daily activities and meet personal needs	Promote self-initiated scheduling and activities that meet deinstitutionalization needs

PERFORMANCE

Skills

Slow reaction time in emergency situations	Develop environmental supports to promote safety
Poor physical endurance	Facilitate scheduling that enhances abilities and allows improvement
Poor visual acuity	Develop environmental modifications that facilitate independent function
Reduced ambulatory stability	Promote safe ambulation
Questionable safety in performing self-care and home care activities	Develop supports that allow optimal independence while providing necessary help
Good interactive skills	Promote involvement in social interactions

Environment

Funding available for an in-home assistant	Obtain the services of an experienced helper through a Medicaid waiver program
Need for equipment in the apartment for safety and independence	Provide appropriate equipment to facilitate safe and independent function
Presence of supportive friends and neighbors	Promote the involvement of these persons in the daily activities of Mrs. Lee

ability to engage in social and physical activities. She worked daily on improving her ability to ambulate with a walker. She began to self-schedule toiletting to prevent "accidents" and use a bedside commode at night.

Outcomes

Mrs. Lee returned to her home and lived there with the above arrangements for 6 months. Occupational therapy intervention resulted in her gradually taking over more household tasks. She began to prepare simple meals, help with cleaning the apartment, go shopping with the chore worker, and assist with the laundry. The chore worker began assuming more of a facilitory role as time progressed. This helper assisted in developing daily schedules of activities and provided supervision to ensure that Mrs. Lee did not overestimate her performance abilities or endurance. Mrs. Lee's incontinence was treated with medications and improved toilet habits. She experienced fewer episodes of incontinence and was able to remain dry throughout the night by scheduling herself for urination every 3 hours. She began to go to the nutritional program with a next-door neighbor on a daily basis after her second month back in her apartment.

Mrs. Lee demonstrated a large number of self-initiated and self-directed activities after her decision to return home was implemented. She began planning for her discharge from the facility and worked on improving her ambulation skills. She sought out individuals with whom she chose to socialize. Mrs. Lee identified specific housekeeping and self-care tasks for improvement and negotiated with the therapist to accomplish her goals.

Mrs. Lee voiced her conviction that her "return home was the turning point for her" and that "if she could do it all over she would not change her decision at all."

Mrs. Lee was discharged from occupational therapy services after 3 months of treatment and active intervention. The in-home helper continued to implement the programming initiated by the therapist and Mrs. Lee continued to participate actively in her personal care, home care and social interactive activities.

Mrs. Lee suffered a massive stroke one evening at her apartment. She was found the next morning by her in-home helper and was admitted to the hospital in a coma. She did not recover consciousness and died of another cerebral infarct after 3 weeks of hospitalization.

THE RESUMPTION OF PURPOSEFUL ACTIONS: MR. MOORE

Mr. Harry Moore is 76 years old and lives in a rural small town with his wife. At assessment, he carried the medical diagnoses of end stage chronic obstructive pulmonary disease, congestive heart failure, adult onset diabetes mellitus controlled by oral agents, and hypertension controlled by diet and medications. Mr. Moore used oxygen 24-hours/day at a rate of 3 liters/minute. He was referred for occupational therapy evaluation of leisure activities and self-care status after he voiced repeated complaints of wanting "to do more for himself."

Performance Evaluations

PERCEPTUAL-MOTOR SKILLS

Mr. Moore's ability to perform motor tasks was severely impaired due to his pulmonary status. Mr. Moore spent approximately 23 of 24 hours/day in bed. He had been functionally bedbound and dependent for the last 2 years.

He was able to sit up in bed with minimal assistance in balancing. He tolerated this posture for 10–15 minutes with minimal shortness of breath. He was able to stand with standby assistance and could walk 5–10 steps while experiencing increasingly severe shortness of breath. He was unable to raise his legs back onto the bed or even lift his feet off the floor without assistance. He could not bend forward, in a seated position past 30 to 40° without loss of ability to breathe and severe bouts of coughing.

Mr. Moore was unable to engage in any activity needing upper arm use for longer than 2–3 minutes due to shortness of breath and general fatigue. He was unable to raise his arms above shoulder height due to shortness of breath.

He got up only for toiletting using a bedside commode next to the hospital bed in his sleeping area. The remainder of the house was assessible to wheelchair use, but due to Mr. Moore's reluctance to get up, he rarely left his immediate surroundings although he had a wheelchair available to him.

PROCESS SKILLS

Mr. Moore was evaluated using the FROMAJE Mental Status Evaluation and the Set Test. Mr. Moore was found to have moderate deficits in judgment, especially regarding safety in emergency situations and the appropriateness of behavior. He had difficulties with recent and immediate recall on the FROMAJE which was confirmed by his wife's observations. He was slightly disoriented regarding his immediate environment, having problems describing the layout of his home and the use of various rooms. He also had problems in performing several daily activities especially in deciding on the order and steps needed to complete tasks, either verbally or by physical actions. He needed repeated verbal prompting to complete tasks with more than one step. He demonstrated more severe deficits in areas of reasoning with a poor ability to explain relationships between cause and effect, such as not eating causing increased weight loss and constant bedrest leading to increased weakness in his legs. He was unable to explain why one would go to a grocery store and why one would wear a coat in cold weather. The results of the Set Test indicated that Mr. Moore may be suffering more from depression than dementia.

COMMUNICATION/INTERACTION SKILLS

Mr. Moore demonstrated limited skills in social interactions. He was able to communicate needs in short simple sentences only, secondary to his poor breath control. Mr. Moore appeared to suffer from mild presbycusis. He misheard much of the conversation held in a normal manner but, he had minimal difficulty hearing conversations if the volume was raised slightly, the speed was slowed, and the pitch was lowered. He made frequent derogatory comments about himself and his helpers. He did not have many visitors and refused to spend time with people when they did visit.

Mr. Moore had presbyopia and used reading glasses to read printed material. His vision did not affect his ability to take his medications correctly, however, his mental confusion made self-medication unsafe regardless of his ability to visually perceive the information.

Habituation Evaluation

ROLES

Mr. Moore's roles were identified by taking an occupational history. Mr. Moore identified the roles of husband, hard worker, "breadwinner" and family man as being very important

to him and ones that he had filled successfully in the past. He indicated that he felt he currently filled none of these roles, but saw himself as dependent, helpless and worthless.

Mr. Moore had worked for one company as a cement mix maker from the ages of 17 to 32. He was promoted to a block construction supervisor. He held this position until his retirement at age 62. He had worked the first shift throughout his career and indicated that "mornings were now the hardest part of the day since he couldn't do a thing for himself." He indicated that he enjoyed his work and regarded his "early retirement" as an unpleasant experience, since it was due to his physician's orders. He stated several times that he believed his medical conditions had worsened considerably since he "started being at home all the time with nothing to do all day long."

Mr. Moore was the 6th of 12 children. He was raised on a sharecropping farm in a rural area. He completed the third grade. He worked with his family in farming, planting and harvesting tobacco and soybean crops until he left home at age 17 to work for the gravel company.

He lived alone in a small apartment near his workplace for 7 years. He stated that he spent most of the time with his male friends in traveling, drinking, card playing, and baseball games.

At age 24 he met his future wife after he suffered an injury at work. She worked as his home care nurse during his convalescence. They dated for 1 year. He gave up much of his time with his friends and became a "solid citizen." They were then married and purchased a small house in the rural town, where they still reside. They tried for several years to have children but were unable to do so. When Mr. Moore was 47 years old they took in their goddaughter after her parents died. His wife stopped working at that time.

At age 60, Mr. Moore stated that he "began drinking some, again" due to his frustrations of failing health and his physician's recommendations that he retire early. After retiring, Mr. Moore spent most of his time visiting with older friends in his home. He stopped drinking after two episodes of diabetic shock. He still had friends who visited, but found that most of his visitors were churchgoers and he lost interest in their visits due to "his worsening breathing and general feelings of purposelessness and worthlessness among all those worthy people." He stated that he felt as though he had become a burden on his wife and he "wished that he could just get it over quickly."

Volition Evaluation

VALUES

The values identified as important to Mr. Moore were hard work and being a good family and churchgoing man. His current failure to meet his personal standards of performance in these areas had resulted in feelings of worthlessness and helplessness.

Temporal Orientation

Mr. Moore expressed no interest or awareness of the future. He was unable to express any positive feelings about what the future held in store and indicated that he was only "playing a waiting game with the Lord."

INTERESTS

Mr. Moore identified the activities of his youth as baseball games, card playing and car rides. After his marriage, Mr. Moore identified his time with his wife in social activities with other couples as pleasurable. The church became a central location for these activities including socials, picnics, bible studies, dances, and revivals. During his middle years Mr. Moore developed an interest in woodworking. He remodeled the kitchen and did some hand carving. He pursued his woodworking interest until his illness worsened. He stated that he "just sits in his bed all day long doing nothing." Mr. Moore was unable to identify any current interests. He did indicate that he would be interested in learning how he could "go on and get it all over with."

PERSONAL CAUSATION

Mr. Moore's statements about himself and his current state of health indicate feelings of external control and lack of control over any aspect of daily activities. He did not recognize his own role in the gradual decreases in physical activities, social interactions or decision making processes.

Output: Occupational Performance

The results of Mr. Moore's self-care evaluation indicated extreme dependence in all areas due to his physical and mental conditions. He was able to feed himself, if set up in bed. This was a slow process due to his shortness of breath and general fatigue. He was able to wash his face, but his wife completed all other bathing tasks in his bed. He was able to help his wife with his dressing, but was not able to put on clothing without full assistance. He needed help to toilet himself. He required help in completing any self-care tasks due to breathing difficulties, mental confusion, lack of interest in these tasks, and general fatigue by his own report and that of his wife.

Environmental Supports

SOCIAL SUPPORTS

Mr. Moore's wife provided all of Mr. Moore's physical care. She was willing to modify her routine to help her husband change his behavior. She was also willing to accept help from other sources and allow Mr. Moore to struggle more in performing self-care tasks, if it was necessary. Her goddaughter was willing to continue providing financial support and help with changing daily routines.

PHYSICAL ENVIRONMENT

The entire home environment was accessible to Mr. Moore by wheelchair, if the oxygen was detached. If an extended length of tubing was used, Mr. Moore could gain access to the screened-in porch as well as the rest of the house. Mr. Moore had all of the adapted equipment needed for safe function.

Goals and Treatment

GOALS

The primary goals for Mr. Moore were to develop his sense of personal causation and worth, improve his involvement in daily self-care and leisure activities, and to involve him in decision making.

TREATMENT

The following actions were taken to meet these goals. To develop leisure skills and promote self-initiation of activities, soap carving was used. This activity used old skills to begin a new leisure skill. Mr. Moore completed three carvings between the therapist's first and second visits, 1 week later. The objects carved were well done and finished as per the therapist's instructions.

The therapist also had Mr. Moore play a card game (Spades) to test out memory skills and mental manipulation skills in a familiar activity. Mr. Moore won two out of the first three games. Mr. Moore was then encouraged to play with an older male friend. Mr. Moore demonstrated few problems in concentration and voiced enjoyment with his success and "his ability to play as well as ever."

The therapist then worked with Mr. and Mrs. Moore to develop a daily schedule of out-of-bed activities. This involved setting up card games in the living room. This necessitated a change to a portable liquid oxygen system. Mr. Moore enjoyed the card games sufficiently after the first session that he was waiting for his visitor at the card table for the next session.

He was also instructed on using an electric razor while seated in a chair in front of a large portable mirror using the over-bed tray for elbow support and to facilitate forearm mobility. A universal cuff was used to help hold the razor in the correct position and to allow Mr. Moore to be independent in shaving and with little change in demand for oxygen or in breathing style.

The therapist negotiated with Mrs. Moore to set up visiting sessions on the front porch in the afternoons to get Mr. Moore out of the house and to encourage casual callers to stop by when they walked down the street. A wheelchair was used to get Mr. Moore in and out of the house to prevent overexertion and severe shortness of breath.

The therapist also contacted the physician to obtain a referral for nursing services and home health aide services to: (*a*) monitor medications and Mr. Moore's physical condition, (*b*) assist in daily performance of personal care therby reducing Mr. Moore's feelings of dependence on his wife; and (*c*) to develop a schedule with two to three choices to be made by Mr. Moore daily on the follow through on personal care tasks and out-of-bed activities.

Table 17.3 summarizes the initial occupational status of Mr. Moore and general treatment goals and interventions used.

Outcomes

Seven months after the initial referral, Mr. Moore is carving animals and small objects from balsa wood. He spends at least 3–4 hours a day carving. He plays cards daily with a variety of old, and some new, friends from a local church.

He shaves himself, but still requires help with almost all other self-care tasks. He develops the daily schedule for the aide based on his needs and what had been done the day before. His FROMAJE scores improved dramatically. His affect was brighter and he was able to identify several aspects of his daily routine that he found pleasurable. He is currently selling his carvings for small amounts of money at the local senior citizens center.

Mr. Moore reported that he "felt more like the man of the house," since he was now making some of his own decisions and did not have to always rely on his wife to take care of everything. He noted that he thought his breathing had gotten better. Even though he still required oxygen 24 hours/day the rate had dropped to 2 liters/minute.

MAINTAINING THE STATUS QUO: MRS. COOK

Mrs. Cook is a 62-year-old widowed woman hospitalized for uncontrolled congestive heart failure. She was initially seen for evaluation in an acute care hospital and was then seen in her home after her discharge. She had experienced another episode of uncontrolled congestive heart failure within 2 days of her return home.

Mrs. Cook carried the medical diagnoses of severe rheumatoid arthritis, congestive heart failure, chronic obstructive pulmonary disease, asthma, anemia, glaucoma with left eye enucleation, and a history of two myocardial infarctions in the past 4 years.

By her physician's report, Mrs. Cook was noncompliant with her medications and was a chronic overmedicator. Mrs. Cook reported that she had problems in complying with medications "due to difficulties remembering which medications were to be taken at what frequencies, and which were for what diseases." She complained of increased feelings of anxiety and depression stemming from her worsening hearing loss and lessening ability to take care of herself. The review of her medical chart indicated that when she became anxious her pulmonary disease became uncontrollable. This resulted in her increasing her intake of medications to improve her breathing. Her misuse of medications had resulted in five hospitalizations in the past 2 years for problems with her chronic obstructive pulmonary disease and congestive heart failure. She was using nine prescribed medications. She was also using 2 liters/minute of oxygen for 6–8 hours/day.

Performance Evaluation

PERCEPTUAL-MOTOR SKILL

The arthritis was severe in her upper extremities, hips, knees, and feet. The severity of her rheumatoid arthritis made her hands generally dysfunctional for all daily activities.

Mrs. Cook was able to ambulate for short distances. She walked with great difficulty due to flexion contractures bilaterally in her hips and knees and multiple deformities in her feet and ankles. She was unable to use a walker or canes due to the involvement of her hands

Table 17.3.
Mr. Moore: Occupational status, goals and interventions

Current occupational status	Goals and interventions
VOLITION	

Personal causation

| Lack of belief that any personal actions can alter disease processes or purposeless existence | Initiate activities that promote physical well-being by active participation |
| | Reinforce positive outcomes of voluntary participation in selected activities |

Values

Incongruency between stated values and current performance	Seek values clarification and resolution
Lack of involvement in activities that foster a sense of temporal orientation	Provide new activities that encourage optimal performance and meet personal standards
	Use new leisure pursuits to develop temporal orientation skills

Interests

| Lack of identified interests | Use past valued leisure skills to promote involvement in new occupations |
| Has past leisure skills that are adaptable to current performance skills | |

| **HABITUATION** | |

Roles

| Inability to successfully fill valued roles | Clarification of expectations of success in fulfilling roles |
| | Reallocation of roles that are valued between Mrs. and Mr. Moore |

Habits

| Demonstrates totally dependent behavior 24 hours/day | Reorganize daily routines to include time out of bed and active participation in some self-care and leisure tasks |
| Totally uninvolved in activities | Promote and reinforce participation in planning and decision making |

| **PERFORMANCE** | |

Skills

Physically dependent with poor endurance and mobility	Involve patient in tasks that are within range of his physical abilities
Mentally confused, unable to follow directions	Use familiar leisure skills to foster improved mental function through involvement in successful activities
Oxygen dependent	Mobilize the oxygen system
Impaired communication skills	Modify verbal cues to match needs and minimize environmental interference

and shoulders. She used a wheelchair in the apartment for most activities. She had adapted many of her appliances and furniture to make it possible for her to continue to use them. She was able to move throughout her home using appropriate safety techniques. Her general endurance was poor and she tolerated gross motor activities for less than 5–10 minutes.

PROCESS SKILLS

Mrs. Cook's mental status was evaluated using the FROMAJE and the Set Test. The results demonstrated that Mrs. Cook showed minimal deficits in mental abilities in a structured setting. There was no indication that her ability to make safe and appropriate judgments was impaired. She was able to follow simple written instructions that were given for medications if they were written in large letters and placed in a well illuminated area. After some trial and error, she followed through on suggestions for new ways to perform tasks, given at the initial evaluation session.

COMMUNICATION/INTERACTION SKILLS

Mrs. Cook had difficulty hearing conversations. She wore bilateral hearing aids, but continued to mishear information and tended to avoid noisy environments and conversations with more than one or two people. Mrs. Cook looked forward to having visitors come to her apartment, but she rarely made arrangements for visits to other apartments in the building.

Habituation Evaluation

ROLES

Mrs. Cook identified the roles of friend, mother and church member as being very important to her throughout her lifetime. She stated that she had felt a loss of the roles of mother and church member recently due to the worsening of her abilities that prevented her from fulfilling those roles to her satisfaction. Mrs. Cook was widowed 15 years ago. She noted that she felt she had recovered well from her husband's death, but "wished that she had taken more time to let him know how much she loved him while he was alive."

HABITS

Mrs. Cook had established a daily routine that permitted her to vary her tasks depending on her general physical and mental well-being. She noted that recently, she was able to do less and less and had let many household tasks and personal care tasks "slide" for a period of 3–4 weeks. These activities included hair care, dressing, laundry, calling for groceries, and sponge baths. Her one daughter, who lives in the area, visits Mrs. Cook on Sundays to take her to church once a month and to maintain active family ties.

Mrs. Cook received weekly visits from several older women in the apartment building. She identified these visits as pleasurable, but indicated that she still missed her old friends and family members since moving to this apartment building. Mrs. Cook said that she often felt "trapped in her apartment because of her difficulty breathing and her inability to use her hands to help herself much." She stated that she had become inactive in most church activities and missed those groups a great deal.

WORK HISTORY

Mrs. Cook worked as a threader in a cotton mill for 30 years from age 17–50. She quit after her arthritis got too severe for her to handle the job. She expressed no regrets about stopping work except for her loss of income and need to go through the disability determination process and become a Medicaid recipient.

Volition Evaluation

VALUES

Mrs. Cook stated that her Baptist beliefs and upbringing formed the basis of what she valued. Living within a budget and having no debts were also identified as important. She valued friendship, family ties and Christian fellowship above independence and physical well-being.

Mrs. Cook stated that she "couldn't do ANYTHING anymore." She indicated that she "doesn't want to be a burden on anyone and wants to stay in her apartment as long as possible." Mrs. Cook also noted that she would like to get out of her apartment more often, but that she was "afraid to get too far from her oxygen and that she couldn't get up or down steps without help." This resulted in social isolation which she disliked and made her feel "less of a worthwhile Christian woman."

PERSONAL CAUSATION

Mrs. Cook viewed herself as only partially responsible for her health status and her living situation. She indicated that she felt that many of the problems she was now experiencing were "due to things that happened to her while she was growing up and over which she had no control." She felt that whatever happened to her next would be due to her physician's recommendations and the therapist's ratings. She noted that she did not want to be placed in a nursing home, but that she would go if it were necessary.

INTERESTS

Mrs. Cook had done various handcrafts until about 8 years ago when her arthritis had gotten to the point where she felt she could no longer use her fingers to manipulate materials. Mrs. Cook still enjoyed reading and spent several hours a day reading romance novels and current fiction. Due to difficulty holding books, she could only read for 10–15 minutes and had great difficulty turning pages. She stated that she did not care for television and volunteered that she watched the news during the evenings "so it wasn't so quiet around the house."

Environmental Supports

PHYSICAL ENVIRONMENT

Mrs. Cook was living in government subsidized apartments for the elderly. She had lived there for 4 years after she was "forced to give up her house in her old neighborhood due to continued rent increases." She had made many adaptations to her apartment to make it possible for her to perform most of her own housekeeping and personal care tasks.

SOCIAL SUPPORTS

Many of the people living in the apartment building were older and knew Mrs. Cook for several years. All of these people were willing to work with the therapist and Mrs. Cook to increase the amount of interaction, if desired.

Output: Occupational Performance

Due to the severe joint deformities and muscular weakness in Mrs. Cook's upper extremities she is generally unable to use her hands for any functional activities. She can feed herself using built up light weight plastic utensils if the food is properly positioned and prepared. It takes her approximately 1–1½ hours to complete each meal due to poor hand use, impaired breathing capacity and "little interest in food." She weighs about 87 pounds

and has shown a weight loss of 1–2 pounds/month for the last 2 years.

Until this most recent hospitalization she had been doing most of her own self-care, although it took a long time and she frequently found herself taking more pain medications to relieve her discomfort after completing the tasks. During the assessment, Mrs. Cook expressed concern about her continued ability to take care of herself given the gradual decline she has experienced over the past year.

Mrs. Cook's apartment was neither clean nor orderly. She expressed dissatisfaction with her housekeeping abilities and concerns that she would soon have to go into a nursing home if she did not improve.

Table 17.4 summarizes Mrs. Cook's occupational status at the time of the assessment and the goals and intervention strategies implemented.

Goals and Treatment

GOALS

Mrs. Cook was able to identify her personal goals for occupational therapy, when options were presented by the therapist. Mrs. Cook identified her objectives as improving and maintaining her current living situation. She wanted to improve her ability to perform tasks in the areas of daily personal care and home care without becoming sick and having to be hospitalized. She wanted to increase the number of social interactions, by having more visitors and getting out to other apartments at least once every other day. She also wanted to become involved in at least one pleasurable leisure activity each day.

TREATMENT

The therapist met with the physician and obtained a home health aide and nursing service referral for the immediate posthospitalization period. The purpose of this referral was to facilitate the establishment of a comprehensive medication regime to be followed and monitored by the nurses and aides. The system used large printed calendars with sample pills attached and clear and simple explanations of the drug action, frequency of intake and a checklist to be completed as the drugs were ingested. A secondary purpose of the referral was to provide necessary assistance with self-care and house care tasks, and to prevent overexcitement and fatigue while Mrs. Cook adjusted to her home setting once again and became familiar and comfortable

Table 17.4.
Mrs. Cook: Occupational status, goals and interventions

Current occupational status	Goals and interventions

VOLITION

Personal causation

Belief in ability to modify the existing situation	Use this strength to initiate a plan that improves function in other subsystems
Feelings of guilt/responsibility for problems with medication adherence	Provide modifications to minimize compliance difficulties

Values

Desire to remain at home	Develop resources to promote safe function in the home
Strong lifelong Christian value system and inability to fulfill expectations of this value system	Clarify personal expectations of performance and roles
Not meeting personal standards on home care and cleanliness	Provide support to get needed assistance in the home

Interests

Difficulty following up on interests due to chronic diseases	Modify equipment to allow participation in interests
Lack of opportunity to join in social activities	Provide physical and social supports to facilitate social participation

HABITUATION

Roles

Gradual loss ability to fulfill valued roles	Explore and work on reintegration of roles into daily routines
High expectations of performance	Clarify and modify expectations

Habits

Well adapted routines to meet previous abilities	Restructure daily plans to meet new demands and changing chronic conditions
Continued physical deterioration resulting in need to change current schedules	Use communication skills to help modify habit patterns and meet new needs

PERFORMANCE

Skills

Inability to use hands in self-care and home care tasks	Provide adaptations to environment that promote function
Worsening chronic problems	Provide help in minimizing negative effects of the disease processes
Difficulty hearing	Ensure use of hearing aid to optimize auditory abilities
Poor visual acuity	Modify written information to meet needs and allow processing of visual information

with her new drug regime. The nurses were also helpful in monitoring Mrs. Cook's blood gas values and cardiac status during the change in activity programming.

The therapist worked with the medical equipment suppliers to obtain a portable oxygen system that could be easily used by Mrs. Cook to leave her apartment as well as improve mobility in the home.

Mrs. Cook followed up on the therapist's recommendation to contact the local Friendly Visitor Program sponsored by the Council on Aging. Within two weeks a visitor was identified who met the requested characteristics and this woman began making weekly visits to Mrs. Cook's apartment and provided telephone reassurance on weekends and in the late evenings.

Mrs. Cook worked with the therapist to become a recipient of home delivered noon meals 5 days a week at a cost of 60 cents/day. Mrs. Cook made all the arrangements after the therapist made preliminary calls concerning eligibility for the program and cost for the meals. After further discussion with Mrs. Cook, her daughter, her physician and the home health aide, the therapist worked with a social worker to obtain permanent Title XX homemaker services through the local department of social services to replace the initial aide service at the conclusion of Medicare Home Health coverage. This service was made available after 2 months to provide 2 hours of help per day, Monday through Friday. The tasks to be completed by the homemaker included assistance with personal care, shopping, house cleaning, laundry, and transportation to and from physician appointments and trips to the store.

The therapist used therapy sessions three times per week for the immediate 6 weeks after her hospitalization to work with Mrs. Cook on energy conservation, work simplification techniques, and designing and providing modified equipment to enable Mrs. Cook to bathe herself, prepare simple meals, dress herself, toilet herself with improved safety and less discomfort, and move about the apartment with decreased feelings of shortness of breath and anxiety.

The therapist also used these sessions to work on the development of leisure skills and to develop a regular social interaction schedule. The therapist worked with Mrs. Cook to develop a book holder that enabled her to read for longer periods and made turning pages easier. A modified embroidery hoop and special needle made it possible for Mrs. Cook to use lateral pinch to do light crewelwork for short periods. She was encouraged to intersperse this activity with other grosser activities to prevent hand fatigue.

The therapist scheduled some of her sessions at times when Mrs. Cook had arranged for some old friends to be at her home. This time was used to devise an activity that would become a routine activity and encourage regular involvement by Mrs. Cook in a group. After members of the group completed interest checklists and discussed the results, bridge was selected as an ongoing activity. This was something they all had enjoyed in the past but had stopped playing due to the lack of regular partners and various changes in vision and/or physical abilities that made the game difficult. The therapist provided some modified equipment to three out of four members of the group which made it possible for all of the women to resume playing the game. The group established a weekly bridge game that generally lasted 2 hours. The location of these sessions rotated to various apartments and Mrs. Cook was accompanied by her homemaker to her friends' residences without problems using her portable oxygen system.

Outcomes

Mrs. Cook has continued to maintain her accomplishments in all areas of occupational performance. She has remained out of the hospital for 9 months. She continues to do her own bathing, toiletting, dressing, and feeding. She has had no recurrences of her pulmonary disease or congestive heart failure being "out of control."

Mrs. Cook has chosen to have two hand surgeries done to realign joints and improve her hand function. She received additional occupational therapy services after these surgeries for splinting and mobilizing her hands and to ensure that her self-care abilities were not compromised during the postoperative period.

Mrs. Cook continues her weekly bridge games and has started to join her friends once a month for lunch in the communal dining area. She has completed several needlework projects and, with the surgical improvement in her hand function, has also taken up counted cross-stitch.

Mrs. Cook has recently negotiated the installation of a LifeLine unit to alleviate her concerns about not being able to contact help in an emergency. She states that she "is doing just fine and just hopes that she'll be able to keep it up for another few years."

SUMMARY

These case examples illustrate complexities and unique aspects found when treating older adults. Occupational therapists working with these individuals must be able to use microscopic to macroscopic vision provided by the model of human occupation when assessing the older adults and their ecosystems. Careful evaluation enables the therapist to formulate effective intervention strategies that meet the occupational needs and goals of the older adults being treated.

CHAPTER 18

Mental Retardation

Mike Lyons, Gary Kielhofner and Marian Kavanagh

The mentally retarded person, by definition, is characterized by significantly subaverage intellectual functioning and concurrently experiences decrements in adaptive behavior (37). The label of mental retardation encompasses a disparate group of individuals presenting widely varying profiles of abilities and deficits due to inherited traits, neurological trauma, environmental factors, and/or unknown agents encountered during the developmental period (0–18 years). Mentally retarded persons are typically categorized into four groupings on the basis of measures of cognitive and adaptive functioning: mildly, moderately, severely, and profoundly retarded (37).

OCCUPATIONAL DYSFUNCTION AMONG MENTALLY RETARDED PERSONS

Dysfunctions in occupational behavior among mentally retarded persons are manifested to varying degrees in difficulties in acquiring and maintaining work, play and self-care behaviors. For example, mildly retarded individuals' occupational dysfunctions may first become highly visible during the school years when they have difficulty meeting the expectations of the student role and perhaps in adulthood when they have difficulty assuming and maintaining the worker role. On the other hand, occupational dysfunction in the profoundly retarded individual will become apparent much earlier with correspondingly greater repercussions throughout life.

Performance

The predominant concern of research and intervention into the adaptation problems of mentally retarded persons has been with the performance subsystem. Mentally retarded persons experience perceptual-motor, process, and/or communication/interaction skill deficits to varying degrees. These deficits constrain performance of work, play, and self-care behaviors.

PERCEPTUAL-MOTOR SKILLS

It has been noted that cognitive impairment is accompanied by decreased capacity for accurate movement (18). As the degree of mental retardation increases, there is frequently an increase in perceptual-motor errors on tests of proficiency which are interpreted as signaling an increase in "organicity" (61).*

Due to the complex interplay of variables influencing perceptual-motor performance, there are differences to be found not only between, but also within, groups categorized by degree of intellectual impairment. For example, a person with a given etiological factor may have dissimilar perceptual-motor characteristics from others of a similar cognitive level but whose retardation may be of different etiology (18).

Fitness

Studies with mildly, moderately and severely retarded school age children suggest that they are consistently less physically fit than their nonretarded age peers (30, 49, 86, 87, 98). However, some evidence is available that, for mildly retarded students at least, those who receive regular and systematic physical education demonstrate physical fitness comparable to their age norms (11, 110).

Physical Development

Performance on motor tasks is influenced in large measure by the status of a person's physi-

---

* Secondly, studies have concentrated on collecting data from the mildly retarded, principally children, or from Down's syndrome children who are generally placed in the moderately-severely retarded category and who represent a large and relatively uniform subgroup of that category (45). Thus, generalization of findings to the mentally retarded persons, per se, must be undertaken cautiously, keeping these limitations in mind. However, a number of tentative conclusions can be drawn regarding the perceptual-motor development of retarded persons.

cal growth and development. Retarded children and adults have consistently been found to be markedly delayed in their physical development when compared with nonretarded persons (92). What is more, findings indicate a strong trend towards more deficient physical growth with increased severity of intellectual impairment (90), particularly where there is an association of retardation with organic factors (versus undifferentiated or cultural-familial factors) (20).

Motor Performance

It has been suggested that the structure of motor abilities among samples of retarded persons is similar to that of nonretarded persons, at least among those who are mildly retarded (85). Generally higher correlations exist between intelligence and motor proficiency with retarded as compared with nonretarded subjects (14, 62, 71).

Retarded children and adults have consistently been found to be markedly less proficient than nonretarded persons in gross and fine motor performance. Studies of children indicate that retarded persons are particularly deficient in static and dynamic balance (86, 106, 116). Little is yet known regarding the course of development among retarded persons in this area or about the relationship between severity of retardation and proficiency on measures of balance (9).

Most available studies on the fine motor development of retarded persons have focused on the performance of adolescent and adult populations, apparently because of the vocational implications of manipulative abilities (82). Deficiencies in the development of fine motor skills for retarded *adolescents* and *adults* appear to be of approximately the same magnitude as for gross motor abilities with a moderate correlation between measures of intelligence and manipulative dexterity (86, 115, 118). It has been suggested, however, that for retarded *children* fine motor abilities are more impaired than gross motor abilities since motor development proceeds from gross to fine (9).

Vestibular Function

One factor underlying the motor proficiency of mentally retarded persons, which has received only limited attention, is that of sensory awareness and responsivity. Recently, interest has been centered upon the vestibular system for its apparent influence on such areas as attention, social-emotional behavior, language, and motor skills. Specific perceptual-motor problems of mentally retarded persons in the areas of postural balance and eye-hand coordination have been interpreted as possible signs of vestibular dysfunction (96). The presence of a vestibular disorder has not been conclusively demonstrated, although Shuer et al. (96) found that a sample of mildly mentally retarded adults demonstrated attenuated nystagmus, indicative of vestibular dysfunction. Studies utilizing vestibular stimulation with subjects of varying age and severity of retardation have shown gains in motor performance (52, 79) suggesting a relationship between vestibular dysfunction and decreased motor proficiency in mentally retarded persons.

Motivation

Findings from studies on the physical and motor development of retarded persons may have failed to take account of the possible influence of volitional factors (9). Many retarded individuals exhibit higher expectancies for failure and less incentive to achieve than the nonretarded(67). Furthermore, retarded children perform better on motor tests when provided with motivational incentives and various motivational incentives have different effects on retarded and nonretarded boys in performing motor tasks (107, 119).

All in all, the literature suggests that motor performance of retarded persons is most impaired on measures which require: (*a*) high incentive motivation for optimum performance, (*b*) conceptual understanding of movement patterns demanding a sequence of responses, and (*c*) movement patterns requiring simultaneous or sequential integration of various senses and parts of the body. Furthermore, limited evidence indicates that the gap between retarded and nonretarded persons in motor performance may widen with age (9).

PROCESS SKILLS

The ability to process information in a rapid manner is important to satisfactory performance of many tasks. A systematic characterization of the rapid information processing skills of mentally retarded individuals has yet to emerge (109). It has been proposed that there are four stages to information processing: short-term sensory storage, perceptual encoding into a more permanent form, central processing (including decision making), and selection of a response. Research into information processing abilities of mentally retarded persons has concentrated almost exclusively on the mildly retarded.

A series of studies on the functional properties of short-term sensory storage of mildly retarded adults strongly suggests that this aspect of information processing in mentally retarded persons does not operate in a functionally or qualitatively different manner from that of nonretarded individuals (83).

Once information has been registered in sensory storage, it must be encoded into a more permanent type of memory; otherwise, the information would be lost. It has been proposed that initial perceptual processing of retarded persons is slower than that of their nonretarded age peers (114). However, this finding has been disputed since subjects are asked to recall alphanumeric stimuli, with which retarded subjects are likely to be less familiar (93, 109).

Investigation of the central processing phase which involves manipulation of the encoded information and decision making, has yielded varying results regarding skill decrements in retarded persons. Compared to peers of equal chronological age, mentally retarded individuals have displayed slower comparison rates in same-different classification judgements (103). However, the retarded subjects have performed similar to equal mental age peers, which appears to indicate that the performance difference is due to developmental immaturity rather than low intelligence per se (109). On the other hand, mentally retarded subjects have been found to scan short-term memory at rates slower than mental age-matched controls (24, 44). However, this result occurs only with alphanumeric stimuli, again suggesting that it may only reflect a differential familiarity with the task stimulus materials. Overall, however, there are substantial indications that mentally retarded persons are less efficient in the central processing phase than nonretarded persons.

With regard to the response selection phase, it has been suggested that the inferior performance of mentally retarded persons on reaction-time tasks is related to mechanisms in the response phase (4, 81). An approximate linear negative relationship between intelligence and reaction time has been observed within the subaverage intelligence range (2).

Thus, while the results are somewhat inconclusive, it appears that, of the four proposed stages of information processing, central processing and response selection are the two areas which detrimentally influence the performance of mentally retarded persons.

Attention

A related aspect of process skills which affects performance of retarded persons is that of attention. Available evidence suggests that mentally retarded persons experience deficiencies in selective attention (125). In other words, they have difficulty attending to relevant information while screening out irrelevant material. This attending process involves multiple levels of attention including: maintenance of a level of arousal to attend, scanning the stimulus field and selecting relevant stimuli, quickly shifting attention to changing relevant stimuli, and maintenance of attending behavior over extended time (77).

In addition to difficulty in the selection of relevant stimuli, a prestimulus arousal deficiency or attentional lag appears to be a serious problem for retarded persons (2). Many of these individuals display an abnormal resistance to change in certain autonomic states. The source of this arousal deficiency has not been made entirely clear. However, it appears that some fundamental property of neural organization either has not been acquired or has been disrupted (2).

The implications of such attentional deficits for performance, in unfamiliar situations in particular, are serious. Not only does the retarded person appear to have difficulty acquiring the initial information relevant to task performance but also is unable to use feedback to properly evaluate the consequences of actions (1). The number of stimulus elements required to produce a given response is negatively correlated with intellectual ability (111). Therefore, it appears that retarded persons require more stimulus elements to be able to respond appropriately than would be necessary with nonretarded persons.

Cognitive Style

A further area of consideration with respect to process skills of mentally retarded persons is cognitive style which refers to the individual's characteristic method of approach to problem solving (34). One important aspect of cognitive style is conceptual tempo, the degree to which an individual reflects upon the differential validity of alternative solutions in problem situations where several potential responses exist simultaneously (50). A person who takes relatively longer to respond and makes fewer errors in problem-solving situations involving response uncertainty is called reflective, whereas one who responds more quickly and commits more errors is called impulsive.

Measures of reflection/impulsivity typically correlate significantly with tests of general intelligence. An impulsive cognitive style (such as is often reported for mentally retarded persons) produces a maladaptive approach which frequently results in poor performance over many tasks. For the mentally retarded person it may produce a low rate of success on tasks which are specific prerequisites to more complex behavior (35).

In summary, the literature on process skills of mentally retarded persons suggests that skill deficits exist in such areas as maintaining an optimal level of prestimulus arousal, selective attention, cognitive tempo, processing of information in the memory, and response selection. These deficits result in less efficient processing of incoming information by retarded persons, adversely affecting occupational performance. The literature offers little insight into process skill deficits among more severely retarded persons. It appears that process skill deficits are more severe in the presence of not only a reduced cognitive capacity but also a complex of other interacting factors. Finally, it cannot be overlooked that deficits in process skills may be related to a paucity of experience among retarded persons. As will be noted later, retarded persons, for a variety of reasons, may develop in restricted and otherwise unfavorable environmental circumstances.

COMMUNICATION/INTERACTION SKILLS

There are a number of components which appear to be essential to interpersonal competence: (a) social inference or how an individual perceives and interprets social situations, (b) referential communication or the selection by the speaker of the most appropriate words or gestures to communicate to a listener based on recognition of his or her viewpoint and informational needs, (c) prosocial behavior or actions that are intended to aid or benefit others, (d) interpersonal goals and motivational orientation or having specified social goals and the urge to pursue these goals through particular lines of action, and (e) interpersonal strategies and social problem solving or strategic, self-initiated actions directed to attainment of interpersonal goals.

Social Inference

Individuals must be sensitive to and make accurate inferences from various cues and stimuli in the social environment in order to appropriately define social goals and pursue effective lines of communication. Mentally retarded children tend to be sensitive to, and compliant with, adult cues, and with externally provided rules and norms for appropriate social behavior. Thus, in a structured setting where the cues are frequent and rules and norms explicit, less ability to perceive and interpret social situations is required to respond appropriately. However, in less structured and less well defined situations the mentally retarded person may fail to adequately or accurately read available social cues and thus may not respond in an appropriate or effective manner (113).

Referential Communication

Communication skills are important in the social acceptance of retarded persons (6). However, the extent of vocabulary may be less important to effective communication than the manner in which vocabulary is used (104). There is evidence that retarded persons may use language in an idiosyncratic manner thus reducing communication effectiveness (64).

Although not all forms of social behavior depend on the utilization of social-cognitive skills, some prosocial behaviors such as generosity, altruism, sympathy, and sharing do require an appreciation of the other's need. In one study, older nonretarded childen were shown not to be more helpful than younger nonhandicapped or retarded children. In fact, retarded childen have been observed to exceed the helping behavior of normal peers (99). Retarded children have also been found to be more cooperative than normal children (70). This cooperativeness may be the result of overreliance on, or heightened sensitivity to, compliance with directives for appropriate behavior from an authority figure (113).

Interpersonal Strategies

One reason for less effective interpersonal problem solving by mentally retarded persons is that they might possess a more limited repertoire of interpersonal tactics (113). While they may be aware of the more conventional kinds of behaviors required in certain social situations, they may lack knowledge of more sophisticated and effective kinds of strategies. The most frequent interpersonal tactic adopted by retarded children and young adults appears to be asking, a relatively primitive social tactic (12, 36, 122).

Interpersonal Goals

Individuals who are heavily burdened by failure, as retarded persons often are, may not translate desired responses from others into interpersonal tasks or goals (121). Such individuals will tend to avoid pursuing interpersonal goals that may risk disrupting a current relationship. Further, they may not employ lines of action which could optimize their social outcomes because of the potential costs of not succeeding. In addition, individuals who attribute social outcomes to external forces outside their control will be unlikely to view interpersonal goals as achievable through their own independent actions. Thus, mentally retarded persons may also have volitional tendencies that inhibit their freedom to be interpersonally competent (113).

It appears that retarded persons as a group are more likely than nonretarded persons to experience interpersonal difficulties. Social competence is incidentally learned, yet retarded persons may have neither the quantity nor quality of experiences sufficient for incidental learning of socially competent behaviors (121). Mentally retarded persons need opportunities to interact freely with others, to take the risks and make the choices which foster socially competent behavior (113).

Habituation

The formation of adaptive patterns of occupational behavior depends on interaction with appropriate external environments. Mentally retarded persons, for whatever difficulties experienced in acquiring patterned behavior, also appear negatively affected by the environments in which they must function and which shape habits and roles.

ROLES

Successful manipulation and management of ongoing social interaction depends on the ability to accurately assume roles, to understand others' and to recognize how one's own actions influence the perceptions and responses of other participants in a social exchange situation.

Role-Taking Ability

Role taking requires one to acquire knowledge about what others are seeing, thinking and feeling (113). Mentally retarded children are generally significantly more egocentric (and therefore less adept at role taking) than their nonretarded chronological age peers on measures of perceptual, affective and cognitive role taking (36). However, it appears that the developmental sequence of role-taking skills of retarded persons, although delayed, is similar to that of nonretarded persons (48).

In a study comparing role-taking abilities of above-average, average and retarded children on a social guessing game, it was found that, at lower psychometric levels, mental age is more critical than chronological age in development of role-taking skills (21). However, at higher psychometric levels, chronological age is more important, suggesting the importance of social experience. Interestingly, a study of orthopaedically handicapped children found that they demonstrated inferior role-taking ability to non-handicapped children of comparable age and intelligence (117). This study also suggests the importance of *experiencing* varied roles and perspectives in the development of social competence (104).

Role Deviance

There is ample evidence that retarded persons desire to hold normal adult roles such as those of spouse, worker, home maintainer, organizational participant, and hobbyist (3, 25, 26, 56, 57). Unfortunately, the desire to enter and hold these roles is not matched by the ready availability of such roles to the retarded person and, in many cases, by sufficient skills and habits of the retarded person to fulfill these roles. More commonly, retarded persons are denied access to normal adult roles and are cast in a social deviant or invalid role (8, 22, 23, 42, 58, 124). Expectations for nonproductivity or incompetence are characteristic of this role (27, 68). These negative expectations include inability to hold a job; inability to care for personal needs; inability to control sexual and aggressive impulses; and tendencies to perform unusual, unacceptable behaviors (42). In addition to the general deviant role ascribed to retarded persons in society, specific deviant roles related to various institutional settings have been noted. For example, in the state hospital, there is a status of "low grades" recognized by other inmates and by staff (7, 72). This role represents the lowest of the social hierarchy, reserved for those persons who are most alienated and incompetent and who can often be expected to engage in repulsive behavior. Furthermore, an informal role of "troublemaker" may also be assigned to persons with acting out or aggressive behavior (58).

Retarded persons have been observed to take on very unusual roles. For example, Goode (33) describes a middle-aged Down's syndrome man who became, for all practical purposes, a "pet" to the cook in a residential facility. While the expectations of this role included demeaning acts such as "barking" on request and being patted on the head, the role had benefits that were otherwise scarce in the facility.

The dynamics of such deviant roles which lead to behavioral aberration can only be appreciated if the perspective of the retarded person is taken. Persons engage in role-relevant behaviors because roles carry with them status and a sense of personal identity. For the retarded person whose deviant role overshadows other roles, it may be difficult or impossible to accrue the benefits of normal role behavior. For example, a retarded worker with physical anomalies may not be able to gain recognition, status or identity from co-workers.

In general, society does not look favorably on retarded persons assuming such roles as spouses, parents and workers. Questions concerning the actual abilities of retarded persons to fulfill roles with substantial demands for judgment do sometimes present difficult ethical dilemmas for all concerned. However, the tendency of society is to err in the direction of underestimating the role capacity of retarded persons and therefore to make fewer roles available to them (3).

Roles as Life Organizers

Retarded persons not only experience a lack of roles but may also lack the experiences of normal role transitions (56). Life role change for the average person involves progression through a series of life roles. The retarded person may become trapped in the invalid role thus having neither an appreciation of past role incumbency or an expectation for future roles. Instead, normal life roles may be seen as highly desirable but unattainable (56, 57). This may lead to either an acceptance of various deviant statuses or a search for a compromise role such as the "trustee" role in an institutional setting.

Although many retarded persons seem to lack almost entirely any occupational roles, some retarded persons do have roles which, at least partially or during some part of their life span, organize their daily lives. Due to the deinstitutionalization movement, related legislation and policies and the existence of agency-sponsored programs in the community, a larger number of retarded persons continue to live with their families well into their adult years. Thus, the roles of family member and, in some cases, home maintainer may serve to organize at least a portion of their time each day. It appears that retarded adults do have some responsibility, albeit usually at a low level, for caring for personal or family needs when living in the family unit (54).

Since roles are first experienced in the context of the family, the degree to which family members nurture and expect competence in the player and family member roles can be important for later competence. For example, it was shown that families which refused to accept the retarded status of one of their members contributed to better outcomes for the retarded person's career than those families who accepted the family member's retarded identity and presumably lowered their expectations for performance (76).

HABITS

The formation of an adaptive habit structure is dependent on a person's access to and, interaction with, various social environments which allow the human system to shape its own behavior to the features and expectations of those environments. Although there is great variation in the habit patterns of retarded individuals, they often exhibit routines that are at variance with the temporal and interpersonal ambience of the larger culture (3, 25, 56). In large measure, these maladaptive habits appear to be related to limitations in environmental interaction.

Social Appropriateness of Habits

When engaging in typical routines of behavior such as greetings, ordering food in restaurants, shopping or riding a bus, individuals are guided by internalized norms which define typical and appropriate interactions and behaviors. Retarded individuals appear to lack an inner sense of the routines involved in such settings. As a result, they tend to stand out and be at variance with the ambience of public settings (25, 58). Such deviation is not limited to behavior but also includes such features as appropriateness of dress or grooming.

Some of the difficulty with internalizing habits to guide routine behavior may stem from learning difficulties of retarded persons. However, it appears that these individuals have, in many instances, internalized patterns of behavior that are ecologically specific to the subcultures of various institutions in which they live (25, 58). For example, Goode (33) documents how a Down's syndrome man was able to grasp the meaning of privacy, but did not include practices related to privacy of self and others in his routines because the residential facility in which he lived was not one where privacy was attainable. His overtly inappropriate public behaviors were more like that of a foreigner unaccustomed to the norms of a new setting than someone who simply was not capable of grasping and internalizing such guides to behavior. Another example of an ecologically relevant, although socially deviant, habit is that of a retarded gentleman in Los Angeles who was observed walking down the street on the edge of the curb instead of the sidewalk. When queried about his behavior, he explained that persons routinely dropped small change while putting money in parking meters and in Los Angeles, where ivy grows around many of the meters, persons simply don't bother to retrieve their dropped change. This man, whose income was severely limited, could accrue some money this way. Similarly, observed habits of gorging food during meals and of hoarding belongings on one's person were found to be related to environmental conditions of scarce food and frequent stealing (57).

Temporal Organization of Behavior

Retarded person' habits of time use are similarly affected by conditions in their environments. Retarded individuals may structure their time use at variance with societal norms; their routines are often characterized by passivity and low levels of activity (56). Limited resources in living settings and other external constraints may limit access to activities. Engagement in activities is often separated by long periods of waiting for opportunities (56). Such waiting, which is generally considered a waste of time by members of mainstream society, may actually be perceived by retarded persons as positive, purposeful activity in view of the limited and unpredictable availability of resources. The person who patiently waits in such an ecology may accrue more benefits. On the other hand, such habits of inactivity and passivity are not adaptive and valued in many other settings.

Rigidity/Flexibility of Habits

Many retarded persons who have had limited experience in a small number of highly structured environments tend not to do well in mildly unfamiliar or unstructured environments. They will often import routines from familiar settings to new settings, with negative consequences. Such persons may be easily upset or disorganized when familiar routines are withdrawn or changed in a setting. These traits also appear to reflect limited experience more than they reflect innate deficits of the retarded individual.

Habits of Passivity and Dependence

Retarded persons may exhibit routines of behavior characterized by a purposeful demonstration of incompetence or inability to elicit help from others around them (58). For example, in observations of classroom behavior of retarded adults, it was found that many of these persons had learned that the most efficient way to accomplish some tasks was to make a public demonstration of incompetence which invariably evoked helping behavior from others. Thus, retarded persons routinely demonstrated that they could not perform simple tasks such as tying a shoe or zipping a coat—when in fact, they could do so, albeit with some difficulty. A more generalized habit of exhibiting confusion and helplessness in the face of new situations and tasks appears to have the same underlying dynamic. Thus, retarded persons may habitually deal with frustration or difficulty by requesting help and by the demonstration of inability to encourage caretakers or other persons in the environment to rescue them. In some cases, it appears that retarded persons go so far as to use incompetence as an exploitive behavior by doing such things as ordering food when they do not have money, secure in the knowledge that someone will rescue them (58).

Because retarded individuals do have genuine difficulty performing some tasks, caretakers often overcompensate by underestimating their competence and requiring unnecessarily simple routines of behavior (3, 29, 57, 58). As a result, retarded persons may acquire habits which presume a lower level of skill than that of which they are capable.

Habits of passivity and dependence also serve to make the retarded person appear unnecessarily incompetent. For example, habits of walking in groups or holding hands may prevent retarded persons from getting lost or becoming unruly, but these behaviors also create appearances of incompetence and deviance when they are carried over into public settings.

Habits of Appearance Management

At the same time that many retarded persons acquire habits which stigmatize them in public, they may also demonstrate habits aimed at creating positive images of themselves (25). For example, retarded persons may routinely produce the appearance of behaviors they cannot actually do, such as "reading" in public (58). Such persons, who do not have the ability to read or write, may have learned to fake the appearances of doing so while staring into a menu or looking at a list of food items on the wall in a restaurant. To appear to be able to read they would say words which had been learned from listening to others.

Generally, these habits of appearance management are transparent in that they give away their perpetrator (25, 58). A retarded person may examine a menu and then go on to order something not on the menu or read aloud an item from one fast-food chain when in a different franchise store.

In summary, the habit patterns of retarded persons may be manifest as a set of inconsistent, rigid and socially inappropriate though ecologically relevant behaviors. These habit patterns appear to reflect the limited, and sometimes deviant, socialization experiences of retarded persons as much as they reflect innate limitations of ability. There is evidence that retarded

persons can successfully acquire work and leisure habits and socially appropriate routines of interaction if they are exposed to appropriate environmental experiences (40, 59, 120).

Volition

The quality of the mentally retarded person's performance in everyday tasks and situations may be judged from various viewpoints. Frequently, the *least* understood viewpoint is that of the retarded person (33). By and large, there is a paucity of knowledge in this area. However, existing research offers some insight into the influence of volitional factors on the occupational behavior of retarded people.

VALUES

While the values retarded persons hold may be somewhat akin to those of the wider society, there is strong evidence from the literature to suggest that many differences exist also.

Temporal Orientation

It has been proposed that mentally retarded individuals may hold different temporal perspectives than the rest of society (46, 54, 56, 91). This appears to be primarily due to their unique life experiences and circumstances. They typically do not see themselves progressing on a life continuum (56). Furthermore, events in their lives generally occur without the influence of, or reference to, any personal plans or purpose. Thus, they are more likely to exhibit a principal concern with the here-and-now. Consequently, service providers can experience frustration in their efforts to engage these people in goal-setting, planning and even recognizing and responding to a program schedule (60).

Meaningfulness of Activities

It seems likely that many retarded people may seek meaning in their lives in a manner similar to their nonretarded peers. For some, work-related activities are a desired source of meaning and value, viewed as bestowing dignity, worth, status, and a sense of normalcy (15, 25, 112). Others may be preoccupied instead with finding a richness in life through alternative sources such as hobbies, leisure, friends, and family (26, 65). This latter phenomenon in recent years has also increasingly characterized the nonretarded population in many industrialized societies.

Occupational Goals

Available evidence suggests that retarded people do formulate goals although these are perhaps ill-defined and without identified means for attainment. From their own perspective, it would seem likely that the setting of goals is largely a futile exercise since, for many of these people, the attainment of their goals is largely outside their control (46). On the other hand, the act of goal-setting has been demonstrated to have significant effects on behavior when the retarded persons are given the means to actively work towards their goals (28).

Personal Standards

Mentally retarded persons appear to adjust their personal standards of behavior in accordance with societal standards (25, 46). For example, they typically desire to be viewed as normal, worthy human beings who have control over such actions as getting married. On the other hand, there are signs that the personal standards of retarded persons frequently are significantly at variance with those of the wider society. There appears to exist a deliberate code of dependence among some retarded people (33, 58). That is, they appear to recognize and value the use of dependence or helplessness in order to solicit help, favors and so on from others. It appears that this is a response to constraints imposed on these people by the environments which they inhabit, predisposing them to adopt a different set of standards.

PERSONAL CAUSATION

The available literature suggests that many mentally retarded persons possess negative beliefs and expectations about their effectiveness in their environments. This has been attributed to both past experience of failure and present externally controlled circumstances.

Locus of Control

Among mentally retarded persons, there appears to exist a disproportionate tendency to function from an external orientation (100). The underlying reason for this apparent externality is unclear, with some researchers attributing it to low intelligence and overly sheltered experiences at home or within an institution and others relating it primarily to repeated experience of failure (38).

Expectancy of Success or Failure

Mentally retarded persons tend to possess a higher expectancy of failure than their nonretarded peers (39, 66, 69, 97). This, in turn, appears to promote failure-avoidance rather than success-striving behavior (19, 80). It has been postulated that this expectancy of failure is principally a function of persistent failure experiences in the past (55) rather than an inherent feature of mental retardation. The likely outcome of this expectancy is that retarded persons may typically aspire to goals which are well beneath their achievement capabilities (126).

Belief in Skill and Its Efficacy

Retarded persons as a group tend to possess a low belief in their skills and the efficacy of these skills, which negatively affects their task performance and overall social adjustment (10, 16, 127). However, it has been suggested that successful engagement in an activity will lead to an improved self-concept in the mentally retarded individual which leads to a more positive disposition for approaching other tasks (105).

INTERESTS

Until recently, there has been only a limited concern for the interest patterns of mentally retarded persons. In the play sphere, a number of studies have recently been undertaken to determine the level of interest enactment and to make some judgment about retarded persons' interest patterns (17, 74, 75, 88,89, 94). These studies have yielded similar and somewhat dismal results. They reveal a restricted pattern with a predominant involvement in home-based, solitary, frequently sedentary pursuits. Factors identified as constraining interests include a lack of appropriate social and activity-specific skills (13, 17, 53, 73, 78), limited experience and awareness of occupations in which to participate (13), restricted opportunities provided by parents and caretakers (13, 17, 73), lack of local resources to facilitate participation (53, 73), difficulties with transportation (13, 73), prevailing community attitudes (78, 108), and lack of friends with whom to do things (13, 17, 53).

Environment

The characteristics of the environment are key variables in the occupational functioning of retarded persons. For example, it is now ac-

cepted that the environment, along with hereditary factors, influences an individual's intelligence and adaptive behavior (66). The environment of the retarded person is also in a period
of drastic change. Cultural attitudes toward retarded persons may be changing, and policies
such as deinstitutionalization are radically altering where retarded persons live.

CULTURE

The retarded person's occupational functioning is most drastically affected by the attitudes
of the culture toward intelligence. Western cultures place a high value on intelligence so that
an implied deficit in this area is tantamount to
the most serious kind of personal flaw—something that strikes at the very worth of the individual (22, 23, 25). To be found wanting in
intelligence is an experience so devastating that
retarded persons typically prefer to fabricate
excuses for their life circumstances that include
physical deficits, emotional problems, lack of
moral character, and the like (25, 57). Implied
in cultural values and in these persons' internalization of these values is that it is worse to
be grossly stupid than immoral, crazy or even
physically impaired.

The consequence of having an attribute so
negatively valued by the culture is that retarded
persons incur the most severe type of stigma
(25). In fact, retardation is often considered to
be associated in the minds of laypersons with a
host of other deficits such as inability to control
sexual impulses, immorality, a propensity for
criminal behavior and violence. Also implied in
many persons' conceptions of retardation is a
belief that the retarded person is unaware of his
or her own condition, personal emotions and
others' reactions. This belief leads some persons
to justify actions toward the retarded individual,
which they would not consider appropriate to a
person of normal intelligence (60).

Historically, attitudes toward retarded persons have also included the notion that retarded
persons are globally incapable of self-regulation
and self-maintenance and that they represent
biologically inferior specimens of the human
species (42, 125). Such attitudes have justified
both keeping the retarded person from public
view (at home or institutionalized), and preventing the retarded person from reproducing
(through eugenic sterilization) (124). Such extreme measures have been attacked through legislation and court rulings over recent years but
the attitudes underlying them still remain in

large measure unresolved. At best, cultural attitudes appear to be changing toward a more
benign, if patronizing, attitude. Change has been
fueled by the ideology of normalization that
retarded persons become most adaptive when
they have experiences analagous to those of
mainstream cultural members (123). It is also
argued that the retarded person has a right to
these experiences. Thus, normalization stresses
the right and dignity of risk, the importance of
community integration and the need for environments to be as minimally restrictive as possible.

SOCIAL GROUP

Because the retarded individual has less intellectual capacity in comparison with average
persons, his or her performance in the social
group is affected. In turn, others' expectations
of, and responses to, retarded individuals will be
critical to occupational functioning.

The family is the primary and pervasive social
group experienced in childhood. Family members typically react to the news that their child
is retarded with grief, guilt, bewilderment, and
anger. Resolving feelings related to having a
retarded child or sibling are important for all
concerned. The retarded child who is reared in
an accepting family that encourages exploration
and risk and expects and nurtures performance
fares better than one who is rejected or overpro-
tected by family members. In the past, cultural
attitudes led many families to institutionalize
retarded members allowing the affective bond
and any expectations for performance to be dis-
sipated. With changing attitudes, more retarded
persons remain in the home and many persons
previously institutionalized have been released
as adults back to their families. Even retarded
adults who live out of the immediate household
often have close familial ties and rely on their
family members as important supports.

Retarded persons may establish a larger network of social relations in a local community.
For example, such persons as shopkeepers, and
other persons who have occasion to interact with
the retarded person, may take a special interest
in that individual's welfare. For many retarded
persons in the community the assistance of a
benefactor—a person or persons who may or
may not be related to the retarded person—is
important for adaptation (25, 26). The role of
benefactor may include emotional support, help
in problem solving, crisis intervention, and so
on.

Some retarded persons do have access to various social groups, e.g. in classrooms, work settings and the like. It is most often the case that these are special settings geared to specific training and management concerns. These special classrooms, vocational or sheltered workshops and special residential living settings tend to have their own social order which may be at variance with that of the larger society.

For example, one study of a classroom for retarded adults demonstrated that the social system was more concerned with control of behavior and with managing appearances than with teaching skills, autonomy and so on. The apparent result was that retarded classroom members became more helpless than necessary and came to accept the fact that they would have to do things without understanding and for appearance sake (58).

In similar fashion, it has been observed that residential facilities in the community may, in the interests of efficiency and avoiding trouble, prefer a lessened level of community mobility and other activities which increase the risk that a retarded resident might somehow get into trouble (3, 57). Restriction on activity can often take the form of long periods of enforced inactivity (3, 57). For example, in one residential facility, adult residents were required to sleep (or at least stay in bed) for up to 12 hours a day; they were, for a portion of this day, confined to a small room and prevented from answering the front door. In another facility, a manager discouraged residents' venturing into the community by fostering unpredicated fears of being mugged, stabbed, and so on. While such practices may be more extreme than in most residential facilities, the underlying logic of resident management suggests that milder, yet still undesirable, limitations may be placed on retarded persons in many residential settings.

TASKS

Because of the limitations of the retarded person, much emphasis has been put on the simplification of tasks to facilitate competence and success. While on the surface task simplification would appear to be a rational strategy, it has been subject to question by some writers. For example, it has been argued that a more therapeutic environment may be one that places task demands on the retarded person (41).

Benignly motivated overprotection by parents and significant others may deprive retarded persons of opportunities to make and learn from mistakes (41). This represents the psychosocial element of the environment that denies the retarded individual responsibility for, and thus access to, various tasks, such as operating an oven in a home setting or machinery in a shop. In Scandinavian countries where normalization principles were developed, retarded persons are allowed the dignity of risk in community and work experiences (84). The expectation exists that retarded persons travel independently. In industry, they are exposed to the normal tasks and risks of the industrial workplace. Restructuring tasks to demand less competence or to make them fail-safe is viewed as potentially dehumanizing. Retarded workers are expected to follow the same precautions as other workers.

Interventions have often focused on facilitation of learning by breaking tasks into their components and applying behavioral principles of sequencing and chaining and cue redundancy (31, 32). More recently, it has been argued that learning tasks should emphasize principles of contextualized learning (60). That is, the acquisition of skills for task accomplishment may be impeded when the task learning is disembodied from its normal context. An example is learning money handling skills in a classroom where exchange of money does not usually occur as contrasted with learning the skill in stores and restaurants. The principle of contextualized learning stresses that a task is better appreciated in its entirety (i.e. in terms of its requirements, purpose and meaning, and its relation to people and tasks) when it is encountered in a natural setting.

Another aspect of tasks is the ratio of persons in the environment to available tasks. Most people identified as mentally retarded are placed in settings where there is a low ratio of tasks to people (95). When this occurs, retarded persons exhibit a lower level of participation in tasks.

In sum, the availability, the complexity and the manner of presentation of tasks to the retarded person can have effects on what skills for task performance the retarded person acquires. Some accepted principles of simplification and task breakdown may actually be counterproductive to effective learning, although this area requires much further study.

OBJECTS

A number of interesting observations have been made of the availability and arrangement of objects in the environments of retarded persons. State hospitals have been severely criticized for their stark surroundings, often devoid of natural objects related to everyday life (5). Due to the influence of normalization principles, there have been improvements in the physical aspects of institutional environments. However, the changes have frequently been at a superficial level and have failed to reflect a view of the retarded person as having the ability to function competently. Murals, curtains and dormitory-type bedroom furniture are some examples of environmental changes. But as Gunzburg and Gunzburg (40, 41) have noted, environments continue to be designed based on expectations for low levels of functioning, and fail to contain the physical elements necessary to promote social competence, work skills and verbal abilities. Many feel that the presence of normal objects has a positive effect on behavior. For example, in the residential architecture of the Scandinavian institutions, spiral staircases and hanging lamps convey the expectation for responsible behavior and a message of trust.

The mere presence of objects in the physical environment is not enough, however. Their availability for use and the arrangement of objects in space can also have an impact. For example, in a residential facility which was a converted apartment complex, residents had stoves and refrigerators in their rooms but these appliances were not connected and could not be used by residents (5). Having access to objects was also an issue in a classroom where teachers feared that letting retarded persons take coats and other objects with them outside the classroom could result in their being lost. Thus, these personal objects were often confiscated during the day (58). In common areas of residential facilities, chairs and tables were observed to be placed along walls instead of in groups; such arrangement discouraged interaction and instead promoted solitary behavior (57).

The symbolic import of objects also has an impact on retarded persons. For example, retarded persons were observed to collect photographs and letters from the garbage and place them strategically in their residences to give the impression that they had relatives and friends who corresponded with them and shared photographs (25). Similar observations of retarded persons "playing cards" in public, or carrying broken watches as a cover for not being able to tell the time, suggest that retarded individuals make extensive use of objects to counter the stigma they experience (57).

PERSON ENVIRONMENT INTERACTION

It is difficult to generalize about what kind of environments will be optimal for facilitating adaptive occupational behavior of retarded persons. Certain elements of the environment may be desirable for some persons and harmful for others (51). An inference made from the findings of a study of group homes (63) was that no one environment is appropriate or optimal for all retarded persons. Specific elements, such as characteristics of the social environment, proximity to the community and transportation, size of group residing in the home, and type of building (renovated or built specifically as a group home), varied in how they met individual's needs. Sometimes, an element initally designed to accommodate or to control behavior of one or a few persons can become restrictive or demeaning to others who enter that environment.

In some cases, smaller facilities which encourage interaction and replicate family traits have been shown to facilitate higher levels of adaptation (41). In other instances, smaller facilities led to closer supervision, more control over residents and other restrictive practices that decreased opportunities for adaptive learning (3).

Much of the literature stresses the value of highly structured and simplified environments, yet one pilot study suggested that retarded persons functioned least competently in the setting designed to maximize function (a sheltered workshop) and were more competent in unstructured leisure and home settings (54).

Deinstitutionalization policy has stressed geographic placement in the community. Yet, studies show that community facilities with restrictive practices along with communities reluctant to receive retarded members, can result in the same segregation proffered by the large state institution (3, 57). In the end, it appears that optimal environments begin with more positive cultural attitudes toward the retarded person and a concomitant willingness to allow the retarded individual, as much as possible, the same range of environmental interactions as others. Some interactions will be beneficial, others not. However, unless there is the opportunity and an expectation for eventual success, the plight of the retarded person becomes a self-fulfilling prophecy in which environments geared to incapacity evoke more of the same.

Assessment

Mental retardation can only be construed in terms of the presence or absence of a broadly defined set of behaviors that are sufficiently ambiguous to prevent one from being totally confident about when it is appropriate to apply this label to a given individual. This ambiguity is particularly evident in the milder levels of mental retardation. Not only does the label of mental retardation describe an individual but also it says important things about the environment in which that person lives. To an extent, our society creates the condition of mental retardation by its expectations of "normal" behavior and by the occurrence of the means to elicit this behavior (22). Thus, assessment of occupational dysfunction will require measurement of performance not only in terms of the individual's attributes but also against the background of that physical and social environment which that individual inhabits (33, 59).

Traditionally, assessment of retarded persons in rehabilitation and educational settings has been based on the assumption that measuring existing aptitudes and traits can be used to predict subsequent learning, performance and adjustments (43).

Frequently employing standardized tests, assessors then used test scores as a basis for classification and determination of eligibility for services. However, most of these standardized tests were not originally developed with mentally retarded persons in mind. Consequently, these persons' ability to respond to test items in a meaningful way was often seriously impaired. Furthermore, the assumption that assessment outcomes served as valid predictors of future behavior was highly questionable. It would also seem that the content of many of these tests was clearly different from the criterion behaviors that are the focus of program intervention. Experience suggests that the aptitudes and traits so measured do *not* in fact predict performance in real life situations (43).

There has been, therefore, a significant change in the approach to assessment of mentally retarded persons. Rather than rely on measures of traits or aptitudes to infer performance, contemporary procedures emphasize the importance of direct assessment of actual competencies. Furthermore, contemporary assessment approaches require the outcomes of measurement to have direct implications for program planning.

There are extreme differences in typical behavioral repertoires between mildly and profoundly retarded individuals. Many instruments cannot span this distance effectively in terms of either the content or format of measurement.

Therefore, most instruments developed for use with mentally retarded persons can be used most appropriately for only part of this continuum.

To identify the needs of (and therefore specific service priorities to be adopted for) each mentally retarded person requires the intelligent selection of suitable measuring tools to be used. In addition to collecting formal assessment information, it is very useful to collect information informally, such as by interview and by review of historical data. Once information on current performance has been collected and interpreted in the areas of concern, it is then possible to ascertain the need for intervention, by considering the gap, if any, between actual and desired performance of occupational behaviors (desired, that is, both by society and by the retarded individual).

There are a number of approaches to assessment of occupational function in mentally retarded persons: direct testing of criterion behaviors in real or simulated settings; observation accompanied by a rating scale of behaviors; measurement of knowledge and subjective factors relevant to criterion behaviors. Direct testing requires the evaluee to exhibit some behavior according to the specific request of an examiner. The retarded individual's competencies are evaluated against the criterion of the competencies required by the environments of concern (e.g. workplace, home, school). The assessment provides a catalogue of the behaviors that have been mastered already and of those still unmastered. Use of a rating scale with observation requires judgements to be made by an examiner or a third person who describes the behavior of the evaluee. The evaluee may or may not be directly observed or required to perform.

Knowledge measurement is the least commonly accepted and used of the three approaches. This is seemingly due to the belief that these cognitively less competent people possess little understanding of real-life situations, much less a knowledge of self or an appreciation of personal competencies. However, research has demonstrated that knowledge is a necessary, though not sufficient, prerequisite for adequate performance in vocational, community, personal, or academic settings (43). Those retarded persons who know more tend to perform better. Furthermore, it is clear that when retarded individuals fail to maintain performance after training, or fail to generalize learned skills from one setting to another, it is often the result of lack of appropriate knowledge, rather than lack of skill (43).

Each type of assessment has its strengths and weaknesses. In comparison with direct testing, ratings are more susceptible to errors of judgment on the part of the rater, although they can provide a better estimate of typical examinee performance over time and they help to overcome reading, writing and verbal difficulties experienced by retarded persons. Tests, on the other hand, have a weakness in that they usually permit only a limited number of opportunities to respond to test items, leading possibly to an underestimate of the retarded person's capabilities because of slowness to respond or atypical nature of response.

Perhaps the most confounding factor for knowledge measures is that those individuals who have restricted experience and more limited powers of abstraction would be expected to have more difficulty imagining what responses they would make to the abstract questions presented. A greater difficulty does not mean, however, that such questions cannot be raised. Indeed, they should be raised where possible so that a comprehensive picture of the retarded person's own perspective can be gained. It is the format of the questions that must be adapted to the capacities of the retarded respondent to reply (be it in the form of verbal question/answer with the less retarded person, or concrete choice-making using limited response options with the more severely retarded person).

Knowledge assessment, of course, covers the range from knowledge of how and where to apply one's skills, to knowledge of self. It is the latter, i.e. insight into one's personal aptitudes, attributes, interests, and feelings (volition), which has been given the least consideration in assessment of a retarded person's needs, and yet is highly significant in influencing the state of occupational function by its governance of skills and routines.

A number of studies with mildly, moderately, and even severely retarded persons (101, 102) have supported the belief that retarded individuals can respond in a meaningful way to questions about their attitudes, abilities, and needs. Such investigation is not, of course, without its difficulties. For example, acquiescence (i.e. giving a socially desirable rather than an accurate response) has been identified as a problem to be dealt with, particularly when yes-no questions are asked. It appears that the degree of acquiescence depends both on the topic and on how it is framed. Moreover, it presents a greater problem among the more severely retarded. Thus, it

would seem that yes-no questions, while they have the advantage of readily yielding responses from most mentally retarded persons, should be avoided as a means of data gathering. Two suggested alternatives are pictorial and force-choice response formats.

Thus, assessment of the mentally retarded individual must, to be comprehensive, provide the clinician with data on the status of all subsystems as well as on the environment and on the interaction of the individual with his/her environment. Table 18.1 provides a range of useful evaluation procedures for each component of the human open system relevant to occupational function. Assessment of volitional factors is limited both by the difficulties of the retarded person in expressing his or her values, interests and feelings of efficacy and by the very preliminary status of the science of assessing these variables. Some of the recommended assessments will only be relevant to more articulate persons, and their use must be circumscribed with careful judgment on the part of the therapist concerning the reliability and validity of a particular administration of the assessment to a given individual. Because formal procedures can lack both relevance and sophistication, the therapist will always rely heavily on participatory experience with, and observation of, the retarded person in order to arrive at a description and explanation of the retarded person's occupational status.

Treatment

Most frequently, dysfunction in work, play, and self-care behaviors of mentally retarded adolescents and adults has been related to skill and, to a lesser extent, habit deficits. Thus, intervention aimed at remediation has been focused on skill training and habit acquisition. Perceptual-motor, process and communication skill deficits are tackled with varying degrees of effort according to the behavioral context (e.g. perceptual-motor skills may receive greater attention than communication skills in relation to development of work behaviors while the reverse may apply with behaviors associated with social recreation).

Behavioral methods have been widely used as a method for training skills in mentally retarded persons. A variety of techniques associated with behavioral approaches and falling under the category of task analysis appear to have utility in enhancing skill acquisition. These include such

Table 18.1.
Occupational status, recommended assessment procedures and treatment considerations for the retarded person

Occupational status	Recommended assessments	Treatment considerations
VOLITION		
Personal Causation		
Tendency to view actions and events as beyond personal control, resulting in lack of self-initiated behavior	Tennessee Self Concept Scale Locus of Control Scale Observation	Provide opportunities for success experiences which are attributable to person's own actions
High expectancy of failure leading to avoidance rather than success-striving behavior.		Encourage participation in decision-making and planning of routines with increasing responsibility for initiating action
Little belief in personal skill or efficacy of skills		Develop realistic appreciation of personal attributes
Values		
Predominantly concerned with here-and-now, with limited future perspective	Time Reference Inventory Expectancy Questionnaire Interview (with individual and significant others) Observation	Clarify aspirations for the future expressed in concrete terms.
Typically ill-defined goals which are not actively worked towards		Assist person to formulate and undertake steps to work towards goals
Meaning in life is sought and found in ways of which little is presently known. Some variation of personal standards from "norm," e.g. code of dependence of some persons		Consider person's own perspective (e.g. sources of meaningfulness in daily life, and personal standards influencing action) before drawing conclusions as to person's needs and initiating intervention strategies
Interests		
Frequently poor discrimination due to lack of experience	Interest Checklist or Occupational Interest Sort Reading-Free Vocational Interest Inventory Observation	Provide guided opportunities for exploration of interests, particularly leisure options
Restricted pattern with a predominant involvement in home-based, solitary, frequently sedentary pursuits		Consider physical and social barriers to interest enactment and investigate ways around these
Potency constrained by limitations of skills, awareness, opportunity, facilities, and friendships		
HABITUATION		
Roles		
Limited availability of normal adult roles (e.g. worker, spouse, home maintainer)	Role Checklist Occupational History Social and Prevocational Information Battery Observation	Create/exploit opportunities in the environment (at home and elsewhere) to explore various adult roles
Frequently cast into roles of invalid and/or social deviant		Identify status of skills and habits that support roles of adulthood
Limited appreciation of role requirements		

Table 18.1.—_Continued_

Occupational status	Recommended assessments	Treatment considerations
**Habits**		
Routines characterized by passivity and low levels of activity Rigidity/inflexibility of habits (so that person becomes upset or disorganized when familiar routines are changed) Limited "inner sense" of appropriate social routines required in various settings	24-hour Log through interview and observation Social and Prevocational Information Battery Adaptive Behavior Scale Adaptive Functioning Index	Construct balanced daily/weekly routines of activity in keeping with person's desires (volition), abilities (performance) and environmental demands Gradually introduce variations in routine to facilitate greater adaptability Increase person's responsibility for organizing own routine

PERFORMANCE

Occupational status	Recommended assessments	Treatment considerations
**Perceptual-motor skills**		
Less physically fit than "normal" age peers. Delayed physical development Less proficient in gross and fine motor performance than "normal" age peers	Adaptive Behavior Scale Adaptive Functioning Index	Identify and focus intervention on skills that support adult occupational roles
**Process skills**		
Slower to manipulate information, make decisions, and select desired response Problems with selective attention and evaluation of feedback More impulsive than reflective in approach to problem solving	Social and Prevocational Information Battery Valpar #17 Prevocational Readiness Battery Observation	Take account of person's learning style and, where necessary, employ such techniques as task analysis (to break tasks into easier segments for learning) and modeling (to allow imitation of complex patterns of behavior)
**Communication/interaction skills**		
More limited repertoire of interpersonal strategies Tendency to inaccurately or inadequately "read" available social cues Limitations in receptive and expressive language skills		Instruct (formally and informally) in methods of communication/interaction related to occupational role performance Modify instructional procedures to account for language difficulties

ENVIRONMENT

Occupational status	Recommended assessments	Treatment considerations
**Psychosocial press**		
Social stigma attached to intellectual deficiency leading to lowered community expectations for performance and fewer opportunities to exercise independence of action	Interview (with person and family) Observation (outside clinical setting, particularly at home) Occupational History	Educate family and significant others towards adoption of a realistic set of attitudes and expectations about person's abilities

Table 18.1.—_Continued_

Occupational status	Recommended assessments	Treatment considerations
		Provide opportunities for demonstration of extent of abilities and for risk taking without threat to own or other's well-being.
Physical press		
Design of physical environments inhabited by retarded persons frequently inhibits exploration of skills and development of competencies	Adaptive Functioning Index Home Life Survey	Facilitate development of social contacts (potential benefactors) within the wider community Break down barriers through exposure (make retarded persons "visible") and public education

tactics as prompting, fading, modeling, chaining, and shaping behavior. Behavioral techniques, however, tend to rely on extrinsic motivators (reinforcers) as motivations for learning. Such an approach is not consistent with the argument which underlies the motivational view of the model—namely, that an intrinsic urge to explore and master underlies learning. In terms of the model, reinforcers are best viewed as feedback informing the retarded persons of the value, consequences and utility of action. Modifications and shaping of behavior occur as this information is incorporated into the system in the throughput process, but learning does not occur because consequences motivate behavior. Rather, the retarded person learns because of a fundamental desire to explore and master. This orients the therapist to look not for reinforcers of behavior, but rather for circumstances that provide avenues for exploration and mastery and to examine environmental conditions to make sure that optimal levels of arousal are present. (As noted earlier the retarded person, for a variety of reasons, is often under- or overaroused.) At the same time this approach does not preclude the use of various task analysis techniques to modulate the arousal potential of tasks and objects and to simplify the process of acquiring skills.

The intrinsic motivation perspective coupled with the recognition that the volition subsystem governs decisions to enter into exploratory and mastery tasks and environments makes it clear that skills acquisition for the retarded person is not just a matter of the performance subsystem. The retarded person's values, feelings of efficacy and interests must be considered prime movers in the learning process.

In addition to volitional factors, it is also necessary to recognize the importance of habituation components of habits and roles in intervention. The roles of personal caretaker, home maintainer, and player can be important to retarded persons at all levels of functioning. Too often the idea that the more severely handicapped person can successfully inhabit such roles is overlooked by others. Occupational therapists can have an impact in this area not only through providing opportunity to perform in these roles, but also through helping relatives, other staff and a variety of persons in the social milieu of the retarded person to perceive the retarded person in these roles. The worker role is also available to some retarded persons in both sheltered workshops and competitive employment. However, as with any worker role, work itself does not assure satisfaction (65); the activities in which the retarded person engages as part of a worker role must be relevant to the volitional traits of that person. Successful performance in the worker role also requires not only that the retarded person learn relevant work skills, but a variety of social and other skills which support work role success. For the retarded person who does not have access to work, either permanently or for extended periods of time, alternative volunteer, amateur and hobbyist roles must be considered.

Since the maladaptive habits of retarded persons often reflect unusual institutional regimens and circumstances, particular attention should be paid to organization of the routine activities of the variety of settings in which a retarded person might reside. This includes not only how time is used but how various behaviors of the retarded person are managed in the setting. For example, destructive behavior should not be addressed not by removing all objects from the environment but by focusing on replacing destructive habits with more adaptive routines. When environments become understimulating, risk free and overly regimented, they encourage habits of passivity and helplessness. The systematic inclusion of opportunities for self-regulated action, risk and stimulation in the environment is, perhaps, the most important single interventive strategy with retarded persons.

Without a balanced perspective on the sources of occupational dysfunction in mentally retarded persons in which volition, habituation, performance, and environment are all acknowledged for their influence, intervention to remediate dysfunction is in danger of producing little more than a "ritual" of socially desirable behaviors "performed" by the mentally retarded individual to "the tune of others."

Many of the mentally retarded persons referred to occupational therapy will present a history of few interests, many failure experiences, little opportunity or encouragement to establish goals and work towards them, arrested occupational role development, poor habit formation, and multiple skill deficits in an environment where competition for work and the privileges bestowed by money and status have been overwhelming. In other words, most mentally retarded persons have experienced a deprived past, inhabit a stagnating, dependent present, and anticipate a vacuous future. Without the help of benefactors (e.g. parent, nonretarded friend), it will be difficult if not impossible to achieve and maintain a state of occupational function in adult life.

Therefore, intervention must be multifaceted in nature. Choice of skills to develop will be dependent on the demands of the environment with regard to occupational role performance as well as on the interests and aspirations of the individual. Level of past experience will determine the level of arousal at which intervention will commence. In all probability, most mentally retarded individuals with a paucity of experience to draw upon will need to do at least some exploration before striving for competence and ultimately achievement in occupational role (be it that of worker, home maintainer, volunteer, hobbyist, etc.). Strategies of treatment for each

subsystem are noted in Table 18.1. Because of the heterogeneity of retarded persons and the multiplicity of potential strategies for remediation, the approaches noted in the table are intended as a list of suggestive strategies and should orient the reader to the process of selecting logical approaches to remediation. They certainly do not exhaust the possibilities for intervention. The next section of this chapter illustrates through two cases how various strategies are employed together in a holistic approach to the retarded person.

A PROFOUNDLY RETARDED STATE HOSPITAL INMATE: ROBERT

Robert is 28 years old and has a diagnosis of profound mental retardation. He is of slight-to-medium build and has a seizure disorder for which he receives anticonvulsive medication. His seizures are documented as petit mal, but occasionally they have grand mal features.

Robert was referred by the interdisciplinary team for an occupational therapy evaluation. Maladaptive behaviors noted in the referral included disrobing in public, physical agression and spitting when staff touched or tried to interact with him.

Robert has lived in an institutional environment since age 4 when he was diagnosed as autistic and mentally retarded. He received treatment and evaluation at several facilities as a child and was admitted at age 12 to the state facility where he now resides. He has spent most of his time since admission on a unit designated for inmates with behavior disorders where he has physically attacked others and damaged his own and public property.

Initial Evaluation

At the time of initial evaluation, Robert was withdrawn, sitting or standing in one position for long periods, and did nothing but sit and watch others. He was difficult to reach or contact and exhibited stereotyped behaviors, such as rocking his body and sitting with his knees under his chin.

The goals of the ongoing evaluation were: to determine any interests or any behaviors which Robert seemed to value, to determine Robert's arousal responses to various environmental conditions, to identify any occupational roles and/or habits, to assess self care skills and play skills, and to assess the hospital environment to determine available objects and tasks which might facilitate competent behavior.

Because Robert had very poor expressive and receptive communication skills, use of conventional assessment tools for these purposes was not feasible. Therefore the occupational therapist utilized chart review and participant observation. Informal observations were made of Robert's behavior throughout the day in the various environments he occupied within the hospital. Program and direct care staff were interviewed concerning their observations, interactions with and attitudes about Robert.

VOLITION

Robert appeared to value interactions with others. He made eye contact and sometimes smiled in response to being touched or when someone spoke to him. He would occasionally reach out to touch the evaluator or hold her hand. These behaviors were observed, to a much lesser extent, with the direct care staff on the unit. It was also observed that direct care staff did not frequently approach Robert, except to stop agressive behavior.

Robert usually preferred to be alone, or at least some distance away from the other residents. This may have been a reflection of the potential of being attacked by other residents. Robert did appear to have some interests. He liked going out of doors, walking about, touching the grass and feeling sunshine on his face. He liked playing in water and taking showers. Interests were determined by noting the frequency with which Robert tried to enact certain behaviors or activities and by any positive affective response to them, such as smiling or laughing.

HABITUATION

The major role available to Robert, and to which he conformed, was that of the deviant or defective. Within the social structure of the unit he appeared to be regarded as a "low grade" resident. He had no friend or player role.

Robert routinely performed daily tasks of feeding and undressing himself. He slept in a bedroom or on the floor about 25% of the time. At other times, he sat with his knees drawn up to his chest, spacing himself as far away from other residents as possible. He frequently slapped, spit at, or threw spit at staff or residents who came within a foot or two of him. Occasionally Robert walked around the day area of the unit with no apparent aim. He was aware of the times for meals and performed some routine behavior at mealtime, such as waiting in the cafeteria line to be served.

Table 18.2.
Robert's typical day

6:30	Staff wake Robert and supervise/perform hygiene and dressing
8:15	Breakfast (30 minute maximum). Residents are sent back to living unit as soon as they finish meals
8:45	Return to unit. Medications are given sometime during this period
10:45	Robert and other residents are usually on the unit, in the day areas or bedrooms. Occasionally, they go outside or to the small recreation room in the building
12:30	Lunch
1:00	Return to unit as described for breakfast. Same as in the morning, except residents are not usually taken outside
3:00	Shift change for staff
5:30	Dinner
6:00	Return to unit. Medications are given sometime in this period
7:30–10:30	Baths are given to residents sometime in this period and staff put residents to bed. Robert frequently gets out of bed and staff return him when he is found later in the evening

A typical day for Robert is outlined in Table 18.2.

PERFORMANCE

Robert had effective use of upper and lower extremities. There was no evidence that he had difficulty seeing or hearing. However, Robert did not seek out sensory information and appeared to have poor sensory processing abilities. He could walk alone, up and down stairs by alternating feet, and ran without falling often. He sometimes walked on tiptoes. Robert had a pincer grasp and could lift a cup or glass to drink, and threw a ball overhand.

Robert fed himself using a spoon, with some spilling. He drank neatly from a cup unassisted. He ate very fast, sometimes dropping food on the floor, chewed with his mouth open and sometimes swallowed food without chewing.

Robert cooperated while being bathed by another. He did not wash his hands or face, made no attempt to brush his teeth and frequently resisted having his teeth brushed by another. Robert occasionally had toilet accidents during the day. He could lower his pants and sit on the toilet without help.

Robert did not care for or choose his own clothing. He was unaware of torn, backwards, or inside-out clothing. He could remove his shoes, socks and shirts, but he often did so at inappropriate times. He sometimes tore his shirts. He did not prepare his own bed at night and required assistance to go to bed.

Robert had no speech. He smiled or laughed to express happiness. He occasionally responded when another person spoke to him. He did not respond to simple directions. Robert did not interact with staff or residents in a socially acceptable manner. Robert had no money handling skills nor domestic or vocational skills. He would not engage in individual or group goal directed tasks or activities.

ENVIRONMENT

The environment which Robert occupied day-to-day was limited to four areas within the Behavior Disorders building (day areas, a small recreation room, bedrooms, and a dining room) and the outside area immediately adjacent to the building. The staff-to-resident ratio was poor in this building and staff had little time or training to develop programs.

The design of this building imposed the following kinds of restrictions. There was minimal staff-resident contact, minimal contact with *any* resident not living on the same wing of the building, and few opportunities to experience novel environments.

The four areas on the wing which Robert occupied were stark, barren and generally unarousing, with a notable lack of objects. On the other hand, the social environment marked by physical outbursts and assaults could often be overarousing. Residents were usually prohibited from entering their bedrooms during the day. Residents from Robert's wing were taken to the small recreation room or outside the building only once or twice weekly. This recreation room was essentially the same as the day areas except for having more windows. That is, it contained hard plastic chairs and a few mats and tables. The recreation room was not used for any particular purpose or for any regularly scheduled activities, except to contain residents away from the living area.

The living area, with bedrooms and bathrooms, was the larger and more complex area which the residents could occupy. Although there were two day areas on the wing, residents were usually confined to only one area and it was therefore crowded, with residents required to be in close proximity to each other.

Staff sometimes brought objects, such as pegboards, bingo games or other fine motor activities, into the living area. Though two benches were the only equipment outside the building, most residents seemed to enjoy a chance to leave the unit.

Treatment Rationale and Goals

Robert was an individual whose cognitive deficits and impaired sensory processing were compounded by an environment which lacked the elements necessary to facilitate exploratory behavior and the development of personal competencies. Table 18.3 summarizes Robert's occupational status. He exhibited an almost complete lack of exploratory behavior and was functioning at a helplessness level. His typical behaviors appeared to be a response to the under- and overarousing aspects of his environment. These were the aggressive and/or hyperactive behaviors of other residents which were intentional or inadvertent sources of injury to Robert, the lack of staff initiating goal-directed activities, the lack of purposeful group or individual action by other residents, and the side effects of medication, sleepiness and lethargy.

In this environment, protecting oneself was efficacious. Robert appeared to accomplish this through his negative interpersonal behaviors and maintenance of a large personal space. As he was cast into an extremely deviant role by staff, they made no attempts to facilitate productive behavior in the form of play, learning self-care skills, interpersonal exchanges or assisting with unit maintenance. Robert had few interests and he was constrained from enacting those he did have. Robert had failed to develop images of socially acceptable versus unacceptable behavior due to the complexity and inconsistency of environmental cues. The low staff to resident ratio meant that staff preferred residents to be inactive and passive.

This maladaptive cycle was exacerbated by Robert's aggressive behavior. Only if it decreased could he have access to less restrictive environments, thus increasing his exposure to opportunities for exploration. To accomplish this, Robert initially needed to feel some degree of safety in the treatment environment and eventually his living environment. Novel stimuli were introduced to elicit exploratory behavior. Treatment was performed in a playful spirit allowing Robert to define some of the boundaries (that is, time limits, choice of objects, spontaneous variations in the play, etc.). Once interest began to replace the negative "survival" behaviors, work on developing

Table 18.3.
Robert's occupational status, treatment objectives and strategies

VOLITION

No apparent values or goals formed	Allow expression of present interests.
No recognition of social desirability of behaviors	Use of clear cues to facilitate development of images of socially desirable and undesirable behaviors
Little interest or opportunity to enact interests	
Very poor sense of personal causation due to unpredictability of events and lack of opportunity for exploration	Exploration of other activities/objects with properties to stimulate simply play behavior
	Engage in simple games, e.g. peek-a-boo, catch, to develop interest in interaction
	Vary games, objects, activities to maintain interest
	Allow Robert some control of limits of interaction, contiguous with overall treatment strategies, to enhance sense of internal locus of control

HABITUATION

Lacks occupational roles to provide expectations for productive behavior; cast in deviant role	Enhance process of habit formation by setting up routine schedule for self-care, unit tasks, leisure activities, therapy sessions, and medication administration
Lacks habits of personal care	
Inactivity, maintaining fixed postures or repetitive performance of stereotyped behaviors are routine for him	Train direct care staff as to purpose of said schedule and necessity for adherence
Shows recognition of some routines, such as meals	

PERFORMANCE

Has deficits in perceptual-motor, communication/interaction and process skills	Increase adaptive interactional skills by providing clear cues for behavior in a playful context and by using simple games in which interaction can be practiced
Is able to ambulate and perform some self-care	
	Encourage interaction with simple objects with varied stimuli such as colors, shapes and textures to enhance perceptual-motor skills

ENVIRONMENT

Lacks human and nonhuman objects to simulate interest or action	Provide a variety of objects in the environment (e.g. different textures and shapes)
Restricted to essentially one environment which is relatively unchanging, has crowded areas and little personal space	Recommend changes in the unit, such as providing sections with carpeting, large tumble forms (to play with, sit in or under, use for games, etc.), Nerf toys
Threatening events, such as attacks by others, are unpredictable	Use both day areas on the wing
	Set up recreation room with equipment described above
	Take residents outside more often and in smaller groups to allow exploration beyond immediate grounds
	Heighten staff's awareness of arousal qualities of objects and activities described and relation to production of adaptive behavior routines

391

interactive play skills and self care skills and routines began. Consultation with unit staff was used to demonstrate that Robert could have occupational roles with expectations for playful and productive behavior, and that explicit environmental cues had to be used to convey the expectations of these roles.

The long-term treatment goal was to facilitate Robert's competence in caring for personal needs, in helping to maintain his living area and as a participant in leisure and cultural activities. The initial goal was to decrease his aggressive behaviors during treatment sessions, to increase exploratory behaviors, to discover activities Robert enjoyed which could be made available within the present milieu, and to develop Robert's ability to interact with the therapist through responding appropriately to given cues. Specific strategies of treatment are noted in Table 18.3.

Treatment Description and Outcomes

Treatment began as 15-minute sessions, scheduled three times weekly and implemented by the occupational therapist. Robert was observed for approximately 5 minutes prior to the treatment. The therapist recorded Robert's behaviors and relevant environmental cues during this observation period. This observation period had three purposes. First, it enabled the therapist to determine Robert's level of arousal prior to the beginning of treatment. This level ranged from very lethargic (e.g. sleeping) to very agitated (e.g. spitting and slapping). Second, the therapist could observe the climate of the immediate surroundings, such as whether it was crowded, whether nearby residents were agitated or noisy or whether housekeeping or maintenance staff were working on the unit. This information was used to determine whether treatment could be done on the ward or if Robert needed to be taken to a quieter or less crowded environment. Further, an examination of the environmental elements sometimes gave a clue to Robert's present level of arousal and, over time, led to a better understanding of the relation of the environment to Robert's behavior. Finally, it enabled the therapist to monitor any positive or negative changes in the physical and psychosocial elements of the environment.

Treatment consisted of the presentation of various types of objects in an attempt to arouse Robert's curiosity and elicit exploratory behaviors. Objects presented were selected for their properties of providing sensory information upon simple physical manipulation. Examples were a fuzzy animal which squeaked when squeezed, a mirror which revolved within a plastic ring, a bright colored hard rubber ball with short flexible spines and a rhythm instrument which clanged when shook. Materials were carried to the unit in a bag or box which Robert was also allowed to explore. Initially the therapist touched Robert's hands, arms, face, and other body parts with some of the objects. His reaction ranged from accepting and noticing the stimulation to reaching for the object and poking, shaking or pounding it against himself. Usually after a short period Robert would throw the object several feet away from himself.

After approximately eight sessions, Robert demonstrated a preference for the "spiny" ball. He would hold it longer and play with the spines. Eventually he would throw it away from himself. Attempts were made to gradually shape this into a game of catch. The therapist would retrieve the ball and roll it along the floor back to Robert. He would hold it awhile then throw it again. Robert would often throw the ball purposely away from the therapist, then laugh mischievously following this. The therapist returned the ball to Robert, gradually rolling it to a point slightly further away from where he was sitting. This type of interaction gave Robert an opportunity to influence the behavior of another in a socially appropriate and accepted manner. In addition, *he* was the initiator in this playful interaction—the actor, rather than the pawn.

At times, Robert began to slap or spit at the therapist. Utilizing the principle of providing clear environmental cues of expectations for behavior, the therapist consistently stopped the interaction, firmly stated, "No, Robert"; moved approximately 8–10 feet away from him; and remained there until the negative behaviors ceased. Then she would walk back to him and reinitiate the interaction.

The following brief incidents illustrate Robert's response to treatment. After 3 months in treatment, Robert's aggressive behaviors had significantly decreased during the treatment sessions. Aggressive behaviors were being replaced with adaptive interactions when clear cues were provided. For example, in one session the therapist moved away from Robert because he was slapping her. When he ceased the behavior, he made eye contact with her, then rose and walked towards her reaching out for the object she held. During one session, no aggressive behaviors occurred over a 15-minute period.

Several specific objects and activities were identified as ones Robert liked. Activities included the game of catch and having the fuzzy animal brought close to, and then lightly touch, various parts of his face. Objects of interest to him included the spiny ball, terrycloth and soft objects, and rhythm instruments which made soft noises. Information about Robert's interests, gathered both in the assessment phase and after treatment began, were shared with program and unit staff through interdisciplinary meetings. At these meetings, the occupational therapist presented the response to treatment and began encouraging staff to view Robert as able to act competently within occupational roles. She discussed the importance of schedules, routines, and the use of consistent and clear communication of expectations.

The therapist also served as a role model for other direct care staff. The following incident is an example. At the beginning of one session, the therapist wished to move to a less crowded location. A direct care aide grasped Robert's arm to begin having him follow her. The therapist intervened, showing Robert one of his favorite objects. He voluntarily followed the therapist to the other day area. Such incidents helped change staff views about Robert and how they should interact with him.

At this point staff have observed a decrease in Robert's aggression on the unit. It is also reported that Robert has begun to approach staff to initiate adaptive interactions. Treatment is being continued in the same manner with further investigation of appropriate play activities, including gross motor, physical fitness activities, and leading to the introduction of self-care materials, such as a tooth brush and washcloth.

CASE STUDY: Peter

Peter is a 24-year-old man who is mildly mentally retarded. He was referred to an Australian government-run rehabilitation center for assessment and guidance.

Assessment

HISTORY

Peter lives with his mother and father and is the younger of two brothers (his brother with whom he frequently disagrees, has recently moved away from home). He is epileptic but his seizures are well controlled by medication. He attended local schools through primary and high school with consistently extremely poor results. From his report, he did not have many friends at high school and was the brunt of many "dirty tricks." Upon leaving school at age 17, he worked for 5½ years in a sheltered workshop/laundry. He left

due to disagreements with some fellow workers, although he had been happy there prior to these recent disagreements. He was seeking alternative employment at the time of referral to the rehabilitation center.

Peter's occupational functioning was assessed using a selection of instruments including Adaptive Functioning Index, Role Checklist, 24-Hour Log, Time Reference Inventory, Expectancy Questionnaire, Interest Checklist, and Locus of Control Scale. To compensate for Peter's reading difficulties, all instrument items were presented to him verbally.

ADAPTIVE FUNCTIONING INDEX

The "social education test" revealed that Peter has a functionally adequate grasp of directional, amount and conservation concepts, is proficient in time telling, possesses no significant motor impairments and has satisfactory numerical and money handling skills. The most notable areas of difficulty for Peter are in knowledge of community facilities, and in reading social cues (the latter which he has identified as being of personal significance).

From the residential checklist completed with Peter and his parents, it is apparent that while he helps with minor household tasks on occasions, Peter has no responsibility for, and thus little experience of, such tasks as doing laundry, ironing, room cleaning, food preparation, and shopping. He handles his own money responsibly and budgets for his own needs. Although he is quite able to use public transportation independently, he does so infrequently and only in the company of other family members apparently because of his mother's fear (somewhat reflected by him) that he will have a seizure while travelling alone. (However, seizures are rare and have never occurred on the occasions where he has traveled by public transport with or without his family). With regard to interpersonal behavior, Peter appears pleasant, friendly, cooperative, and appropriate in his interactions. He possesses a pronounced stutter which, while it does not interfere grossly with his communication, is still a hindrance and an apparent source of embarassment to him in social interactions.

Vocationally, reports from Peter's former employers suggest that he is a conscientious (tending towards being overly meticulous), punctual, hard working person who presents well in the work setting. However, he is a slow worker and has some difficulty in working without considerable structure and direction. He had generally enjoyed good relations with staff and fellow workers until recent times when he disagreed repeatedly with several new male employees at the workshop. Among his co-workers, he possessed only one friend whom he sometimes saw on weekends.

24-HOUR LOG

Since Peter is attending the rehabilitation center 5 days a week, he completed logs for typical weekends. These are characterized by a lack of routine. Much time appears to be spent in purposeless waiting for something of interest to happen. Long periods of inactivity may be punctuated by time spent playing videogames by himself or with his workmate on the occasions that he visits. Sometimes he may watch television or talk to his mother while she does her work. Occasionally, he will help with chores around the house or in the garden if he is specifically requested to do so. However, he does not have regular homemaking responsibilities to fulfill. In essence, much of his time on weekends is passively spent, with little organization or sense of purpose.

ROLE CHECKLIST

Peter perceives that his roles as a worker and as a participant in an organization (both of which are moderately valued by him) have been disrupted for the present. He is maintaining the roles of hobbyist, friend and family member and has recently adopted the role of home maintainer which he plans to continue (all of these roles are moderately valued by him). Interestingly, the only role which he values highly, that of a student, has been lost. Details of his evaluations are shown in Table 18.4.

INTEREST CHECKLIST

From the checklist, it is apparent that Peter has difficulty discriminating his interests. He reports a strong interest in 34 (over half) of the 60 activities listed and a mild interest in a further 14 of the remaining 26. He has experienced the majority of the activities on the checklist at some time. Currently, he is participating in 10 different activities of interest at least once a month. However, these activities are primarily homebased, and tend to provide limited opportunity for active expression of interpersonal interaction. Peter maintains that he does not have the time to do other activities that he has indicated he would like to engage in. Yet from his 24-Hour Log it is apparent that he has a good deal of "empty" time on the weekends. During con-

versation about his interests, Peter remarked that he frequently takes an interest in those things that his mother likes, a rather atypical attitude for a person 24 years of age in our society. It would seem that Peter has not as yet developed the means whereby choices are made among alternative activities according to interest, and whereby these choices are acted upon and maintained over time motivated by interest.

TIME REFERENCE INVENTORY

Peter exhibits a strong orientation to the past in his responses, most notably in relation to the negative items of the inventory. He appears to view the past as a time of difficulty with the belief that things are getting better. It would seem, however, that there is limited

Table 18.4.
Peter's role checklist responses

Role	Past	Present	Future
Student	X		
Worker	X		X
Volunteer			X
Caregiver			X
Home Maintainer		X	X
Friend	X	X	X
Family member	X	X	X
Religious participant			
Hobbiest/amateur	X	X	X
Participant in an organization	X		X

Role	Not at all valuable	Somewhat valuable	Very valuable
Student			X
Worker		X	
Volunteer	X		
Caregiver		X	
Home maintainer		X	
Friend		X	
Family member		X	
Religious participant	X		
Hobbiest/amateur		X	
Participant in an organization		X	

thought of, or reference to, the future at this stage.

EXPECTANCY QUESTIONNAIRE

Peter's responses on the questionnaire suggest a preoccupation with work. He possesses only vague notions of a future in which he will be working or looking for work. He sees that the options are "work or starve." He considers that there will probably be little change in the future so that he will be doing similar work of a routine nature as in the past and present. He states that work is important to him primarily for the money he hopes to earn. While not being very optimistic, he considers that if he had plenty of money, he would like to own his own business. In all, his expectations of the future are narrow and vague, but with some realism about his restricted options.

LOCUS OF CONTROL QUESTIONNAIRE

From the questionnaire, it is apparent that Peter does not possess a strong sense of internal control over his life. At the same time, on the internal-external continuum, he does not present a view of being externally controlled. On the whole, given an understanding of his life experience thus far, it seems that his "middling" perception of control is probably a fairly realistic one.

In addition to assessment by formal means, information on Peter was obtained via a social worker interview with Peter and his parents. This, combined with informal comments made by Peter during assessment, complemented the existing picture of the physical and psycho-social environment which Peter inhabits. Peter does not live the "normal" life of a 24-year-old man. Besides being dependent on his parents for meeting his physical needs, he appears to be quite dependent for emotional fulfillment also, in particular on his mother. It seems that his mother encourages this and that while he willingly accepts this, at times he expresses resentment of it also. His mother apparently believes him to be somewhat of an incompetent person (e.g. because of his epilepsy he should not ride the bus alone) who should not be encouraged to become more independent. He, therefore, has few role demands or responsibilities placed on him in the home environment. His academic failures in a role which he sees as very valuable and his fears of the unknown without his mother support this dependence in his own mind. The sheltered workshop has been the other principal environment in which he has

been required to function and, of recent times, this has been an unhappy situation. It is the environment from which he has drawn his friendships and considerable personal gratification in the past but his disagreements there have forced him to withdraw from it. He has only one male friend (and no female friends), a former co-worker whom he sees intermittently on weekends. In all, it would appear that Peter maintains a poor fit with his physical and social environment when viewed against the expectations of society for performance by a 24-year-old man.

Occupational Status

Peter could be viewed as moving within a maladaptive cycle (Table 18.5). At 24 years of age, his interests are neither clearly developed nor strongly enacted in leisure or vocational domains. He values work and the money it brings and yet he cannot find well paid employment and is presently without even sheltered employment. His view of the future is vague and his aspirations lack definition. He has a history of failure in academic pursuits (on which he places a very high value) with an associated poor sense of internal control. His home environment supports this by encouraging dependence and, to a lesser degree, incompetence.

His most valued role, that of a student, has been terminated upon leaving school and the valued roles of worker and organization participant have been disrupted, at least temporarily. The environment has done little to support the continuation of valued roles or the exploration of new ones (e.g. opportunities for further academic endeavors are not available; there are few work options available and his knowledge of these is limited; he is not being encouraged to explore the home maintainer role). The habit routines which support occupational roles (other than work) have not been internalized for skills to be organized into the necessary action patterns. Instead, much time is spent aimlessly waiting for something worthwhile to happen.

Skills themselves, while moderately developed through school and work experiences, have frequently not been rehearsed and sufficiently applied across all areas necessary for independent functioning at the level expected of a 24-year-old person by the social environment.

Intervention

See Table 18.5 for details of intervention strategies. Peter is attending the rehabilita-

Table 18.5.
Peter's occupational status and strategies for intervention

Occupational status	Intervention strategies
VOLITION	

Personal Causation

| Does not possess a well developed sense of personal control; his environment does not promote internal control | Provide opportunities for accomplishment and feedback on results of actions; attempt to influence environment to support this |

Values

| Mostly oriented to the past which is viewed in fairly negative terms; more positive outlook on present and future though expectations are narrow and ill-defined | Engage client in setting concrete, short-term, realistic goals and steps to work towards; and gradually clarify long-term aspirations |

Interests

| Poorly developed discrimination of interests, and a narrow pattern of home-based, solitary leisure pursuits; pursuits may be a function more of environmental factors than of strong personal choice | Explore leisure and vocational interests to develop discrimination and selective enactment of a broader range of interests |

HABITUATION

Roles

| Has lost the only role in his life that he perceives as *very* valuable (that of a "student"); valued roles of "worker" and "participant in an organization" have been disrupted, although several other valued roles are maintained | Provide opportunities to resume or adapt valued roles |

Habits

| Free time is very poorly structured with little purposeful organization of time on weekends—much time spent waiting for something to happen | Assist with structuring of time usage according to needs |

PERFORMANCE

| Existing skills are not being adequately exploited and developed by application in all areas of performance relevant to independent adult functioning; thus, performance deficits are exacerbated by limited experience in applying skills | Provide opportunities to acquire and rehearse skills pertinent to various vocational and independent living situations |

ENVIRONMENT

| Independence is discouraged—few responsibilities placed on him in home environment and fear of failure to cope in strange situations is passively encouraged; very limited network of social supports beyond family | Attempt to bring about change of attitude in family through education as to client's needs and existing competencies; expand opportunities for interaction with age peers |

tion center on a full weekly program of 5 days but continuing to reside with his parents. The overall plan of intervention is for Peter to begin at an exploratory level of occupational functioning where he can investigate and im-

plement any necessary changes to his occupational life-style, progressing to competence and, ultimately, to achievement in the roles he is endeavoring to fulfill. This will require thorough examination of interests and values, restoration of confidence in abilities, exploration of roles and their requirements, adjustment of habits to accommodate a fresh understanding of volition and roles, development of new skills and refining of existing ones, and facilitation of environmental changes to support occupational functioning. It is anticipated that this process will be initiated at the center but will be continuing beyond the time when Peter ceases to attend the center.

To explore and refine his interests as they are manifested in work and leisure, Peter will undertake work experience in various center workshops, quite different from his only vocational experience to date. In accord with his stated preferences he will move among four areas: a metal workshop which includes motor body repair; a wood workshop; an outdoor area with yard work and gardening duties; and a light trades area for dissembly/assembly of a small mechanical apparatus. These vocational areas with their tasks graded according to cognitive and motor complexity offer not only exploratory possibilities but also opportunities for acquisition of skills necessary for performance in varied work environments and clear feedback as to success of action. Initially, on the easier tasks, there is limited risk of failure. However, with increasing complexity of tasks and reducing supervision and structure, succeess becomes much more reliant on client application and aptitude. All vocational areas encourage development of habits appropriate to the worker role. For Peter, the greatest concern is with facilitation of greater self-direction and adaptability in various work environments.

To further his leisure exploration, Peter has selected: to join a center-organized bowling group which meets once a week out of hours at a community bowling alley; to take leatherwork classes in the center craft area; and to participate in a camping/bushwalking program which involves weekend excursions once a month. These leisure activities also provide opportunities for regular social interaction with other male and female young adults.

With his interest in cooking and his need to advance his independent living skills, Peter has enrolled in center-run, limited duration, courses in food preparation and community survival. In both of these, the emphasis is on learning by *doing*. In the food preparation classes, participants are able to occasionally invite a family member to come and join them in a meal they have prepared—an opportunity for Peter's mother to view his competence in action. In the community survival course run parallel with the other, participants plan menus, shop for groceries, devise budgets, use public transport regularly, navigate through city streets, and use such public facilities as telephones, post office, and banks.

Peter is to be encouraged to plan his time usage on weekends and to seek from his parents some homemaking duties for which he would have a weekly responsibility. Thus, his weekends could be spent in cleaning his room, doing some yardwork, taking some food preparation responsibilities, doing some of his laundry, and participating in one leisure activity preferably outside his home (e.g. going to a movie, skating, riding his bike to visit his former workmate, going for a walk, going to a football match with his father, playing video games or pool at a fun parlor).

Experience in formulating and working toward short-term goals will be facilitated in various ways including: participation in setting personal production targets each week in work areas; saving for desired goods and events with careful budgeting in the community survival course; participation in planning his own program at the center in line with perceived needs; menu planning and budgeting prior to grocery shopping for food preparation classes. Peter will also be encouraged to think about and discuss with his social worker and occupational therapist such issues for his future as: work, living independently and social relationships, including marriage.

Finally, he will be able to attend remedial tutoring sessions at the center to assist his reading—furtherance of the student role to improve a skill that he holds to be important. He will also be attending speech therapy at the center twice a week to learn to cope with his stutter. His family will be encouraged to attend family support and information nights run at the center on an "ad hoc" basis by a social worker and occupational therapist, with an accent on coping with disability and optimizing independent functioning.

Outcomes

After 2 months attendance at the center, Peter has progressed in various ways. In the work areas, he has discovered that metal work and woodwork are not to his liking, compounded by the difficulty he has experienced in becoming proficient with the manipulative demands of such tasks. He is a slow but meticulous worker in the light trades tasks and likes the outside nature of yard work. Due to the economic climate with limited job prospects and also to Peter's difficulties in acquiring employable work speeds and being self-directed, it appears likely that he may only be able to find such employment in a sheltered environment, at least for an interim period. To supplement his income, the possibility of his doing several hours of mail box advertising deliveries on weekends is being examined.

In the leisure arena, Peter is planning to join a bowling league for disadvantaged young adults to further improve his proficiency; he is doing leatherwork projects on weekends at home; and he has been camping once and hopes to go again. He is now catching the bus home from the center each day with another rehabilitee, instead of being driven to and from by his father. He is happy about his progress in reading and hopes to join an adult literacy course run by a technical college when he leaves the center.

Peter's proficiency in the food preparation area is improving although he has not, as yet, prepared a weekend meal at home. This is seemingly due to his mother's mixed feelings about such an undertaking. It has been proposed to his parents that they attend an upcoming course for parents of retarded persons on "moving towards independence," run by a state government agency for mentally retarded persons. On the weekend, Peter reports that he is doing some cleaning of his own room as well as helping his father in the yard. He and his former workmate are keeping in contact, visiting each other at home. They plan to go on some outings also.

Peter is still a long way from thinking clearly about his future. It is difficult for him to grasp the ramifications of the constraints he faces, on the one hand, and the possibilities that could be, on the other. Yet, he is discovering something more of himself and the world he lives in. He is closer to developing a "fit" with his environment—progress on the road from occupational dysfunction to function.

SUMMARY

This chapter illustrated use of the model to examine occupational dysfunction in the mentally retarded person and as a guide to assessment and intervention. Because of the extreme heterogeneity of mentally retarded persons, particular aspects of discussions will have more-or-less relevance to specific individuals, and the assessments and strategies of treatment will be forthcoming from careful consideration of the individual in question and his or her functional and dysfunctional patterns.

References

1. Baumeister AA, Hawkins W, Holland J: Motor learning and knowledge of results. *Am J Ment Defic* 70:590–594, 1966.
2. Baumeister AA, Kellas G: Reaction time and mental retardation. In Ellis NR (ed): *International Review of Research in Mental Retardation.* New York, Academic Press, 1968, vol 3.
3. Bercovici SM: *Barriers to Normalization.* Baltimore, University Park Press, 1983.
4. Berkson, G: An analysis of reaction times in normal and mentally deficient young men. 3. Variation of stimulus and response complexity. *J Ment Defic Res* 4:69–77, 1960.
5. Blatt B, Kaplan F: *Christmas in Purgatory: A Photographic Essay on Mental Retardation.* Boston, Allyn & Bacon, 1966.
6. Blount WR: A comment on language, socialization, acceptance, and the retarded. *Ment Retard* 7:33–35, 1969.
7. Bogdan, R., Taylor, S., DeGrandpre, B., Haynes, S.: Let them eat programs: attendants perspectives and programming on wards in state schools. *J Health Soc Behav* 15:142–151, 1974.
8. Braginski DD, Braginski BM: *Hansels and Gretels—Studies of Children in Institutions for the Mentally Retarded.* New York, Holt, Rinehart, & Wilson, 1971.
9. Bruininks RH: Physical and motor development of retarded persons. In Ellis NR (ed): *International Review of Research in Mental Retardation.* New York, Academic Press, 1974, vol 7.
10. Burke D, Sellin D: Measuring the self-concept of ability as a worker. *Except Child* 39:126–132, 1972.
11. Carter JL: The status of educable mentally retarded boys on the AAHPER Youth Fitness Test. *J Health, Phys Educ, Rec* 34:8, 1966.
12. Chan K, Smith D, Reid H: *Interpersonal Tactics of Mentally Retarded and Normally Achieving Children.* Paper presented at the annual meeting of the Western Psychological Association, Seattle, 1977.
13. Cheseldine S, Jeffree D: Mentally handicapped adolescents: their use of leisure. *J Ment Defic Res* 25:49–59, 1981.
14. Clausen J: *Ability Structure and Subgroups in Mental Retardation.* Washington, D.C., Spartan Books, 1966.
15. Cleland C, Swartz J: Work deprivation as motivation to work. *Am J Ment Defic* 73:703–712, 1969.
16. Collins H, Burger G, Doherty D: Self-concept of EMR and nonretarded adolescents. *Am J Ment Defic* 75:285–289, 1970.
17. Coyne P: Developing social skills in the developmentally disabled adolescent and young adult: a recreation and social/sexual approach. *J Leisur* 7:70–76, 1980.
18. Cratty B: *Motor Activity and the Education of Retardates* Philadelphia, Lea & Febiger, 1974.
19. Cromwell RL: A social learning approach to mental retardation. In Ellis NR (ed): *Handbook of Mental Deficiency.* New York, McGraw-Hill, 1963.
20. Culley WJ, Jolly DH, Mertz ET: Heights and weights of mentally retarded children. *Am J Ment Defic* 68:203–210, 1963.
21. DeVries R: The development of role-taking as reflected by behavior of bright, average, and retarded children in a social guessing game. *Child Dev* 41:759–770, 1970.
22. Dexter LA: Towards a sociology of the mentally

defective, *Am J Ment Defic* 61:10–16, 1956.

23. Dexter LA: Research on problems of mental subnormality, *Am J Ment Defic* 64:835–838, 1960.

24. Dugas JL, Kellas G: Encoding and retrieval processes in normal children and retarded adolescents. *J Exp Child Psychol* 17:177–185, 1974.

25. Edgerton RB: *The cloak of competence: stigma in the lives of the mentally retarded.* Berkeley, Calif, University of California Press, 1967.

26. Edgerton R, Bercovici S: The cloak of competence: years later. *Am J Ment Defic* 80:485–497, 1976.

27. Farber B: *Mental Retardation: Its Social Context and Social Consequences.* Boston, Houghton Mifflin, 1968.

28. Flexer R, Bihm E, Shaw J, Sigelman C, Raney B, Jansson D: Training and maintaining work productivity in severely and moderately retarded persons. *Rehabil Counsel Bull* 25:10–17, 1982.

29. Floor L, Rosen M: Investigating the phenomenon of helplessness in mentally retarded adults. *Am J Ment Defic* 79:565–572, 1975.

30. Francis RJ, Rarick GL: Motor characteristics of the mentally retarded. *Am J Ment Defic* 63:792–811, 1959.

31. Gold MW: Stimulus factors in skill training of retarded adolescents on a complex assembly task: acquisition, transfer, and retention. *Am J Ment Defic* 76:517–526, 1972.

32. Gold MW, Barclay CR: The learning of difficult visual discrimination by the moderately and severely retarded. *Ment Retard* 11:9–11, 1973.

33. Goode DA: Who is Bobby? Ideology and method in the discovery of a Down's syndrome person's competence. In Kielhofner G (ed): *Health Through Occupation: Theory and Practice in Occupational Therapy.* Philadelphia, FA Davis, 1983.

34. Gow L, Ward J: Effects of modification of conceptual tempo on acquisition of work skills. *Percep Mot Skills* 50:107–116, 1980.

35. Gow L, Ward J: Extension of the use of measures of cognitive style to moderately-severely retarded trainees in a field setting. *Percep Mot Skills* 55:191–194, 1982.

36. Greenspan S: Social intelligence in the retarded. In Ellis NR (ed): *Handbook of Mental Deficiency, Psychological Theory, and Research,* ed 2. Hillsdale, N.J., Erlbaum, 1979.

37. Grossman HJ (ed): *Manual on terminology and Classification in Mental Retardation.* Washington, D.C., American Association on Mental Deficiency, 1973.

38. Gruen GE, Ottinger DR, Ollendick TH: Probability learning in retarded children with differing histories of success and failure in school. *Am J Ment Defic* 79:417–423, 1974.

39. Gruen G, Zigler E: Expectancy of success and the probability learning of middle-class, lower-class, and retarded children. *J Abnorm Psychol* 73:343–352, 1968.

40. Gunzburg HC, Gunzburg AL: *Mental Handicap and Physical Environment.* New York, Macmillan, 1973.

41. Gunzburg HC, Gunzburg AL: "Normal" environment with a plus for the mentally retarded. In Canter D, Canter S (eds): *Designing for Therapeutic Environments.* New York, Wiley, 1979.

42. Guskin SL: Social psychologies of mental deficiency. In Ellis NR (ed): *Handbook of Mental Deficiency.* New York, McGraw-Hill, 1963.

43. Halpern AS, Lehmann JP, Irvin LK, Heiry TJ: *Contemporary Assessment for Mentally Retarded Adolescents and Adults.* Baltimore, University Park Press, 1982.

44. Harris GJ, Fleer RE: High speed memory scanning in mental retardates: Evidence for a central processing deficit. *J Exp Child Psychol* 17:452–459, 1974.

45. Henderson S, Morris J, Ray S: Performance of Down syndrome and other retarded children on the Cratty Gross-Motor Test. *Am J Ment Defic* 85:416–424, 1981.

46. Heshusius L: *Meaning in life as experienced by persons labeled retarded in a group home: a participant observation study.* Springfield, Ill, Charles C Thomas, 1981.

47. Hourcade J: Effect of a summer camp program on self-concept of mentally retarded young adults. *Ther Rec J* 11:178–183, 1977.

48. Houssiadas L, Brown LB: The coordination of perspectives by mentally defective children. *J Genet Psychol* 110:211–215, 1967.

49. Howe CE: A comparison of motor skills of mentally retarded and normal children. *Except Child* 25:352–354, 1959.

50. Kagan J: Reflection-impulsivity: the generality and dynamics of conceptual tempo. *J Abnorm Psychol* 71:17–24, 1966.

51. Kahana E: A congruence model of person-environment interaction. In Whitney PG, Byerts TO, Ernst GF (eds): *Theory Development in Environment and Aging.* Washington, D.C., Gerontological Society, 1975.

52. Kantner R, Clark D, Allen L, Chase M: Effects of vestibular stimulation on nystagmus response and motor performance of the developmentally delayed infant. *Phys Ther* 56:414–421, 1976.

53. Katz S, Yekutiel E: Leisure time problems of mentally retarded graduates of training programs. *Ment Retard* 12:54–57, 1974.

54. Kavanagh MR: *Person-Environment Interaction: The Model of Human Occupation Applied to Mentally Retarded Adults.* (Unpublished research project, Virginia Commonwealth University, 1982.)

55. Keogh B, Cahill C, MacMillan D: Perception of interruption by educationally handicapped children. *Am J Ment Defic* 77:107–108, 1972.

56. Kielhofner G: The temporal dimension in the lives of retarded adults. *Am J Occup Ther* 33:161–168, 1979.

57. Kielhofner G: An ethnographic study of deinstitutionalized adults: their community settings and daily life experiences. *Occup Ther J Res* 1:125–141, 1981.

58. Kielhofner G: "Teaching" retarded adults: paradoxical effects of a pedagogical enterprise. *Urban Life* 12:307–326, 1983.

59. Kielhofner G, Miyake S: The therapeutic use of games with mentally retarded adults. *Am J Occup Ther* 35:375–382, 1981.

60. Kielhofner G, Takata N: A study of mentally retarded persons: applied research in occupa-

tional therapy. *Am J Occup Ther* 34:252–258, 1980.

61. Kodman F: Perceptual-motor learning with moderately retarded persons. *Percep Mot Skills* 53:25–26, 1981

62. Kral P: Motor characteristics and development of retarded children: success experience. *Educ Train Ment Retard* 7:14–21, 1972.

63. Landesman-Dwyer S, Stein JG, Sackett GP: A behavioral and ecological study of group homes. In Sackett GP (ed): *Observing Behavior. vol 1, Theory and Applications in Mental Retardation.* Baltimore, University Park Press, 1978.

64. Longhurst TM: Communication in retarded adolescents: sex and intelligence level. *Am J Ment Defic* 78:607–618, 1974.

65. Lyons MJ: *Employment and Personal Adjustment of Mentally Retarded Persons: Towards an Emic Perspective of the Relationship.* (Unpublished master's thesis, Virginia Commonwealth University, 1983.)

66. MacMillan D: Motivational differences: cultural-familial retardates versus normal subjects on expectancy for failure. *Am J Ment Defic* 74:254–258, 1969.

67. MacMillan DL: The problem of motivation in the education of the mentally retarded. *Excep Child* 37:579–586, 1971.

68. Macmillan DL: *Mental Retardation in School and Society.* Boston, Little, Brown, 1977.

69. Macmillan DL, Keogh BK: Normal and retarded children's expectancy for failure. *Develop Psychol* 4:343–348, 1971.

70. Madsen MC, Connor C: Cooperative and competitive behavior of retarded and non-retarded children at two ages. *Child Dev* 44:175–178, 1973.

71. Malpass LF: Motor skills in mental deficiency. In Ellis NR (ed): *Handbook of Mental Deficiency.* New York, McGraw-Hill, 1963.

72. Marden PW, Farber B: High-brow versus low-grade status among institutionalized mentally retarded boys. *Soc Prob* 8:300–312, 1961.

73. Matthews PR: Why the mentally retarded do not participate in certain types of recreational activities. *Ther Rec J* 14:44–50, 1980.

74. McConkey R, Walsh J, Mulcahy M: The recreational pursuits of mentally handicapped adults. *Int J Rehabil Res* 4:493–499, 1981.

75. McDevitt S, Smith P, Schmidt D, Rosen M: The deinstitutionalized citizen: adjustment and quality of life. *Ment Retard* 16:22–24, 1978.

76. Mercer J: Career patterns of persons labeled as mentally retarded. In Friedson E, Lorber J (eds): *Medical Men and Their Work: A Sociological Reader.* Chicago, Aldine-Atherton, 1972.

77. Mercer C, Snell M: *Learning Theory Research in Mental Retardation: Implications for Teaching.* Columbus, Ohio, Charles E. Merrill, 1977.

78. Mitic TD, Stevenson CL: Mentally retarded people as a resource to the recreationist in planning for integrated community recreation. *J Leisur* 8:30–34, 1981.

79. Montgomery P, Richter E: Effect of sensory integrative therapy on the neuromotor development of retarded children. *Phys Ther* 57:799–806 (a), 1977.

80. Moss JW: *Failure-Avoiding and Success-Striving Behavior in Mentally Retarded and Normal Children.* Ann Arbor, Mich, University Microfilms, 1958.

81. Mulhern T, Baumeister AA: Effects of stimulus-response compatibility and complexity upon reaction times of normals and retardates. *J Com Physiol Psychol* 75:450–463, 1971.

82. Neeman RL: Part 2: Manipulative dexterity and perceptual-motor abilities of mentally retarded adolescents and young adults. *Am J Occup Ther* 25:309–312, 1971.

83. Pennington FM, Luszcz MA: Some functional properties of iconic storage in retarded and nonretarded subjects. *Mem Cogn* 3:295–301, 1975.

84. Perske R: The dignity of risk and the mentally retarded. *Ment Retard* 10:24–26, 1972.

85. Rarick GL: The factor structure of motor abilities of educable mentally retarded children. In Jervis GA (ed): *Expanding Concepts in Mental Retardation: A Symposium.* Springfield, Ill, Charles C Thomas, 1968.

86. Rarick GL, Dobbins DA: *Basic Components in the Motor Performance of Educable Mentally Retarded Children: Implications for Curriculum Development.* Washington, D.C., U.S. Office of Education, 1972.

87. Rarick GL, Widdop JH, Broadhead GD: Physical fitness and motor performance of educable mentally retarded children. *Except Child* 36:509–519, 1970.

88. Redding SF: Life adjustment patterns of retarded and non-retarded low functioning students. *Except Child* 45:367–368, 1979.

89. Reiter S, Levi A: Leisure activities of mentally retarded adults. *Am J Ment Defic* 86:201–203, 1981.

90. Roberts GE, Clayton BE: Some findings arising out of a survey of mentally retarded children. Part 2: Physical growth and development. *Develop Med Child Neurol* 11:584–594, 1969.

91. Roos P, Albers R: Performance of retardates and normals on a measure of temporal orientation. *Am J Ment Defic* 69:835–838, 1965.

92. Rundle AT: Anthropometry: a ten-year survey of growth and sexual maturation. In Richards BW (ed): *Mental Subnormality: Modern Trends in Research.* London, Pitman Medical & Science Publishing, 1970.

93. Ryan M, Jones B: Stimulus persistence in retarded and nonretarded children: a signal detection analysis. *Am J Ment Defic* 80:298–305, 1975.

94. Rynders J, Johnson R, Johnson D, Schmidt B: Producing positive interaction among Down syndrome and nonhandicapped teenagers through cooperative goal structuring. *Am J Ment Defic* 85:268–273, 1980.

95. Schoggen P: Ecological psychology and mental retardation. In Sackett GP (ed): *Observing Behavior, vol 1, Theory and Applications in Mental Retardation.* Baltimore, University Park Press, 1978.

96. Schuer J, Clark F, Azen S: Vestibular function in mildly mentally retarded adults. *Am J Occup Ther* 34:664–670, 1980.

97. Schuster S, Gruen G: Success and failure as

determinants of the performance predictions of mentally retarded and nonretarded children. *Am J Ment Defic* 76:190–196, 1971.

98. Sengstock WL: Physical fitness of mentally retarded boys. *Res Q Am Assoc Health, Phys Ed, Rec* 37:113–120, 1966.

99. Severy LJ, Davis KE: Helping behavior among normal and retarded children. *Child Dev* 42:1017–1031, 1971.

100. Shipe D: Impulsivity and locus of control as predictors of achievement and adjustment in mildly retarded and borderline youth. *Am J Ment Defic* 76:12–22, 1971.

101. Sigelman C, Budd E, Spanhel C, Schoenrock C: When in doubt, say yes: acquiescence in interviews with mentally retarded persons. *Ment Retard* 19:53–58, 1981.

102. Sigelman CK, Schoenrock CJ, Spanhel CL, Hromas SG, Winer JL, Budd EC, Martin PW: Surveying mentally retarded persons: responsiveness and response validity in three samples. *Am J Ment Defic* 84:479–486, 1980.

103. Silverman WP: High speed scanning of nonalphanumeric symbols in cultural-familially retarded and nonretarded children. *Am J Ment Defic* 79:44–51, 1974.

104. Simeonsson RJ: Social competence. In Wortis J (ed): *Mental Retardation and Developmental Disabilities. An Annual Review*. New York, Brunner/Mazel, 1978.

105. Simpson H, Meaney C: Effects of learning to ski on the self-concept of mentally retarded children. *Am J Ment Defic* 84:25–29, 1979.

106. Sloan W: Motor proficiency and intelligence. *Am J Ment Defic* 55:394–406, 1951.

107. Solomon AH: Motivational and repeated trial effects on physical proficiency performances of educable mentally retarded and normal boys. *IMRID Behavioural Science Monograph*, NO. 11. Nashville, Tenn, George Peabody College for Teachers, 1968.

108. Stager S, Young R: Intergroup contact and social outcomes for mainstreamed EMR adolescents. *Am J Ment Defic* 85:497–503, 1981.

109. Stanovich KE: Information processing in mentally retarded individuals. In Ellis NR (ed): *International Review of Research in Mental Retardation*. New York, Academic Press, 1978, vol 9.

110. Stein JU: Physical fitness of mentally retarded boys relative to national norms. *Rehabil Lit* 26:205–208, 1965.

111. Stevenson H, Knights R: Effects of visual reinforcement on the performance of normal and retarded children. *Percept Mot Skills*, 13:212–222, 1961.

112. Talkington L, Overbeck D: Job satisfaction and performance with retarded females. *Ment Retard* 13:18–19, 1975.

113. Taylor AR: Social competence and interpersonal relations between retarded and nonretarded children. In Ellis NR (ed): *International Review of Research in Mental Retardation*. New York, Academic Press, 1982, vol 11.

114. Thor DH: Discrimination of succession in visual masking by retarded and normal children. *J Exper Psychol* 83:380–384, 1970.

115. Tizard J, O'Connor N, Crawford JM: The abilities of adolescent and adult high-grade male defectives. *J Med Sci* 96:889–907, 1950.

116. Turnquist DA, Marzlof SS: Motor abilities of mentally retarded youth. *J Health, Phys Educ, Rec* 25:43–44, 1954.

117. Volpe R: Orthopaedic disability, restriction, and role-taking activity. *J Spec Educ* 10:371–381, 1976.

118. Wagner EE, Hawver DA: Correlations between psychological tests and sheltered workshop performance for severely retarded adults. *Am J Ment Defic* 69:685–691, 1965.

119. Wagner HD: *The Effects of Motivation and Repeated Trials on Physical Proficiency Test Performance of Educable Mentally Retarded Girls*. (Doctoral dissertation, George Peabody College for Teachers) Ann Arbor, Mich, University Microfilms, 1968.)

120. Wehman P, Hill M, Goodal P, Cleveland P, Brooke V, Pentecost J: Job placement and follow-up of moderately and severely handicapped individuals after three years. *J Assoc Severe Handicap* 7:5–16, 1982.

121. Weinstein EA: The development of interpersonal competence. In Goslin DA (ed): *Handbook of Socialization Theory and Research*. Chicago, Ill, Rand McNally, 1973.

122. Weiss D, Weinstein E: Interpersonal tactics among mental retardates. *Am J Ment Defic* 72:653–661, 1967.

123. Wolfensberger W: *The Principle of Normalization in Human Services*. Toronto, National Institute of Mental Retardation, 1972.

124. Wolfensberger W: *The Origin and Nature of Our Institutional Models*. Syracuse, NY, Human Policy Press, 1975.

125. Zeaman, House BJ: A review of attention theory. In Ellis NR (ed): *Handbook of Mental Deficiencies, Psychological Theory, and Research*, ed 2, Hillsdale, NJ, Erlbaum, 1979.

126. Zigler E: Research on personality structure in the retardate. In Ellis NR (ed): *International Review of Research on Mental Retardation*. New York, Academic Press, 1966, vol 1.

127. Zisfein L, Rosen M: Self-concept and mental retardation: theory, measurement, and clinical utility. *Ment Retard* 12:15–19, 1974.

WORKBOOK:
Applying the Model of Human Occupation

Roann Barris, *Editor*

Contributors:

Sally Cubie
Gary Kielhofner
Ellen Kolodner
Ruth Levine
Ann Neville

Workbook

Introduction

Introduction

The exercises in this workbook were developed with two primary purposes in mind: to provide resources for assimilating and illuminating material covered in the text, and to give readers the opportunity to see the relevance of this material to their own lives as well as those of their clients.

The workbook is divided into two major sections. The first part parallels the theoretical and developmental chapters of the text, and emphasizes application of the material in these chapters to oneself. The second part corresponds to the chapters on general and specific clinical applications. Here, the reader will have a chance to practice occupational analysis, program development and treatment planning using cases provided in the workbook or individually selected cases from clinical experiences.

SECTION A:
Applying the Model to Yourself

Exercise One

Values

OBJECTIVE: to explore the concept of values
and its relationship to your current daily life

STEP ONE: On the table that follows list five activities from the past few weeks (or the past few months) that stand out in your mind as very important or valuable. Don't try to figure why or how they are valuable now; just list those activities which come immediately to mind. You might, for instance, recall a quiet dinner with an old friend, baking a cake with your mother's favorite recipe, taking your children roller skating, finishing a term paper or some work project, balancing your checkbook after having put it off for several weeks, and so on.

Activities Table

Valuable activity	Rate each time frame according to the meaning/importance this activity has for you		
	Past. Nostalgia; old familiar activity that always makes me remember good times; something a significant other taught me in the past	Present. For the here and now; to get the most out of the moment	Future. In order to have things be better in the future to accomplish a goal, etc.
1.			
2.			
3.			
4.			
5.			
Totals:			

Exercise One—Continued

STEP TWO: After you have listed five activities you will complete three sets of ratings pertaining to the time frame, meaning and standards of performance for each activity. Fill in each box by entering the appropriate number:

0 = **This was not relevant/true for this activity**
1 = **This was somewhat relevant/true for this activity**
2 = **This was very relevant/true for this activity**

Add up the total scores for each column. You can compare what dimensions of values influenced your recollection of these as valuable activities. For example, you might find they were all future oriented or that you were very concerned with outcomes. On the other hand, you might find that each activity had its own particular reasons for being valuable, and that no overall pattern characterizes the activities.

Activities Table—*Continued*

Rate each of the following dimensions concerning your feelings about why this activity is important or meaningful					Rate each of the following as to how it would be as a gauge of your performance		
Personal awareness. Openess to new possibilities	Personal satisfaction. To be good to myself, to fill a need, etc.	Because others value this, or need this to be done	Personal competence. To develop or improve my abilities	To receive recognition for accomplishment	I used my abilities as best I could	Was it successful; did I accomplish what I intended?	My consideration of others and their needs; that I helped someone, or was sensitive to their feelings, and so on

Exercise Two

Interests

OBJECTIVE: to identify and explore your strong interests and qualities of these interests

STEP ONE: On the table that follows list your 10 strongest interests.

STEP TWO: Place a check in the column that best describes your frequency of participation, the social nature of your participation, your motives, and whether this interest is work, play or self-care.

STEP THREE: Count the checks in each of the frequency columns and record these numbers in the spaces for totals to determine the potency of your interests. How many times did you check each? If you did not engage in some of these interests frequently, do you know why? For example, does time for school leave less free time, or did a lack of economic resources or other people prevent you from participating?

Interests Table

Strong Interest	Check the column that best describes the *frequency of participation* in the last year				
	Daily	Weekly	Monthly	Yearly	Never
1.					
2.					
3.					
4.					
5.					
6.					
7.					
8.					
9					
10.					
Totals:					

Exercise Two—Continued

STEP FOUR: Now add up the "Alone" and "With others" columns. These give you an indication of whether your interests tend to be solitary or social. Were the two columns about equal? If they were not, can you explain why? For instance, is your work/school mostly with others so that you like to be alone when you recreate?

STEP FIVE: Now add up the total for the three columns under motivation. Overall, were your interests more or less equally divided among these categories? Or, do your interests tend to fall in one category? How do your achievement-related interests differ from your exploration interests? You may find it useful to refer back to Chapter 5 where these levels of function are discussed.

STEP SIX: Add up the "Work," "Play" and "Daily Living Tasks" columns. This gives you an indication of your patterning of interests. Are all your interests related to just one area?

Interests Table—*Continued*

Check whether this interest is *social or solitary* in nature		Check the column that best describes your *motivation* for engaging in this interest			Check one or more columns that best describes this interest		
Alone	With others	Exploration	Continuance	Achievement	Work	Play	Daily Living Tasks

Exercise Three

Belief in Skill

OBJECTIVE: to examine a component of personal causation—belief in skill—and its relationship to the pattern of occupations in your daily life

STEP ONE: Beside each activity below enter the code that best describes how well you think you do it. If you have never done the activity, rate how well you think you *would* do it after having some experience with it. Don't consider whether you'd like to do it or not; just indicate what you think your abilities would be. Use the following code:

G = I am (would be) good at this
O = I am (would be) okay at this
P = I am (would be) poor at this

1. Archery   _____

2. Ask someone for help   _____

3. Lead a discussion group   _____

4. Plan a party   _____

5. Exercise   _____

6. Balance a checkbook   _____

7. Run in a race   _____

8. Give helpful criticism to others   _____

9. Find resources in a new city   _____

10. Participate in a job interview   _____

11. Thread a needle   _____

12. Decide between two job offers   _____

13. Roller skate   _____

14. Budget money for the year   _____

15. Introduce myself to strangers   _____

Exercise Three—Continued

STEP TWO: Now, using the following key, enter scores for each activity by the appropriate number.

P = 1
O = 2
G = 3

1. _____   2. _____   4. _____

5. _____   3. _____   6. _____

7. _____   8. _____   9. _____

11. _____   10. _____   12. _____

13. _____   15. _____   14. _____

Total: _____   _____   _____

STEP THREE: Add up the scores in each column to find a total. Your first score represents your belief in your perceptual-motor skills; the second, your belief in your interpersonal/communication skills; and the third, your belief in your process (planning and problem-solving) skills. In looking over these scores, consider the following questions: Are your three scores equal or very similar? Do your current leisure interests overlap with the category(ies) in which you have your highest score? Do the scores reflect your own ideas about your abilities?

Exercise Four

Roles and Habits

OBJECTIVE: to examine the pattern of roles and habits in your daily life

STEP ONE: On the following tables list the major activities for a typical weekday and weekend day.

Weekday Role Table

List activities	Student	Worker	Volunteer	Caregiver	Home maintainer	Friend	Family member	Religious participant	Hobbyist/amateur	Participant in organizations	Other _____	Nonrole related
9:00												
10:00												
11:00												
12:00												
1:00												
2:00												
3:00												
4:00												
5:00												
6:00												
7:00												
8:00												
9:00												
10:00												

Exercise Four—Continued

STEP TWO: For each activity check the role which this activity fits. Some activities may not fit into any role and be just a habit. If this is the case, check the "Nonrole" column. (You may want to consult Chapter 2 which gives a more complete description of the roles that are listed.)

Weekend Role Table

List activities	Student	Worker	Volunteer	Care giver	Home maintainer	Friend	Family member	Religious participant	Hobbyist/amateur	Participant in organization	Other___	Nonrole related
9:00												
10:00												
11:00												
12:00												
1:00												
2:00												
3:00												
4:00												
5:00												
6:00												
7:00												
8:00												
9:00												
10:00												

Exercise Four—Continued

STEP THREE: In the first part of this exercise you observed how tasks are tied into certain roles. Roles organize other habits related to meeting expectations or standards of performance. List your present roles in the next table. Now think about the demands each role makes for certain standards of performance, e.g. self-care, clothing requirements, time use, and so on. Rate each role on the scale of 1–5 for each of the dimensions given in the table.

STEP FOUR: Add up the total scores for all roles. Compare which roles have more demanding standards and which are more informal and less demanding. A high number for several roles may indicate potential role conflict in your life, as this would mean that each of your roles is very exacting and demanding, and relatively distinct from your other roles.

Exercise Four—Continued

Habits Table

Role	5 4 3 2 1	Impeccable grooming vs Casual, lax, grooming	Uniform dress vs Nonuniform, wear what you want	Rigid schedule (same hours always) vs Flexible schedule	Routine performance vs Variable performance	Punctuality, promptness required vs Punctuality not required	Total

Exercise Five

Contexts of Daily Life

OBJECTIVE: to examine the pattern of novelty and routine in the settings of your daily life and the relationship between these settings and your work, leisure and daily living tasks

STEP ONE: In the chart make a list of the settings you usually enter on a typical *weekday* (for example, office, restaurant, classroom, and so on). Then make a similar list for the settings you enter on a *weekend* day.

Settings Table

Settings	Familiar	Novel
Weekday		
Weekend day		

416

Exercise Five—Continued

STEP TWO: Each column of the chart asks you to rate the settings on your list according to a particular quality. For example, is each setting familiar to you (you've been there often and know what to expect) or novel? Put a check in the columns that apply to each place.

STEP THREE: Consider the following questions. Were some places more arousing than others? What caused these places to be arousing to you—your role in that setting? other people? the tasks carried out there? the objects in the setting? Were your weekday and weekend day similar in the amount of novelty or familiarity of the settings?

Settings Table—*Continued*

My role here is:		Tasks I perform here are:			This place is:	
Important	Unimportant	Daily Living	Work	Leisure	Exciting	Boring

Exercise Six

Arousal and Environmental Layers

OBJECTIVE: to explore the concept of arousal and how the four environmental layers—objects, tasks, social groups, and culture—contribute to your own feelings of arousal

Arousal refers to feelings of excitement and stimulation generated by an interaction between a person's previous experiences and attributes of the environment. Novelty, complexity, and unfamiliarity are conditions that often contribute to increasing levels of arousal. This exercise involves four steps, each corresponding to one of the layers of the environment. For each part, you will consider why some situations or settings are more or less arousing for you.

Exercise Six—Continued

STEP ONE: Think of several *objects* that you find arousing and several that are unarousing. Generally, arousing objects may be things that you don't use too often or that your prefer not to use, while unarousing objects may be things that you interact with frequently. After you identify these objects, record them in the spaces below and answer the questions above each column.

Objects Table

Object	Is this object simple or complex?	Is it always used the same way (rigid use) or is it fairly malleable (flexible use)?	Is this object plentiful or relatively scarce?	What does this object mean to you? (For example, is it a status symbol?)
List three unarousing objects:				
List three arousing objects:				

Exercise Six—Continued

STEP TWO: Think of both an arousing and an unarousing *task* that you have performed recently. Then, on the dimensions below, place an X between each pair of characteristics at the point on the line which best describes the task. For example, if the unarousing task is extremely simple, place the X close to the word "simple." If, however, it is moderately complex, place the X closer to the word "complex." Do the same for each dimension for both tasks. Then connect the Xs to create a profile of the arousal level for each task. Do you generally prefer tasks that are more similar to the arousing task or the unarousing task? Which of the two tasks is more representative of the kinds of things you do everyday? In each task, what contributed to the presence or absence of arousal?

Tasks Table

Unarousing task: _____   Arousing task: _____

Simple ——————— Complex		Simple ——————— Complex
Time-limited ——————— Ongoing		Time-limited ——————— Ongoing
Whenever you want ——————— Certain times only		Whenever want ——————— Certain times only
Flexible rules ——————— Rigid rules		Flexible rules ——————— Rigid rules
Playful ——————— Serious		Playful ——————— Serious
Cooperative ——————— Competitive		Cooperative ——————— Competitive
Public ——————— Private		Public ——————— Private

Exercise Six—Continued

STEP THREE: Now compare two *organizations or groups* of which you are a member. Choose groups that differ in the degree of arousal they induce in you. To determine why one group is more arousing than the other, fill in the following chart.

Social Groups Table

Description	Arousing group:	Unarousing group:
How many people belong?		
What is its function?		
What do you do to become a member?		
Is this group highly vulnerable to things that happen outside it?		
What kinds of networks exist among members?		

In comparing the two groups, consider the following questions: Is the size of the group a source of arousal for you? Is the function? Was the group difficult to join, thereby making membership a source of arousal? Does this group expect members to be similar? If so, do your expectations of not being like other members lead to your arousal? Is the group vulnerable to outside forces, thus making its activities more consequential and arousing? Are the networks in the group complex, making it difficult to "learn the ropes"?

Exercise Six—Continued

STEP FOUR: The highest level of the environment is *culture*. Because people are often members of more than one cultural group, arousal may be created when these cultures differ in their values, use of time, space, and so on. Identify two cultural groups to which you belong* and try to answer the questions in the table for each one. Are your answers discrepant for these two cultures? Are the demands of one culture more arousing to you than those of the other?

---

* For example, American, Irish, Catholic, Jewish, rural farm culture, urban professional, and so on.

Culture Table

Description	Cultural group	Cultural group
What are some highly valued activities?		
What are the cultural meanings of these activities?		
Do you participate in these activities?		
Does anything happen if you don't? Why or why not?		

Exercise Six—Continued

Cultural Table—*Continued*

Description	Cultural group	Cultural group
What are some activities not approved by this culture?		
Have you or do you ever do these?		
Are there ever any consequences? What are they?		
Does this culture emphasize doing one thing at a time? keeping busy?		
Do you associate certain places with this culture? which?		
Does this culture emphasize tradition and ritual?		
How are norms usually taught? (informally, technically or formally)		

Exercise Seven

The Development of Your Occupational Life-Style

OBJECTIVE: to examine the relationship of occupational roles to life stages and events in your own life

STEP ONE: On the time line below, list up to 10 of your major life events in a developmental sequence. These events might include starting elementary school, going to college, your first job, marriage, and so on.

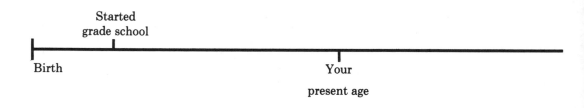

STEP TWO: Using the life events from the time line, list on the following form the occupational roles that were/are taken on or given up with each event. For example, in marriage, the roles of caregiver and home maintainer might be assumed; in graduation from college, the role of student might be left.

Exercise Seven—Continued

Occupational Roles

Event	Roles left	Roles assumed

Is there always an even exchange between roles assumed and roles left? Do certain life events leave you with a deficit of roles? A surplus? Are there any life events that seem to have been a response to having an imbalance in roles?

STEP THREE: Choose one role that has been particularly meaningful to you, and in which you have been involved for a long period of time. Examine how the task expectations, your habits, your ability to perform in this role, and so on, have changed over time. For example, in a work role, some changes over time might include moving from the position of trainee, to staff position, to supervisor; along with these changes the individual may have felt a steady increase in confidence and competence to perform; finally, increasing commitment to the role may have led the person to allocate more time to this role and less time to some other pursuit.

SECTION B:
Clinical Application of the Model

Exercise Eight

Occupational Analysis

OBJECTIVE: to practice an approach to occupational analysis which is based on the model of human occupation

STEP ONE: Review Chapter 12 and the analysis of meal preparation as an occupation. The work sheets for this exercise follow the format used in that chapter.

STEP TWO: Choose an occupation that is personally meaningful to you, either because you use it in the clinic, because it is a special interest of yours or because it is something you plan to use one day. Now answer the questions included on the sheets entitled *Occupational Analysis*.

STEP THREE: The work sheets entitled *Clinical Occupational Analysis* ask you to envision using the occupation in a clinic setting. Complete the three parts to this stage of analysis.

STEP FOUR: The *Occupational Relevance Scale* and the *Occupational Content Form* allow you to summarize the results of the Occupational Analysis and the Clinical Occupational Analysis. After completing this step, do you think that this is an occupation you will use (or continue to use) in the clinic?

Exercise Eight—Continued

Occupational Analysis

I. **Environmental analysis.** What press is created by objects, tasks, social groups and culture in this occupation?

   A. **Objects:** What objects are used in this occupation, and what are their characteristics (availability, complexity, flexibility, symbolic meanings)?

   B. **Tasks.** What action sequences must be carried out? What are important task characteristics (complexity, rigidity, degree of playfulness, temporal requirements, social nature)?

   C. **Social groups/organizations.** What social groups/organizations use this activity?

   D. **Culture.** What is the cultural significance of this activity?

Exercise Eight—Continued

Occupational Analysis—*Continued*

II. **Volitional analysis.** How does this occupation activate personal causation, values and interests?
   A. **Personal causation.** Does it provide experiences of personal effectiveness, through skill use relevant to everyday life? Does it provide experience in management of external and internal control? Are outcomes predictable?

   B. **Values.** What are inherent performance standards? What awareness of time (past, present, future) and of time use is developed in this occupation? What other values may be enacted?

   C. **Interests.** Does it provide variety? Is it likely to be familiar to many people? Is it widely available?

Exercise Eight—Continued

Occupational Analysis—*Continued*

III. **Habituation analysis.** How does this occupation organize behavior into habits and roles?

A. **Roles.** Is this occupation important in performance of the following roles: worker, caregiver, home maintainer, family member, friend, student, volunteer, organization participant, religious participant, hobbyist/amateur, other? Explain briefly.

B. **Habits.** Describe the primary habit systems which organize behavior in this occupation.

Exercise Eight—Continued

Occupational Analysis—*Continued*

IV. **Performance analysis.** In the performance of this occupation, how are perceptual-motor, process and interpersonal skills used?

Under each skill category, list the primary habit systems identified in step III, and describe the relevant aspects of the activity.

A. **Perceptual-motor:**

B. **Process:**

C. **Communication/interaction:**

Exercise Eight—Continued

Occupational Analysis—*Continued*

V. **Output analysis.** How is this occupation used in work, play and/or daily living tasks?

   A. **Work:**

   B. **Play:**

   C. **Daily living tasks:**

Exercise Eight—Continued

Clinical Occupational Analysis

I. **Exploratory learning.** What arrangements of object, task, social group, and cultural context will encourage skill learning?

Skill Sequence (graded behaviors to be learned for this skill)	**Occupational environment** (object, task, social group, cultural context)
A.	A.
B.	B.
C.	C.
D.	D.
E.	E.

Exercise Eight—Continued

Clinical Occupational Analysis—*Continued*

II. **Competence learning.** How can the occupation be practiced as part of daily routines? Identify practice routines using the occupation in work, play and daily living tasks.

   A. **Daily living tasks:**

   B. **Leisure:**

   C. **Work:**

III. **Achievement learning.** How can the occupation be used in role performance?

   Occupational role: ⎯⎯⎯⎯⎯⎯⎯⎯⎯⎯⎯⎯⎯⎯⎯⎯⎯⎯

   Occupation: ⎯⎯⎯⎯⎯⎯⎯⎯⎯⎯⎯⎯⎯⎯⎯⎯⎯⎯⎯

   A. **Standards of performance.** Describe standards of performance for this role using this occupation.

   B. **Trial enactment.** Identify a graded sequence for trial enactment of the role.
      Stage 1. Planning:

      Stage 2. Implementation:

      Stage 3. Feedback:

Exercise Eight—Continued

Occupational Relevance Scale

Occupation: _____

Evaluate the occupation on the following factors. Place check mark in appropriate column.

	High	Moderate	Low
Performance/output			
Uses a variety of skills (perceptual-motor, process, interpersonal)	————	————	————
Important in work, play and daily living tasks	————	————	————
Behavioral organization			
Used in many roles	————	————	————
Generates practical habit patterns	————	————	————
Motivation			
Allows a wide range of choice	————	————	————
Is highly valued in the dominant culture	————	————	————
Environmental press			
Can be easily practiced in ordinary settings	————	————	————
Can generate various levels of arousal	————	————	————

Exercise Eight—Continued

Occupational Content Form

Occupation: _____

Evaluate the occupation on the following factors. Place check mark opposite appropriate description.

Output
In which area(s) of output is the occupation used?

    _____ Work

    _____ Play

    _____ Daily living tasks

Production
What skills are frequently used in the occupation?

    _____ Perceptual-motor

    _____ Process

    _____ Interpersonal

Habituation
For which roles is the occupation useful?

_____ Caregiver	_____ Volunteer
_____ Worker	_____ Family member
_____ Friend	_____ Hobbyist
_____ Student	_____ Home maintainer

    _____ Organization participant

    _____ Religious participant

    _____ Other _____

Volition
Which aspects of volition does it develop?

    _____ Exploring personal/social values

    _____ Developing interests

    _____ Experiencing personal effectiveness

Environment
In which social groups is it often enacted?

    _____ Solitary   _____ Friends

    _____ Family   _____ Community

In what settings is it usually practiced?

    _____ Home   _____ Workplace

    _____ School   _____ Neighborhood

    _____ Other _____

Exercise Nine

Treatment Planning

OBJECTIVE: to integrate information presented in chapters on treatment planning and applications by applying it to a case study

STEP ONE: For this exercise, either select one of the cases included here or choose one from your own practice (this may be a patient you are no longer treating but for whom you still retain evaluation materials). Before starting, you may wish to reproduce the work sheets for this exercise in order to have blank copies for future use. Although this exercise involves judgment and there are no "right" answers, suggested answers are included as a guide for comparison.

After deciding which case you will use, formulate a list of clinical questions that will establish a treatment plan based on sound clinical reasoning. In developing these questions, you may wish to refer to the table "Evaluation Outline" that appears on p 438 which includes some questions from Chapter 11, Treatment Planning, as well as alternative questions that reflect the American Occupational Therapy Association (AOTA) Uniform Terminology.

Read the presenting information below for the case you choose, and record your clinical questions on *Work Sheet 1*. Then compare your questions with those listed in *Part A* of the case you chose. On the basis of this comparison, add any questions you now feel should be a part of your list.

CASE 1: Mrs. Duffy

Presenting Information

The patient, Mrs. Duffy, is a 73-year-old woman whose second husband died approximately 8 years ago. He suffered from a heart condition and gradually became housebound for a year before he died. Mrs. Duffy feels guilty regarding his death as she granted permission for a biopsy, after which her husband died. She had her first major depressive episode after his death. She was treated as an outpatient and placed on medication. She has no friends at this time and quit her job as a bookkeeper prior to hospitalization. Mrs. Duffy was talking about suicide to her sons; this precipitated her current hospitalization.

CASE 2: Tim

Presenting Information

Tim is a 25-year-old young man who was in good health on duty with the U.S. Army in Europe when he was involved in an automobile accident. Tim does not remember the circumstances of his accident, but he was found severely injured, breathing on his own, but unable to move any part of his body below the neck.

The diagnosis is complete quadraplegia with cervical fractures of C_5 anterior on C_6. He also sustained an open laceration of the left lower extremity, left upper thigh and a transverse contusion across the abdomen with questionable internal injuries. He was stabilized medically and transported to a hospital in Europe. Gardner Wells tongs and 20 pounds of traction were employed to reduce the C_5, C_6 fracture, and he was placed on a Stryker frame.

Medical examination showed good ($4/5$) cervical trapezius bilaterally, and trace ($1/5$) deltoid on the left. Touch sensation below the nipple line was absent symmetrically. Pinprick sensation was absent below the clavicles symmetrically. Pinprick sensation was intact for deltoid, biceps, forearm area, and thumbs bilaterally and there was residual sensation in the C_7 dermatome in the hand. There was no evidence of sacral sensation and sphincters were flaccid.

Exercise Nine—Continued

A CT scan revealed multiple fractures through the bodies of C_5 and C_6, through the posterior elements of C_5 and C_6 and a fracture through the facet of C_6 on the right. Eighty pounds of traction unlocked the right facet. Six weeks after the injury, he was transferred to a Spinal Cord Injury Unit in the United States for a rehabilitation program. Since treatment goals vary over the course of rehabilitation for Tim, you will be asked in this case to evaluate and to set goals and treatment plans at a particular point.

Upon transfer to the Rehabilitation Unit, Tim was placed in a halo brace and vest to stabilize the fractures. Manual muscle testing at this time revealed *good* sternocleidomastoid and *good* trapezius, and spinal accessary bilaterally. Patient had *trace* supraspinatus bilaterally, *poor* infraspinatus on right, *trace* infraspinatus on left, *trace* anterior deltoid, middle deltoid, posterior deltoid, rhomboids and biceps on the right and *poor* teres minor on the right. On the left patient had *0* anterior deltoid, *trace* posterior, middle deltoid, *trace* rhomboids, teres minor and biceps. Sensation evaluation revealed sensation present at C_6 level dermatome. Pinprick and 2-point discrimination are present at C_7.

PHASE II. Five months after the injury, the halo traction was removed as the patients' cervical spine demonstrated stability on x-ray. Muscle strength was increasing due to decreased edema, stabilization of the cervical spine, and the therapy program. Areas of increasing muscle strength were: *fair* triceps and wrist extension on the right and *poor+* wrist extension on the left. Tim was able at this point to drive his electric wheelchair with an assistive device. With a ball bearing feeder attached to his wheelchair and a setup for meals he can feed himself. Tim is practicing with the ball bearing feeder and practicing wheelchair mobility.

It is at this phase, and with the above performance subsystem data, that you are evaluating the patient for further treatment goals and strategies.

STEP TWO: Use your revised list of questions to determine how you will evaluate the patient. You may find it helpful to review the Instrument Library in the Appendix. Keep in mind that one assessment may answer several questions.

Record your assessment choices in the second column of *Work Sheet 1*. When through, refer to *Part B* of the case and compare your choices with the instruments that were actually used. (If this is your own case, what instruments did you use in practice? Are they the same as the ones you now listed?) If the answers you listed are different from the ones used in the case, check to see if your choices adequately cover or reflect your clinical questions. Different patterns of instruments can yield similar information, so your instruments may vary while still being appropriate.

STEP THREE: Review the results of the assessments which are summarized in *Part C* of the case (or the results of evaluations you administered to your own client). Use *Work Sheet 2* to summarize the patient's assets and liabilities. Then integrate this data into a model or theory of dysfunction in this client, and briefly summarize this theory in the appropriate space.

Now, check your responses by comparing them with *Part D* of the case study.

STEP FOUR: You have formulated clinical questions, assessed the patient, listed assets and liabilities, and developed an explanation of the occupational dysfunction in this patient. It is now appropriate to establish an intervention plan. On *Work Sheet 3*, record goals and treatment methods in the appropriate columns. These goals and methods should reflect the patient's own goals and the status of each subsystem.

To compare your answers with those used in the case, refer to *Part E*. (If you used your own case, would you make any changes in what you did?)

Now that you have completed one case study, you may wish to try the other workbook case or to select one from your own experience to practice further.

Exercise Nine—Continued

Evaluation Outline

Occupational behavior model	Uniform terminology
VOLITION	
Does the person feel in control and expect success or failure in various life situations?	What is the status of the person's psychosocial skills, such as self-concept?
What occupations are meaningful for this person?	
What standards of performance guide his/her actions?	
What goals does this person have?	
Can this person identify interests and does he/she enact them? What is the pattern?	What interests does the person evidence?
What is this person's orientation to time? (consider use and beliefs)	

Exercise Nine—Continued

Evaluation Outline—*Continued*

Occupational behavior model	Uniform terminology
HABITUATION	
What roles has this person internalized?	What are the person's life roles?
Does the person identify an imbalance, conflict, or loss of roles?	Is there a balance to these roles?
PERFORMANCE	
How does the person problem-solve, plan & organize behavior?	What is the person's functional status in: physical daily living sensory motor cognitive & psychosocial skills?

Work Sheet 1. Clinical Questions and Assessments

Use this worksheet to organize a list of clinical questions that will help you to develop a treatment plan.

Model component	Clinical questions	Assessment instruments
Volition Personal causation:		
Values:		
Interests:		
Habituation Roles:		
Habits:		

Performance
Skills:

Environment
Current:

Expected:

Exercise Nine—Continued

Work Sheet 2. Patient Status

Use the space below to identify the patient's assets and liabilities, and to propose a theory or explanation of dysfunction in this person.

Model component	Assets	Liabilities
Volition Personal causation:		
Values:		
Interests:		
Habituation Roles:		
Habits:		

Exercise Nine—Continued

Work Sheet 2—*Continued*

Model component	Assets	Liabilities
Performance Skills:		
Environment Current:		
Expected:		

Explanation/theory of the dynamics of dysfunction:

Exercise Nine—Continued

Work Sheet 3. Intervention Plan

Establish a plan for intervention by recording treatment goals and methods in the appropriate columns below.

	Goals
Volition	
Habituation	
Performance	
Environment	

Exercise Nine—Continued

Work Sheet 3—*Continued*

Methods

Exercise Nine—Continued

CASE 1: MRS. DUFFY

PARTS A and B: CLINICAL QUESTIONS AND ASSESSMENTS FOR MRS. DUFFY

Model component	Part A Clinical questions	Part B Assessment instruments
Volition		
Personal causation	Does Mrs. Duffy feel in control of her life? Does she derive feelings of efficacy from her daily activities? Does she view herself as capable or incapable?	Internal/External Scale Occupational History (OH) Unstructured activity interview (AI)
Values	Does Mrs. Duffy value her daily activities? What sources of meaning exist for her in daily life?	OH, AI
	What is her temporal orientation?	Time Reference Inventory
Interests	What are her interests? Does she enact these interests? Does she have a balance of social, solitary, passive, active, and other types of interests?	AI Interest Checklist
Habituation		
Roles	What roles has Mrs. Duffy internalized? Why has she given up the worker role? Has she recently given up or been deprived of any other roles? Does she have a balance among her roles?	Role Checklist (Part I)[a]
Habits	Do Mrs. Duffy's habits support her roles? Does she use her time well? Or does she spend a long time getting little done?	AI
Performance		
Skills	Are Mrs. Duffy's cognitive, interactional, and motor skills intact? Are her skills relevant to her roles and interests?	OH Clinical observation
Environment		
Current	Where is Mrs. Duffy living now? What are the expectations of others in her environment for her to be productive? Does her environment provide the physical resources she needs to be productive?	OH
Expected	Will she be returning to this same environment? If her environment is unsatisfactory, how easily can it—or parts of it—be changed?	OH

[a] Part II was not available when Mrs. Duffy was evaluated.

Exercise Nine—Continued

PART C: ASSESSMENT RESULTS FOR MRS. DUFFY

Occupational History

Mrs. Duffy is a highly skilled bookkeeper, but interrupted this work role to raise her two sons. Although she has been recently working part-time, she quit her job prior to her present hospitalization. During her previous depressive episode in which she was treated as an outpatient, she was able to maintain her worker role.

In the past, Mrs. Duffy was very concerned with keeping her home clean and neat. She related that, "If you smoked a cigarette I would empty the ash tray immediately." However, since her depression 8 years ago, she has slowly neglected her apartment. Her apartment is roach infested, has holes in the walls, and is cluttered with boxes full of her late husband's clothing and various other items. She lives in a "bad" neighborhood and does not feel safe leaving her apartment.

Mrs. Duffy had a very active social life when her husband was alive. They dined out frequently and had many friends whom they visited. Mrs. Duffy's two sons are from her first marriage; she also has six grandchildren. She spends her weekends with one or the other son and highly values her relationship with them and her grandchildren. One of her sons has been attempting to rent an apartment for her close to his home. Mrs. Duffy's role as caregiver and family member to her grandchildren were the only roles about which she expressed any enjoyment or excitement during the occupational history interview.

Time Reference Inventory

SCORING SUMMARY

	Past	Present	Future	Totals
Positive (first 10 items)	10	0	0	10
Negative (second 10 items)	0	10	0	10
Neutral (third 10 items)	10	0	0	10
Total	20	10	0	30

Average years projected into future = 0 (mean for normals is 9.6)
Average years projected into past   = 51.4
Average age focus   = 52 (her present age is 73)

Exercise Nine—Continued

Interest Checklist

PRESENT INTERESTS

	Number of like very much	0
	Number of like	14
	Number of indifferent	66
	Number of dislike	0
	Number of dislike very much	0

PAST INTERESTS

	More	25
	Same	55
	Less	0

PATTERNS OF INTEREST

The activities she like included music, spending time with her children, laundry, TV, and knitting. However, none of her interests were strong interests; nor did she indicate strong dislikes for activities. This lack of potency of interests did not seem to be a problem in the past, as she indicated stronger degrees of interest in 25 activities prior to her depression. Just before her hospitalization, Mrs. Duffy had suspended participation in all her interests except for television and family-related activities.

Mrs. Duffy's current interest pattern reflects a focus on solitary activities such as reading, watching television and listening to music, except when activities involve her family. Mrs. Duffy enjoyed more household-related tasks and socially oriented activities such as concerts and dancing prior to her depression. Her pattern of interests has narrowed with her diminished discrimination and potency.

Role Checklist

Role	Past	Present	Future
Student			
Worker	X		X(maybe)
Volunteer			
Caregiver	X	X	X
Home maintainer	X		X
Friend	X		X
Family member	X	X	X
Religious			
Participation			
Hobbyist/amateur	X		
Participant in organizations			X

Exercise Nine—Continued

Unstructured Activity Interview

Mrs. Duffy indicated that her daily routine was very limited prior to her hospitalization. In a typical day she woke up between 5 and 6:30 a.m., stayed in her pajamas, made tea, went back to bed, got up again, paced in her apartment and "looked through the peephole." She felt unsafe in her neighborhood, but would sometimes go out in the afternoon to get something to eat. She rarely cooked and did little, if any, housework. Her weekends were spent with her sons and her grandchildren.

Internal/External Scale

Mrs. Duffy scored a 16 which indicates a high external orientation.

Observations During Assessment

Mrs. Duffy required three 45-minute sessions to complete the battery of tests. Overall, she was cooperative but had difficulty concentrating and was unable to complete any of the tests independently. She needed much support and reassurance. The second day she was overtly more depressed, complaining of dizziness, how difficult it was to get dressed (although she showered and dressed in 10 minutes while I waited), and how little sleep she got due to her roommate. She made an interesting slip when she said, "I'm dizzy, I'm busy, I'm dizzy."

Exercise Nine—Continued

PART D: MRS. DUFFY'S OCCUPATIONAL STATUS

Model component	Assets	Liabilities
Volition		
Personal causation		Strong belief in external control
Values	Values family and caregiver roles. Prior to depression, had high performance standards	Is not oriented to future; views past more positively than present
Interests	Although not strong, did identify past interests. Continued to participate in family-related interests before hospitalization	Indifferent to many activities in present; enacting few interests and most of these were solitary
Habituation		
Roles	Maintained roles of family member and caregiver; had achieved in worker role in past	Has lost worker, home maintainer, friend, and hobbyist roles.
Habits		Habits totally disrupted prior to hospitalization; large blocks of time doing nothing, or pacing
Performance		
Skills	Motor skills intact	Unable to concentrate, cannot plan or make decisions
Environment		
Current	Family is supportive and nearby	Neighborhood is unsafe. Apartment was neglected, is dirty and roach infested. Lives alone
Expected	Son wants to find new apartment for her to move to	

Exercise Nine—Continued

Explanation/Theory of the Dynamics of Dysfunction

Mrs. Duffy was an intelligent woman attempting to cope with her husband's death. The disruption in her life-style, initiated by his death, had been associated with a progressive decline in her participation in occupational roles.

In the past, Mrs. Duffy led an active social life, had many friends, was a meticulous housekeeper, and despite her age, maintained a part-time job as a bookkeeper. All of these roles had deteriorated. She felt unable to change her life situation and had given up all responsibility for worker and home maintainer roles. Although her future orientation was extremely limited, she did indicate several roles she saw in the future for herself. She also had been able to maintain the roles of family member and caregiver, albeit on a limited basis.

Mrs. Duffy's routine prior to hospitalization was extremely maladaptive. Her only adaptive occupational behavior related to her weekends when she visited her sons and grandchildren. In summary, Mrs. Duffy appeared to be fluctuating between incompetence and helplessness. However, her minimal role maintenance and a few interests had kept her from having a total disruption in all subsystems.

Exercise Nine—Continued

PART E: INTERVENTION PLAN FOR MRS. DUFFY

Model subsystem	Goals	Method
Volition	Enable patient to assume control while in hospital	Give Mrs. Duffy self-transportation privileges; encourage her to use hospital facilities (such as library) on her own; involve in planning treatment program; provide positive feedback on skills
	Examine future goals	Focus on ways to resume worker role
	Reactivate past interests	Provide connections with caregiver role and past interests, e.g. knitting a birthday gift for grandchild
Habituation	Explore possibilities for resuming interrupted roles	Contact organizations related to interests, call former employer, join cooking group in occupational therapy
	Improve use of time; take responsibility for self-care habits	Resume daily living routine in small increments in hospital; carry over leisure activities from occupational therapy to free time
Performance	Increase capacity for independent work and decision making	Involve in decisions regarding treatment; encourage her to take responsibility for planning use of free time
Environment	Explore possibility of moving; if not feasible, then examine ways to improve current apartment	Involve family in activities related to either relocation or reorganizing apartment

Exercise Nine—Continued

CASE 2: TIM

PARTS A AND B: CLINICAL QUESTIONS AND ASSESSMENTS FOR TIM

Model component	Part A Clinical questions	Part B Assessment instruments
Volition		
Personal causation	How much control does Tim feel he has over his present life situation? Is there evidence of a previous level of control over life goals and plans?	Occupational History (OH) Clinical observations Activity Record (AR)
Values	What did Tim like to do in his free time? What things and events does he value? What are important activities now? Is there a major change in the value of daily occupations? What are his goals for the future?	OH, AR (for a day prior to accident and a day in the hospital)
Interests	What is his past level of participation and enjoyment of occupation? In the past was he able to discriminate among interests? What is his interest pattern? What is his current level of participation in activities?	AR Interest Checklist (modified)
Habituation		
Roles	What are his perceived past, present and future roles? Was there a balance of roles prior to accident? What roles were disrupted by the accident?	OH Role Checklist
Habits	How did he organize time prior to the accident? How is his time organized in the hospital? Are hospital routines supportive of his anticipated future roles?	AR, OH
Performance		
Skills	What are his perceptual-motor skills? What are his communication/interaction skills? What are his process skills? What potentials does he have for skills necessary to attain occupational goals and fulfill occupational roles?	Manual muscle testing, sensory testing, and passive/active range-of-motion evaluation and activities of daily living evaluation as summarized under phase II description. Other evaluations would include observation of problem-solving and communication/interaction skills to determine adequacy for roles and goals

Exercise Nine—Continued

PART C: ASSESSMENT RESULTS FOR TIM

Occupational History Data

Prior to his accident, Tim worked full time as an Army section chief in radio operation and repairs. He was stationed in Germany. He had joined the Armed Forces because he wanted a change from his college major in music. In the Army, he was offered three career options and chose electronics. He was satisfied with his choice. He worked at his present job for the past 7 years. He liked the trouble shooting and problem-solving aspects, but disliked the long hours. At times, he would work in the field for 72 hours. Prior to joining the Army, he had part-time jobs during college, working in gas stations. He related no role models or guidance from parents regarding his career choice. However, his job history does reflect competence and his feelings of personal causation in work.

In college, Tim studied the trumpet, piano and guitar. He liked school and enjoyed studying and learning new things. While in the Army, he continued using his musical talent and skills as a hobby. He was a disk jockey, and also played in many bands in Europe. His paralysis prevents his playing any of these musical instruments. Tim had a highly organized schedule before (one largely determined by the Army, although he shows good use of free time). Now, he is controlled by the rehabilitation schedule and reports disliking this feeling of external control.

In the future, Tim sees himself working as a biomedical engineer. He would like to design equipment for maximizing the independence of quadriplegic patients (e.g. television, tape players and computers). Currently, his parents (who are supportive of his goals) are checking school entrance requirements and wheelchair accessibility, but Tim has not concretized his goal beyond this point. He does appear to derive a strong sense of purpose from this goal and to be very committed to it. Tim made his career decision 2 months after the accident in the hospital. At that time he questioned what he would do for the rest of his life. He feels that his strengths to pursue this goal are his stubbornness and his willingness to try new challenges. He is not able to spell out particular obstacles or requirements for himself to return to school and for the actual work by being an engineer. His experimentation with the role has been through designing adaptive equipment for himself and others. He has done this successfully with the equipment being fabricated by a therapist or by other patients. He demonstrates a good ability to communicate his ideas orally as he has not yet attempted drawing or drafting.

His plans or goals for the future involve the following:

1. Going to school
2. Learning how to drive
3. Living with his parents
4. Getting married (his present girl friend is pregnant and a wedding is planned)

One year from now, he sees himself in school with part-time work, and 5 years from now, in business for himself and taking care of his wife and child.

Exercise Nine—Continued

Results of the Interest Checklist

Patient indicated his level of interest on 68 activities of the interest checklist for the past 10 years. No other categories of the checklist were completed since it was determined to be too stressful for a first meeting. The following is a breakdown of the results.

Number of strong interests: 36
Includes the following categories of activities:

Physical Sports: Football, bowling, swimming, auto racing, hunting, cycling, pool, exercise, fishing, driving, camping, walking

Social/Recreation: Playing cards, dancing, holiday activities, chess, visiting, traveling, parties, concerts, dating, table games

Activities of Daily Living: Car repair, cooking/baking, shopping

Manual Skills: Car repair, model building

Cultural/Educational: Languages (Austrian, German, Spanish), reading, classical music, collecting coins, concerts

Number of some interest: 22
Gardening, writing, pets, mending, barbecues, wrestling, housecleaning, pottery, home decorating, clubs, singing, clothes, handicrafts, attending plays, home repairs, woodworking, child care, tennis, science, leatherwork, photography, painting/drawing

Number of no interest: 10
Includes: laundry/ironing, politics, scouting, hairstyling, basketball, sewing/needlework, church activities, golf, and speeches

The three most important interests for this patient are:

1. Bowling
2. Driving
3. Auto repair

Also notable is that, while hospitalized, Tim has participated in wheelchair sports and bowling.

Exercise Nine—Continued

Results of the Role Checklist

Role	Past	Present	Future	Value
Student	X	X[a]	X	Very valuable
Worker	X		X	Very valuable
Volunteer	X		?	Somewhat valuable
Caregiver	X		X	Somewhat valuable
Home maintainer	X		X	Somewhat valuable
Friend	X	X	X	Very valuable
Family member	X	X	X	Very valuable
Religious participant	X		?	Somewhat valuable
Hobbyist/amateur	X	X	X	Somewhat valuable
Participant in organizations	X	X[b]	X	Somewhat valuable

[a] He considers his current rehabilitation program to be school—thus, the present student role.

[b] Veterans Association.

Exercise Nine—Continued

Activity Record

Tim filled out an activity record for a typical day prior to his accident and for his present rehabilitation schedule in order to determine changes.

Results of the Activity Checklist

Percentage of time spent:	Prior to accident	In hospital
Doing things one does well	78	26
Doing things very important	68	23
Doing things valued a lot	100	23
Doing things enjoyed a lot	83	20

Remarkable aspects of his present schedule are long periods of time spent waiting for nursing services or therapies and several hours spent watching television each day. The waiting time is not only negatively experienced, but also contributes to feelings of helplessness. He does not particularly value or find interesting the time in the evening spent watching television.

Exercise Nine—Continued

PART D: TIM'S OCCUPATIONAL STATUS

Model variable	Strengths	Liabilities
Volition		
Personal causation	Feels some sense of control since he is able to help out in dressing, and is able to feed himself when set up with ball bearing feeder. Historically, he has had personal causation and appears to be attempting to reinstate control through future goals	Feels controlled by hospital routine and staff. Much time spent "waiting" especially in the morning. Poor grooming may contribute to a sense of helplessness. Personal causation is at risk if he encounters unforeseen obstacles to goal attainment after discharge
Interests	He is able to discriminate among interests and has numerous strong interests (bowling, driving, and auto repair are most important). He continues participation in many interests despite hospitalization and is motivated to pursue other interests	Interference of many past interests due to performance subsystem limitations
Values	He considers rehabilitation therapies to be enjoyable and meaningful and he enjoyed and found meaning in activity prior to hospitalization. He has a definite long-term goal for the future; he would like to be a biomedical engineer. Two roles relating to this goal, student and worker, are highly valued by Tim	Much time spent "waiting" especially in the morning (contrary to his values of using time well). Much time in evening is spent watching TV and this is not a valued activity. He has not clearly formulated necessary intermediate objectives for attaining long-term goals
Habituation		
Roles	He identifies five continuous roles: 1. Student (he views rehabilitation program as form of school) 2. Friend 3. Family member 4. Hobbyist 5. Participant in organizations He plans to enter the student, worker and caregiver roles. He had good role balance prior to accident.	He has three major role disruptions—worker, caregiver, and home maintainer. He does not appear to have a clear sense of role obligations for some roles or any specific plans for meeting those obligations. For example, he has not anticipated what will be necessary skills and habits for the student worker and caregiver roles, each of which the plans to enter in the future

Exercise Nine—Continued

PART D:　TIM'S OCCUPATIONAL STATUS—*Continued*

Model variable	Strengths	Liabilities
Habits	He previously had good habit patterns. He has established routine in hospital	Tim's habits related to grooming are poor. Tim has not established habits related to student or worker role. All of his time in the evening is spent watching TV. He has too much waiting time over which he has no control
Performance		
Skills	He is mobile in the electric wheelchair. Tim is generally becoming stronger in upper extremities and is able to move his arm to his mouth. He is beginning to hone wrist extension. He is able to feed himself when set up in ball bearing feeder. Tim has good communication/interaction skills and is a good problem solver, using this latter ability to think of adaptations for himself and others	Overall muscle strength is trace to poor and passive range of motion is within normal limits. Sensation present at C_6 level dermatome. Pin prick and 2-point discrimination are present at C_7 level. He has a severe loss of hand function, limiting all activities of daily living skills

Explanation/Model of Tim's Occupational Status

Tim is a previously competent individual whose injury and subsequent quadriplegia has severely limited his perceptual motor skills. Fortunately, he has good communication/ interaction and process skills which he is beginning to use to compensate for the losses. Tim's success in problem solving to creatively design adaptive equipment has encouraged his belief in his abilities to become a biomedical engineer. Tim appears to have the intellectual capacity to pursue this goal, but has not developed explicit goals to attain the necessary status as an engineering student nor has he explored many of the skills needed for both the student and engineering role. His appraisal of these role and goal demands needs to become more specific, along with his understanding of his abilities and limitations and the necessary adaptations to bridge any gaps. Additionally, Tim has a highly structured routine imposed by the rehabilitation program and he has not prepared for postdischarge when he must organize his own time. The arrangement he will have with his parents and his wife and yet unborn child remains to be worked out. Thus, while he is currently functioning at an exploratory level, beginning to reinstate some skills and to formulate life plans, he needs to proceed to a competency level where he would acquire the necessary organization of behavior to enter role performance upon discharge.

Exercise Nine—Continued

PART E: INTERVENTION PLAN FOR TIM

Model variable	Goal	Methods
Volition		
Personal causation	To increase feelings of control. To avoid possible threats to control in future. To encourage realistic assessment of skills possessed and needed for goals and roles	Share with patient the results of the battery of tests reviewing strengths and liabilities. Planning and practice for student and worker roles
Interests	To increase and maintain participation in interests	Explore ways patient could use "waiting" time in pursuit of interests
Values	To increase amount of time spent in meaningful activity. To more clearly specify short-term goals pursuant to his long-term goals of school and work	Explore time in the evening watching TV (not a valued activity). Would patient like to change time spent watching TV? Collaborative review of goals and planning for goal attainment
Habituation		
Roles	To be able to incorporate disrupted roles into new life-style as a disabled person. To clarify expectations of student and worker role along with special difficulties he might encounter	Explore roles of student, worker, home maintainer and caregiver with patient and the expected role behaviors. Explore with Tim necessary adaptations for resuming these roles (e.g. helping in care of child). Related to worker role, explore career as a biomedical engineer. Simulate prevocational tasks related to this job. Refer to vocational rehabilitation
Habits	To be able to make a transition from routines in hospital to routines necessary for personal goals. To encourage necessary daily living skills for these roles	Establish a routine in hospital that more closely resembles school or work routines. Obtain further information about grooming. Will family member of aid assist? Set up schedule with patient to improve self-care and time use and graduate over time to allow increasing responsibility
Performance		
Skills	To maintain and increase muscle strength. Utilize good process skills. To graduate from ball bearing feeder to universal cuff. Increase wheelchair mobility	Participate in occupations of interest. Participation in occupations that incorporate problem-solving skills and expected role behaviors of student and worker (i.e. using books, drafting equipment with adaptations). Practice using universal cuff. Involve patient in wheelchair sports

Exercise Ten

Program Development

OBJECTIVE: to use the model of human occupation as the basis for developing, expanding,
or revising an occupational therapy program

This exercise involves a synthesis of the theory and applications that have preceded
it. There are no answers or feedback for the exercise, but the program illustrations in
Chapter 13 can serve as a review. To begin the exercise, decide what setting you are
planning to apply this to; if you are a student, your fieldwork setting may be a good
choice. Also, determine whether or not you want to review an existing program using
this guide in order to identify possible changes, or to start a new program where none
has existed.

STEP ONE: Identify characteristics of the population in this setting. Use the following
framework to describe performance deficits and etiology, typical occupational behavior
and environmental characteristics, and the nature of occupational dysfunction.

Performance Deficits

Major pathological conditions or conditions for which population is at risk	Causes	Areas of occupational performance skill deficits (typical referral reasons)

Desired/Typical Occupational Life-styles

Volitional characteristics	Typical roles and habit patterns	Skills needed/used in everyday life	Environmental characteristics (objects, tasks, groups, cultural values)

Exercise Ten—Continued

Nature of Occupational Dysfunction

Typical level of Dysfunction. (inefficacy, incompetence, helplessness)

Type of Dysfunction.
Volition:

Habituation:

Performance:

How does environment contribute to, or maintain, dysfunction?

How do usual life-style or behavior patterns contribute to, or maintain, dysfunction?

Anticipated length of time to reverse occupational dysfunction.

Exercise Ten—Continued

STEP TWO: This step involves a delineation of program goals, resources needed, specific therapeutic procedures, and the sequencing of the program.

General Program Goals

Volition:

Habituation:

Performance:

Environmental Interaction:

What constraints and resources are available to affect attainment of these goals? Use the next form to identify these.

Exercise Ten—Continued

Service Delivery System

Constraints	Resources
Staffing	
Space	
Budget	
Time	
Other services and relationship of occupational therapy to these	

Exercise Ten—Continued

Therapeutic Program Description

Evaluations to be used

Occupations/program content (Will these be enacted in groups? In individual treatment sessions?)

Program sequence (Program should reflect changing expectations and emphases from initial intake phases through predischarge and termination. Will there be links between this program and programs in other settings?)

Appendix: Instrument Library

The following pages contain information concerning various assessments which can be used with the model of human occupation. This instrument library is intended as a reference tool to provide information on instruments indicated or mentioned in earlier chapters. Additionally, it can be used to locate appropriate assessments for different age groups and for specific variables in the model. For this purpose a preliminary chart, which lists all the assessments indicating variables from the model on which they provide information, is presented. Each instrument is then listed alphabetically and the following information is provided: 1) instrument title, 2) type of assessment or means of administration, 3) content of the assessment, 4) basic information concerning reliability and validity of the assessment, 5) the intended or appropriate population(s), 6) relevant references, and 7) instructions on how to obtain the assessment if it is not reproduced in a published source. Several individuals who are developing assessments have graciously agreed to be contacted with requests for copies of, and information about, the assessments on which they are working. Persons contacting these individuals should expect to reimburse them for duplication and mailing costs. Additionally some assessments must be purchased from various agencies which have responsibility for marketing them. Prices were not given here since they are subject to change and could lead to more confusion in the long run. It is hoped that this instrument library will be an asset to therapists and students wishing to identify potential assessments and to have a quick reference source.

Instrument Library: Preliminary Chart

Domain	Component	Item	Activity Questionnaire	Adaptive Functioning Index	Adolescent Feminine and Occupational Development Questionnaire	Adolescent Role Assessment	American Association on Mental Deficiency Adaptive Behavior Scale	Arthritis Hand Assessment	Assessment of Preterm Infant Behavior	Asset: A Social Skills Program for Adolescents	Automatic Thoughts Questionnaire	Bay Area Functional Performance Evaluation	Bayley Scales of Infant Development
VOLITION	Value	Time orientation											
		Meaningful activity	X										
		Personal goals											
		Personal standards			X	X							
	Personal causation	Internal-external											
		Expectancy/success									X		
		Belief in skill	X	X									
		Belief in efficacy											
	Interests	Discrimination											
		Pattern											
		Potency (enactment)	X										
HABITUATION	Roles	Perceived incumbency				X	X						
		Internalized expectations				X	X						
		Balance/conflict											
	Habits	Degree of organization	X	X	X								
		Social appropriateness		X	X		X						
		Flexibility/rigidity	X										
PERFORMANCE	Skills	Interact/communicate				X	X		X	X		X	X
		Processes				X	X					X	X
		Perceptual-motor				X	X	X	X			X	X
ADAPTATION	Cycle	Trajectory (history)				X							
		Personal satisfaction											
		Environmental satisfaction		X									
ENVIRONMENT	Press	Psychosocial											
		Physical											
	Fit	Person-environment interaction											
POPULATION	Age	Child					X		X				X
		Adolescent	X		X	X	X			X			
		Adult	X	X			X	X			X	X	
		Elderly	X	X							X	X	

Behavior Setting Observations

Bruininks-Oseretsky Test of Motor Proficiency

Environmental Questionnaire

Expectancy Questionnaire

Fromage Mental Status Evaluation

Functional Assessment

Functional Status Index

Group-Interaction Skills Survey

Home Life Survey

Hopelessness Scale

Instrumental Activities of Daily Living

Interest Checklist

Internal-External Scale

Jebson-Taylor Test of Hand Function

Klein-Bell Activities of Daily Living Scale

Let's Talk Inventory for Adolescents

Leisure History Interview

Leisure Satisfaction Scale

Locus of Control Scale

Miller Assessment for Preschoolers

Monitored Work Evaluation

Neonatal Behavioral Assessment Scale

Occupational Case Analysis Interview

Occupational Functioning Tool

Instrument Library: Preliminary Chart—Continued

	1. Occupational Picture Interest Sort	2. Occupational Questionnaire	3. Occupational Role History	4. Occupational Therapy Functional Screening Tool	5. Parachek Geriatric Rating Scale	6. Performance Activities of Daily Living Evaluation	7. Piers-Harris Children's Self-Concept Scale	8. Play History	9. Pleasant Events Schedule	10. Preschool Play Scale	11. Preschool Rating Scale	12. Reading-Free Vocational Interest Inventory
VOLITION												
Value — Time orientation			X	X								
Value — Meaningful activity		X	X	X				X				
Value — Personal goals			X	X								
Value — Personal standards			X	X								
Personal causation — Internal-external			X	X				X				
Personal causation — Expectancy/success			X	X				X				
Personal causation — Belief in skill		X	X	X			X	X				
Personal causation — Belief in efficacy		X	X	X			X	X				
Interests — Discrimination	X		X	X								
Interests — Pattern	X	X	X	X				X				X
Interests — Potency (enactment)	X	X	X	X				X	X			
HABITUATION												
Roles — Perceived incumbency			X	X								
Roles — Internalized expectations			X	X								
Roles — Balance/conflict			X	X								
Habits — Degree of organization		X	X	X				X				
Habits — Social appropriateness		X	X	X				X				
Habits — Flexibility/rigidity		X	X	X				X				
PERFORMANCE												
Skills — Interact/communicate			X	X	X			X		X	X	
Skills — Processes			X	X	X	X		X		X	X	
Skills — Perceptual-motor			X	X	X	X		X		X	X	
ADAPTATION												
Cycle — Trajectory (history)			X					X				
Cycle — Personal satisfaction			X									
Cycle — Environmental satisfaction			X									
ENVIRONMENT												
Press — Psychosocial			X	X				X				
Press — Physical			X	X				X				
Fit — Person-environment interaction			X				X	X				
POPULATION												
Age — Child	X	X	X				X	X		X	X	X
Age — Adolescent	X	X	X					X				X
Age — Adult	X	X	X	X		X			X			
Age — Elderly				X	X				X			

Instrument											
Revised Gesell and Armatruda Developmental and Neurologic Examination	X				X X X	X				X	
Riley Motor Problems Inventory	X				X						
Role Checklist	X X X						X	X			X X
Role Performance Scale	X			X	X X X	X X X	X X				
St. Luke's A.M. Day Center Initial Vocational Screening Form	X X			X	X X X	X X X	X X X	X X X			X X
Self-Attitude Questionnaire	X									X	
Self-Directed Search	X X							X X	X X X		
Self-Esteem Scale	X X								X		
Set Test	X				X						
Social and Prevocational Information Battery	X X			X X	X X	X	X X				
Social Climate Scales	X X X	X	X								
Southern California Postrotary Nystagmus Test	X			X							
Southern California Sensory Integration Tests	X			X							
Test for Auditory Comprehension of Language	X			X							
Time Reference Inventory	X										
Valpar No. 17 Prevocational Readiness Battery	X X			X X X						X X	
Vineland Social Maturity Scale	X X X			X X X	X X						

Instrument Library: Description

Title	Content	Reliability and validity	Population	References/sources
Activity Questionnaire (self-administered paper and pencil inventory)	The activity questionnaire is a modified version of the occupational questionnaire designed to gather additional information for the physically disabled person. Thus, it not only gathers data on volitional aspects of everyday activities (personal causation, value and interest) but also on pain, difficulty and fatigue	No published assessment of the reliability or validity of the assessment is available, although studies are planned	Adolescents and adults with physical disabilities	Available from: Occupational Therapy Service, Department of Rehabilitation Medicine, Clinical Center, Building 10, Rm 5D37, National Institutes of Health, Bethesda, Md 20205
Adaptive Functioning Index (question/answer by examinee, plus observational rating)	Combination of results from (1) social education test, (2) vocational checklist, (3) residential checklist, reflects performance in areas of perceptual-motor, process and communication skills, and habits related to adjustment in social and vocational environments. Subtest scores from each of the three sections yield a profile of the examinee, from which goals for intervention can be formulated	No details available on reliability or validity	Mildly and moderately retarded adolescents and adults	Available from: Nancy J. Marlett, Vocational and Rehabilitation Research Institute, 3304 33rd Street N.W., Calgary 44, Alberta, Canada. Hughes M, Hardman E: Final report of the adaptive functioning index project at Koomarri Training Centre, Canberra. A.C.T., 1975. In *Rehabilitation Research and Development Digest*. Australian Department of Social Security, 1976 (instrument not reproduced here)
Adolescent Feminine and Occupational Development Questionnaire (self-administered multiple choice)	Responses to items indicate developmental level of female in the areas of personal causation (autonomy of decision-making), internalization of family and friendship roles, general habits and global values.	Content validity based on a literature review; clinical use with 30 adolescents provided relevant treatment planning information. No examination of reliability presented	Female adolescents (emotionally disturbed population)	Pezzuti L: An exploration of adolescent feminine and occupational behavior development. *American Journal of Occupational Therapy* 33:84–91, 1979

Instrument	Description	Reliability/Validity	Population	Reference
Adolescent Role Assessment (semistructured interview)	The instrument is not designed to yield a total score. A major limitation with it is its traditional view of the feminine social role. Focuses on role development and internalization in the areas of school, family and friends. Questions concerning childhood play, school performance, family responsibilities, peer interactions, work-related goals, and fantasy provide information about trajectory and current organization of roles. Scoring criteria for responses are given, so a profile of functioning is obtained	No reliability data are reported and clinical use suggests that varying interpretations of the rating criteria are likely. Content validity is based on a literature review	Adolescents with psychosocial dysfunction	Black M: Adolescent role assessment. *American Journal of Occupational Therapy* 30:73–79, 1976
American Association on Mental Deficiency Adaptive Behavior Scale (observation-based rating scale)	The scale is divided into two parts: developmental adaptation and social adaptation. The developmental section evaluates skills and habits in 10 behavior domains such as independent functioning, physical development and language development. The social adaptation part is composed of 14 domains related to maladaptive behavior (e.g. antisocial behavior or untrustworthy behavior). The instrument yields a numerical score for each domain; these scores can be compared with norms developed from a reference group	There has been rather extensive examinaton of both reliability and validity of this measure. Overall data suggest the instrument has acceptable stability. Factor analytic studies support validity of the domains. There is also evidence of concurrent and predictive validity	Originally designed for use with mentally retarded persons, but has been used with emotionally disturbed individuals. The instrument is considered relevant to both children and adults	Available from: Fogelman CJ: AAMD Adaptive Behavior Scale (1974 revision) American Association on Mental Deficiency, Washington, D.C.

Instrument Library: Description—Continued

Title	Content	Reliability and validity	Population	References/sources
Arthritis Hand Assessment (standardized test, administered by an occupational therapist)	This instrument documents specific upper extremity and hand deformities seen in patients with various types of connective tissue disease. Range of motion, degree of joint deformity, ADL status, main functional hand limitations, measurements of pinch, grip and sensation are all included in this assessment	No reliability or validity studies of this instrument have been reported	Most applicable to an adult population with connective tissue disease	Melvin JL: *Rheumatic Disease: Occupational Therapy and Rehabilitation* Philadelphia, FA Davis, 1982
Assessment of Preterm Infant Behavior (standardized test)	Measures the preterm infant's behavioral organization in four systems; physiological responses, motor capacities, state control, and self-regulation. Tests a variety of maneuvers which range from distal sensory input through high amounts of direct tactile and vestibular input and attentional/interactive abilities. Also examines the degree and kind of facilitation necessary to bring out the examiner to bring out the infant's best performance	Reliability and validity measures not reported in manual. Training and testing for interobserver reliability is recommended for use of test and is required for research	Premature infants who are in open isolettes or cribs in room temperature and room air	Als H, Lester BM, Tronch E, Brazelton TB: Manual for the assessment of preterm infant behavior. In Fitzgerald, et al. (eds): *Theory and Research in Behavioral Pediatrics.* New York, Plenum, 1980, vol 1 Als H, Lester BM, Tronick E, Brazelton TB: Towards a research instrument for the assessment of preterm infants behavior. In Fitzgerald, et al. (eds): *Theory and Research in Behavioral Pediatrics.* New York, Plenum, 1980, vol 1
ASSET: A Social Skills Program for Adolescents (comprehensive skills training program, including an integrated assessment component)	The following communication/interaction and process skills are covered: giving positive feedback, giving and accepting negative feedback, resisting	Based on large body of behavioral research which indicates that the skills identified are important to delinquent youths and that training	Adolescents. Specifically tested on juvenile delinquents. Further research is in progress with a wider range of youths	Hazel JS, Schumaker JB, Sherman JA, Sheldon-Wildgen J: *Leader's Guide-Asset: A Social Skills Program for Adolescents.* Norman Baxley &

Instrument	Description	Reliability/Validity	Population	Reference
(continued)	peer pressure, problem solving, negotiations, following instructions, and conversational skills. Pre- and posttraining questionnaires are included for self- and parental evaluation in all eight skill areas. Pre- and posttraining checklists for all areas are also included for the leader to assess the skill level	ing is deemed effective. Preliminary evidence suggests trained delinquents receive fewer recorded offenses after training		Associates, 1981. Distributed by Research Press, 2612 N. Mattis Ave., Champaign, Ill 61820 Hazel JS, Schumaker JB, Sherman JA, Sheldon-Widgen J: The development and evaluation of a group skill training program for court-adjudicated youths. In Upper D, Ross SM (eds): *Behavioral Group Therapy, 1981, An Annual Review.* Champaign, Ill, Research Press
Automatic Thoughts Questionnaire (ATQ-30) (30-item, self-report, paper-pencil inventory of negative beliefs. Each item rated on a scale from 1–5 in relation to how often the thought occurred in the past week)	Four factors were identified in this questionnaire of negative cognitions: perceptions of personal maladjustment and desire for change, negative self-concept and negative expectations, low self-esteem, and giving up/hopelessness. Related to the model, the questionnaire measures sense of personal causation—specifically beliefs about success/failure.	High reliability coefficients reported for split half and internal consistency. Good concurrent validity reported	Adults. Instrument developed and tested using undergraduate college students	Hollon SD, Kendall PC: Cognitive self-statements in depression: development of an automatic thoughts questionnaire. *Cognitive Therapy and Research* 4:383–395, 1980
Bay Area Functional Performance Evaluation (task performance and observation rating scale)	The task-oriented subtest involves five parts: a shell-sorting task, bank deposit slip, house floor plan, block design, and draw-a-person. The social interaction scale is a rating of behavior. Together, the two subtests provide informa-	Interrater reliability with the test developers was excellent; it was much lower, although acceptable, with newly trained raters. Instrument has face validity, and correlations with Functional Life Scale, Geriatric Rating Scale, and	Has been used with psychiatric adult inpatients and geriatric clients	Bloomer J, Williams S: *The Bay Area Functional Performance Evaluation.* San Francisco, Langley Porter Institute, 1979 DiTullio FM: *An Investigation of Concurrent Validity of the Bay Area Functional*

Instrument Library: Description—*Continued*

Title	Content	Reliability and validity	Population	References/sources
	tion about cognitive, affective, interpersonal, and perceptual motor skills necessary to the performance of daily living tasks. Scores can be compared with norms for high, middle and low functional capacity	Global Assessment Scale suggest concurrent validity as well		*Performance Evaluation with a Geriatric Population* (unpublished research project, Virginia Commonwealth University, 1980)
Bayley Scales of Infant Development (standardized test)	Measures developmental status in the first 2½ years of life. Scale is divided into three parts: (1) Mental scale: assesses cognitive, perceptual skills, beginning communication; (2) Motor Scale: assesses degree of control of body, coordination of gross and fine motor skills; and (3) Infant Behavior Record: notes child's social and objective orientations towards environment	Reliability measures: split-half coefficients. Mental scale median 0.88. Interobserver reliability (% of agreement) mental scale 89.4%; motor scale 93.4%. Test-retest reliability (% of agreement) mental 76.4%; motor 75.3%. Correlation with Binet IQ test reported. Training recommended for examiners.	Normal children from 2–30 months of age	Bayley N: *Manual for the Bayley Scales of Infant Development.* New York, The Psychological Corporation, 1969 Examination materials available from same source
Behavior Setting Observations (general guidelines for environmental observations)	Behavior setting refers to a physical milieu characterized by a recognizable pattern of behavior (e.g. a classroom). Observations of a behavior setting can focus on: typical roles of persons in setting, expected behaviors, temporal boundaries of the setting, mechanisms for	This is not a standardized method, so reliability and validity cannot be described. However, behavior settings have been used as a unit in a variety of environmental studies	Focus of observation is environment, rather than specific persons	Barker RG, Wright HF: *Midwest and Its Children: The Psychological Ecology of an American Town.* Hamden, Conn, Archon Books, 1971 (1955) Wicker AW: *An Introduction to Ecological Psychology.* Monterey, Calif, Brooks/Cole, 1979

Instrument	Description	Reliability/Validity	Population	References
	maintaining the existence of setting and countering deviant behaviors, how many people are usually involved, objects that are essential to the setting			
Bruininks-Oseretsky Test of Motor Proficiency (individually therapist-administered test)	Eight subtest areas, consisting of 46 items, cover gross and fine motor skills, including balance, coordination, visual-motor, strength, speed, and dexterity. A composite, gross motor and fine motor score are yielded and raw scores can be converted to percentiles, stanines, and age-equivalent scores, based on normative data from 800 school children	Test-retest reliability is satisfactory and interrater reliability, for untrained raters, is high. Test has internal consistency and some concurrent validity	Developed for use with children, ages 4.5–14.5; can be used with learning disabled and retarded children	Bruininks RH: *Examiners Manual, Bruininks-Oseretsky Test of Motor Proficiency.* American Guidance Service, 1978 Ziviani R, Poulsen A, O'Brien A: Correlation of the Bruininks-Oseretsky Test of Motor Proficiency with the Southern California Sensory Integration Tests. *American Journal of Occupational Therapy* 36:519–523, 1982
Environmental Questionnaire (semistructured interview)	This interview focuses on characteristics of the subject's living environment, and the subject's perceptions of constraints and positive qualities in the setting. Questions attempt to uncover preferences for, and press for, involvement in daily living tasks and leisure activities. The yield is qualitative; data are not quantified in any way	Apart from the exploratory study describing the development of the instrument, it does not appear to have been used in research. The instrument has face validity	Psychiatric clients living in the community	Dunning HD: Environmental occupational therapy. *American Journal of Occupational Therapy* 26:292–298, 1972
Expectancy Questionnaire (structured interview)	This brief interview asks respondents to indicate responses to the question "What do you expect to be	No reliability or validity data have been reported	Children, and appears appropriate for adolescents and adults	Farnham-Diggory S: Self, future, and time: a developmental study of the concepts of psychotic, brain

Instrument Library: Description—Continued

Title	Content	Reliability and validity	Population	References/sources
	doing . . . ?" The question is completed with various phrases (e.g. 1 year from now, 10 years from now) in order to get an indication of the person's orientation to the future and whether or not he/she has identifiable goals. Responses from the questionnaire are typically categorized into types of goals			damaged, and normal children. *Monographs of the Society for Research in Child Development*, 31:(1, Serial No. 103), 1966
FROMAJE Mental Status Evaluation (informal interview)	Provides data on mental functioning. This is a mental status screening tool that assesses functional safety (F), reasoning ability (R), orientation (O), memory skills (M), arithmetic skills (A), judgment (J), and emotional stability (E). Ratings of 1 to 3 are given in each area. Ratings indicate severe to no impairment of performance. A profile of abilities is obtained and a global score is determined that indicates some degree of dementia or depression if the score falls within certain ranges	There are no published data on the reliability of this instrument. Validity studies with other mental status and orientation tools indicate the areas tested are appropriate	Verbal adults	Tool and instructions found in: Libow LS: A rapidly administered, easily remembered, mental status evaluation: FROMAJE. In Libow LS, Sherman FT (eds): *The Core of Geriatric Medicine: A Guide For Students and Practitioners.* St. Louis, Mosby, 1981
Functional Assessment (interview)	The assessment consists of an interview of a patient to determine functional ca-	The instrument has been studied and there is evidence of interrater agree-	Adults who have polyarticular disabilities	Convery FR, Minteer MA, Amiel D, Connett KL: Polyarticular disability: a func-

Instrument	Description	Reliability/Validity	Age Group	Reference
(continued)	pacity for 19 activities of daily living and mobility items. Questions for different levels of function for each area are spelled out. Dependent on the respondent's answers, one of four ratings, from independent to unable, is given. The interview is based on the previous week	ment and of concurrent validity		tional assessment. *Archives of Physical Medicine and Rehabilitation* 58:494–499, 1977
Functional Status Index (therapist-scored rating scale based on standardized interview)	This evaluation measures an arthritis patient's functional status by the degree of assistance required to perform 18 different activities of daily living. The interviewer asks the patient to indicate the degree of help, amount of pain and degree of difficulty for specific activities of daily living. The patient's responses are based on the degree of functional impairment experienced over the last several days before the evaluation	The evaluation has been studied and acceptable levels of internal consistency, interrater reliability and test-retest reliability were found. Additionally, it was found to correlate with clinical judgment indicating concurrent validity for the tool	Older adults suffering from arthritis	Jette AM, Dennison OL: Inter-observer reliability of a functional status assessment instrument. *Journal of Chronic Disease* 31:573–580, 1978
Group-Interaction Skills Survey (structured observation, checklist)	Provides information on group interaction skill. Five developmental subskills are listed in terms of the ability to participate in the following groups: parallel, project, egocentric-cooperative, cooperative, and mature groups. Evaluation involves structured obser-	There are no published data on reliability and validity	No designated age group	Mosey AC: *Activities Therapy.* New York, Raven Press, 1973, pp 92–93 Mosey AC: *Three Frames of Reference for Mental Health.* Thorofare, NJ, Charles B. Slack, 1970

Instrument Library: Description—Continued

Title	Content	Reliability and validity	Population	References/sources
	vation of patients in a collaborative activity and checking component behaviors for each subskill. Ability to participate at a group level is assumed if all components are checked			
Home Life Survey (form completed by an observer familiar with the subject's home life)	This instrument is designed to measure person-environment fit by determining the degree of responsibility assumed in the home environment. The four areas covered are meals, dressing, family activities, and chores	There are no reliability or validity data on the instrument as yet; it is still in early developmental stages. The instrument was developed for a pilot study and appears to have promise	Adult, mentally retarded persons, but would appear to have wider applicability to other disabled adults and adolescents	Available from: Marian Kavanagh, M.S., O.T.R., 106 Seneca Rd., Richmond, Va 23226
Hopelessness Scale (Self-report, paper-pencil scale)	Three factors identified related to hopelessness are affect or feelings about the future, lack of motivation and future expectations. Related to the model, this scale measures personal causation: specifically, belief in skill, belief in efficacy of skill and belief in success/failure for the past and the future. Each true/false response is given a score of 0 or 1. A high score indicates a high degree of hopelessness or a lowered sense of personal causation	High reliability coefficients reported for internal consistency. Also highly significant inter-item correlations. Good concurrent validity reported. Several hypotheses were tested and confirmed supporting construct validity	Appropriate for use with adults	Beck AT, Weissman A, Lester D, Prexler L: The measurement of pessimism: the hopelessness scale. *Journal of Consulting and Clinical Psychology* 42:861–865, 1974

Instrument	Description	Reliability and Validity	Population	References
Instrumental Activities of Daily Living (observation, interview and performance)	Provides data on the person's ability to perform various self-care activities. Eight general activities are identified and subdivided in levels of complexity. The person is rated on the ability to perform tasks within each area. Points are given for independent function on tasks. A score is totalled	There are no data available on the reliability of this instrument. Validity studies comparing this test with others indicate it is an appropriate tool to measure these areas of self-care	Older adults in institutions, also appropriate for community-based elderly	Instrument and instructions appear in Lawton M, Brody E: Assessment of older people: self-maintaining and instrumental activities of daily living. *Journal of Gerontology* 30:179–186, 1970 Lawton M: The functional assessment of elderly people. *Journal of the American Geriatrics Society* 21:465–481, 1971
Interest Checklist—modified (self-administered, paper and pencil inventory)	The interest checklist originally developed by Matsutsuyu (1967) contained 80 items for which the respondent indicated casual, strong and no levels of interest. Respondents were also asked to add additional interests and to narrate their leisure histories. The checklist was modified by Scaffa (1981) and further modified by Neville and Kielhofner (1983). In its most recent modified form, the items remain the same, but respondents indicate interest for the past 10 years and past year, indicate current participation (yes or no) and indicate whether they would like to pursue the interest in the future (yes/no)	Reliability of the instrument (a 5-point scale replaced the 3-point scale for this study) was studied and found to be high. No assessment of the 3-point version or modified scales has been done.	Adolescents and adults. The modified version may be too complex for confused or cognitively-limited persons	Matsutsuyu, J: The interest checklist. *American Journal of Occupational Therapy* 32:628–630, 1967 Neville A, Kielhofner G: *Modified Interest Checklist* (unpublished workbook, National Institutes of Health, 1983) Rogers J, Weinstein J, Figone J: The interest checklist: an empirical assessment. *American Journal of Occupational Therapy*, 32:628–630 Scaffa M: *Temporal Adaptation and Alcoholism* (unpublished masters project, Virginia Commonwealth University, 1981)

Instrument Library: Description—*Continued*

Title	Content	Reliability and validity	Population	References/sources
Internal-External Scale (forced-choice pencil-and-paper questionnaire)	Measures belief in internal or external control over events. Originally believed to be a unidimensional scale, more recent research suggests three dimensions: fatalism (does fate determine one's consequences), social system control (can one effect change in society) and self control. Yield of instrument is single score—norms for both versions of instrument are available	Revised, multidimensional version has good internal consistency for the three dimensions and low inter-correlations among dimensions. Discriminant, concurrent and construct validity for earlier version	Older adolescents and adults	Reid DW, Ware EE: Multidimensionality of internal versus external control: addition of a third dimension and nondistinction of self versus others. *Canadian Journal of Behavioral Science* 6:131–142, 1974 Schlegel RP, Crawford CA: Multidimensionality of internal-external locus of control. *Canadian Journal of Behavioral Science* 8:375–387, 1976 LeFaut HM: *Locus of Control: Current Trends in Theory and Research.* Hillsdale, NJ, Lawrence Erlbaum Assoc, 1976 (instrument reproduced here) Rotter J: Generalized expectancies for internal versus external control of reinforcement. *Psychological Monographs*, 80:1–28, 1966 (contains original instrument)
Jebsen-Taylor Test of Hand Function (standardized test)	This evaluation is a measure of timed motor coordination for seven hand activities: (1) writing a short sentence, (2) turning over 3 × 5 inch cards, (3) picking up small objects and placing in a container, (4)	Reliability data have been gathered on the assessment and norms are available for age and sex.	Adults aged 20–94	Jebsen RH: An objective and standardized test of hand function. *Archives of Physical Medicine and Rehabilitation* 50:311–319, 1969

Instrument	Description	Reliability and Validity	Population	Reference
	stacking checkers, (5) simulated eating, (6) moving empty large cans and (7) moving weighted large cans. The evaluation determines the degree of coordination impairment in an individual with upper extremity dysfunction	Interrater reliability examined initially by having 20 patients rated independently by occupational therapists and rehabilitation nurses. Further reliability data are to be obtained. Predictive validity was supported through a phone call follow up several months after discharge	Physically disabled adults	Klein RM, Bell B: Self-care skills: behavioral measurement with Klein-Bell ADL scale. *Archives of Physical Medicine and Rehabilitation* 63:335–338, 1982
Klein-Bell Activities of Daily Living Scale (occupational therapist observes performance and scores results)	This scale consists of 170 behavioral items categorized into areas of bathing/hygiene, eating, dressing, mobility, elimination and emergency telephone use. Items are scored "ACHIEVED" (behavior is performed without verbal or physical assistance from another person) or "FAILED" (assistance is needed)			
Leisure History Interview (semistructured interview)	This interview format, modified from an activity interview developed by Buchenholz, traces the pattern of leisure activities engaged in from childhood through the present. Activities are identified for various time intervals; then favorite activities are examined in depth. Qualitative data yield descriptions of themes and trends relevant to volition and habituation	Reliability and validity have not been investigated	Adolescents	Buchenholz, B: Activity analysis: a technique in the study of adolescents. *American Journal of Psychotherapy* 18:594–605, 1964 Available from: Roann Barris, Ed.D., OTR, University of Wisconsin-Madison, Occupational Therapy Program, 1300 University Ave, Wisc 53706

Instrument Library: Description—Continued

Title	Content	Reliability and validity	Population	References/sources
Leisure Satisfaction Scale (paper-and-pencil Likert-type scale)	Six subscales consist of a total of 51 items describing types of satisfactions or needs that are met through leisure. These satisfactions reflect feelings of intrinsic motivation, challenge, intellectual stimulation, social affiliations, relaxation, physiological needs, and aesthetic concerns. There are no guidelines for interpreting scores—information is used qualitatively	High alpha coefficients suggest internal consistency. Instrument has face and content validity; other validity not examined	Adolescents and adults	Beard J, Ragheb M: Measuring leisure satisfaction. *Journal of Leisure Research* 12:20–33, 1980
Let's Talk Inventory for Adolescents (structured interview format)	Standardized evaluation of communication skills. After being given brief background information, subjects are asked to respond to stimulus pictures. Verbatim response records (or audiotapes) are analyzed relative to length and complexity of response, intent and audience appropriateness. Means for children with normal language development are provided. Suggested intervention strategies are available (Wiig, 1982a)	Studies support its reliability and validity. The test-retest correlation compares favorably with other similar language tests. Internal consistency of items and content validity are both good. Interrater reliability correlations were consistently high, and the instrument was found to have diagnostic validity	Preadolescents and adolescents (ages 9 through young adulthood)	Wiig EH: *Let's talk: Developing Prosocial Communication Skills.* Columbus, Ohio, Charles E. Merrill, 1982a Wiig, EH: *Let's Talk Inventory for Adolescents.* Columbus, Ohio, Charles E. Merrill, 1982b
Locus of Control Scale (orally administered, forced choice format)	Adapted from Bialer-Cromwell Children's Locus of Control Scale (Bialer, 1961) to 23 forced choice	Mixed results obtained from studies of reliability (test-retest, split-half, internal consistency) and validity	Mildly mentally retarded adolescents and adults	Floor L, Rosen M: Investigating the phenomenon of helplessness in mentally retarded adults. *American*

Instrument	Description	Reliability/Validity	Population	Reference
	response pairs, the scale explores the extent to which subjects view outcomes as internally/externally controlled (measure of personal causation). Sum of responses indicative of an internal orientation gives a gross indication of relative position on an internal/external continuum	(construct) of the Bialer scale; however, no validity/reliability data available on Floor and Rosen's adapted format		*Journal of Mental Deficiency* 79: 565–572, 1975
Miller Assessment for Preschoolers (Standardized test)	This is a screening tool of 27 core items designed to be used by educational and clinical personnel to identify children in need of further evaluation. The test includes items classified as sensory and motor abilities, cognitive abilities and combined abilities	Interrater reliability on 40 children ranged from 0.84 to 0.99. The percentage of scores which remained the same on 90 children over a 1- to 4-week interval ranged from 72–94%	Children 2 years 9 months to 5 years 8 months	Miller LJ: *Miller Assessment for Preschoolers.* Littleton, Colo, The Foundation for Knowledge in Development, 1982
Monitored Work Evaluation (occupational therapist tests the patient and completes the evaluation)	This is a four-part evaluation staged at different post myocardial infarct (MI) phases. The interview with the patient results in a job (task) analysis to determine the type of evaluation suitable for the patient's situation. A Walk and Carry Test at 3 weeks post-MI and 2 months post-MI determines selected hemodynamic responses to work tasks that require a combination of dynamic and static exercise	There are no published data on the reliability or validity of this instrument	Adults in the various stages of recovery from an MI or coronary artery bypass surgery	Sheldahl LM, Wilke NA, Tristani FE, Kalbfeisch JH: Response of patients after myocardial infarction to carrying a graded series of weight loads. *American Journal of Cardiology,* 52:698–703, 1983 Harrington KA, Smith KH, Schumacher M, Lunsford BR, Watson KL, Silvester RH: Cardiac rehabilitation: evaluation and interventions less than 6 weeks after myocardial infarction. *Archives of Physical Medicine and Rehabilitation* 62:151–155, 1981

Instrument Library: Description—Continued

Title	Content	Reliability and validity	Population	References/sources
Neonatal Behavioral Assessment Scale (standardized test)	Measures an infant's available interactive responses to the environment. Contains 27 behavioral items and 20 elicited responses. Scores are grouped into four behavioral dimensions of newborn organization: (1) interactive capacities; (2) motoric capacities; (3) organizational capacities-state control; (4) organizational capacities-physiological response to stress	Interobserver reliability ranges from 0.85–1.00. Test-retest reliability—mean of all items 0.592 with agreement by one criterion and 0.783 with agreement by two criteria. Training and testing for reliability recommended for use; required for research	Full-term newborn infants from 3 days to 1 month	Available from: Nancy Wilke, OTR, Cardiopulmonary Rehabilitation Center, Veteran's Administration Medical Center, 5000 West National Ave, Wood, Wisc 53193 Brazelton T B: *Neonatal Behavioral Assessment Scale. Clinics in Developmental Medicine No. 50.* Philadelphia, Lippincott, 1973 Sameroff A (ed): *Organization and Stability of Newborn Behavior: A Commentary on the Brazelton Neonatol Behavior Assessment Scales.* Monograph of the Society for Research in Child Development, Serial No. 177, vol 43, Nos. 5–6. Chicago, Child Development Publications, the University of Chicago Press Training films available from: Educational Developmental Corporation, 10 Mifflin Place, Cambridge, Mass 02138
Occupational Case Analysis Interview and Rating Scale (semistructured in-	This interview format corresponds to the case analysis method developed by	A study of interrater reliability suggests that reliability of components ranges from	Short-term adult psychiatric population, to be used in discharge planning	Cubie S, Kaplan K: A case analysis method for the model of occupation.

	Description	Reliability/Validity	Population	References/Availability
terview with ordinal rating)	Cubie and Kaplan (1982). Questions cover each component of the model and a rating scale is used to quantify the responses. Scores are obtained for each component as well as global assessment of the system dynamic, history of the system, context, and system trajectory	fair to excellent; overall reliability is excellent. Instrument has face and content validity; other studies of validity have not been done		American Journal of Occupational Therapy 36:645–656, 1982 Kaplan K: Short-term assessment: the need and a response. Occupational Therapy in Mental Health, 4:29–43, 1984
Occupational Functioning Tool (interview and observation protocol with rating scale)	This is a screening tool for institutionalized subjects. It provides ratings of personal causation, values, interests, habits, roles, and skills. A 5-point scale is used to make each rating, following the completion of an interview	Test-retest reliability appears acceptable; interrater reliability is substantial. Demonstrated concurrent validity with Life Satisfaction Index-Z and discriminated between community residents and institutionalized subjects	Institutionalized subjects	Available from: Gary Kielhofner Dr.P.H., OTR, Associate Professor, Department of Occupational Therapy, Sargent College of Allied Health Professions, Boston University, University Road, Boston, Mass 02215
Occupational Picture Interest Sort (Combination sorting procedure, interview and rating scale to be filled out by the therapist)	The instrument gives data on the discrimination, pattern and potency of interests. In a simple two-step process, respondents sort pictures of persons engaged in various activities into "like" and "dislike" categories, later sorting the "like" pictures into two piles representing stronger and milder interests. The therapist then asks questions regarding participation in ten strong interests to obtain a potency score. Finally, the therapist completes a rating scale based on observation of the re-	The authors of the instrument examined both reliability and validity in a small study. Test-retest reliability for the sort and interrater reliability for the scale appear acceptable. There is some evidence of concurrent validity. The carefully posed photographs used as stimuli would appear to enhance the instrument	Mildly and moderately retarded individuals. Would appear useful for any population with cognitive and/or reading problems	Shakun R: The Assessment of the Reliability of the Occupational Picture Interest Sort for Mentally Retarded Adults (unpublished masters project, Virginia Commonwealth University, 1984) Scott MB: The Validity of the Occupational Picture Interest Sort for Mentally Retarded Adults (unpublished project, Virginia Commonwealth University, 1984) Available from: Mary Beth Scott M.S., O.T.R, 4115 Windsor St, Pittsburgh, Pa 15217

Instrument Library: Description—Continued

Title	Content	Reliability and validity	Population	References/sources
Occupational Questionnaire (paper-and-pencil self-report; can also be completed with assistance)	spondent during the administration; this scale measures discrimination. Respondent reports on time use for each half-hour period of waking time. Ratings are made of type of activity (work, play, rest, or daily living task), feelings of competence during activity, feelings of pleasure, and worth of activity to individual. Thus, it provides data on habits, values, potency of interests, and feelings of efficacy. Percent scores and summed rating scores can be obtained	Percent agreement ranged from adequate to good in one study of reliability. Some concurrent validity evidence.	Adolescents and adults; alternate versions for special diagnostic groups have been developed	Riopel N: *An Examination of the Occupational Behavior and Life Satisfaction of the Elderly* (unpublished master's research project, Virginia Commonwealth University, 1981) Available from: Gary Kielhofner Dr.P.H. OTR, Department of Occupational Therapy, Sargent College of Allied Health Professions, Boston University, University Road, Boston, Mass 02215
Occupational (Role) History (Interview with optional rating scale)	The occupational history originally developed by Moorhead (1969) was a lengthy history designed to obtain qualitative data on the occupational life-style of the respondent. Florey and Michelman (1982) developed an abbreviated interview based on the original, and labeled it the occupational role history. Harlan (1983) further revised the interview to be suitable to a physically disabled population and devised a rating scale based on the history. All three histories are inter-	The latest version of the history with the rating scale has been examined empirically and interrater and retest reliability both appeared good. Authors of the interview were all careful to build content validity into the instrument A major study is now underway at Boston University, Department of Occupational Therapy to develop a standardized occupational history	Adolescents and adults	Moorhead L: The occupational history. *American Journal of Occupational Therapy* 23:329–334, 1969 Florey L, Michelman S: Occupational role history: a screening tool for psychiatric occupational therapy. *American Journal of Occupational Therapy* 32:301–308, 1982 Harlan B: *Determining the Reliability of the Occupational Role History When Used with Physically Disabled Persons* (unpublished

Instrument	Description	Reliability/Validity	Population	Reference
Occupational Therapy Functional Screening Tool (interview-based rating scale)	views that yield qualitative information about the person's occupational strengths, weaknesses and life experiences. This instrument is a modification of the Occupational Functioning Tool. The interview has been changed to be more appropriate for an acute care physically disabled population. The rating scale remains the same. The tool is used only as a screening tool to identify areas of problems within the human system	Previous work done on the Occupational Functioning Tool would suggest that this tool would be reliable and valid. However, the instrument in modified form has not been empirically studied	Physically disabled adults	masters thesis, Virginia Commonwealth University, 1983) Available from: Occupational Therapy Service, Department of Rehabilitation Medicine, Clinical Center, Building 10, Rm 5D37, National Institutes of Health, Bethesda, Md 20205
Parachek Geriatric Rating Scale (checklist completed by caregiver or therapist)	Provides data on the person's general physical status, self-care skills and social behavior. There are ten items rated in a dependent to independent (1–4) scale. The ratings produce a profile of the individual's areas of abilities and disabilities. The areas assessed are: ambulation, eyesight, hearing, toilet habits, eating, hygiene, grooming, room care, individual response, and group activity participation	There are no published reliability studies. There is a significant correlation between the Parachek and a longer measure of geriatric functioning	Institutionalized older adults	Miller ER, Parachek JR: Validation and standardization of a goal-oriented, quick screening geriatric scale. *Journal of the American Geriatrics Society* 22:224–237, 1974 The tool and instructional manual are available from: Center for Neurodevelopmental Studies, Inc., 8621 North 3rd Street, Suite A, Phoenix, Ariz 85020
Peformance Activities of Daily Living Evaluation (performance evaluation)	Provides data on performance skills in the area of self-care skills. Six general activities are evaluated.	There are no data available on reliability of this instrument. Validity studies have been done using other	Institutionalized and community-based older persons	Katz S, Ford AB, Moskowtiz RW, Jackson BA, Jaffe MW: Studies of illness in the aged, the index of

Instrument Library: Description—*Continued*

Title	Content	Reliability and validity	Population	References/sources
	Each performance is rated on a 1–3 scale for independence of performance. The areas of assessment are bathing, dressing, toileting, transfers, continence, and feeding. Ratings in each area are compiled to reach a general rating of performance abilities	evaluations of self-care and the instrument appears to be valid for institutionalized populations		ADL: a standardized measure of biological and psychosocial function. *Journal of the American Medical Association* 185:94–107, 1963
Piers-Harris Children's Self-Concept Scale (self-administered paper and pencil questionnaire)	This recently revised scale measures self-concept in the following domains: (1) behavior, intellect and school status; (2) physical appearance; (3) attribution of anxiety; (4) popularity; (5) happiness; and (6) satisfaction. The scale yields a total score as well as scores for the above clusters	Test-retest reliability based on a 3-week interval was estimated at 0.73	Standardized on over 1000 children in grades 4 through 12 but subsequent research has shown it to be reliable with children as young as 5 years. The adapted form for younger children requires that the examiner assist the child in reading the items	Piers EV, Harris DB: *Piers Harris Children's Self-concept Scale* (rev). Los Angeles, Calif, Western Psychological Services, 1984
Play History (parent/caretaker interview with optional rating scale)	The play history is an interview of the parent or caretaker which seeks to determine the developmental level of a child's or adolescent's play and the adequacy of the play environment and play experiences over the course of development. Five major play epochs are examined and four elements (materials, actions, people, and set-	In a small study the instrument demonstrated good interrater reliability for the rating scale and acceptable test-retest reliability. Preliminary evidence of concurrent and discriminant validity was also provided in the study	Children and adolescents	Takata N: Play as a prescription. In Reilly M (ed): *Play as Exploratory Learning.* Beverly Hills, Sage, 1974 Takata N: The play history. *American Journal of Occupational Therapy,* 23:314–318, 1969 Behnke C, Menarcheck-Fetkovich M: Examining reliability and validity of the play history. *American*

Instrument	Description	Reliability/Validity	Use	References
(continued)	ting) are examined within each epoch. The interview yields rich qualitative data on the play experiences and play environment. In addition, a rating scale has been devised to quantify judgements about adequacy of experiences and environment			*Journal of Occupational Therapy* 38:94–100, 1984 (a revised copy of assessment available from these authors)
Pleasant Events Schedule (paper-and-pencil questionnaire)	Instrument lists 320 events or activities to be rated by respondent as to frequency of occurrence and enjoyability. Items are social, nonsocial, sex-role related, sexual, stimulus-seeking, outdoorsmanship, and crafts related. A shorter form provides 86 items. Instrument yields an obtained pleasure score (potency of interests)	Reasonable stability over time; concurrent validity between self-report and a close observer's report; construct validity is suggested by relationships between this instrument and improvement in depressed persons, locus of control and success-failure expectancies	Screening tool for depressed adults	MacPhillamy JD, Lewinsohn PM: *Manual for the Pleasant Events Schedule.* Eugene, Ore, Department of Psychology, University of Oregon, 1976 MacPhillamy DJ, Lewinsohn PM: The Pleasant Events Schedule: studies on reliability, validity, and scale intercorrelations. *Journal of Consulting and Clinical Psychology* 50:363–380, 1982
Preschool Play Scale (rating scale based on observation(s) of children in free play)	The preschool play scale is designed as an assessment of the child's developmental level of play. Fourteen categories of play are observed and rated (play age 0–1 to 5–6). These are used to obtain domain scores (participation, imitation, material management, and space management) and an overall play age	Two studies with samples of normal and handicapped children support good test-retest and interrater reliability for domain scores and overall play age. The same studies provided evidence of concurrent validity	Preschoolers	Bledsoe N, Shephard J: A study of reliability and validity of a preschool play scale. *American Journal of Occupational Therapy* 36:783–788, 1982 Harrison H: *Examining the Reliability and Validity of the Preschool Play Scale with a Disabled Population* (unpublished masters thesis, Virginia Commonwealth University, 1984) Knox S: A play scale. In

Instrument Library: Description—Continued

Title	Content	Reliability and validity	Population	References/sources
Preschool Rating Scale (observer rating scale)	This rating scale is designed to assess a preschool child's personal social development. Five areas are assessed: coordination, verbal expression, auditory understandings, orientation, and social relations	Average interrater correlation coefficient estimate was 0.74. Discriminant analysis indicating that the PRS can classify children as typical or nontypical provided predictive validity	Children aged 2½ years to 6½ years. Norms available for 1040 children in six 6-month age groups	Reilly M (ed): *Play as Exploratory Learning*, Beverly Hills, Sage, 1974 Available from the Center Preschool Services Franklin Institute Research Laboratories, Philadelphia, Pa
Reading-Free Vocational Interest Inventory (self-administered paper and pencil test which does not require reading abilities)	This instrument is a test of vocational preferences or work interests. Various job categories are illustrated in line drawings in triads. The respondent indicates preference by circling the most desirable of each of the three illustrations. The instrument, when scored, indicates the degree of interest in various vocational areas such as building trades, clerical work, animal care, etc	There is evidence of acceptable test-retest reliability. There is also evidence of internal consistency in the instrument. There is evidence of concurrent validity and the instrument was found to appropriately identify persons already in chosen areas of work	Retarded persons, especially the educable mentally retarded person at the high school level	Available from: EDMARK Associates, 13241 Northup Way, Bellevue, Wash 98005
Revised Gesell and Amatruda Developmental and Neurologic Examination (standardized exam)	Developmental assessment of the preschool child. Revision of the Gesell Developmental Schedules. Measures the quality and integration of five areas of behavior: (1) adaptive skills, (2) gross motor skills, (3) fine motor skills,	Description of the method by which the test was revised is in the manual along with discussion of the revised norms. Interobserver reliability for individual test items (percentage of agreement) overall 93.7% for age levels: *r* values	Normal infants from 1 week to 36 months of age	Knobloch S, Stevens F, Malone A: *Manual of Developmental Diagnosis*. Hagerstown, Md, Harper Row, 1980 Knobloch H, Pasamanick B (eds): *Gesell and Amatrudas Developmental Diagnosis*, ed 3. Hagerstown,

Instrument	Description	Reliability/Validity	Population	Reference
	(4) language skills, and (5) personal-social skills	range from 0.84–0.99. Validity measures described in text		Md, Harper Row, 1974 Available from: Mr. Nigell Cox, 69 Fawn Dr, Cheshire, Conn 06410
Riley Motor Problems Inventory (standardized test)	The purpose of this test is to provide a quantified system of observation of neurological signs from which the examiner can determine the need for referral and measure the motor component as a factor in any related syndrome. The three descriptive categories of the test are oral motor, fine motor and gross motor	Research validity was ascertained by comparison of the RMPI with the Bender Gestalt Visual Motor Test and the Human Figure Drawing Test (see manual). Test-retest on 24 children over a 13-week to 4-month interval was 0.77. Interrater reliability among 15 clinicians scoring videotapes of five children was 0.91	Test has normative data for children aged 4 through 9	Riley G: *Riley Motor Problems Inventory*. Los Angeles, Western Psychological Services, 1976
Role Checklist (paper-and-pencil self-report checklist)	Instrument lists ten roles with occupational components and a category for "other." Respondent indicates past, present and future intentions related to performance of each role. Part II of the checklist asks for degree of valuation of each. Thus, it measures perceived incumbancy, role balance, and values related to occupational roles. Number of past, present and future roles can be calculated, as well as number of discontinued or interrupted roles	Test-retest reliability ranges from fair to high for individual roles; is substantial for overall part I and part II scores. Preliminary research suggests discriminant and concurrent validity. Instrument has face and content validity	Adolescents and adults	Oakley F: *The Model of Human Occupation in Psychiatry* (unpublished master's research project, Virginia Commonwealth University, 1982) Available from: Fran Oakley M.S. OTR, 9301 Autoville Dr., College Park, MD 20740
Role Performance Scale (semi-structured interview and rating scale)	This instrument was developed to record long-term role performance history	A detailed manual has been developed to standardize administration. Reliability	Adult psychiatric clients	Available from: Good-Ellis, M., Fine, S. B., Spencer, J. H., Jr., M.D., Department

Instrument Library: Description—Continued

Title	Content	Reliability and validity	Population	References/sources
	and to assess levels of role functioning. Role performance in work (or equivalent), education, home management, rehabilitation programs, family, social relationships, leisure, self-management, and health care is examined. Operationally defined scales rate each role from 1–6. Roles can be rated for various time segments, and an average level of functioning score can also be obtained	and validity are currently being examined		of Therapeutic Activities, The Payne Whitney Clinic, 525 East 68th St, New York, NY 10021
St. Luke's A.M. Day Center Initial Vocational Screening Form (self-administered questionnaire)	Questions cover work and educational history, and development of occupational behavior during childhood and adolescence through present. Yields information about skills, interests, meaningful activity, occupational goals	No data on reliability or validity are available	Adults and adolescents in psychiatric day treatment	Available from: Cheryl Salz and Suzanne White, St. Luke's Hospital, 114th St. and Amsterdam Ave, New York, NY 10025
Self-Attitude Questionnaire (self-administered questionnaire)	Examines the adolescent's perceptions of self-devaluing experiences in school, family and with peers; degree of valuation of normative and contranormative structure; feelings of defenselessness and vulnerability; attempts at avoiding responsibility; and awareness of deviant acts	Information on reliability is not available. Instrument has been used in research to support the hypothesis that negative self-attitudes will correlate with deviant behavior	Designed for research with adolescents, focusing on antecedents of delinquent behavior	Kaplan HB: Antecedents of deviant responses: predicting from a general theory of deviant behavior. *Journal of Youth and Adolescence* 6:89–99, 1977. (includes questionnaire items) Kaplan HB: Antecedents of negative self-attitudes:

Instrument	Description	Comments	Population	Reference
	among peers. Thus, it looks at feelings of efficacy, belief in self and moral values			membership group devaluation and defenselessness. *Social Psychiatry*, 11:15–25, 1976
Self-Directed Search (self-administered and self-scored questionnaire)	Measures belief in various areas of skill, pattern and discrimination of interests, and abilities. Answers are categorized in six occupational areas (realistic, investigative, artistic, social, enterprising, conventional). Individual obtains a three-letter code which correlates with some of 500 occupations that are included in the test booklet	A high degree of internal consistency, and moderate to high test-retest reliability. Predictive validity measured over a 3-year period was low	Adolescents and adults for vocational evaluation. Not useful with individuals who are very disturbed, uneducated or illiterate	Holland J: *The Self-Directed Search Counselor's Guide.* Palo Alto, Calif, Consulting Psychologists Press, 1982
Self-Esteem Scale (pencil-and-paper strongly agree/strongly disagree scale)	Ten statements describe positive and negative feelings about oneself. Because these items include feelings of competence and efficacy, it measures an aspect of personal causation. Yield is either a total score or a nominal ranking of high, medium or low	Used as a Guttman scale, reproducibility and scalability coefficients are good. Adequate internal consistency, moderate test-retest. Has discriminative and concurrent validity	Adolescents, but has been used with older age groups as well	Rosenberg M: *Society and the Adolescent Self-Image.* Princeton, Princeton University Press, 1965
Set Test (informal question and answer)	Provides differentiating data on dementing versus depressive mental disorders. This is a short, gross screening tool that uses fund of information to determine the general type of mental impairment present. Four common categories of ten items each	There is no published data on the reliability of this instrument. Validity studies have been done using diagnoses determined by geriatricians. These studies indicate the Set Test is a valid screening tool	Older adults suspected of having dementing or depressive disorders	Issacs B, Kennie AT: The Set Test as an aid to the detection of dementia in old people. *British Journal Psychiatry* 123:467–470, 1973 Issacs B, Aktar AJ: The Set Test: a rapid test of mental function in old people.

Instrument Library: Description—Continued

Title	Content	Reliability and validity	Population	References/sources
	are requested. A point is awarded for each correct response. Scores below a certain level indicate dementia rather than depression as the probable mental problem			*Age and Aging* 1:222–226, 1972
Social and Prevocational Information Battery (orally administered, mostly true/false choice)	Scores from the nine tests within the SPIB reflect knowledge related to roles, habits and skills considered important for adaptation within postschool environments: employment, economic self-sufficiency, family living, personal habits, and communication. Three scores are derived for each test and for the total battery: raw scores, percentage correct and percentile rank	Internal consistency reliability: 0.78–0.82 for 9 tests and 0.94 for total battery; test-retest reliability: 0.62–0.79 for tests and 0.90 for battery. Moderate predictive validity re community adjustment (correlation 0.58) indicated	Mildly mentally retarded adolescents and young adults (an adaptation, SPIB-T, has been designed for use with the moderately retarded	Available from: Andrew S. Halpern, Paul Raffeld, Larry Irvin, and Robert Link, California Test Bureau/McGraw-Hill, Del Monte Research Park, Monterey, Calif 93940 Irvin L, Halpern A, Reynolds, W: Assessing social and prevocational awareness in mildly and moderately retarded individuals. *American Journal of Mental Deficiency* 82:266–272, 1977. (Instrument not reproduced here)
Social Climate Scales (true/false self-administered questionnaires)	These scales measure staff and residents' perceptions of desirable values, attitudes and behaviors in various settings. They can be completed in terms of "real" conditions and "ideal" conditions. In the real form, they measure social press; in the ideal form, they provide a picture of values. Each social climate scale yields several	These are generally stable scales that have been factor analyzed. Most have been examined for discriminative validity and are sensitive to changes in the environment	Psychiatric ward and community programs, work, school, family, and sheltered care settings	Moos RH: *Evaluating Treatment Environments: A Social Ecological Approach.* New York, Wiley, 1974 Moos RH: *Evaluating Educational Environments.* San Francisco, Jossey-Bass, 1979. Moos RH, Lemke S: *Multiphasic Environmental Assessment Procedure: Preliminary Manual.* Palo Alto,

Instrument	Description	Reliability/Validity	Population	References
Southern California Postrotary Nystagmus Test (standardized test)	dimension scores which can be compared with norms for other settings. This test measures one aspect of vestibular system processing by providing information on quality and duration of postrotary nystagmus	Test-retest reliability after an interval of 1 week was 0.83 on 42 children. Several other studies report similar results; Keating found correlations between SCPNT and electronystagmography	Children aged 4.0–8.11 years. Normative data on 111 boys and 115 girls from Los Angeles, Calif	Social Ecology Laboratory, 1979. Ayres AJ: *Southern California Postrotary Nystagmus Test Manual.* Los Angeles, Calif, Western Psychological Services, 1975. Deitz JC, Siegner CB, Crowe TK: The Southern California Postrotary Nystagmus Test: test-retest reliability for preschool children. *Occupational Therapy Journal of Research* 1:165–177, 1981. Keating NR: A comparison of duration of nystagmus as measured by the Southern California Postrotary Nystagmus Test and electronystagmography. *American Journal of Occupational Therapy* 33:92–97, 1979. Kimball JB: Normative comparison of the Southern California Sensory Integration Tests: Los Angeles vs. Syracuse data. *American Journal of Occupational Therapy* 35:21–25, 1981
Southern California Sensory Integration Tests (standardized tests)	This group of 17 tests was designed to identify patterns of sensory integrative dysfunction. The tests	Reliability of tests that were later published as the SCSIT varied depending upon age of child and spe-	Children aged 4.0–8.11 years. Normative data on 1,004 children from Los Angeles, Calif	Ayres AJ: Patterns of perceptual-motor dysfunction in children. A factor analytic study. *Perceptual and*

Instrument Library: Description—Continued

Title	Content	Reliability and validity	Population	References/sources
	minimize the need for verbal directions or responses and are designed to be used as a group. The SCSIT will be replaced with a new set of tests called the Sensory Integration and Praxis Tests, which will be available in 1986	cific test. When used as a group, the tests have adequate reliability. Some tests (motor accuracy) have sufficient reliability to be used independently. Tests were found to discriminate at the 0.01 level between a group of children with suspected brain dysfunction and a normal control group. Further construct validity was established through repeated factor analyses		*Motor Skills* 20:335–368, 1965 Ayres AJ: *Southern California Sensory Integration Tests Manual*, Revised 1980. Los Angeles, Calif, Western Psychological Services, 1980 Numerous other studies in occupational therapy literature
Test for Auditory Comprehension of Language (standardized test)	This test measures the auditory comprehension of language structure and assigns the child to a developmental level of comprehension. Performance on specific items also allows determination of areas of linguistic difficulty	Validity was demonstrated by correlation between test scores and age, discrimination between children who have disorders and those who do not and detection of improved language function. Test-retest reliability is reported at 0.94 for the English version and 0.93 for the Spanish version	Children aged 3.0–6.11	Carrow E: *Test for Auditory Comprehension of Language*. Texas, Learning Concepts, 1973
Time Reference Inventory (self-administered paper-and-pencil test)	Measure provides an indication of orientation to time and the significance of past, present and future events. Yield includes the number of positive, negative and neutral events in past, present and future; average number of years	Reliability and validity have not been reported	Has been used to study temporal orientation of alcoholics and mentally retarded adults	Roos P, Albers R: Performance of alcoholics and normals on a measure of temporal orientation. *Journal of Clinical Psychology* 21:34–36, 1965 Roos P, Albers R: Performance of retardates and

Instrument	Description	Population	Reliability/Validity	Availability
	projected into the past and future; and age at which individual has focused most of his/her concerns			normals on a measure of temporal orientation. *American Journal of Mental Deficiency* 69:835–838, 1965
VALPAR No. 17 Prevocational Readiness Battery (primarily "hands-on" assessment)	Using a work example format, data is gathered on perceptual-motor, process and communication/interactional skills reflecting ability to function in competitive employment and associated independent living situations. Scores on the 14 subscales are combined to provide a profile. Points derived from the subscales are compared to norm tables for identification of functional skill deficits	Mildly and moderately mentally retarded persons	Currently no reliability or validity information appears to be available, although the instrument appears to have face validity	Available from: VALPAR Corporation, 3801 East 34th St, Suite 105, Tucson, Ariz 85713. Botterbusch KF: *A Comparison of Commercial Vocational Evaluation Systems*. Menomonie, Wisc, Materials Development Center, 1980 (instrument not reproduced here)
Vineland Social Maturity Scale (structured interview administered to parent or guardian)	The scale gives information relevant to skills and habits. It assesses actual behavior in a variety of daily living situations and reflects independence in social relations, occupation, locomotion, communication, self-help, and self-direction. Main use of the scale is as a screening tool to detect developmental delays	Mentally retarded population from birth to 30 years	There are no reported data on reliability; the n scale was developed so as to manifest content validity based on known information about behavior in various developmental stages. The instrument was standardized using a moderately large sample	Available from: American Guidance Service, Inc., Publisher's Building, Circle Pines, Minn 55014

Glossary

Adaptive behavior	Behavior indicative of the ability to meet one's need to explore and master and the variable physical and psychosocial demands of one's environment
Alopecia	Loss of hair; baldness
Alphanumeric stimuli	Arabic numerals and alphabetic letters used in research to study discrimination, memory and other cognitive functions of the brain. Characters conveying information by using both letters and numbers
Amyotrophic lateral sclerosis (ALS)	A chronic progressive disease of unknown etiology involving deterioration of motor neurons in the cortex, medulla, and spinal cord. Symptoms may include hyperreflexia, spasticity, muscle weakness and atrophy—beginning in the upper extremities and spreading throughout
Arousal	An internal state of excitement in an organism, with physiological and subjective manifestations
Asymmetrical tonic neck reflex	Reflex stimulated by turning head to side. Response is a tendency toward increase in extensor tone on face side and increase in flexor tone on skull side
Ataxia	Factor of muscle coordination; irregularity of muscle action
Atrophy	A wasting away; a diminution in a size of a cell, tissue, organ or part.
Autonomic dysrefexia	In spinal cord injury (SCI) patients (above T_7) a disturbance in the autonomic nervous system causes the blood pressure to rise secondary to either visceral or bladder distension. This can be a life threatening situation for a (SCI) patient. Symptoms may include restlessness, headache, skin flush, cold sweat, and/or excessive spasticity
Availability	The presence or absence of objects in the environment
Belief in the efficacy of skill	The belief that one's abilities are useful and relevant in one's life situation
Belief in skill	A person's conviction that he or she has a range of important abilities
Bronchopulmonary dysplasia	Chronic lung disease due to damage to the lungs and bronchioles caused by the respirator
Cardiomyopathy	A disease of the myocardium that usually results in fibrosis of hypertrophy
Catecholamines	A group of chemicals whose common properties include the ability to stimulate those functions of the body not under conscious nervous control
Catheterization	Process of introducing a flexible tube into the bladder through the urethra in order to empty the bladder of urine
Centralization	The process of developing leading parts which govern lower, more primitive components of a system

Cervical spondylosis · Condition which involves compression of the spinal cord and/or spinal nerve roots due to narrowing of the intervertebral canal by osteoarthritic changes in the vertebrae

Chemotherapy · Treatment by the systemic administration of chemicals

Circularity · The cyclical pattern of function in an open system involving intake, throughput, output, and feedback

Closed system · A system which does not interact with its environment or exhibit properties of life

Collative properties · Discrepancies between a person's past experiences and present perceptions of the environment (e.g. novelty, surprise, complexity)

Colostomy · The surgical creation of an opening between the colon and the surface of the body

Commanding · The process of giving control signals to lower level components of a system in order to achieve a (higher) purpose not inherent in the lower components

Communication/interaction skills · Abilities for sharing and receiving information and for coordinating one's behavior with that of others in order to accomplish mutual activities and goals

Competence · The quality of being able or having the capacity to respond effectively to the demands of one or a range of situations

Complexity · The potential for continual discovery of ways to use or experience the environment

Concrete operational thought · The cognitive stage described by Piaget which occurs between 7 and 11 years. Mental abilities during this stage are internalized actions. Characteristics include reversibility of thought, and ability to focus on, and relate, several dimensions of a problem simultaneously

Congestive heart failure · A condition which occurs as a result of damage to the myocardium caused by rheumatic fever, congenital heart defects, heart attack, atherosclerosis or high blood pressure. Now, the heart muscle lacks strength to circulate the blood flow throughout the body and the blood flow is inadequate to meet all the body's needs resulting in edema, kidney retension and pulmonary edema

Conservation · Concept which involves the understanding of qualitative and quantitative relationships remaining the same, despite irrelevant changes

Constraining · The process of limiting the commands which can be given by a higher level system

Coping · The active psychosocial process through which persistent efforts are made to overcome and solve the problems and dilemmas of the person or those imposed by the environment

Corollary discharge · Internal feedback from active movement, contributes to awareness and monitoring of movements

Coronary artery disease · A disease that occurs when one or more of the three coronary arteries is partially or totally obstructed by one or more atherosclerotic plaques

Cultural familial	Etiological designation of retarded persons where there are no identified hereditary or physical agents responsible, and in which the individual is mildly retarded, has no pathological cerebral condition, and has one or more relatives who have impaired intellectual functioning
Culture	The beliefs and perceptions, values and norms, and customs and behaviors that are shared by a group or society and passed from one generation to the next through both formal and informal education
Cup arthroplasty	A surgical technique for remodeling the acetabulum and the femoral head and covering the head with a metal cup used in treatment of arthritis of the hip
Decentration	A process of differentiation which occurs throughout development. There is a realization of the separateness of things along with an understanding of the existence of self. This process also contributes to the ability to focus on more than one aspect of a situation
Decubiti	Ulcer/bed sore that develops in SCI patients secondary to prolonged periods of sitting (especially on areas with boney prominences) which cut off blood supply and cause tissue breakdown
Degree of organization in habits	The degree to which one has a typical use of time which supports competent performance in a variety of environments and roles and provides a balance of activity
Dependent edema	Swelling in lower extremities due to gravitational pull on a poor vascular system
Deviant	Differing from an accepted normal or acceptable standard
Differentiation	The process of becoming more heterogeneous, of developing parts with different characteristics
Discrimination of interests	The degree to which one differentiates a liking or expectation of enjoyment in certain occupations
Ecological variables	Events that either directly or indirectly threaten one's survival or well-being
Electrolarynx	An electronic hand-held device which creates a mechanical sound that can be formed into words when the laryngectomee moves his/her mouth as a normal speaker would
Entropy	The tendency of closed systems to wear down and become more homogeneous
Enucleated eye	Removal of the eye from the socket
Environment	The objects, persons and events with which a system interacts
Environmental control unit	A system affording centralized control over a number of preselected environmental devices. The latter may include lights, bed controls, radio, television, calculator, page turner and/or alarm system. Control switches may be operated using a mouthstick, breath control (sip and puff), tongue movements, or by hand
Equifinality	The property of an open system whereby it can achieve a final goal or status through alternative routes and from different initial conditions

Esophageal speech	A low pitched sound which is produced when a laryngectomee forces air back into the esophagus and expels it, causing the esophageal and pharyngeal walls to vibrate. This sound (controlled belch or burp) is then shaped into words by moving the mouth as a normal speaker would
Eugenic sterilization	Movement undertaken to prevent retarded persons from reproducing based on the premise that mentally defective individuals will produce like offspring. Laws were passed in some states allowing sterilization without due process consideration; this was a common practice in many large, rural institutions
Exacerbation	Increase in severity of a disease or any of its symptoms
Expectancy of success or failure	The person's anticipation of future endeavors and whether their outcomes will be successful or not
Feedback	The process of returning to the system information concerning output and its consequences
Flexibility	The degree to which objects lend themselves to manipulations and changes by the user
Formal learning	The transmission of cultural norms in situations where right and wrong ways of doing something are so taken for granted that explanations are not given
Function	The dominant purpose of the group or organization
Functional play	Play consisting of repetitive actions, sometimes referred to as exercise or practice play. This may occur throughout development whenever a new skill is acquired
Futurity	The quality or state of being future oriented
Habits	Images guiding the routine and typical ways in which a person performs
Habituation subsystem	A collection of images which trigger and guide the performance of routine patterns of behavior
Hemipelvectomy	Amputation of the entire leg and half of the pelvic bones
Hierarchy	The arrangement of parts of a system into interconnected lower and higher components in which higher components command lower ones and in which lower ones constrain the higher
Informal learning	The transmission of cultural norms through imitation of role models, trial and error, and other intuitive processes that tend to be difficult to describe or pin down
Instrumental values	Values that are specific and goal oriented
Intake	The importation of energy and information from environment
Interests	Dispositions to find occupations pleasurable
Internal versus external orientation	The individual's conviction that outcomes in life are related to personal actions (internal control) versus the action of others, fate or luck (external control)
Internalized expectations	Images that one holds of what others expect one to do by virtue of being in a role

Internalized roles	Images that persons hold of themselves as occupying certain statuses or positions in social groups and of the obligations or expectations that accompany being in these roles
Kernig's sign	A reflex contraction and pain in the hamstring muscles when attempting to extend the leg after flexing the thigh upon the body
Kyphosis	Abnormal backward curvature of the spine
Laryngectomy	Removal of the entire larynx or part of it (i.e. hemi laryngectomy)
Leading part	A component of a system which has command over several lower parts
Leukemia	A disease of the blood-forming tissues, characterized by an abnormal increase in leukocytes and amount of bone marrow. There are several types of leukemias
Lipofusin	A class of fatty pigments
Mastectomy	Surgical removal of the breast
Meaningfulness of activities	An individual's disposition to find importance, security, worthiness and purpose in particular occupations
Mechanistic thinking	The tendency to see all phenomena as machine-like in their operations
Melanoma	A malignant tumor, usually developing from a nevus and consisting of black masses of cells with a marked tendency to metastasis
Meningitis	An infection of the meninges (the protective membranes covering the brain and spinal cord) usually occurring due to entry of bacterial or vial organisms via the bloodstream into the central nervous system
Metastasize	To spread to some other part or parts of the body
Minimally restrictive environments	A principle of the normalization movement which means an individual should live in an environment which provides him the greatest access to persons and objects as can be safely provided considering the limits of his disability
Modularization	The process of generating patterned interconnections of component structures that allow them to function as a semiautonomous whole
Monitored task evaluation	A series of tasks graded to produce a gradual increase in cardiovascular work load while engaged in activities. During the evaluation, the patient is continually monitored for heart rate, blood pressure response, EKG, ischemia, and symptoms
Moro reflex	A normal newborn reflex elicited by backwards displacement of the head and characterized by abduction and extension of the arms and legs, followed by adduction and flexion
Multiple myeloma	A malignant neoplasm of plasma cells usually arising in the bone marrow and manifested by skeletal destruction, pathological fractures and bone pain
Myopathy	Any disease or abnormal condition of striated muscle

Nasal cannula	Short tubes inserted in the nasal passages and attached by a tube to the machine that supplies oxygen
Nature of work and play	The meaning and value of work and leisure, the activities that are considered acceptable forms of each, and the extent to which a culture dichotomizes these behaviors
Negative entropy	The ability of the open system to build itself up and become more complex by differentiation
Neuronal model	Within the brain, a copy or symbolic representation of something in the environment
Normative	Conforming to norms
Norms	Shared expectations about behavior
Novelty	The experience of completely new events
Object complexity	The level of skill and learning required for use
Objects	The materials and artifacts which we use and interact with daily
Occupational goals	Objectives for personal accomplishments or for future occupational activities or roles
Old-old	Persons 75 years of age or older
Open system	A composition of interrelated structures and functions organized into a coherent whole that interacts with an environment and that is capable of maintaining and changing itself
Organic factors	Genetically determined conditions or vulnerability to certain environmental agents and/or damage to the central nervous system which results in mental retardation
Organicity	Dysfunction in the nervous system related to demonstrable changes in the brain's structure. Degree of dysfunction related to organic or biological factors (i.e. due to disease, injury or malformation of the central nervous system)
Organizational size	The number of persons involved in a social group
Osteoarthritis	A chronic disease involving the joints. Characterized by destruction of articular cartilage and overgrowth of bone
Ostomies	A general term referring to any operation in which an artificial opening is formed between two hollow organs or between one or more such viscera and the abdominal wall
Osteosarcoma	A sarcoma derived from, or composed of, any tissue which is concerned in the growth or repair of bone
Output	The action of the system directed at the environment
Palliative	Tending to lessen the pain, or severity of, without curing
Paraplegia	Paralysis in lower extremities and lower portion of the trunk
Pattern of interests	A configuration of occupations one is disposed to enjoy
Perceived incumbency	The belief that one has the status, rights and obligations of a role and that others also perceive one to be in the role
Perceptual motor skills	Abilities for interpreting sensory information and for manipulating self and objects
Performance subsystem	A collection of images and biological structures and processes

which are organized into skills and used in the production of purposeful behavior

Permeability of boundaries	Ease of membership and insularity of group
Personal causation	A collection of beliefs and expectations which a person holds about his or her effectiveness in the environment
Personal standards	Commitments to performing occupations in moral, excellent, efficient or otherwise socially sanctioned ways
Plasmapheresis	Laboratory procedure that exchanges blood plasma in patients with rheumatoid arthritis. It is hoped that the patient's immunologic response to the arthritis will be more effective with plasma exchange. This is an experimental procedure reserved for patients with rheumatoid arthritis whose disease is uncontrolled by traditional medicine management
Postural mechanisms	Responses used for posture, equilibrium and locomotion
Potency of interests	The degree to which interests are based on past experiences and influence present action
Presbycusis	Hearing loss associated with old age.
Presbyopia	A visual condition of old age involving defective accomodation and inability to clearly focus for near vision
Press	Environmental expectations for certain behaviors
Prestimulus arousal deficiency	A deficit in attention to the important dimensions of a task when they are of low intensity requiring a simpler task or more pronounced cues to elicit the desired response
Process skills	Abilities directed at managing events or processes in the environment
Psychophysical variables	The physical characteristics of the setting and their intensity or quality
Purposefulness	The open system characteristic of seeking to accomplish goals
Quadriplegia	Tetraplegia or paralysis in all four limbs and part of trunk
Quality-of-life	Positive feeling states captured by concepts like happiness, well-being and hope
Radical neck dissection	A block dissection of either or both sides of the neck which includes removal of the lymphatic tissue between the mandible and the clavicle, as well as the jugular vein and the sternocleidomastoid muscle. It may also include sacrifice of the spinal accessory nerve
Radiation therapy	The treatment of disease by ionizing radiation
Reaction time	Period of time taken to produce a desired action in response to a stimulus event
Reductionism	The study of phenomena by examining their constituent parts and the cause-and-effect relations between the parts
Remission	A diminution or abatement of a symptom or disease; also a period during which such a diminution occurs
Resonation	The impact of changes or disturbances at one level of a

system on other levels, often involving a transformation of energy or information as an effect is mediated across each level

Rigidity/flexibility of habits

The degree to which a person is able to change routines of behavior to accommodate periodic contingencies

Role balance

Integration of an optimal number of appropriate roles into one's life

Role blurring

The sharing of skills and purposes among different professionals

Rules

The internal organization of a task; standards of performance

Sarcoma

Any of various malignant tumors that begin in connective tissue

Seriousness/playfulness

The context and consequences of task performance

Seropositive rheumatoid arthritis

Results of laboratory studies indicate that this kind of rheumatoid arthritis is more severe with errosive changes at the joints than seronegative rheumatoid arthritis

Skills

The abilities that a person has for the performance of various forms of purposeful behavior

Social appropriateness of habits

The degree to which one's typical behaviors are those expected and valued by the environments in which one performs

Social dimension

The public or private nature of a task, and the degree to which it is cooperative or competitive

Social groups and organizations

Collective units of individuals, including informal social groupings (e.g. a lunch table group at work), naturally occurring groups and formalized organizations developed for the explicit purpose of achieving some goal

Sociodramatic play

Higher level of symbolic play, consisting of at least two players. Actions and verbalizations involve imitative and make-believe elements

Somatomotor adaptive response

A motor action in response to sensory input, enabling mastery of the body and environment. Effectiveness of the response is dependent on sensory integration

Space/time dimension

When and where play and work occur

Spasticity

A state of hypertonicity, or increase over a normal tone of muscle, with heightened deep tendon reflexes

Spontaneity

The ability to initiate action without external agency

Steady state

A set of dynamic conditions which an open system seeks to maintain

Stoma

Any opening on a free surface

Structural complexity

The degree of hierarchical and lateral networks in a group

Structure

The patterned arrangement of components

Stryker frame

A specialized bed which rotates around a longitudinal axis and allows for the safe repositioning of spinal cord injured patients every few hours, in prone or supine, to avoid pressure areas and the development of decubiti

Subluxation	An incomplete or partial dislocation
Surprise	Unexpected events
Symbolic meaning	The power, status, prestige, independence, interests, and so on, communicated by objects
System	A set of objects with interrelationships that allow them to function collectively toward an identifiable purpose
Task	The sequence of actions engaged in to satisfy either societal requirements or internal motivations to explore and be competent
Task complexity	The level of skill and the number of steps required to execute the task
Technical learning	The transmission of cultural norms in situations where right and wrong are determined by reasoning and logic
Temporal boundaries of tasks	The degree to which a task is time-limited or continuous, and seasonal or discretionary
Temporal orientation	The way in which an individual interprets and views his or her own placement in time: it includes the degree of orientation or concern with passt, present or future, and beliefs about how time should be used
Temporality	Quality or state of being aware of time
Tenodesis	In the quadraplegic patient, this term refers to the movement of active wrist extension, facilitating grasp or pinch in the fingers due to the pull on the flexor tendons crossing the wrist and extending into the fingers. Mechanical or externally controlled tenodesis can be achieved by the use of a battery power wrist/hand orthosis that positions the wrist in extension
Terminal values	Values that are general and serve as guiding life principles
Throughput	The transformation of imported information and energy to another form and its incorporation into the structure of the system resulting in structural maintenance and change
Total hip replacement	A surgical procedure used in treating severe arthritis where the acetabulum and the femoral head are replaced by metal components
Transient ischemic attacks (TIAs)	Small strokes or undetected cerebral vascular accidents
Transmission of knowledge and values	How a culture passes on beliefs and norms from one generation to the next
Ulcerative colitis	Inflammation of the colon with ulceration of the mucosa. Causes pain, passage of watery stools or colic
Values	Images of what is good, right and/or important.
Volition subsystem	An interrelated set of energizing and symbolic components which together determine conscious choices for occupational behavior
Young-old	Persons under 75 years of age

Index